P9-AFM-599

Health care reform is at the top of our national agenda. But the terms of the debate—cost, access, insurance—disguise the larger crisis in health care delivery. In this comprehensive collection of nearly sixty essays, researchers, activists, health care professionals, and members of the Health/PAC board analyze our national health care system, and offer policy suggestions and options for reform.

Covering topics ranging from rising health care costs, to women and AIDS, to community health projects, *Beyond Crisis* is a clear, in-depth analysis of American health care problems and solutions. Offering expert analyses of the current crisis, the Clinton administration's reform proposals, and models for alternative systems (such as Canada's National Health Service), this book is an invaluable guide for concerned citizens, nurses, doctors, health managers, and health policy analysts. For anyone who recognizes that the American health care system costs too much, accomplishes too little, and reaches too few, *Beyond Crisis* is a powerful and timely call to arms.

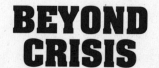

BEYOND CRISIS

CONFRONTING HEALTH CARE IN THE UNITED STATES

NANCY F. McKENZIE, Ph.D., is Executive Director of the Health/Policy Advisory Center. Founded in 1968, Health/PAC is an independent and influential national organization that focuses on health care delivery in America. Dr. McKenzie is the editor of *The Crisis in Health Care: Ethical Issues* and *The AIDS Reader: Social, Political and Ethical Issues,* both Meridian anthologies.

BEYOND CRISIS

CONFRONTING HEALTH CARE
IN THE UNITED STATES

A HEALTH / PAC BOOK

EDITED BY
NANCY F. McKENZIE, Ph.D.

Foreword by Barbara Ehrenreich

A MERIDIAN BOOK
Riverside Community College
Library
4800 Magnolia Avenue
Riverside, California 92506

RA 395 .A3 B48 1994

Beyond crisis

MERIDIAN
Published by the Penguin Group
Penguin Books USA Inc., 375 Hudson Street,
New York, New York 10014, U.S.A.
Penguin Books Ltd, 27 Wrights Lane,
London W8 5TZ, England
Penguin Books Australia Ltd, Ringwood,
Victoria, Australia
Penguin Books Canada Ltd, 10 Alcorn Avenue,
Toronto, Ontario, Canada M4V 3B2
Penguin Books (N.Z.) Ltd, 182–190 Wairau Road,
Auckland 10, New Zealand

Penguin Books Ltd, Registered Offices:
Harmondsworth, Middlesex, England

First published by Meridian, an imprint of Dutton Signet, a division of
Penguin Books USA Inc.

First Printing, March, 1994
10 9 8 7 6 5 4 3 2 1

Copyright © Health/PAC, 1994
All rights reserved

ⓜ REGISTERED TRADEMARK—MARCA REGISTRADA

LIBRARY OF CONGRESS CATALOGING IN PUBLICATION DATA
Beyond crisis : confronting health care in the United States / edited
   by Nancy F. McKenzie.
      p.   cm.
   "A Health/PAC book."
   ISBN 0-452-01108-6
   1. Medical policy—United States.   2. Medical care—United States.
   3. Medical economics—United States.   I. McKenzie, Nancy F.
RA395.A3B48   1993
362.1'0973—dc20   93–16007
                                                       CIP

Printed in the United States of America
Set in Times New Roman
Designed by Leonard Telesca

Without limiting the rights under copyright reserved above, no part of this publication may be reproduced, stored in or introduced into a retrieval system, or transmitted, in any form, or by any means
(electronic, mechanical, photocopying, recording, or otherwise), without the prior written permission of
both the copyright owner and the above publisher of this book.

BOOKS ARE AVAILABLE AT QUANTITY DISCOUNTS WHEN USED TO PROMOTE PRODUCTS OR SERVICES.
FOR INFORMATION PLEASE WRITE TO PREMIUM MARKETING DIVISION, PENGUIN BOOKS USA INC., 375
HUDSON STREET, NEW YORK, NEW YORK 10014.

Thanks to the Health/PAC Board and their past and new articles contained herein. Special appreciation to Dave Kotelchuck and Sally Guttmacher; to Art Levin and Hal Strelnick, who both provided continuing support, references, special writing, and innumerable critical comments. I am indebted, in addition, to Sharon Lerner; Ellen Bilofsky, for her editorial work on most of the *Bulletin* articles contained here; Martin Cozza; and Karen Hysmith. My thanks go to Rosemary Ahern, my editor, who seems to like the challenge of making sense of my writing and of extending her patience to both the glorious issues and the inglorious details involved in a work like this.

Finally, I acknowledge the many people providing care to themselves and to others who offered their thoughts, their time, credulity, and patience to my attempts at translation.

CONTENTS

SECTION II THE CRISIS IN PROVIDER INSTITUTIONS: ISSUES AND
             AREAS FOR REFORM

SECTION V TOWARD ADEQUATE POLICY IN HEALTH CARE
                DELIVERY

FOREWORD

Barbara Ehrenreich

This book illustrates a fine old radical principle: Things are often simpler than they seem. In the media, "health reform" has become a mind-numbing swarm of issues and marginally distinguishable options. We are told that the way ahead is difficult and murky, that only experts can possibly make it out, that, despite our current extravagant expenditures on health care, real reform will require "painful sacrifice" on the part of average citizens. The majority preference—for a Canadian-style system of national health insurance—has been brushed aside as naive and unsuited to American reality. Other nations have functioning systems of public health care; our case is made out to be uniquely baffling and complex.

There *is* something uniquely paradoxical about the American health care system: We spend more on it, per capita and as a percentage of GDP, than any other nation, and we get far from our money's worth in return. Seven hundred sixty-eight billion dollars a year are pumped into the American health care system, yet 37 million Americans have no insurance at all; millions more are inadequately insured; and our mortality rates, especially for the poor and people of color, compare unfavorably with those of many third world nations. American infant mortality is higher than that of Costa Rica, and Harlem is a deadlier place for a man to live in than Bangladesh. Somehow, our vast expenditures do not translate readily into "health."

The system, in the conventional formulation, "doesn't work." This understanding is a huge advance over the denial characteristic of the Reagan and Bush administrations, when our leaders routinely praised American health care as "the best in the world." But it also misses the point. There is a far starker analysis implicit in the pages that follow: that the American health care system "works" just fine—if you acknowledge that delivering health care is not its primary goal.

Central to Health/PAC's analysis is the insight that the American health care system is highly successful in at least one thing: making money for the private interests that dominate it. Physicians are among the most highly paid professionals in America. Drug and medical equipment companies generate steady, and sometimes spectacular, profits for their investors. Hospitals are increasingly likely to be part of giant profit-making chains, and even legally non-profit facilities generate invisible surpluses in the form of handsome salaries and perks for their top doctors and administrators. Anyone who thinks the health care system "doesn't work" should take a look at an investment guide to the medical industry.

Health care, in other words, is only a by-product of the American health care system. Yes, the system does provide care—for millions. But it far more reliably and consistently provides wealth and security for a small elite.

The trouble is, we all pay for it. Through Medicaid and Medicare, the public sector plays a major role in funding private health care. Three hundred ninety billion dollars, or 51 percent of money spent on health care, originates as taxes and represents the potential power of the public. Yet as Health/PAC's studies have repeatedly shown, the public sector effectively subsidizes the private, profit-making side of health care—most notably, by underwriting the care of millions who are too old, too poor, or too sick to be profitable to care for on their own. And throughout our current debate over health care reform, private forces have lobbied energetically to maintain their comfortable and protected status.

In the 25 years that have passed since a young economist named Rob Burlage founded Health/PAC, nothing has happened to alter this basic analysis. If anything, the dimensions of what even Richard Nixon discerned as a "crisis" in 1969 have grown catastrophically. Costs continue to escalate, bringing ever more desperate and punitive attempts at control: Insurers—public and private —have become a dominant presence on the medical "team," making what can be life-or-death decisions. Dozens of public hospitals have been closed in the interests of budget-cutting. Employers by the droves are wriggling out of long-standing health insurance guarantees for their workers and retirees.

Health care is not, of course, the only factor determining health. Lifestyle, environment, and standard of living all play their part and, tragically, these other conditions have deteriorated for countless Americans just as the health care system has withdrawn further and further from the business of providing care. We may smoke less than we did 25 years ago, but we also work, on the average, far harder, with diminishing time for sleep or family life. And, while 25 years ago we prided ourselves on the "conquest" of infectious diseases, AIDS and tuberculosis now rage at epidemic force.

One of the saddest measures of deterioration is the diminishing status of health care as a political issue for the poor. When Health/PAC began its work in 1968, health care was, along with education and welfare, a key issue mobilizing the urban poor. Today, health care has been all but overshadowed by more immediate needs—for mere shelter, for example, and protection from gunfire in the demoralized, economically moribund inner cities.

But perhaps the scariest feature of the health crisis of the 1990s compared to that of the 1960s is that the health system itself has become hazardous to our collective health. Escalating health costs add a massive dead weight to the federal deficit, inhibiting efforts to reform health care or do anything else that might improve the general health, like cleaning up the environment or rebuilding the inner cities. Health costs also hobble the private economy, and are an important factor contributing to the corporate downsizing that has eliminated so many jobs. The problem, then, is not just that the health system "doesn't work" or works to the wrong ends—it has become a blight on the entire economy, a huge, bloated, parasitical growth.

As Health/PAC's analysis shows, the "managed competition" reform proposed by the Clinton administration does not even begin to address the problem. The Clinton proposal originates in the fanciful assumption that consumers are to blame for ''overutilizing'' health services and otherwise failing to control costs. In fact, Americans *under*utilize health care compared to the people of other industrialized nations and have little control over the costs or the nature of the services they do use. It's the doctor—or, increasingly, the insurance company—who determines whether a headache merits nuclear magnetic resonance imaging or just an aspirin. Health care is one case in which we have seen the enemy—and it isn't us.

The solution Health/PAC points us toward is both conceptually simple and politically daunting: Take the profit out of health care. This is a matter of empirical evidence, not ideological bias. Marketplace medicine has had its chance, and it has failed. Attempts to squeeze more care per dollar out of a system that is fundamentally dedicated to something other than care can do nothing but fail. Besides, many of our most urgent needs—for preventive care and care for the poor—will never be profitable and will inevitably be neglected in a profit-driven system.

So, then, where will the incentive come from to provide care for a nation of 250 million people, the great majority of whom will never be entirely profitable to serve? We have a hard time imagining anything getting done without the incentive of personal or corporate gain. Yet most other nations manage, somehow, to provide health care or health insurance in a nonprofit fashion, through the public sector. We are not so congenitally different from the British, the Swedes, or our neighbors in Canada.

Health/PAC reminds us that America boasts a tradition other than individualism and profit-seeking. It is a tradition of mutual help and organizing for change: union struggles for safe workplaces and health benefits; people with AIDS acting up for care and cure; women confronting a sexist medical system; poor people organizing for community uplift; health workers advocating for low-income communities. And finally there is Health/PAC itself—a tiny band of thinkers and activists whose vision of a just and caring health system should inspire us all.

INTRODUCTION

Nancy F. McKenzie

It is not possible to set a new health care system in front of the American people and say, "Take it, it's better than the one you have." Individuals must struggle for these changes, and policymakers must take responsibility for ensuring that debates about the health care system and its institutions reflect the true issues and are accountable to American citizens. Only a social movement around health care issues will bring true reform. Even with a new administration the issue is really what the American people can bring about. What was true of Roosevelt is true of President Clinton: "I agree with you, now make me do it."

As this anthology should indicate, the crisis of health care delivery is so multiple as to be beyond crisis. In fact, we should agree with former Surgeon General Koop, who said that the system is approaching "chaos." Without a large social movement coalesced around the promise of *substantial* reform, it is unrealistic to expect that health care costs won't continue to rise 15 percent a year; that basic care will not continue to diminish and become more and more unavailable; that there will not be more outcries about the poor, the disabled (including the elderly), and the seriously ill "costing too much." And it is folly to think that the American health care system will ever have any real public health policy. This anthology has been compiled to address the basic lack of knowledge that we all have with respect to the real health care system in the United States.

Beyond Crisis contains six sections, which attempt to outline the extent and areas of the health care system that are in "crisis," as well as offer the innovations that have come from patients, providers, and communities. It offers options for an adequate health care system in the United States, and analysis of the current national reform agenda.

Each section is preceded by an introductory essay by either the editor of the anthology or a Health/PAC Board member. The introductions are intended to orient the reader to the material, as well as offer a position on the topic of the section. Each section also includes a voice reading or readings. These are first-person essays and editorials which personalize the crisis before us and allow individuals to speak beyond the often numbing language of professional policy.

A substantial portion of this reader is made up of *Health/PAC Bulletin* articles published in the last 10 years. The *Bulletin* is the journal of the Health Policy Advisory Center—a non-profit health advocacy center that has been in existence for over 25 years. Health/PAC thinks of itself as the only "Health PAC that is not a PAC." But, as is obvious from the articles contained here, Health/PAC does represent individuals. It does have a constituency, made up of those individuals who have *no* vested interest in the health care system in the United States, who are most in need and least served in a for-profit health care system. Other articles and readings help fill out the story of health care in America.

There is no preferred way to read this anthology. It is designed to be a comprehensive treatment of the health care delivery system in the United States as it approaches both its darkest hours and a genuine dawn of the possibility for reform. One can begin with the national reform debate in Section VI or with the current health crisis in Section I. Each section can be read on its own.

Health Care Delivery in the United States

The United States health care system is "beyond crisis" not only because we have allowed our system to be driven by the twin incentives of profit and technological innovation, but because we entered the age of "non-government" in 1980 and have been suffering its effects for the last 12 years. We are paying for this tragic myopia with a health crisis of staggering proportions. We have reached the point where our institutions have become murderous of the poor, and wholly undemocratic for the rest of us. The readings in the first section of this anthology, "Health Status in the United States: Communities at Risk," drive this point home and position it as the first and foremost issue of health care reform in the United States.

The crisis of the system can be seen by the continuum of disarray beginning with health care financing and ending in the undermining of patient and civil rights and of our democratic institutions. The continuum includes five "crises," and these make up the conceptual core of the anthology. They are:

Crisis in Costs

By the year 2000, each family will pay $16,000 a year for health care. Our current system costs $800 billion, with 15 percent inflation per year. (Section I, "Health Status in the United States: Communities at Risk," offers in-depth articles on the cost issues, and Section II, "The Crisis in Provider Institutions," goes on to tie these costs to the larger issues of access.)

As we look at the offerings for change in the health care system currently being discussed, the superficial quality of the options is shocking and seems to be fueled by the desire of employers to contain costs, of the business community to socialize health care costs for corporations, and to subsidize the insurance industry. "Managed competition" is not designed to respond to our health care needs. If it were, it would be neither as complicated as it is nor as purely fiscal in nature. (For a more far-reaching analysis of President Clinton's plans for reform, see Section VI, "Proposals for a National Agenda.")

While consumers and corporations express their outrage over the costs of health care and fear that city and state budgets cannot carry the multiple health needs of the poor, the changes currently offered for legislation suggest that the "system cure itself." This attitude is reminiscent of the failed "trickle-down" economic theory. As Arthur Levin points out in Section VI, "Proposals for a National Agenda," just as in previous years of "reform," the real question is who will gainsay the demanded new changes and who can resist changes in the status quo of health care delivery. A status quo in which the health care industries—insurance, pharmaceutical, corporate, and academic hospitals—make enormous profits, including our Congressional representatives who accept sizeable contributions from the health lobbying political action committees (PACS). (See "What's Blocking Health Care Reform?" p. 592, in Section VI.)

Health care delivery is the sixth largest industry in the United States and the third largest employer. Between 1980 and 1990, 40 percent of all PAC money to members of Congress came from health PACS.

The cost of health care in the United States is part of the crisis of health care. But, while important, it disguises even larger problems.

The Crisis in Access

The crisis in costs is fed by the crisis in access to health care in the United States. Health care costs are due to an unregulated market in health care goods, and can only be remedied by federal control of health care provision. But there is still the question of the efficiency of that provision. And more insurance or tax breaks will not solve the problem. *Parts of the health care system are unworkable at any price.*

From anyone's vantage point, an ounce of prevention is still worth a pound of cure. That 50 million people are uninsured or so underinsured that they can't seek basic health care is a very complicated fact about access to health care. Lack of insurance does not mean that individuals forego health care altogether. Nor does it follow that the insured seek more care, or more use of physicians "unnecessarily." The treatment of health care services as a consumer item so distorts the reality of health needs—needs that include a livable environment, workplace safety, and early preventive and diagnostic care—as to be patently absurd.

Individuals most in need of health care too often forego seeing a provider because they are forced to, and they eventually reach a point where their condition worsens and they are in need of highly costly acute care. When they seek later care, they do so at hospitals rather than at doctors' offices, with the consequent lack of quality care that the emergency room offers and at the cost of emergent, or crisis, care. While such costly care may be good for a hospital's finances, it is not good for individual or state and city budgets. Here begins the perception that the "poor" are pushing up the costs of health care to all other income groups. Here begins the mad scramble of moderately well-off individuals for some sense of future security in health insurance plans that try to cut costs, remain almost unintelligible, and do not adequately serve patient needs.

The question of access points to the logic of health care delivery in the United States, that increasingly eliminates everything "healthy" that cannot be made into a commodity item—things like housing, nutrition, a long-term approach for care, and involvement of the patient in his or her own health-restoring regimens. Section III of this anthology, "The Changing Medical/Industrial Complex: The Bottom Line vs. the Public Agenda," seeks to address the structural incoherence of the health care system. And it is the section that analyzes this incoherence as a part of the analysis developed by Health/PAC in 1968. In this version, Hal Strelnick, M.D., offers an introduction to the readings by outlining the major industries and their effect upon treatment as well as medical education.

The issue of the costs of health care disguises the lack of rationale of third-party payments for health care, as well as the inadequacy of the configuration of health care delivery in the United States—the preponderance of acute-hospital-based delivery, and the resultant lack of access to basic care that one in five Americans experiences. The history of cost-containment in public programs and the lack of governmental incentives toward basic care provision in the private sector have made our system so lopsided that money, time, talent, and energy all tend to move toward the most refined and technique-intensive care, at the loss of the most basic, rudimentary, and common-sense care.

For the poor, the lopsidedness is particularly disastrous. Loss of clinics, closing of hospitals in poor neighborhoods, Diagnosis Related Groups, Medicaid rationing, Oregon's Health Rationing Plan and now Medicaid Managed Care all contribute to limiting patient use of basic care, with long-term, high-cost consequences. Only a small portion of doctors choose to provide primary care—family practice services, internal medicine, obstetrics/gynecology—and a small percentage of those will provide it to poor patients. Public entitlements are so disproportionate in their payment fees that those few physicians who could provide basic care are opting out of Medicaid and Medicare programs altogether. The institutional exclusion of the sick also occurs in the private arena. Lack of access to physicians occurs because so few physicians wish to practice in poor communities. A recent study in New York City that I was associated with showed a total of 27 primary-care physicians for 1.7 million people in the City's 9 lowest income communities.[1] In New York State, only 15 percent of physicians take Medicaid payment in their private practices. And nationally 50 percent of all admissions to the hospital are through the emergency room because so many individuals lack physicians.

Finally, the lack of access is increasing as 100,000 individuals a month are dropped from insurance rolls and as the insurance industry redlines illness. Ninety-nine percent of insurance companies report prohibiting insurance for people with AIDS. This is becoming true for many chronic illnesses and shows a disturbing trend that favors the well and makes insurance a cost for cost financing. Given that health insurance now moves toward no-risk patients, or charges so much for sickness that many individuals are "self-payers" for their health care, it is clear why many call for the end to all third-party payment for health care delivery. (See "Excluding More, Covering Less: The Health Insurance Industry in the U.S." in Section III, p. 310; also see "Liberal Benefits, Conservative Spending: The Physicians for a National Health Program Proposal" in Section VI, p. 666.)

The Crisis in Equity

We are currently suffering the effects of the skewed health financing policy of the last thirty years. The Reagan/Bush era saw the economic rout of everyone but the very rich, and the dismantling of public programs, preventive care, basic physician education and training, and the failure to oversee health insurance. All have created an empty portal of care before a Legion of Need.

The Legion of Need is outlined as follows:

- One in 4 Americans lived in poverty some time in 1991, the largest income disparity on record since 1940.
- Three-fourths of Americans live in an urban setting and federal aid to cities has declined by 50 percent.
- Cuts in "Safety Net" programs between 1980 and 1990 have been substantial:
    14 percent in maternal health
    40 percent in community clinics
    35 percent in health programs for children and the elderly
    75 percent in housing assistance.
- The maternal mortality rate of women of color is three times that of white women. One-third to one-half of these deaths are unnecessary and could easily be avoided using preventive measures, given that they are primarily attributable to lack of prenatal care.[2]
- Because they come so late to treatment, only 30 percent of women diagnosed with breast cancer at Harlem Hospital live five more years, compared to 70 percent of white women and 60 percent of black women nationwide.[3]
- "A child in Chile or Malaysia is more likely to celebrate his first birthday than a black baby throughout much of the Mississippi Delta."[4]
- Black men in central Harlem are less likely to reach age 65 than men in Bangladesh. Inner-city areas like Harlem are "analogous . . . to natural disaster areas."[5]
- After controlling for differences in age, sex, race, and specific disease, the uninsured are 1.2 to 3.2 times more likely to die during a hospital stay than the insured.[6]
- 50 percent of individuals with AIDS are homeless.

Crisis in Public Health

In the United States over the past 20 years, health care provision increasingly has been defined by the provision of medical services alone. Simultaneously, public and preventive programs have been systematically de-funded and dismantled. The predictable result is that the American health care system is now besieged by public health issues it is unequipped to handle. In 1988, it was syphilis. In 1989–90 it was measles, due to a national shrinking of childhood immunization programs. In 1991, and for at least the next 20 years, it is tuberculosis.

After a century of decline in the United States, tuberculosis is increasing, and strains resistant to multiple antibiotics have emerged. This excess of cases is attributable to changes in the social structure in cities, the human immuno-deficiency virus epidemic, and a failure in certain major cities to improve public treatment programs.[7]

Americans are familiar with tuberculosis, which is emblematic of struggling populations, through knowledge of earlier historical periods when it was cor-related with poverty in American cities and was a disease of the elderly poor. Recent visibility has come from other, less-developed countries, as well as from poor immigrants to the United States.

In the past 10 years, however, we have developed a tuberculosis epidemic of staggering proportions, largely involving individuals between the ages of 22 and 44. Despite the preventability and curability of TB, cases in New York City, for example, have doubled since 1985, to 50 cases per 100,000 in 1991 (the national incidence is 10 cases per 100,000). New York's Black and Latino com-munities have 45 times the national average, comprising 80 percent of cases.

While many point to the high incidence of HIV, it remains true that only three-quarters of new TB cases can be related to HIV infection.[8]

The response to the current TB epidemic reveals not only the inadequacy of the health care system to intervene in a growing number of epidemics, but also the limitations of the current debate on health care reform. The re-emergence and flourishing of this 19th-century disease is only the latest wave of health disasters to batter a population increasingly lacking in housing, employment, and public and primary health care. (This is highlighted in Section IV, "Com-munity Response and Innovative Policy.") The current debate ignores the fact that the public and primary health care infrastructures, which could be expected to treat TB patients, have been dismantled and abandoned.

Tuberculosis is not news to African Americans. They have suffered dispro-portionately from tuberculosis since the early 1900s. And it was not until after World War II that medical theorists in the United States surmised that African Americans' genetic makeup ("weak lungs") was not the cause of their dispro-portionate suffering but rather their poverty, their working conditions, their *lack of access to basic health care.*

As opposed to the poor today, in the Great Depression individuals still had some connection to health care provision. The current tuberculosis epidemic is emblematic of what happens in a country that privileges acute care delivery over basic care, over public health, over common human decency; a country that in 1980 went into denial about the reality of its economic and housing policies, and its public responsibilities.

Nothing in the history of the United States revealed . . . public duplicity in such bold relief as our health-related conduct during the 80s. It was a period of national fantasy, an escape from reality. Directed by a president who be-lieved that "homeless people live on the street because they want to," the scenario called for more money for weaponry of questionable utility at the expense of services to the hungry, homeless, disabled, poor, women, children and others. Decades of public health advances were rescinded in a few years and there was hardly a whisper of outrage. The American people, their elected representatives, their professional organizations, and their leaders of every kind, let it happen.[9]

Crisis in Democracy

In 1968, Barbara Ehrenreich and John Ehrenreich in *American Health Empires: Power, Profits, Politics* told Americans that there was no "system" of health care in the United States. For 25 years individuals have witnessed and, finally, accepted that their health care system is wholly profit-based; that the pieces of health care that they receive, or (significantly) don't receive, are commodities like all others in a highly developed global economy; and that arguments about decency, justice, and responsibility are wholly inappropriate in the arena of profit margins and utilization. Like a phantom limb, discussions of health care as a social good kicks in at times but, by and large, it is the amputated discourse it became in 1970.

In 1994, most middle-income Americans expect a health care system that responds to public needs about as much as they expect an adequate public transportation system. Yet individuals also know that something larger, deeper, and more awful is happening to them and to their friends, and even to strangers across a divide of region and culture. "Medicine" or "health care" is becoming a metaphor for neglect, for a civil rights struggle, for what might be monstrous about American life devoid of a belief in the common good. What once were their caretakers have receded behind institutions that betray a collusion with darker, more mean-spirited forces. Commodification is one thing. The commodification of medicine, they know, is quite another.

Unlike the grave consequences of the commodification of other parts of everyday life—housing, food, clothing, transportation—the commodification of health care has a de-civilizing effect upon the culture that owns it. The political milieu that allows health care to be a part of a free market tacitly agrees to tolerate its effects, not only in the delivery of medical services, but in the lack of regard for preventing disease and injury. Viewed in this light, it is not surprising that the United States shares with South Africa the fact that it has no public health care system.

The ramifications of a capitalist health care system are wide and cover everything from the lack of governmental concern with work safety to the "arbitrage" brokering of cancer treatments. The society that allows life-insurance policies on individuals with AIDS to be listed in stock portfolios is the same culture that is likely to have diseases of the developing world in developed world cities.

Medicine is both product and rescue, both use and care. It is both a part of basic resources and the safety net when resources fail. Illness has its own duality. It is both fact and condition. It is an economic and social/political process that focuses on the vulnerability of the individual body. Illness is both about an individual person, and about a society. Once illness is truncated from its social basis and regarded in solely medical terms, it becomes bio/medical, and no standard remains by which to measure healthy or ill *societies*.

In such a reversal of social and individual causes, there is no longer any way in which to talk of prevention. The logic of "illness" moves understanding toward acute conditions and away from any larger unit of social or even environmental analysis.

To be sick in America is to be in a continuum of jeopardy—to be invisible in the sea of "undeserving sick," to risk one's livelihood to pay for health care, to endure endless situations of disrespect, or to be subjected merely to the irritating arrogance of providers become patriarchs.

To be sick and poor is to become a pariah. Whether one begins poor and gets sick or whether one begins sick and gets poor as a result, sickness and poverty go hand-in-hand in America and it is difficult to distinguish them. It is unsettling to note how similar Dickens' portraits of disease-infested London slums are to the present-day reality of New York City, ravaged by a new epidemic of tuberculosis.

Everyone feels the continental shift when the doctor becomes the purveyor; when medicine becomes the corporation and the moral arbiter. And this does not happen overnight, or directly. Western culture has long warned against the power of the person who heals, for in healing is the ability to harm. Hippocrates, however, was correct when he stated that the ability to heal is civility itself— if rightly used.

The American health care system is not made up simply of individual doctors who may "harm or heal," however. As this anthology illustrates, it is made up of institutions and entire agencies that function as business managers, executing the financial directives of those providers or regulators. If the institutions in America had a strong health agenda, individual practitioners would not be entrepreneurs. Opportunism and the exploitation of individuals occur within institutions and behind the technical jargon of advanced education. When this happens, as it has in the management mentality for all areas of American life, it is a loss, but not a direct danger. In health care it is a direct danger.

The HIV epidemic taught America that getting a fatal disease can change one's class status. The same is true for cancer, kidney disease, or any disabling condition. One has only to look at our elderly sick, our homeless, our mental health infrastructure, our disability medicine, our tuberculosis programs, or our drug treatment programs, to see that poverty begets disease, disease begets poverty, and *both* serve as sources of stigmatization within a national health system wholly tuned to profit from or, barring that, exclude those individuals for whom it's supposed to care.

For institutions to become wholly heartless and parasitical upon the vulnerability of individuals as they have in America means that an inversion in values has occurred and every agency or individual meant to help is, at least in part, in complicity with a larger social machine of exploitation. Under Reagan and Bush, this exploitation has taken place in housing, in HCFFA, in NIH, in HHS, in HRA, in insurance. It has occurred in every agency connected to the health of individuals, from social services to primary care. And it has perverted discourse to such an extent that it is almost impossible to articulate the loss in reasonableness, in humaneness, in decency.

As the articles in this anthology attest, the economic development of American medicine has affected not only our concept of health care, its access and its distribution, it has reversed the priorities of care and spent myriad institutional energies *disguising* that fact. The "new federalism" of the 1980s now lends itself easily to calls for "rationing," for decisions about whether our elderly populations are "too old for health care," for "caps" on services to those most in need, to an "apartheid" duality of services—one for the poor and one for the rich—that comes with an ideology that distinguishes, however covertly, the "deserving sick" from the "undeserving sick"—whether that duality is "managed competition" for the employed or Medicaid managed care for the poor.

The Social Darwinism of the last 10 years is entrenched in our culture. And health care policy is no innocent bystander. It profits at every turn and is fast becoming the ultimate gatekeeper. The "health apartheid" that is before us— the general inaccessibility of health care institutions to the poor, the lack of insurance, the structures of institutional churning, the dismantling of Medicaid, the very distinction between the "too old, sick, or poor for health care" and everyone else—are issues of democracy and point to the breakdown of the social contract—between government and individuals, between providers and patients, between citizens and citizen.

There are signs of resistance. The very breakdown of social obligation in our institutions has fostered a new set of "informal" relations of obligation. Whether it is between ACT UP and the FDA, between providers of health care in shelters or in migrant worker camps, between citizens in cities or working at the front line against the invisibility of whole communities, a new health activism is taking place across race and class lines and forging the call for a new shape to the health policies of medicine in the United States. As the system approaches "chaos," individuals with literally nothing left to lose gain sight of their own power to help and be helped. If this new activism can become a true political movement among the coalitions representing those at multiple jeopardy with our health care system, it will be the "civil rights" issue well into the year 2000, and will foster the conceptual core that can articulate adequate health care policy in the United States. These issues are treated in Section V, "Toward Adequate Health Care Policy," as well as in Section VI, "Proposals for a National Agenda."

It is clear that without changes in the financing of health care and the configuration of services; without a national citizens' movement for both 1) a universal, comprehensive, one-tier health financial plan (a national health program) *as well as* 2) the declaration of a state of emergency in our poorest communities and something like an Emergency Health Infrastructure Administration, emphasizing rural and urban preventive and basic care outreach to deal adequately with a wave of health emergencies, the 1990s offers the supreme anti-democratic nightmare.

As the national reforms of the Clinton Administration show, it remains true that health care policy reflects the priorities of the culture and those priorities

are not monolithic. Yet, as the articles in Sections IV, "Community Response
and Innovative Policy," V, "Toward Adequate Health Care Policy," and VI,
"Proposals for a National Agenda," address different solutions, they also point
to the dreams of patients, communities, health care providers, and policy makers
who do still believe in common human decency.

NOTES

1. Community Service Society. "Building Primary Care in Low-Income Communities in New
York City," New York, 1990.
2. I. Emmanuel, et al. "Poor Birth Outcomes of American Black Women: An Alternative
Explanation," *Journal of Public Health Policy*, 10:3, 1989, pp. 299–309.
3. Office of the Comptroller. "Poverty and Breast Cancer in New York City," New York, Oct.
1990.
4. "Forgotten Americans," *American Health*, Nov. 1990.
5. Colin McCord. *New England Journal of Medicine*, 1990.
6. J. Hadley, et al. "Comparison of Uninsured and Privately Insured Hospital Patients," *Journal of the American Medical Association*, 265:3, Jan. 16, 1991.
7. Barry R. Bloom & Christopher J. L. Murray. "Tuberculosis: Commentary on a Re-emergent
Killer," *Science*, Vol. 257, No. 21, August 1992.
8. Brudney & Dobkin. "A Tale of Two Cities: Tuberculosis Control in Nicaragua and New
York City," Seminar in Respiratory Diseases, 1991; also "Resurgent Tuberculosis in New York
City," *American Review of Respiratory Disease*, 144:745, 1991.
9. Harry Sultz, DDS, MPH. "Health Policy: If You Don't Know Where You're Going, Any
Road Will Do," *American Journal of Public Health*, 1991; 81(4):418–420.

HEALTH/PAC AND ITS ROLE IN HEALTH CARE REFORM

Nancy F. McKenzie and Rob Burlage

Health/PAC was founded in 1968 for the purpose of analyzing the "power structure" of American health care. The critical analysis was based explicitly on both the views of progressive health organizers in the local communities of Northeast "inner cities" and in the organizing experiences of the civil rights, anti-war, feminist, and environmental movements of the 1960s.

Health/PAC's founding issue, "Health *Is* the City's Business" (*Health/PAC*, Bulletin No.1, June 1968), chronicled the deepening dominance of New York City's seven academic medical centers over city hospitals, particularly regarding the community initiatives for health centers in Harlem, the Lower East Side, the Bronx, and Brooklyn. These metropolitan (and regional) medical "empires" were shown to be agents of a larger profit-hosting "medical-industrial" complex (made up of hospital capital financing and "high-tech" expansion, pharmaceutical research, and insurance financing on Wall Street). This dominance was not only seen in the huge profits it offered but also in the industries' control of the principles of health care delivery that insured the complex's continuance—its high-tech model of care.

These early *Bulletin* issues were based upon Rob Burlage's "New York City's Municipal Hospitals," released May 1, 1967. This report included a graphic portrayal of community need against outlines of the institutional dominion over neighborhoods. It contained structural and program proposals for reform. An issue of the report was featured in a special issue of *The Milbank Memorial Fund Quarterly*. What had seemed to the media and general public as a philanthropic idea by the academic medical centers of New York to offer health services to the public, got a different and critical treatment, one that even the *New York Times* considered to be a new framework for understanding health systems and for formulating policy and program analysis. The report anticipated and directly influenced the report of Mayor John Lindsay's Commission on Personal Health Services, chaired by Gerard Piel, publisher of *Scientific American*, and the creation by New York State in July 1970 of the City Health and Hospitals Corporation. The groundwork was laid to broaden and deepen a fightback policy against the undermining of public health leadership, community voice, and frontline health workers fighting in New York and across the United States.

A national system analysis was published as *The American Health Empire: Power, Profits, Politics* by Barbara and John Ehrenreich (1970), a best-selling paperback modestly recognized as a "das Hospital" of, and for, the health civil rights movement. It later formed the basis for the treatment of health issues that became the "mark" of Health/PAC, and the *Health/PAC Bulletin*. Almost immediately the *Bulletin* became a journal that progressives could rely upon for a "system-challenging" analysis of health care delivery in the United States.

Health/PAC, as both child and parent of the new and still evolving progressive health movement, attempted openly to develop an appropriate, popular, and locally usable analysis that was neither academic "leftist" nor purely "populist." We sought to be both politically/economically sophisticated enough to understand what drives the "system" and community driven enough to see where and to what extent the system's dominance affected individual patients and frontline health workers, not only with respect to health care access but through institutional arrangements that were wholly disempowering and alienating.

Through the 1970s and 80s the *Health/PAC Bulletin* continued to elaborate on the "empire's" interpretation of health care delivery. It was essential, after the treatment of the academic "empires," to point to the fact that the voluntary hospitals and their affiliated academic health centers were becoming much like the "chain management mentality" of for-profit medicine, and increasingly under corporate control. Louanne Kennedy was the main analyst of these changes. (See "The Losses in Profits: How Proprietaries Affect Public and Voluntary Hospitals," in Section III of the anthology, p. 295.) Kennedy and others, like Tony Bale and Alan Sager and Ronda Kotelchuck, explicitly evolved the "empires'" concept, focusing on profits in the industries and showing the corporate influence of government financing which produced "fiscal reform for Medicare"—Diagnosis Related Groups (DRGs) and prospective payment systems. (See Ronda Kotelchuck's analysis in "And What About the Patients?: Prospective Payment's Impact on Quality of Care," in Section II, p. 190, and "The Threat and Promise of Medicaid Managed Care: A Mixed Review," in Section III, page 321.) The coming of the corporations in health care mirrored the coming of the epidemics of our major urban areas, placing patients in increasing jeopardy and casting physicians as lethal gatekeepers in the most obvious conflict-of-interest positions.

Prognosis Negative, the second Health/PAC book, edited by Dave Kotelchuck, offered a kind of workbook anthology for institutional organizing and promoting community health care efforts across the nation and began Health/PAC's efforts to not only analyze the health care system but to offer education and point the way to activism.

Health/PAC coined the term "medical-industrial complex" in part as a conceptual corollary to the Pentagon's contractors and the era of the Vietnam War, but more important, it served to shift the debate about the need for health care reform from the content of specific health institutional policy interpretations to a complete "systems analysis." Before the appearance of Health/PAC and its analysis of the health "empires," criticism of health care delivery came from Physicians Forum, *Consumer Reports*, and some journalistic and academic analyses. They all emphasized a) organized medicine—your local medical society and its fights against health care reform, as well as the National Health Institutes and the American Medical Association as the main culprits; and b) "the drug company profiteers" highlighted by the Kefauver hearings. No one disclosed the systemic way these interests intertwined with the power of academic medical centers.

Most writings on the health care system after 1978 paid homage to or retorted against what became known as the "the Health/PAC analysis."

Health/PAC Twenty-Five Years Later

The latest round of health reform debate bears striking resemblance to the previous national discussions, while failing to acknowledge the ways in which national life has changed since the 1960s, or the extent to which health care delivery has become as much an issue of infrastructure, as of financing.

It is important to understand that the era of the "new federalism" brought about by a twelve-year-long Republican Administration had direct health consequences, the most dramatic of which has been the *convergence* of high rates of illness due to poverty with a bare bones basic health care delivery system. No sector of basic health oversight or basic health care delivery, or health care costs of public programs was spared—with predictable results.

Beginning in the early 1980s and continuing up until the present, Health/PAC has focused its analytic energies both on the continuing crisis in health care delivery as an elaboration of the "health empires," as well as on interpreting community struggles and the new activism born from them. We have been able not only to glean from community struggles the effects of our major American "empire," but the positive response that can come from both necessity and genuine care. Numerous articles in recent issues of the *Bulletin* discuss and document the evolution of the new "health civil rights" movement. Many are contained in this anthology. Finally, we have also striven to take on the critical truth-telling function that all reform needs in times of political struggle—documenting the ways and manner in which the "medical industrial complex" is both parasitical on illness and the "medicalizer" of social problems.

This anthology speaks to the urgency of making the current health care landscape visible. It encompasses our analysis as well as an articulation of the health activism that is dictated by this greater complexity of crisis.

Health care is no longer a financial access and cost control issue. It is, and reflects, a social crisis of mammoth proportions; an issue of "health security" and social stabilization reminiscent of the movements for social security in the 1930s; and one that calls, as did the 1929 and 1930s Depression, for wholly new institutions and community participation born of an explicit new health civil rights struggle.

It is our hope at Health/PAC that this anthology can be used, as have the other Health/PAC books and *Bulletins*, not only to change the paradigm of health care analysis, but to continue the momentum for reform of the American health care system toward access, equality and community control. We aim precisely with this work to give courage to those fighting on the front lines of the health struggle.

We invite you to join us, as we also continue to seek to join you.

SECTION I

HEALTH STATUS IN THE UNITED STATES: COMMUNITIES AT RISK

INTRODUCTION

Sally Guttmacher
and David Kotelchuck

One measure of the effectiveness of a country's health care delivery system is the health status of its people. Health care doesn't determine the types and distribution of disease in a society, but it has obvious impact on the rates of mortality from illness and the severity of the illness. Also, the extent of death and disfunction from illness in various subpopulations in a society gives us insight into how well its health care system is working—who is receiving and benefiting from medical care, and who remains outside the system.

International Comparisons

A look at this country's national health statistics reveals a disturbing decline in the health status of our citizens relative to those in other industrial and developing countries. Two signal health statistics, infant mortality and life expectancy at birth, reveal this quite clearly. Their values, as those of many useful national health statistics, reflect both the impact on health of the national economy, and the equity of distribution and delivery of health resources among members of that society.

Infant Mortality

In an earlier book, *Prognosis Negative: Crisis in the Health Care System,*[1] Health/PAC traced the relative decline of U.S. infant mortality rates between 1955 and 1973 compared to those of 20 other industrial countries. During this time period, the nation's infant mortality rate dropped from 8th to 15th among these 20 countries, even as the U.S. rate improved in absolute terms—falling from 26.4 infant deaths per 1,000 live births in 1955 to 17.7 per 1,000 live births in 1973.[2]

In the ensuing 15 years, this trend has continued, based on currently available United Nations data.[3] Of the 20-nation group, the U.S. dropped from 15th in 1973 to a tie for 17th in 1988 (Table 1), ranking above only the troubled Czechoslovakia and the no-longer-existent USSR. The U.S. infant mortality rate of 10 deaths per 1,000 live births in 1988[4] is more than twice that for Japan, the country with the lowest national infant mortality rate. If the U.S. had the same infant mortality rate as Japan in 1988, a majority of infants who died in the U.S. that year would have been saved, sparing the lives of over 20,000 infants that year alone. In view of the enormity of this loss, the Bush Administration's assertion that the U.S. infant mortality rate has been falling in recent years gives little comfort, since half of these personal tragedies may have been preventable.

(Note: It is of interest, especially in view of the current U.S. national debate over adopting a health care system similar to that enacted in Canada in 1971 (see Ref.5, as well as Section VIII), that in the 15-year period from 1973 to 1988, Canada surged dramatically from 12th to 6th place among the 20 selected industrial nations in infant mortality, while the U.S. continued to fall (Table 1). Between 1955 and 1973 Canada had remained essentially stationary relative to the other countries.)

Life Expectancy

During the last 15 years, the life expectancy of U.S. females at birth has continued to increase. But as in the case of infant mortality, progress in the U.S. has not kept pace with that in other industrial countries. Thus between 1972 and 1987–88, U.S. female life expectancy dropped from 5th to 9th place among 15 selected industrial nations,[6] as indicated in Table 2.

Females born in Japan in 1988 could expect to live fully three years longer on average than those born in the U.S. This reflects both the lower infant mortality in Japan, as well as the lower death rates at other ages. Note also that while U.S. female life expectancy was falling relative to other countries during this time period, female life expectancy in Canada was rising from 6th to 4th place among the 15 selected nations.

Only in male life expectancy at birth has the U.S. held its position in recent years relative to other nations. It has remained in the same place among the 15 selected nations between 1972 and 1987–88, albeit at a relatively low 11th-place ranking (Table 3). Canada meanwhile, suffering from similar, if not related, economic malaise as the U.S., has still improved its standing from 7th to 4th place among these 15 nations.

These national health care statistics are a reflection of the declining U.S. economy, lack of implementation of known preventive measures, and this society's stagnation in health care delivery. But when we look at the health care problems facing vast subgroups within our population, such as poor and underemployed Americans, children, female-headed households, Black, Latino, Native American and Asian-American populations, we see how badly we are failing as a society to provide adequate health care to all our people. A look at the AIDS epidemic and the shameful lack of governmental response to it, despite a loss of 200,000 lives in the U.S.[7] and counting, further confirms this observation.

Differences in mortality and morbidity among the many different subgroups within U.S. society are highlighted by such parameters as race, class, gender, and citizenship status. As Health/PAC has noted previously, the U.S. health care system did not create distinctions in care by race, class, and gender, but it does reflect and thereby reinforce them.[1] And we know that some of these parameters themselves are deeply intertwined, such as race and class.[8,9] But let us look briefly at these parameters separately and the differentials in mortality and morbidity that follow from them.

Table 1
Infant Mortality Rates for
20 Selected Countries

(Deaths/1000 Live Births)

1955			1973			1988		
Rank	Country	Rate	Rank	Country	Rate	Rank	Country	Rate
1.	Sweden	17.4	1.	Sweden	9.6	1.	Japan	4.8
2.	Netherlands	20.1	2.	Finland	10.1	2.	Sweden	5.8
3.	Norway	20.6	3.	Norway	11.3	3.	Finland	5.9*
4.	Australia	22.0	4.	Netherlands	11.6	4.	Netherlands	6.8
5.	N. Zealand	24.5	5.	Japan	11.7	4.	Switzerland	6.8
6.	Denmark	25.2	6.	Switzerland	12.8	6.	Canada	7.2
7.	U.K.	25.9	7.	France	12.9	7.	W. Germany	7.5
8.	U.S.	26.4	8.	Denmark	13.5	8.	France	7.7
9.	Switzerland	26.5	9.	E. Germany	16.0	9.	Norway	8.0
10.	Finland	29.7	10.	N. Zealand	16.2	10.	Australia	8.1
11.	Canada	31.3	11.	Australia	16.7	10.	E. Germany	8.1
12.	Czech.	34.1	12.	Canada	16.8	12.	Denmark	8.3*
13.	Ireland	36.8	13.	Belgium	17.0	13.	U.K.	9.0
14.	France	38.6	14.	U.K.	17.5	14.	Australia	9.2
15.	Japan	39.8	15.	U.S.	17.7	14.	Ireland	9.2
16.	Austria	40.7	16.	Ireland	17.8	16.	Belgium	9.7*
16.	Belgium	40.7	17.	W. Germany	20.4	17.	N. Zealand	10.0*
18.	W. Germany	41.7	18.	Czech.	21.2	17.	U.S.	10.0
19.	E. Germany	48.8	19.	Austria	23.7	19.	Czech.	11.9
20.	USSR	—	20.	USSR	26.3	20.	USSR	24.9

* 1987 Data

Sources:
United Nation Demographic Yearbook, 9th Ed., 1957, pp. 200–09; *Ibid.*, 25th Ed., 1973, pp. 256–62; *ibid.*, 41st Ed., 1989, pp. 342–50.

Health by Social Class

European industrial countries such as Britain and Sweden have long classi-fied and analyzed death and illness statistics by social class based on occupation, but the United States does not do so.[9,10] Thus, to conduct such an analysis for the U.S., one must depend on so-called surrogate variables, each of which only partially reflects aspects of social class or socioeconomic status, such as income, education, and occupation as reflected (inadequately) on death certificates.[10]

In Britain and Sweden and other countries where mortality rates are analyzed according to social class, relative risks of mortality for manual (blue-collar) workers have persisted at levels 15 to 45 percent greater than those for non-

Table 2
Life Expectancy at Birth (Female)
for Selected Countries

1972			1987–88		
Rank	Country	Rate	Rank	Country	Rate
1. Sweden		77.41	1. Japan		81.30
2. Norway		76.83	2. Switzerland		80.70
3. Japan		75.92	3. Sweden		80.15
4. Denmark		75.90	4. Canada		79.79
5. U.S.		75.20	5. Norway		79.55
6. Canada		75.18	6. Australia		79.46
7. Switzerland		75.03	7. Austria		78.63
8. E. Germany		74.19	8. W. Germany		78.37
9. Australia		74.18	9. U.S.		78.30
10. Austria		74.10	10. U.K.		77.64
11. USSR		74.00	11. Denmark		77.60
12. U.K.		73.81	12. N. Zealand		77.27
13. N. Zealand		73.75	13. E. Germany		75.91
14. W. Germany		73.44	14. Hungary		74.03
15. Hungary		72.05	15. USSR		73.78

Table 3
Life Expectancy at Birth (Male)
for Selected Countries

1972			1987–88		
Rank	Country	Rate	Rank	Country	Rate
1. Sweden		71.97	1. Japan		75.54
2. Norway		71.09	2. Sweden		74.16
3. Denmark		70.70	3. Switzerland		73.90
4. Japan		70.49	4. Canada		73.02
5. Switzerland		69.21	5. Norway		72.75
6. E. Germany		68.85	6. Australia		72.03
7. Canada		68.75	6. Austria		72.03
8. N. Zealand		68.44	8. U.K.		71.90
9. Australia		67.92	9. W. Germany		71.81
10. U.K.		67.81	10. Denmark		71.80
11. U.S.		67.40	11. U.S.		71.50
12. W. Germany		67.24	12. N. Zealand		71.03
13. Austria		66.80	13. E. Germany		69.81
14. Hungary		66.28	14. Hungary		66.16
15. USSR		65.00	15. USSR		65.04

Sources:

United Nations Demographic Yearbook, 25th Ed., 1973, pp. 94–100; *ibid.*, 41st Ed., 1989, pp. 130–140.

manual (managerial, professional, sales, and administrative) workers, and these differences are observed for most major causes of death.[11,12] These would be expected to persist in the U.S. as well. This has been observed for occupational, educational, and income differentials in the classic 1973 study by Kitigawa and Hauser, who concluded that, "Socioeconomic differences in mortality were evident no matter which indexes of socioeconomic level were employed."[13] More recently this was observed for U.S. heart disease and cerebrovascular mortality by income, education, and occupation, according to calculations based on specially collected 1986 U.S. government data.[14]

If U.S. data relating mortality and social class is scant, it is relatively abundant for morbidity and social class, as measured by the surrogate parameters of income, education, and occupation on death certificates. Two key sources of government data on health, illness, and insurance coverage and social class are the third edition of *Health Status of Minorities and Low-Income Groups* by the Health Resources and Services Administration (HRSA), 1990,[15] and *Health Characteristics by Occupation and Industry: United States, 1983–85* by the National Center for Health Statistics (NCHS), 1989.[16]

Table 4 presents a list of health-related variables, all of which have been shown to vary with personal or family income, either directly (e.g., number of dental visits per person per year) or inversely (e.g., percent of adults without teeth). The extent of these disparities is presented in the information source shown. Clearly, based on these results, lower personal and/or family income is associated with poorer health status and less health insurance coverage.

However, because of the limitations of income as an indicator of social class, especially during periods of great unemployment, one can examine the relationship of health status and level of education, considered by some a better indicator of social class than income.[17] But this variable presents a similar pattern of relationship to health status as that presented in Table 4 for personal or family income.[15,16]

Similarly, current occupation, as indicated in health interviews, portrays a pattern of better health in professional, sales, and clerical workers than for skilled, semi-skilled, and service workers and laborers.[16] This is further strengthened by considering health status in terms of occupation and industry *of longest employment*, again based on health interviews.[18] Whatever appropriate variable is used as a surrogate for social class—income, education, or occupation—persons of higher socioeconomic status have better health, greater access to health services, and longer lives.

Health by Race/Ethnicity

Statistics collected on the United States population indicate obvious differences in the health status of the major racial/ethnic groups. Because the genetic makeups of the various groups are so similar, it is misguided to argue that the differences are a result of biological distinctions. As one group of public health professionals has said, "The fact that we know which race we belong to says more about our society than our biology."[19] Rather, the differences in health between racial/ethnic groups in the United States reflects the society's social

Table 4
Income-Related Health Variables

Health Category	Health Variable*	Info Source†
Health Status	Self assessment of health as fair or poor (all ages)	HSM, p. 71
	Respondent assessed health status (from poor to excellent)	HCOI, p. 44
Health Conditions and Disabilities	Limitation of activities due to chronic conditions	HCOI, p. 56
	Eight or more bed days in last year	HCOI, p. 68
	Specific health impairments/1000 elderly persons: Visual, hearing, back, loss of extremities	HCOI, p. 306
	Incidence of all acute medical conditions in past year	HCOI, p. 92
	Percent hospitalized in last year	HCOI, p. 80
	Percent with 6 or more physician contacts in last year	HSM, p. 334
	Heart Disease mortality	HSM, p. 135 & 144
	Cancer mortality	HMS, p. 135 & 144
Preventive Health	Percent women with Pap smear in last year	HSM, p. 51
	Percent women with breast exam by health professional in last year	HSM, p. 51
	Percent persons who had blood pressure checked in last year	HSM, p. 61
	Percent persons who currently smoke cigarettes	HSM, p. 77
	Percent distribution of total number good health habits	HSM, p. 73
Dental Health	Percent adults (45 years or more) without teeth	HSM, p. 230
	Number dental visits per person per year (all ages)	HSM, p. 233
	Interval since last dental visit	HSM, p. 233
	Number dental visits per child (2–16 years)	HSM, p. 232

Table 4
Income-Related Health Variables *(cont.)*

Health Category	Health Variable*	Info Source†
	Percent children (2–16 years) who had dental visit within last year	HSM, p. 232
	Percent persons (all ages) who have never visited a dentist	HSM, p. 233
Health Insurance	Percent persons with hospital insurance coverage	HCOI, p. 108
	Percent persons with doctor or surgical insurance coverage	HCOI, p. 108
	Percent of uninsured workers (under 65 years)	HSM, p. 364
	Percent workers (under 65 years) *not* obtaining health insurance from their own jobs	HSM, p. 365

* For all adults (ages 18 years or older), unless otherwise noted. Elderly persons are ages 65 years or older.

† HSM = *Health Status of Minorities and Low-Income Groups: Third Edition*, HRSA, 1990. (Ref.15)

HCOI = *Health Characteristics by Occupation and Industry: U.S., 1983–85*, NCHS, 1989. (Ref.16)

organization, which in turn is guided by a system of beliefs or ideology. Racism, which is a system of social relations in which one racial group justifies its domination over the other on ideological grounds, continues to have a strong influence on social organization in the United States.[20] The fact that health status in the United States varies by race and ethnicity is a consequence of our history of racism, and the integration of racist values into our economic and social system. Thus, for example, people who are not white in the United States, if they are lucky enough to find work, are more likely to be tracked into poorly paying and "riskier" jobs, which are less likely to offer health insurance.

Because even "scientific" thinking is informed by the prevailing ideology, statistics are frequently interpreted as showing racial differences in a biological sense instead of economic or class differences as an explanation for the variation in health status between racial/ethnic groups. On the other hand, many scientists have argued that race is meaningless as an explanation for variation in health. Only a few diseases have been linked to genetic traits like skin color, and the physical differences between members of different racial groups tend to be less than the genetic variation within the groups. In addition, researchers have recently called into question the statistics upon which we base our analysis of racial/ethnic differences. They have pointed out serious inconsistencies in the manner in which race and ethnicity are coded when data is collected in the U.S., and argue that scientific principles for defining and validating these categories are also lacking.[22]

Although race or ethnicity is not sufficient to explain racial and ethnic differences in health status, racism may help in understanding the etiology of the health differences in subpopulations of the U.S.[20,23] Racism exists both on individual and institutional levels. Thus, to a significant extent, differences in health status between racial and ethnic groups reflect differences in opportunity, income, and thus lifestyle.

Racism perpetuates conditions of poverty and neglect for non-whites residing in the United States. Poverty rates as measured by the proportion of the population living below a specified income, currently about $14,000 for a family of four, are not equally distributed by race or ethnicity in the United States. According to 1988 census data, whereas one-tenth of whites had incomes below poverty, this was true for slightly over a quarter (27 percent) of those of Latino origin and for almost one-third (32 percent) of Blacks. The differences are even more striking for children under 18 years of age. About two-fifths of both Black children (44 percent) and Latino children (38 percent) live below the poverty line compared with less than one-fifth (14 percent) of white children.[24]

Health Statistics Reporting

Currently, most national health statistics are reported for four minority groups in the United States: Asian and Pacific Islanders, African Americans, Latinos, and Native Americans.[25] Combined, these groups make up about a fifth of the population. But because of higher birth rates than whites and greater immigration, it is estimated that by the second decade of the next century, about two-fifths of school-age children will come from minority groups.[26]

African Americans are the largest group and, because they have had many generations to assimilate, socially the most homogeneous of the minority groups. They have the highest mortality rates of any racial or ethnic group in the country, and the gap between their life expectancy and that of whites continues to increase.

Latinos are the second largest and fastest growing minority in the United States, with birth rates three to four times that of non-Latino whites.[27] In addition, during the 1980s Latinos seeking work or political asylum immigrated to the United States in record numbers. Close to 40 percent of the immigrants to the United States during this period were from Latin America. Many of the recent immigrants attracted to this society are forced to reside in an underclass, defined in part by the illegal immigration status of many of its members. Because many are not legal residents, they do not have access to care through Medicaid or other entitlements.[28] The three major subgroups that constitute the majority of the Latino population are Mexican-Americans, Puerto Ricans, and Cuban-Americans. Recently the number of Central and South Americans has increased as well.

Of the three major subgroups, Puerto Ricans appear to be in the worst health, reporting more chronic health problems than Blacks, Mexican-Americans, or Cubans.[29] Despite the fact that rates of poverty between Blacks and Latinos are similar, and except in relation to specific diseases like diabetes mellitus, the latter appear to enjoy better health.

In the discussion which follows, most of the differences will be presented as comparisons between Blacks and whites because, until the 1985 Report of the DHHS Task Force on Black and Minority Health, statistical comparisons were largely between whites and non-whites, over 90 percent of whom were Black. In addition, until 1988, national death certificates did not necessarily include Latino identifiers. Thus the preponderance of comparative data continues to be between Blacks and whites.[30]

Perceived Health by Race/Ethnicity

Most Americans, regardless of race or ethnicity, rate themselves as healthy compared with others of their own age. Blacks, however, are more likely to rate their health as poor compared to whites. When income is taken into account, it is clear that poverty is a more important determinant of perceived health than is race. Blacks and whites alike with incomes below $10,000 were over four times as likely to rate their health as only poor or fair compared to those who had incomes above $30,000.

Educational level also seems to be a determinant of how well people feel. People with more education feel better about their health no matter what their racial or ethnic group, although racial differences in perception of health remain substantial even when you compare people of different racial/ethnic groups with 12 or more years of education. Twice as many Blacks as whites with 12 or more years of education rated their health as only poor or fair (22 percent compared with 9 percent).[25]

Use of physician services, which reflects both health status and access, also varies by race and by income. In general, people who are less healthy see physicians more frequently. When looking at utilization it is important to bear in mind what was noted previously, namely that poor people feel less healthy. Even though they are more likely to live at or below the poverty level, Black children under the age of 18 have fewer physician contacts than white children. Adults with low incomes who rated their health as poor visited physicians less frequently than wealthier people who thought themselves to be in poor health. When the data is adjusted for health status it indicates that Blacks had lower physician utilization rate, 5.6 visits per person compared with whites, 6.5 visits per person.[25]

Mortality by Race/Ethnicity

There has been no substantial improvement in the ratio of Black to white death rates during the past forty years. Mortality rates for African Americans are higher than those of whites and of other minority groups. Thus, whereas life expectancy increased for whites during the latter part of the last decade, it has decreased for Blacks. Infant mortality rates, considered to be the most sensitive overall health status indicator, have been decreasing more rapidly for whites than for Blacks.[26]

By the end of the 1980s the three major causes of death in the U.S. were heart disease, cancer, and stroke. The health status differential between African Americans and other non-whites living in the United States is largely due to differences in deaths from cardiovascular disease and cancer, which are discussed below.

A. Heart Disease

Ischemic heart disease (IHD) is the leading cause of death in the United States, accounting for approximately 500,000 deaths in 1989.[31] Rates of mortality for IHD vary by region in the U.S., with the Northeast having the highest rates and the West the lowest. The highest state rates for men and women are in New York, and the lowest in Hawaii (Men: New York 755.1 per 100,000 compared to 316.4 in Hawaii. Women: New York 462.6 per 100,000 compared to 184.0 in Hawaii).[31] Between 1980 and 1988 death rates for those age 35 or older declined by 24 percent. The decline occurred for both Blacks and whites and both men and women, although the rates declined more rapidly for men than for women and for whites than for Blacks. It is not yet clear what factors have contributed to this, but it appears that declines in the incidence of coronary heart disease (CHD), changes in lifestyle which reduce risk, and better quality medical care have all contributed.

High serum cholesterol and hypertension are conditions which put people at risk for CHD. Latino males and females have a lower prevalence of high serum cholesterol than do whites or Blacks, whose rates appear to be similar. Age-adjusted prevalence rates for hypertension are much higher for Blacks and much lower for Latinos than they are for whites. African-American males are the most likely group to be afflicted with hypertension and have a 23 percent higher prevalence than white males.

Although mortality from CHD has declined, particularly among middle- and upper-middle-class men, it still accounted for 27.5 percent of deaths in the U.S. in 1987.[32] The steady decline in mortality during the past thirty years has largely been due to reductions in risk factors. Increased exercise, a reduced fat diet, and decreased cigarette smoking appear to be the three aspects of lifestyle change which contribute most to this reduction.

Cigarette smoking, the single most avoidable cause of death in the United States, accounted for an estimated 434,000 premature deaths in the United States in 1988.[33] The rate of years of potential life lost before age 65 was twice as high for Blacks as for whites. Smoking is more common in males than females and in African Americans, American Indians, and Latinos than whites. Approximately two-fifths of the men in these groups smoke compared to less than a third of white males. Smoking is about as common in white and Black females, and white women appear to have caught up with white men in terms of the percentage who smoke. Latino men smoke less as they become more acculturated to the U.S., whereas with women it is just the opposite, that is, as Latinas become more acculturated to U.S. ways they smoke more.[29] Although Black adolescents are less likely to smoke than their white counterparts, by adulthood they are more likely to.[33] In addition, Blacks tend to use brands with higher tar and nicotine content.[34] It appears that in the United States the age at which smoking begins has decreased substantially for Black and white women, and that regular smoking behavior is occurring at younger ages. Those who begin smoking at younger ages are at greater risk of becoming heavy smokers and thus of smoking-related morbidity and mortality.

B. Cancer

Cancer incidence and prevalence rates have been increasing in industrialized countries, although cancer mortality rates have risen only slightly since 1973.[35] Between 1983 and 1987 the overall cancer mortality rates per 100,000 were 299.7 for Black males, 212.5 for white males, 161.0 for Black females, and 137.6 for white females. During this period, cancer mortality rates fell by at least 16 percent for those under age 45 and rose by a similar amount for those age 65 or older.[36]

As with prevalence, Blacks appear to have a higher incidence rate of cancer, and shorter survival rates than whites. Whereas incidence may tell us something about the impact of racism upon environmental conditions and which communities are more likely to host toxic dumps, survival rates tell us something about access to medical services and life-extending drugs, and about stressful living conditions.

The most common sites for cancer include the lung, breast (female), prostate, and colon/rectum. The incidence and prevalence of these cancers vary by sex and race/ethnicity. The relative rates of cancer mortality among Black and white Americans between 1983 and 1987 are presented in Figures 1 and 2.

As indicated in Figure 1, the ratio of Black to white rates of cancer mortality for all sites of cancers was 1.3 for this period. That is, Blacks suffered a 30 percent greater rate of mortality from cancer for all sites than whites during this period. (A ratio of 1.0 means equal mortality rates for Blacks and whites.) Note also that of the 24 specific cancer sites for which the mortality ratio is calculated, almost twice as many (14 sites) are greater for Blacks than whites (8 sites). At two sites, lung (females) and urinary bladder, the cancer rates are equal (ratio = 1.0).

In recent years, the overall rate of cancer mortality has worsened for Blacks more significantly than for whites. Between 1973 and 1987, Blacks showed an 11.6 percent increase in mortality rates for cancers at all sites, more than double the 5.1 percent increase for whites (Figure 2). Also, Black rates decreased by a smaller amount or actually increased among all but two of the cancer sites for which the corresponding white rates decreased in this time period. This suggests that progress in the detection, screening, and/or treatment of cancer has had a greater impact on white Americans than on Black Americans during this time period.

1. Lung Cancer Lung cancer, which is largely preventable, is the leading cause of cancer mortality in the United States, accounting for over one-quarter of all cancer deaths in 1990. Approximately two-thirds of lung cancer cases occur in males, and among males it is second only to cancer of the prostate in terms of incidence. It is the second leading cause of death among Black males, after coronary heart disease.

Figure 1

SEER CANCER INCIDENCE AND US MORTALITY RATES, 1983–87

RATIO OF BLACK RATE TO WHITE RATE
ALL AGES

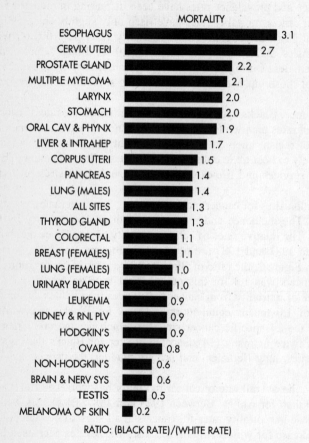

MORTALITY

ESOPHAGUS	3.1
CERVIX UTERI	2.7
PROSTATE GLAND	2.2
MULTIPLE MYELOMA	2.1
LARYNX	2.0
STOMACH	2.0
ORAL CAV & PHYNX	1.9
LIVER & INTRAHEP	1.7
CORPUS UTERI	1.5
PANCREAS	1.4
LUNG (MALES)	1.4
ALL SITES	1.3
THYROID GLAND	1.3
COLORECTAL	1.1
BREAST (FEMALES)	1.1
LUNG (FEMALES)	1.0
URINARY BLADDER	1.0
LEUKEMIA	0.9
KIDNEY & RNL PLV	0.9
HODGKIN'S	0.9
OVARY	0.8
NON-HODGKIN'S	0.6
BRAIN & NERV SYS	0.6
TESTIS	0.5
MELANOMA OF SKIN	0.2

RATIO: (BLACK RATE)/(WHITE RATE)

Source (for Figures 1 and 2):

Cancer Statistical Review, 1973–1987, edited by Lynn A. Gloeker Ries, Benjamin F. Havrey, Brenda K. Edwards. National Cancer Institute, U.S.H.H.S., N.I.H. publication No. 90–2789.

Figure 2

TRENDS IN CANCER MORTALITY RATES
PERCENT CHANGE: 1973–87, SELECTED SITES
WHITES, BLACKS, ALL AGES

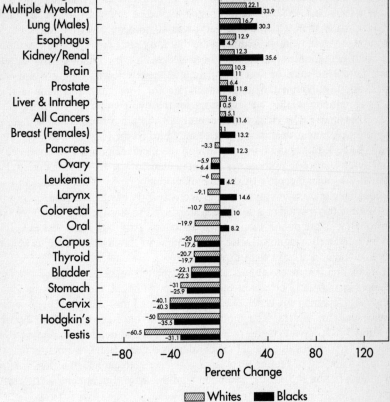

Source:
See Table 1.

Lung cancer incidence ranks third behind breast and colon cancer in women. For females of both races lung cancer incidence has been increasing steadily, largely because of increased cigarette smoking. Based on trend data, it is expected that increases in the incidence of lung cancer among women will continue until 2013.[35] The near doubling of lung cancer incidence rates among Latino men and women between 1970 and 1980 is clearly linked to increased cigarette smoking.[29]

There is a substantial racial difference in terms of incidence and mortality. Between 1977 and 1983 the age-adjusted incidence rate was 40 percent higher for Black males than white males, but it was 10 percent lower for Black women compared to white women. Although the mortality rates from lung cancer among Black and white males has steadily been decreasing, the relative survival rates, which are an indicator of access to care, are slightly lower among Blacks than whites. Also, although the lung cancer rate for Mexican-Americans is much lower than among whites, survival rates for the two groups are about the same.

2. Breast and Cervical Cancer In 1988, breast cancer accounted for 20 percent of all cancer deaths for Black and white women ages 45 to 74.[37] There appears to be a rather dramatic increase in the incidence during the past decade for all adult women in both races. Although some of the increase is due to more sensitive diagnosis because of the use of mammography, there is concern that additional factors are involved in the increase.[35] A slight increase in survival rates during this period has also been attributed to earlier diagnosis. Survival rates for Blacks are poorer than for whites, due in part to the fact that the cancer is more frequently diagnosed later in the course of the disease and thus at a less favorable stage in Blacks than in whites.

Unlike breast cancer, almost all deaths related to cervical cancer are preventable through early detection and follow-up. Although more Black than white women are screened for cervical cancer, the related mortality for Black women is twice that for whites. The mortality rates for both races declined between 1980 and 1987; however, the ratio of Black to white deaths has remained unchanged. The excess in cervical cancer deaths among Black women appears to be due to a variety of factors associated with access to care such as less frequent Pap smears before the 1980s, and poorer follow-up and treatment at the current time.

The AIDS Epidemic

Although heart disease and cancer are the leading causes of death in the United States, the AIDS epidemic represents the most dramatic change in health status of the U.S. population during the last decade. Of all diseases, it perhaps best highlights the inadequacies and unresponsiveness of our health care system.

Since the first case of AIDS (acquired immunodeficiency syndrome) was reported in the U.S. in June 1981,[38] the grim face of AIDS has been ever-changing—in complexion, in gender, in the social classes of its victims. But the epidemic, whomever it strikes, continues unabated.

It took eight years—from June 1981 until August 1989—for the first

100,000 cases of AIDS to be reported in the U.S. and its territories. It took only two years—from September 1989 until November 1991—for the next 100,000 cases to be reported.[7]

The second 100,000 persons diagnosed with AIDS had a larger percentage of female and heterosexual male intravenous drug users—24 percent vs. 20 percent in the first 100,000 cases—and a smaller percentage of homosexual/bisexual men—55 percent vs. 61 percent in the first 100,000 cases. Of the first 100,000 victims, 9 percent were women; of the second, 12 percent—an increase of about 33 percent. Black and Latino persons, always disproportionately hard hit, are now even more victimized by AIDS. Of the first 100,000 victims, 27 percent were Black and 15 percent Latino; of the second 100,000, 31 percent were Black and 17 percent Latino.[7]

If we compare the numbers of persons newly diagnosed with cases of AIDS in 1990 and 1991, the last two years for which these data are currently available, the changing face of AIDS stands out in even sharper contrast. In the single year from 1991 to 1992, the number of AIDS cases among females rose by 15 percent, among Blacks 10.2 percent and among Latinos 11.5 percent.[39]

Among regions of the U.S., the rate of new AIDS cases being reported annually is rising most rapidly in the South among all the major exposure categories—homosexual/bisexual men, females and heterosexual men using intravenous drugs, and persons reporting heterosexual contact with AIDS victims or persons at high risk of HIV (human immunodeficiency virus) infection.[39] Cases are also rising steadily, but at a slower rate, in the West and Midwest. Only in the Northeast, presumably due to better organization of AIDS support and political action groups and greater public education, are the rates of new cases dropping among homosexual/bisexual men and IV drug users (but not for high-risk heterosexual contacts).

There are currently an estimated one million persons infected with HIV in the United States. As of December 31, 1991, a cumulative total of 206,392 persons had been officially diagnosed with AIDS. Of this number, 133,232 persons have died of the disease.[7]

By 1989, HIV infection/AIDS had become, after unintentional injuries, the second leading cause of death among men 25 to 44 years of age, exceeding even heart disease, cancer, and homicide for this age group.[40] Among women in this same age group AIDS was the eighth leading cause of death in 1988, and expected to rise to fifth leading cause of death in 1989.[40]

As expected from their disproportionate percentage of all AIDS cases, Blacks and Latinos make up a disproportionate percentage of all AIDS deaths as well. Of the first 100,000 AIDS deaths, 28 percent were among Black Americans and 16 percent were among Latinos.[40]

These figures on AIDS disease and death, affecting the lives of millions of people in this country, represent an American tragedy. The failure of will by U.S. political leadership at all levels to respond to the epidemic—indeed the refusal by President Reagan for many years even to mention the name of the disease—is a national scandal.[41,42,43]

Based on the numbers of HIV-infected persons in the U.S. population, and the continuing lack of a commensurate response to this crisis by government and the health care system, the AIDS epidemic in the United States will, tragically, almost certainly get worse in the near future.

NOTES

1. Health/PAC (D. Kotelchuck, ed.). *Prognosis Negative: Crisis in the Health Care System*, Vintage, 1976.

2. Health/PAC. *Op. cit.*, pp. 6–9.

3. United Nations. *Demographic Yearbook: 41st Edition*, United Nations, pp. 342–50, 1989. (See also note in Ref.4)

4. U.S. Department of Commerce. *Statistical Abstract of the United States: 111th Edition*, USGPO, p. 77, 1991. (Note: The provisional 1988 value (9.9) listed in the 1989 U.N. Demographic Yearbook (Ref.3) was replaced by the final value (10.0) listed in this source. All other U.N. values listed were final values.)

5. Wolfe, Samuel. "Importing Health Care Reform: Issues in Transposing Canada's Health Care System to the United States," *Health/PAC Bulletin*, 20(2):27–33, Summer, 1990.

6. United Nations. *Op. cit.*, pp. 130–40. (Note: Only 15 countries were selected for comparison here, rather than the 20 countries used in the section on infant mortality, because differences in the years for which such data were reported by different nations limited the number of countries for which appropriate life expectancy comparisons could be made.)

7. Centers for Disease Control (CDC). "The Second 100,000 Cases of Acquired Immunodeficiency Syndrome—United States, June 1981–December 1991," *Morbidity and Mortality Weekly Report (MMWR)*, 41:28–29, 1992.

8. Smith, Davey, and George and Matthias Egger. "Socioeconomic Differences in Mortality in Britain and the United States (editorial)," *American Journal of Public Health*, 82(8):1079–81, August, 1992.

9. Navarro, Vicente. "Race or Class or Race and Class: Growing Mortality Differentials in the United States," *International Journal of Health Services*, 21(2):229–35, 1991.

10. Kitigawa, Evelyn, and Philip Hauser. *Differential Mortality in the United States: A Study in Socioeconomic Epidemiology*, Harvard, Ch.1, 1973.

11. Marmot, M.G., and M.E. McDowall. "Mortality Decline and Widening Social Inequalities," *The Lancet*, 2(8501):274–76, Aug. 2, 1986.

12. Vagero, Denny, and Olle Lundberg, "Health Inequalities in Britain and Sweden," *The Lancet*, 2(8653):35–36, July 1, 1989.

13. Kitigawa and Hauser. *Op. cit.*, p. 152 & Ch. 8.

14. Navarro, Vicente. *Op. cit.*, pp. 230–31.

15. Health Resources and Services Administration (HRSA). *Health Status of Minorities and Low-Income Groups: Third Edition*, Dept. Health & Human Services, 1990.

16. National Center for Health Statistics (NCHS). *Health Characteristics by Occupation and Industry: United States, 1983–85*, CDC, 1989.

17. Kitigawa and Hauser. *Op. cit.*, p. 23.

18. NCHS. *Health Characteristics by Occupation and Industry of Longest Employment*, CDC, 1989.

19. Krieger, Nancy, Diane Rowley, Allen A. Herman, Byllye Avery, and Mona T. Phillips. "Racism, Sexism, and Social Class: Implications for Studies of Health, Disease and Well-Being," Draft, 1991.

20. Rose, G. "Sick Individuals and Sick Populations," *Int. J. Epidemiology*, 14:32–38, 1985.

21. Polednak, A.P. *Racial and Ethnic Differences in Disease*, NY: Oxford Press, 1989.

22. Hahn, Robert A. "The State of Federal Health Statistics on Racial and Ethnic Groups," *J. Amer. Medical Assn. (JAMA)*, 267(2)268–71, 1992.

23. Mullings, L. "Inequality and African-American Health Status: Policies and Prospects," in *Race: Twentieth Century Dilemmas—Twenty-First Century Prognosis*, W. Van Horne, ed., Madison: Univ. of Wisconsin Institute on Race and Ethnicity, 1989.

24. U.S. Bureau of Census. *1980 Census of Population: General Population Characteristics*, Summary PC80-1-B1, USGPO, 1980.

25. NCHS. "Health United States, 1990," U.S. Public Health Service, 1991.

26. Nickens, Herbert. "The Health Status of Minority Populations in the United States," *Western J. of Medicine*, pp. 27–32, July, 1991.

27. Munoz, Eric. "Care for the Hispanic Poor," *JAMA*, 260(18):2711–12, 1988.

28. Guttmacher, Sally. "Immigrant Workers: Health, Law, and Public Policy," *J. Health Politics, Policy and Law*, 9(3):503–14, 1984.

29. Council on Scientific Affairs. "Hispanic Health in the United States," *JAMA*, 265(20):248–52, 1991.

30. U.S. Dept. Health and Human Services. *Report of the Secretary's Task Force on Black and Minority Health*, Executive Summary, Vol. 1, 1985.

31. CDC. "Trends in Ischemic Heart Disease Mortality—United States, 1980–1988," *MMWR*, 41(30)548, 549, and 556, 1992.

32. CDC. "Coronary Heart Disease Attributable to Sedentary Lifestyle—Selected States, 1988," *MMWR*, 39(32):541–44, 1990.

33. CDC. "Differences in the Age of Smoking Initiation Between Blacks and Whites—United States," *MMWR*, 40(44):754–57, 1991.

34. CDC. "Trends in Lung Cancer Incidence and Mortality—United States, 1980–1987," *MMWR*, 39(48):875 and 881–83, 1990.

35. National Cancer Institute (L. A. Gloeckler, B. F. Hankey and B. K. Edwards, eds.). *Cancer Statistical Review 1973–1987*, NIH Publication No. 90-2789, 1990.

36. Davis, Devra Lee, and David Hoel. "Figuring Out Cancer," *International Journal of Health Services*, 22(3):447–53, 1992.

37. CDC. "Mortality Surveillance System Charts," *Monthly Vital Statistics Reports*, 40(8):6–7, 1991.

38. CDC. "Pneumocystis Pneumonia," *MMWR*, 30:250–52, 1981.

39. CDC. "Update: Acquired Immunodeficiency Syndrome—United States, 1991," *MMWR*, 41:463–68, 1992.

40. CDC. "Mortality Attributable to HIV Infection/AIDS—United States, 1981–1990," *MMWR*, 40:41–44, 1991.

41. Shilts, Randy. *And the Band Played On*, N.Y.: St. Martins Press, 1987.

42. Freudenberg, Nicholas. *Preventing AIDS: A Guide to Effective Education for the Prevention of HIV Infection*, Amer. Public Health Assn., 1990.

43. Arno, Peter, and Karyn Feiden. *Against the Odds*, N.Y.: HarperCollins, 1992.

A GUIDE TO THE READINGS
IN SECTION I

The following readings give a statistical picture of those groups of people that can be singled out as being at visible risk of harm in the current chaotic health care system. The first article, "The Uninsured: From Dilemma to Crisis," is one of three articles written by Emily Friedman on the lack of access to poor individuals. (See Section II for her discussion of public hospitals.) This article concerns not only the uninsured but also the underinsured. Friedman points to the narrow coverage many individuals receive from private insurance and the confusing and inadequate public insurance offered by Medicaid, Medicare, and other federal, state, and local supports.

The charts on the costs of health care, the family burdens of insurance, and the costs of private insurance premiums tell their own astounding story of who is at risk of being without health care. The charts on poverty and poverty in women demonstrate precisely who those individuals are likely to be, indicating that the "feminization of poverty" has become the "feminization of pain and suffering."

Neither charts nor articles can adequately tell the stories of individuals who are homeless. Some of these are people who are mentally ill (See "Homelessness" and "People with Chronic Mental Illness" by the Robert Wood Johnson Foundation, pp. 44 and 45). Some are men, women, and children on home relief, ineligible for any other support. Some are families that spend years transiently housed.

The issue of homelessness has become socially and medically complex precisely because individuals who are homeless or only transiently housed are also usually chronically ill and sicker than their more well-off counterparts; being without social supports, they are often discharged directly from a hospital to a public shelter. Yet, the homeless as sick individuals are essentially invisible.

Although health care delivery has become more problematic in cities and housing programs have gone beyond crisis proportions in state budgets gutted by federal withdrawal, states *continue* to cut back on benefits to the poor as a politically painless way of cost containment. We have witnessed this in the "safety net" cuts of the 1980s and early 1990s. The interconnection of health and housing policies was highlighted as issues of the "deinstitutionalized mentally ill" five years ago. And they are still tied to the wholly disruptive lives that those seeking help for serious mental illness contend with. (This is discussed in "Care of the Seriously Mentally Ill: Eight Current Crises," p. 46.)

The conditions of the lives of individuals without homes go far beyond issues of deinstitutionalization. As our tuberculosis and HIV epidemics attest, as do the lack of discharge planning for homeless individuals in hospitals, sickness is as much intertwined with homelessness itself as with previous conditions that made the medically underserved become the housing underserved. The attempt to save costs by cutting public entitlement has been shown to backfire again and again by putting pressure on other public parts of the services system, especially the medical provision offered by public hospitals.

The reemergence and flourishing of tuberculosis is only the latest wave of health disasters to batter a population increasingly lacking housing, employment, and public and primary health care—the basic human services essential for a community's well-being. Fifty percent of individuals with AIDS are homeless, and 20 to 40 percent of homeless individuals are estimated to be HIV antibody positive. Yet, it will not do to continue to list people by disease category, ones that come at the end or as the result of unlivable conditions. This is helpful to neither the individuals, to city and state health strategies, nor to those who advocate for the views of homeless individuals as individuals in need of a multiplicity of medical and housing responses.

There are many individuals with "infectious" diseases and there are also individuals with chronic hypertension, diabetes, asthma, who, left untreated and without respite from lack of housing, are in great jeopardy. We have so neglected our poor that we do not know who these individuals are, or are likely to be. And without such data, policies designed to address housing and/or medical needs cannot be developed.

The "invisible ill" are as much a part of the west coast as the east coast, as Frank Clancy's "Burnout in L.A.," p. 81, attests to. His "Healing the Delta," p. 72, shows the health activism, almost entirely of female providers, for individuals in rural areas of the nation, principally the Mississippi Delta.

The issue of African-American and Latino health status is startlingly portrayed in "Racial Comparison of Health Data," p. 89, and government studies of health care access by the Government Accounting Office reports are contained in this section. From these comparisons we can easily see how women are multiply affected by their lack of access to care and by the dependence upon the health care system. A system that seeks, if they are poor, and particularly if they are African American or Latina, to blame them for their ill health, without understanding the peculiarities of their needs. In "Women—The Missing Persons in the AIDS Epidemic" by Kathryn Anastos and Carola Marte, p. 97; as well as "Abortion: Where We Came From, Where We're Going" by Ellen Bilofsky, p. 105, these issues are addressed.

While it is important for health policy to point out the gendered nature of health research (predominantly for men) and health reproductive technology (for women), and to emphasize the over-determination of women's futures through the medicalization of reproduction, it is always necessary to point to the almost entirely schizophrenic nature of such technologies—e.g., the fact that while they are proffered as state-of-the-art diagnostic tests and indispensable to health or to womanhood, in a for-profit health care system, technological advances are almost always unavailable to low-income women.

The lesson here is that what is a consumer health item and, thus, health promotion for the consumer, is virtually non-existent for the low-income consumer; both in health care terms and in social attitudes. This explains why the

U.S. can have a supportive social climate of motherhood for middle-income women and simultaneously speak disapprovingly of births among low-income women, particularly women of color. The difficulty for women to maintain health insurance for themselves and their children (see the voice piece, "The Insurance Game," p. 109), the callousness of providers, and the fragmentation of health care services makes poor women and their children not only invisible but a group who seek to "disappear" before a system that scapegoats them.

We end this section with the second voice piece by Teresa McMillen, "Too Little, Too Late: A Child with AIDS," p. 111.

THE UNINSURED:
From Dilemma to Crisis

Emily Friedman

Some health policy issues are like bad pennies; despite repeated efforts to re-solve them, they keep coming back. Probably no health policy issue of this century (with the possible exception of insuring and structuring long-term care, which affects far fewer people) has proven as intractable as access to acute care for Americans who lack coverage for the cost of that care. It was a problem for most Americans at one time; after the introduction of private insurance early in the twentieth century, it became a problem more of specific groups, notably the elderly and the poor. Coverage of those who were uninsured was a policy cen-terpiece (largely unrealized) of President Harry S Truman's administration. With the passage of Medicaid and Medicare in 1965, it was thought the issue was largely resolved.

The uninsured, however, like the proverbial poor, seem always to be with us. In fact, their numbers have grown significantly in the past 15 years. Proposals for solutions are rife, but consensus on how to attack the problem has proven, to say the least, elusive. Nevertheless, the dilemma of the uninsured has become a crisis, affecting all aspects of the health care system and many aspects of society.

Who Is Uninsured?

Most estimates place the number of Americans lacking public or private coverage between 31 and 36 million.[1-4] The 1987 National Medical Expenditure Survey found that 47.8 million people lacked insurance for all or part of 1987, with between 34 and 36 million uninsured on any given day and 24.5 million uninsured throughout that year.[1,2]

The US Bureau of the Census found that, from the first quarter of 1986 to the last quarter of 1988, 63.6 million people lacked coverage for at least one month and 31.5 million lacked it in the final quarter of 1988.[3] The Employee Benefit Research Institute reported that, in 1988, 33.3 million Americans had no private insurance and were ineligible for public coverage.[4] Even the more conservative figures represent a significant increase over the 26.6 million un-insured reported in the 1977 National Health Care Expenditures Study.[5]

When examined further, the statistics provide a troubling picture. Although most figures discussed herein are from the 1987 National Medical Expenditure Survey, virtually all other studies have found substantially the same patterns.

In terms of age, those who are 19 to 24 years old are most likely to be uninsured; 20.3 percent of this group were uninsured for all of 1987, and another 18.2 percent were uninsured for part of the year.[1,2] Children younger than 18 years were the next most likely to lack coverage, with nearly one in four uninsured either all or part of the year. The National Center for Health Statistics reports that, in 1988, 17 percent of children under 18 years had neither private insurance nor Medicaid coverage.[6] Given the importance of preventive and early intervention care to the health of the young, these rates are a cause of concern.

Of those aged 25 to 54 years, 19.8 percent were uninsured all or part of the year, as were 13.6 percent of those aged 55 to 64 years.[1,2] (Medicare covers virtually all Americans 65 years or older.) The fact that more than one in eight Americans who are 55 to 64 years old lack coverage at least part of the year is disturbing, in that this group faces a much higher risk of serious health problems than do younger Americans.

Racial and ethnic differences affect rates of coverage. Of non-Hispanic whites, 18.6 percent were uninsured for all or part of 1987, as were 29.8 percent of black Americans and 41.4 percent of Hispanic Americans.[1,2] Studies using differing methodologies going back as far as 1978 have shown that Hispanic Americans are the most likely to be uninsured of any ethnic group.[7] As Hispanics represent the fastest-growing ethnic population group in the nation, their consistently low rate of coverage is a potential warning of worse yet to come.

Men are slightly more likely to be uninsured than women; 23.8 percent of men were uninsured for at least part of 1987 as opposed to 21 percent of women.[1,2] This undoubtedly reflects the fact that virtually all men, regardless of their income, are excluded from eligibility for Medicaid. Also, Medicaid now covers low-income pregnant women with incomes up to 185 percent of the poverty line, as well as many mothers with dependent children. Furthermore, women are disproportionately represented in the poverty population, so, to the extent that Medicaid covers that population, more women than men are likely to be protected.

Income level is also associated with lack of coverage. The uninsured represented 47.5 percent of those with incomes below the poverty line in 1987, 45 percent of those with incomes between poverty and 125 percent of poverty, 36.7 percent of those with incomes from 125 percent to 200 percent of poverty, 17.8 percent of those with incomes 200 percent to 400 percent of poverty, and 8.8 percent of those with incomes above 400 percent of poverty.

The proportion of uninsured varies by state, depending on several factors, including the level of Medicaid coverage in the state, the demographics of the population, insurance practices, overall income, the nature of employment, and state health policy. The National Medical Expenditure Survey found lack of insurance highest in the South (27.4 percent of the population were uninsured at least part of the year) and West (27.2 percent) and lowest in the Midwest (16.7 percent) and Northeast (15.7 percent).[1,2] The Employee Benefit Research Institute found that lack of coverage ranged from less than 10 percent in Massachusetts, Pennsylvania, Michigan, Wisconsin, and Iowa to more than 25 percent in Louisiana, Texas, and New Mexico.[4] However, with so much coverage tied to employment and with states changing Medicaid and other health policies constantly, these figures are volatile.

Many Underinsured As Well

If the policy debate is to be framed accurately in terms of issues of coverage and access, a second group, the underinsured, must also be mentioned. This population is more difficult to define, because it faces risks that are more specific. That is, a patient's diagnosis can determine whether coverage is sufficient or not, and surveys of whether a person has coverage at all are unlikely to reveal such gaps in protection. Where a person receives care, how long the person is a patient, what types of treatment are required, and whether there is a dollar or time limit to coverage all affect the sufficiency of insurance. Nevertheless, a 1985 estimate, based on data projected from the 1977 National Health Care Expenditures Study, was that 26 percent of the nonelderly population, or approximately 56 million people in 1984, were "inadequately protected against the possibility of large medical bills."[8]

To this population, whose major problem is insufficient overall coverage, could be added those whose insurance precludes coverage of a given condition or imposes a waiting period before such coverage becomes operative (which is often the case with pregnancy). Also included are those who are covered by Medicaid but lack access to physician care because of physician reluctance to treat Medicaid clients and those who, insured or not, face difficulty in obtaining obstetric care because of the decreasing number of obstetricians willing to accept new patients (American College of Obstetrics and Gynecology, news release, May 3, 1988).[9-12]

Physician resistance to treating such patients has been ascribed to many causes, including low and delayed Medicaid payments, fears of malpractice litigation, paperwork, cultural or language problems, noncompliance, and other factors, including racial discrimination.[13] Certainly, the prospect of low or nonexistent payment is a disincentive to most providers.

The total number of uninsured and underinsured, even if the latter group has not been sufficiently identified, could easily represent one in every four Americans on any given day.

Erosion of Medicaid

How such a large number of Americans came to be at risk, through lack of coverage or lack of access or both, is a challenging question. Theoretically, coverage of health care costs is available to virtually all Americans through one of four routes: Medicare for the elderly and disabled, Medicaid for low-income women and children (and some men) and those with certain disabilities, employer-subsidized coverage at the workplace, or self-purchased coverage for those ineligible for the previous three. However, as many as 10 million more Americans were uninsured at least part of the year in 1987 than in 1977. What happened?

Of the four routes to coverage, Medicare has aged best. A universal enfran-chisement that is neither means tested nor related to the workplace, Medicare each year covers more Americans for most acute care. Beneficiaries' out-of-pocket costs remain high, however, and coverage for long-term care remains skimpy, especially with the repeal of Medicare catastrophic care coverage.

Medicaid, however, has suffered a more equivocal fate. Although passed by Congress, Medicaid is a state-level program, with each state defining income levels and other standards of eligibility and the federal government subsidizing a certain portion of expenses, depending on the state's overall wealth. Thus, coverage has always varied from state to state, with northern states and some western states offering more generous benefits than southern and other states.

In the early 1980s, both the federal and state governments sought to control or reduce Medicaid expenditures in the face of tax cuts, growing costs, and reduced federal funds for the program. This led to freezes and reductions in both eligibility and provider payments. The result was a basically stable number of beneficiaries despite an increase in the poverty population. Because of Med-icaid's categorical approach to eligibility, certain groups—most low-income men and childless couples, for example—do not qualify. However, there was little growth between 1980 and 1985 even among potentially eligible popula-tions.

Medicaid's fortunes began to change in the late 1980s, as Congress mandated Medicaid coverage of pregnant women (at least for pregnancy-related services) and young children with incomes as high as 185 percent of the poverty line. These mandates were resisted by many states because they required substantial increases in spending; by 1990, the governors of 49 states had asked Congress to refrain from further mandates—a request Congress did not heed as it in-creased child eligibility that year.

Medicaid faces another vexing problem: Although families receiving Aid to Families with Dependent Children constitute between 70 percent and 75 percent of the Medicaid population, three-fourths of Medicaid expenses go to the costs of care for the aged, blind, and disabled, especially patients in nursing homes. Indeed, Medicaid has, perhaps in violation of the intent of Congress, become a form of long-term care reinsurance for the Medicare population. In the absence of either major growth in affordable private long-term care insurance or inclu-sion under Medicare of more extensive long-term care coverage, the stress on the Medicaid program is likely to continue.

As a result of the rather tangled path it has traveled, Medicaid never covered the entire poverty population and was estimated to cover only 38.7 percent of that group in 1983.[14] By 1989, it was estimated that only 40 percent of the poverty population was covered by the program.[15] Although congressional man-dates may boost that figure somewhat, the majority of the poor remain unpro-tected by the program that was designed to cover them.

The Workplace Connection

The third route to coverage—employer-subsidized insurance for workers and often for dependents—has also seen serious erosion in recent years. This was the cornerstone of health insurance in the past—appropriate for a nation steeped in the Puritan work ethic and even more appropriate in an age in which labor shortages of many types are looming. The unspoken agreement was that, if a person was employed, he or she would receive health insurance benefits, subsidized to some degree by the employer or at least priced lower than individual coverage to reflect the fact that the subscriber belonged to an employee group.

However, the workplace is no longer a guarantor of coverage, if it ever was. The National Medical Expenditure Survey found that, in 1987, of the uninsured population, 46.4 percent were working adults, 6.8 percent were nonworking spouses of working adults, and 23.6 percent were children of working adults.[1,2] In other words, 76.8 percent of the uninsured either were employed or were nuclear-family dependents of the employed.[1,2] The Employee Benefits Research Institute found that, in 1988, 85 percent of the uninsured were either workers or family members of workers.[4]

The employed uninsured are unevenly distributed. The National Medical Expenditure Survey found that they were more likely to work part time or to be self-employed and to work in settings with fewer than 100 workers, especially in settings with fewer than 25 workers. In settings with fewer than 10 employees, 26.3 percent of workers were uninsured.[1,2]

Service industries, as opposed to manufacturing industries, were more likely to employ uninsured workers, reflecting both the lack of a tradition of employment-based coverage in the service sector and a much lower level of unionization, which is usually associated with generous health benefits.[1,2] The Employee Benefit Research Institute, using March 1989 data from the Bureau of the Census, found similar patterns.[4]

Thus, the majority of the uninsured are tied, directly or through family relationships, to a workplace that is no longer an automatic source of insurance. In some cases the employer does not offer coverage. In others the coverage is offered but is not affordable or is not purchased by the employee. In still others the employee acquires coverage for himself or herself but not for a dependent spouse or children. All of these possibilities are more likely in small business settings.

Employers are not necessarily the villains. Insurance products for small business are both limited and expensive. According to the General Accounting Office, small businesses have little ability to spread risk over a large number of employees, which results in higher premiums, should an employee incur large costs.[16]

Small businesses also face a far greater likelihood of premiums being based on experience rating rather than on community rating. Small employee groups are also seen by insurers as a higher risk, which means that, compared with larger employee groups, they are subject to more exclusions, medical testing of applicants, and denials of coverage because of health status and are less able to absorb the significant increases in premium prices that have been the pattern of the past two decades.[16]

Indeed, a major element in the crisis of the uninsured is the simple fact that health care costs a great deal more than it once did. The US Department of Health and Human Services reported in 1990 that, for 1989 (the last year for which final data were available), national health care spending increased 11.1 percent, to $604.1 billion (US Dept of Health and Human Services, press release, December 20, 1990). This meant that US spending on health care from 1980 through 1989 increased 128 percent. Insurance premiums reflect those costs plus insurers' own expenses and margins, leading to average increases in premiums that reached 18 percent in 1989.[17] In addition to increasingly selective attitudes toward risk on the part of insurers, insurance is becoming less affordable simply because the cost of the services it covers is doubling every few years.

If small businesses face problems in offering and retaining coverage, the individual insurance market faces collapse. This is the population that insurers characterize as the highest risk, requiring disproportionate administrative costs and usually proving unprofitable.

Medical underwriting, experience rating, refusal to cover those deemed "uninsurable," cancellation of policies on short notice, and high premiums are common if not almost universal barriers for those seeking individual coverage. As a result, for an individual unable to qualify for group or public coverage, obtaining affordable insurance is dependent on having a sufficiently high income and very good health status. This, needless to say, eliminates many of those who are most likely to need coverage, that is, those who are poor, sick, and/or unable to acquire workplace-based insurance.

The working uninsured are a complex population, and even data-based generalities are dangerous. Despite the small-business focus, many of the uninsured work for large firms, as is the case with agricultural and seasonal workers. Some of the uninsured simply choose not to acquire coverage, although they represent a small minority of this population. Some are eligible for either public or private coverage but are unaware of this and thus have never sought it. Although most of the uninsured are poor or near poor, some are middle-class people denied coverage by virtue of poor health status or "risky" jobs. It is a highly heterogeneous population, with multiple reasons for being at risk. Nevertheless, it is safe to say that the original notion of tying coverage to employment is working less well with each passing day. In times of economic downturn, when higher unemployment produces more medical indigence and lower tax revenues to fund public programs such as Medicaid, the fragility of the entire concept of linking coverage to employment becomes painfully clear.

Why a Crisis Now?

Most crises are born of a series of small events that one day reach critical mass. So it has been with the uninsured. The framers of Public Law No. 89–97, which brought Medicare and Medicaid into being in 1965, believed that universal health insurance was just around the corner, yet it failed to materialize.[18] When it was reported in 1980 that 26.6 million Americans lacked coverage, a response might have been expected but was not forthcoming. A large number of efforts—expansion of Medicaid; coverage of children by Blue Cross and Blue Shield plans; state insurance pools for the "uninsurable"; and coverage experiments funded by states, localities, and private sources—have attempted to address at least part of the problem, yet it continues unabated.

Has the issue reached critical mass? If not, it is well on the way to doing so, for at least five reasons.

1. Although coverage is not the sole determinant of health status, it is a key factor in improved health, as Medicaid data have demonstrated.[19] Although availability of care does not guarantee it will be used,[20,21] the uninsured have been shown to receive less care, even if they are able to gain entry to the system.[22] It is thus not unreasonable to assume that medical indigence is associated with lack of care and poorer health status. In other words, coverage does make a difference.

2. The health care system is suffering damage as a result of being asked (implicitly) to provide care for the uninsured who cannot pay. Because the uninsured often do not have access to physicians in private offices, health maintenance organizations, or other settings, they disproportionately seek care at hospitals. As an anonymous physician once observed, "They do not go to the doctor; they go to the institution."

Nevertheless, it was estimated in 1985 that physicians provided $9.2 billion in bad debt and charity care in 1982.[23] A 1988 survey by the American Medical Association found that physicians reported $6.3 billion in uncollected revenues that year (Socioeconomic Monitoring Service data, American Medical Association, 1988).

According to the American Hospital Association, hospitals in 1989 provided $11.1 billion in uncompensated care, an increase of $7.2 billion over 1980.[24] Although not all of this can be attributed to care of the medically indigent, most of it does represent such services. However, not all hospitals are equally affected, because the uninsured are not equally distributed. Teaching hospitals, Veterans Affairs hospitals, public hospitals, children's hospitals, and inner-city hospitals are harder hit, and the load among even these facilities is unequal.[25] Staggering under the pressure of the acquired immunodeficiency syndrome epidemic, drug abuse, increased trauma, problem pregnancies, and other results of social change and social neglect, most municipal and some private hospitals are barely coping with emergency care and are hardly able to provide timely—let alone elective —services to the uninsured. Rural hospitals face problems of their own, because of chronic low occupancy; one or two long stays by uninsured patients can doom a facility.

Care is often theoretically available through public or private clinics and other settings, both funded and voluntary. However, these are often so overloaded that access is illusory. In Chicago, Ill, for example, as of November 1990, pregnant women had to wait 125 days for an appointment with a physician at a public clinic (*Chicago Tribune*, November 25, 1990:§4, p. 1).

Thus, a minority of US hospitals carry the majority of the burden of the uninsured, and that burden is growing. As a result, there is quarreling among hospitals, between hospitals and physicians, and between hospitals and governments as the cost of treating the uninsured increases while subsidies (especially philanthropy) decline. With emergency departments in some cities (including

New York, NY) now the most common source of inpatient admissions, and with nearly 100 hospitals closing each year,[26] more and more hospitals are facing a horrendous choice: caring for all the uninsured and failing, or turning at least some of them away and surviving.

As a result, serious questions are being asked about the level of charity care that hospitals, clinics, physicians, and other providers should be expected to provide. Certainly, those entities holding charitable tax exemptions should be expected to provide some indigent care, although the requirement for such care was removed from the federal tax code in 1969.

Should some hospitals have case loads that are 10 percent or 20 percent uninsured while others have virtually no uninsured patients? Should indigent care provided by hospitals be subsidized largely by a haphazard patchwork of subsidies, tax levies, adjustments in Medicare and Medicaid payments, and other partial measures that are neither reliable nor well organized?

3. Another factor contributing to calls for action on the uninsured is the increasingly uncomfortable situation of employers. The number of employers who do offer coverage is dropping (*Business Week*, November 26, 1990:187), which is not surprising in view of the increasing cost of insurance and the voluntary nature of the arrangement.

The playing field is becoming more unequal: Some employers offer coverage, some do not. Some offer a lavish benefit package, others offer a lean one. Some are self-insured and, because of a federal statutory prohibition, cannot be required by states to offer mandated benefits; others must provide a wide range of benefits that raise the cost of coverage considerably. Whether one has coverage no longer depends on *whether* one is employed but rather on *where* and *by whom*.

Employer discomfiture is being exacerbated by calls for mandated employer coverage of all workers and even of dependents. Only the state of Hawaii has succeeded in legally requiring that most people working more than 19 hours per week be covered by employer-subsidized insurance.

The state of Massachusetts has passed legislation requiring most employers to provide a certain level of coverage to workers or else pay an assessment; it is scheduled to go into effect in 1992. However, the law is being challenged in court, and the newly elected governor of the state has proposed repeal of the employer mandate.[27] Other states are interested in some form of employer mandate, but the federal prohibition on state regulation of self-insured employers under the Employee Retirement Income and Security Act makes it extremely difficult to require these firms to participate (Hawaii has a federal waiver). Employers, anxious about being forced to subsidize expensive benefits but concerned about uninsured workers and unequal benefits, are also seeking a solution.

The uninsured have become a workplace issue in another way. The youngest baby boomer is now 26 years old; nearly 20 years of large numbers of entry-level workers have given way to a much leaner supply. If health insurance benefits are not offered by employers, what will lure new workers? Asking women, for example, to give up Medicaid coverage to become uninsured workers seems questionable in terms of incentives. In a labor-short era, the role of workplace benefits is critical.

4. Another force for a solution is the interrelationship of the uninsured and health care costs. On the one hand, it can be argued that, if health care for the more than 200 million Americans who have at least some coverage is so expensive, we cannot afford to cover the 31 to 37 million who have no coverage. On the other hand, it can be argued that the uninsured represent significant hidden costs. After all, most of them do receive care, at least when their lives are at stake or when they are having babies. Given their compromised or non-existent access to primary and preventive care, however, their point of entry into the system is too often a hospital emergency department. The timing of their seeking care is also often a case of too little, too late.

As a result, conditions that could have been prevented or treated in a cost-effective manner—from measles to carcinoma of the breast to diabetes—become emergencies, with both higher costs and worse outcomes. This, in turn, distorts staffing and practice in emergency services, leading, in the words of a health policy analyst many years ago, to primary care in the emergency setting, equivalent to tending a rose garden with a bulldozer. It is hardly a cost-effective use of health care resources.

The larger economic issue is that most of us pay the hidden costs of medical indigence, one way or another. Every insurance premium includes some of the costs of care of the uninsured. Even self-insured employers pay part of that cost. Paying patients subsidize nonpaying patients. The society as a whole pays the price of prenatal care that is not given, immunizations that are not provided, cancers that are not detected, diabetes that is not monitored, mental illness that is not discovered. The uninsured can be very expensive.

5. The last factor driving the need for action may appear secondary in a health care economy that has become hard edged. Nevertheless, issues of ethics and equity are as important and powerful as the economic or logistical issues. Foremost among these is whether a democracy that thinks of itself as the moral hope of the world can justify grave inequalities in access to health care, which in most countries is considered an essential human need.

It is often pointed out that, among developed nations, only the United States and South Africa have not implemented universal access to care. This is overstated; there are holes in every safety net. However, the holes in our net are more numerous and yawn deeper and wider than in many less-wealthy nations.

We claim that other nations ration care because the insured must wait sometimes; however, in our nation, the uninsured can wait forever. We claim that ours is the best health care system in the world; however, if tens of millions of Americans have little or no access to care, the claim rings hollow.

In addition, a health care system that has become too selective in terms of whom it treats carries with it the seeds of its own destruction. Our system has been built—properly, in my opinion—on a tradition of pluralism, public guarantees and private largesse, and both institutionalized and voluntary giving; a tradition of faith, hope, and charity.

Should the public lose faith in that arrangement (and in recent years we have

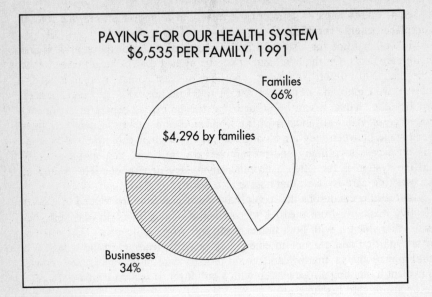

PAYING FOR OUR HEALTH SYSTEM
$6,535 PER FAMILY, 1991

Families
66%

$4,296 by families

Businesses
34%

Source:
Families USA, December, 1991

seen evidence of such a loss of confidence[28,28]), the very basis of the health care system is in jeopardy. Health care providers can hold themselves out as morally superior, but if they are not seen as such by the populace, voluntarism and autonomy can easily be replaced by fiat.

Many of our health status indicators are lagging or beginning to lag behind those in the rest of the developed world—and, indeed, in some of the Third World. Pressure is building to give up on our current system and develop another, based on the Canadian or some other centralized model.[28,29] The moral standing of American health care is on the line. We must produce a workable answer to the crisis of the uninsured, or all of us—health care providers and the society alike—could suffer the terrible and long-term consequences of inaction.

It is to that search for solutions that this issue of *The Journal* has been dedicated.

I acknowledge the assistance provided in the preparation and revision of this article by William H. Dendle III, MPH, Irene Fraser, Ph.D, and Alan Sager, Ph.D.

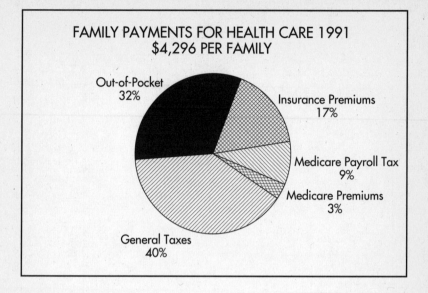

**FAMILY PAYMENTS FOR HEALTH CARE 1991
$4,296 PER FAMILY**

Out-of-Pocket
32%

Insurance Premiums
17%

Medicare Payroll Tax
9%

Medicare Premiums
3%

General Taxes
40%

Source:
Families USA, December, 1991

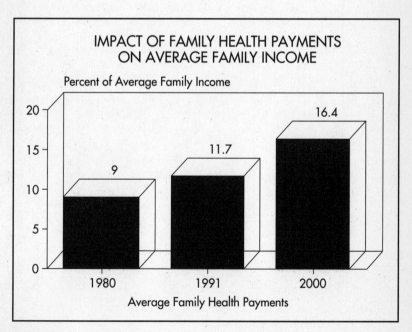

**IMPACT OF FAMILY HEALTH PAYMENTS
ON AVERAGE FAMILY INCOME**

Percent of Average Family Income

9

11.7

16.4

1980

1991

2000

Average Family Health Payments

Source:
Families USA, December, 1991

Figure 1

NUMBER OF PEOPLE WITH PRIVATE INSURANCE, 1960—1990

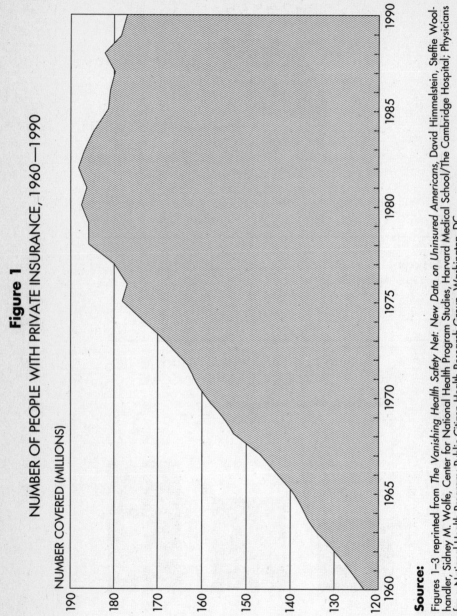

Source:

Figures 1–3 reprinted from *The Vanishing Health Safety Net: New Data on Uninsured Americans,* David Himmelstein, Steffie Woolhandler, Sidney M. Wolfe, Center for National Health Program Studies, Harvard Medical School/The Cambridge Hospital; Physicians for a National Health Program; Public Citizen Health Research Group, Washington, DC

Figure 2

NUMBER OF PEOPLE WITH PRIVATE INSURANCE AND TOTAL INSURANCE PREMIUMS, 1960–1990

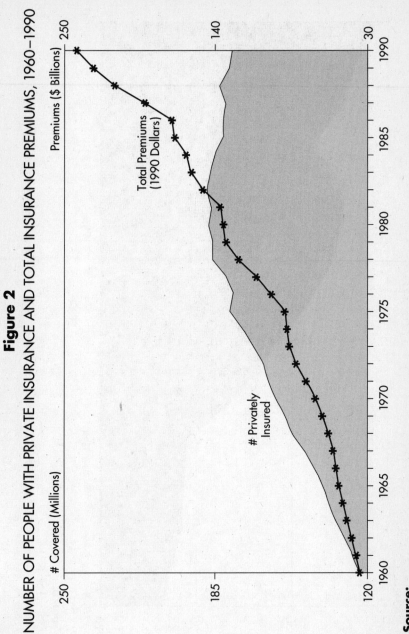

Source:
HIAA/NCHS

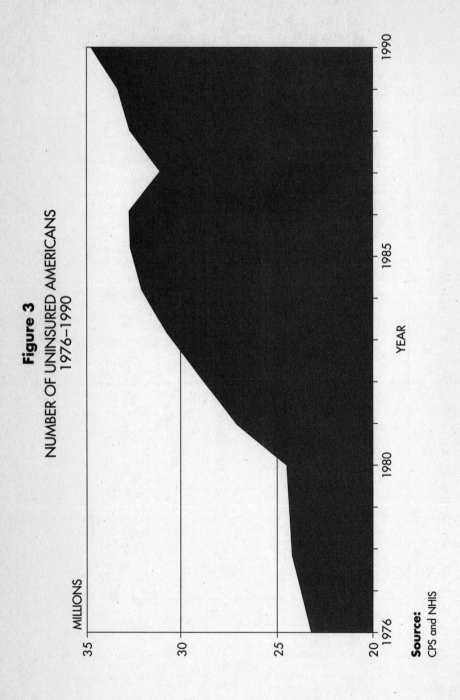

Figure 3
NUMBER OF UNINSURED AMERICANS
1976–1990

Source:
CPS and NHIS

NOTES

1. Short PF, Monheit A, Beauregard K. *National Medical Expenditure Survey: A Profile of Uninsured Americans: Research Findings 1.* Rockville, Md: National Center for Health Services Research and Health Care Technology Assessment; 1989.

2. Short PF. *National Medical Expenditure Survey: Estimates of the Uninsured Population, Calendar Year 1987: Data Summary 2.* Rockville, Md: National Center for Health Services Research and Health Care Technology Assessment; 1990.

3. Nelson C, Short K. *Health Insurance Coverage, 1986–88.* Washington, DC: US Dept of the Census; 1990. Current Population Reports, Household Economic Studies, Series P-70, No. 17.

4. Chollet D, Foley J, Mages C. *Uninsured in the United States: The Nonelderly Population Without Health Insurance, 1988.* Washington, DC: Employee Benefit Research Institute; 1990.

5. Kasper JA, Walden DC, Wilensky GR. *Who Are the Uninsured?* Hyattsville, Md: National Center for Health Services Research; 1980. National Health Care Expenditures Study, Data Preview 1.

6. Bloom B. *Health Insurance and Medical Care: Health of Our Nation's Children, United States, 1988.* Hyattsville, Md: National Center for Health Statistics; 1990. Advance Data From Vital and Health Statistics of the National Center for Health Statistics, No. 188.

7. Treviño FM, Moyer ME, Valdez RB, Stroup-Benham CA. Health insurance coverage and utilization of health services by Mexican Americans, mainland Puerto Ricans, and Cuban Americans. *JAMA.* 1991;265:233–237.

8. Farley P. Who are the underinsured? *Milbank Mem Fund Q.* 1985;63:476–503.

9. Friedman E. Doctors, doctors everywhere: and patients who can't get care. *Health Business.* January 4, 1991;6:1T–2T.

10. Medicaid participation declines. *SMS Rep.* September 1989;3:1–3.

11. Yudkowsky BK, Cartland JDC, Flint SS. Pediatrician participation in Medicaid: 1978 to 1989. *Pediatrics.* 1990;85:567–577.

12. Access to normal obstetrical care: a disturbing trend. *SMS Rep.* January 1989;3:3.

13. Fossett JW, Perloff JD, Kletke PR, Peterson JA. Medicaid patients' access to office based obstetricians. Presented at the 118th Annual Meeting of the American Public Health Association; October 3, 1990; New York, NY.

14. Gornick M, Greenberg JN, Eggers P, Dobson A. Twenty years of Medicare and Medicaid: covered populations, use of benefits, and program expenditures. *Health Care Financ Rev.* 1985; 7(annual suppl):13–59.

15. Swartz K, Lipson D. *Strategies for Assisting the Medically Uninsured.* Washington, DC: Urban Institute and the Intergovernmental Health Policy Project; 1989.

16. *Health Insurance: Availability and Adequacy for Small Businesses.* Hearings before the Subcommittee on Antitrust, Monopolies, and Business Rights of the Senate Committee on the Judiciary, 101st Cong, 2nd Sess (1990) (testimony of Mark V. Nadel, associate director for national and public health issues, Human Resources Division, General Accounting Office).

17. Cerne F. Rate decreases unlikely despite health insurers' healthy profits. *Am Hosp Assoc News.* November 5, 1990;26:8.

18. Friedman E. *The Problems and Promises of Medicaid.* Chicago, Ill: American Hospital Association; 1977.

19. Friedman E. Medicare and Medicaid at 25. *Hospitals.* August 5, 1990;64:38–54.

20. Aday LA. Access to what? for whom? *Health Manage Q.* Fourth Quarter 1990;12:18–22.

21. Piper JM, Ray WA, Griffin MR. Effects of Medicaid eligibility expansion on prenatal care and pregnancy outcome in Tennessee. *JAMA.* 1990;264:2219–2223.

22. Hadley J, Steinberg EP, Feder J. Comparison of uninsured and privately insured hospital patients: condition on admission, resource use, and outcome. *JAMA.* 1991;265:374–379.

23. Ohsfeldt R. Uncompensated medical services provided by physicians and hospitals. *Med Care.* 1985;23:1338–1344.

24. *Medicaid Underpayments and Hospital Care for the Poor: A Fact Sheet.* Chicago, Ill: American Hospital Association; 1991.

25. Friedman E. Hospital uncompensated care: crisis? *JAMA.* 1989;262:2975–2977.

26. Friedman E. Analysts differ over implications of more hospital closings than openings since 1987. *JAMA.* 1990;264:310–314.

27. Massachusetts health care law threatened. *Med Health.* February 11, 1991;45:2.

28. Blendon R. Three systems: a comparative survey. *Health Manage Q.* 1989;11:2–10.

29. Blendon R, Leitman R, Morrison I, Donelan K. Satisfaction with health systems in 10 nations. *Health Aff.* Summer 1990;9:185–192.

POVERTY

Robert Wood Johnson Foundation, 1991

The poverty rate in the United States since the 1960s reflects fluctuations in the nation's economy, as well as federal policies. The chart shows the steep drop in the poverty rate following the mid-1960s' War on Poverty and the further declines that occurred during economic boom cycles in the 1970s. Yet, in the 1980s—generally a period of economic expansion—we see a rise in poverty, which is attributed to a recession early in the decade, a decline in manufacturing jobs, shrinking federal programs that helped people on the brink of poverty, and a greater number of households headed by women than at any other time in our history.

Twelve percent of people ages 65 and over—one in eight—live below the federal poverty level. A greater proportion of elderly than nonelderly Americans are near-poor, with incomes between 100 percent and 125 percent of the poverty threshold. Historically, the elderly were hardest hit by poverty, because they were the most likely to be disabled and without work or income. In more recent times, improved retirement plans, Social Security, Medicare, and other programs all have helped improve the financial status of people 65 and older.

In 1974, the poverty rate among children under 18 began to surpass the poverty rate among the elderly and now exceeds it by a significant margin. About 20 percent of all children—one in five—live in poverty, and 44 percent of black children do.

In 1988, 31.6 percent of blacks lived below the federal poverty level, as did

FEDERAL POVERTY THRESHOLDS

Household Size	1968	1988
One person	$1,742	$6,024
Two	$2,242	$7,704
Four	$3,531	$12,092
Seven	$5,722	$18,248

Note:

Federal statistics classify as poor only those families with incomes below the federal poverty threshold. The poverty threshold varies according to family size, and each year it is adjusted for inflation. For example, the 1988 poverty threshold for a family of four was $12,092. (The median income for households of all sizes was $27,230 that year.) Believing the thresholds are too conservative, some analysts classify people with incomes up to 125, 150 or even 200 percent of federal poverty thresholds as "near-poor."

26.8 percent of Hispanics and 10.1 percent of whites. Poverty is 3 times more common among blacks than whites, mainly because more than half of black families are headed by unmarried women, often with young children. Families headed by women tend to be poorer because women may receive lower wages than men in comparable positions, have fewer chances for advancement, have less education and, therefore, lack skills for higher-paying jobs, have child-care responsibilities that limit their opportunity to work, or do not receive adequate —or any—child support payments.

Poverty is less common among people with more education. In 1988, 20.8 percent of householders who had not completed high school were poor, compared to 3.5 percent of those who had completed one or more years of college.

POVERTY BY AGE, RACE, AND HISPANIC ORIGIN, 1960—1988

Percent of People below Poverty Level

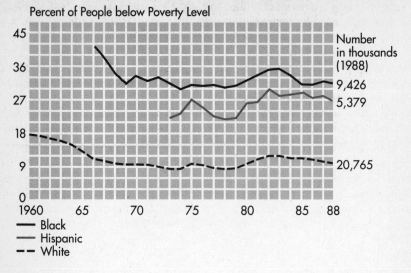

Number
in thousands
(1988)

9,426

5,379

20,765

— Black
—— Hispanic
-- White

Percent of Children and Elderly Below Poverty Level

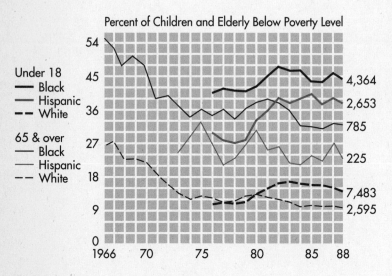

Under 18
— Black
—— Hispanic
-- White

65 & over
— Black
—— Hispanic
-- White

4,364

2,653

785

225

7,483
2,595

Note:

People of Hispanic origin may be of any race.

Source:

US Bureau of the Census. *Money, Income and Poverty Status in the United States: 1988.* Current Population Reports, Series P-60, No. 166. Washington, DC. 1989. Table 18, pp. 58–59, and Table 19, pp. 60–61.

WOMEN IN POVERTY

Ruth Sidel, Ph.D.

This issue of *Democratic Left* on women and politics appears at a critical moment—during a national election and during a time of severe recession when the economic hardship suffered by millions of people in the United States highlights the necessity of rethinking our social and economic priorities. One of the crucial issues largely ignored by virtually all of the candidates in this year of political attention to the "middle class" is the economic status of women and children.

It is important to note that while many women have moved into a wide variety of professional, managerial, and entrepreneurial occupations in the United States during the last quarter century nonetheless a dual labor market continues to exist and the majority of women continue to work in low-paid, low-status jobs doing primarily clerical, service, and sales work. Moreover, while women's wages, particularly those of young women, have risen in recent years, full-time, year-round female workers earn only about 70 percent of the earnings of comparable male workers. This gap is a central factor that keeps a vast number of women—and their children—in poverty in the United States.

Rising Poverty Rates

In 1990, 13.5 percent of the US population—33.6 million people—was officially classified as poor—that is, as living below even the unrealistically-low Federal poverty line. The number of poor people and the poverty rate have declined somewhat since 1983 when over 15 percent of all Americans lived below the poverty line, but the number and rate rose sharply in 1990. Between 1989 and the recession year of 1990, 2.1 million additional Americans, particularly children and the elderly, fell into poverty.

Moreover, the composition of poor families has changed significantly over the past thirty years. In 1959, 23 percent of all poor families were headed by women; by 1989 that figure had risen to 51.7 percent. Today nearly 40 percent of the US poor are children and over half are members of female-headed families.

The situation of families headed by African-American and Latina women is even more bleak. They continue to be at greatest risk of poverty. Among poor black families in 1989, nearly three-quarters, 73.4 percent, were headed by women with no husband present; among poor families of Latino origin, nearly half, 46.8 percent, were headed by women.

Life Chances

In comparing the poverty rate of married-couple families with that of female-headed families, the significant differences in economic status and therefore in life chances become clear. Among white married-couple families, the poverty rate in 1989 was 5 percent; among white female-headed households, the poverty rate was five times higher, or 25.4 percent. While the same differentials are apparent among black families and among families of Latino origin, these groups suffer from the additional burden of significantly higher poverty rates for all households. Among black families, for example, 11.8 percent of married-couple families lived below the poverty line in 1989, while 46.5 percent, nearly half of female-headed families, lived in poverty. The statistics for Latino families are equally disturbing: 16.2 percent of married-couple families lived in poverty, compared to 47.5 percent of female-headed families.

The poverty rate for children continues, as it has since 1975, to be higher than that of any other age group. In 1990 the poverty rate for all children under eighteen was 20.6 percent. In other words, over 13 million— one out of every five American children —lived below the poverty line. In 1989 14.2 percent of white children, 34.9 percent of Hispanic children, and 43 percent of black children lived in poverty. Among children under the age of six, over 5 million, of 22.5 percent, were officially poor.

Stereotyping the Poor

Since the mid-1980s several critical, often life-threatening problems that particularly afflict women and children have added to the extraordinary toll that poverty takes on their health and well-being: The crack epidemic with its alarming number of ''crack babies'' and the subsequent prosecution of poor, usually African-American women for the ''prenatal crime'' of delivering drugs to the fetus; the dramatic escalation of violence on the streets of our cities with people of color all-too-often the victims; the ubiquity of homelessness with a significant percentage of homeless families headed by women; and the continuing existence of hunger, particularly among female-headed families.

But perhaps the most disturbing phenomenon of the early 1990s is the denigration of the poor and the blatant perpetuation of sexist and racist stereotypes. To equate people living in poverty, particularly recipients of Aid to Families with Dependent Children (AFDC), with the ''underclass'' is to brand them unfit, unmotivated, unwilling or unable to do their part to achieve their piece of the American Dream. In reality, such an ''underclass'' comprises but a small segment of the poor. During 1989 in nearly half—48.9 percent—of all poor families at least one member worked full-time or part-time, and in 16.2 percent of poor families at least one member worked full-time year-round. Even among female-headed families, in which all of the familial responsibilities rest on the single parent, 41.6 percent of the householders worked in 1989 and 8.8 percent worked full-time year-round. Popular perception fueled by demagogic leaders also erroneously labels the majority of the poor as people of color and thus, the disparaging of ''welfare mothers'' often becomes coded language for racism.

In fact, two-thirds of all Americans living below the poverty line are white.

Consequently, in these difficult economic times hostility toward the poor has led in many states to particularly punitive cutbacks of AFDC. In 1991 AFDC benefits were reduced more than in any year since 1981. Nine states cut basic benefits below previous levels and several states attempted to tie benefits to approved social behavior. For example, New Jersey recently enacted a far-reaching if short-sighted piece of social policy. The law refuses money to support any additional child born to a mother already receiving welfare. Any such child will therefore have to share the food of the other children, share the clothing grant of other family members and reduce even further the family's standard of living.

What's Needed: A Family Policy

The question of how to provide a decent standard of living for America's poor families remains a topic of debate. A family policy with benefits for all, regardless of income, improves the chances of appropriate legislation passing and reduces the likelihood of both the cutback of benefits and stigma to the recipients. Family policies similar to the one described here are in place in virtually every industrialized country with the exception of the United States.

To arrest the steadily widening gap between rich and poor and to provide a genuine safety net for women and children such entitlements should include comprehensive, accessible, affordable maternal and child health care within a comprehensive health care system for all Americans; paid parental leave at the time of the birth or adoption of a child; first-rate, widely accessible and affordable child care and after-school care; stronger child support legislation; and a higher minimum wage for all workers. Moreover, the United States should seriously consider children's allowances for all families regardless of income.

Targeted Programs

But the policies necessary for middle-class families will not alone be sufficient to help poor women and children overcome the pernicious effects of poverty. Besides universal entitlements, targeted programs for poor families are urgently needed. These include housing subsidies and the construction and rehabilitation of low-income housing; the expansion of food stamp assistance and increased funding for WIC (the Supplemental Food Program for Women, Infants, and Children); and finally, real welfare reform. Every state should pay benefits that will bring families at least up to the poverty line and should offer training programs and employment counseling to those recipients who are able and choose to take advantage of them.

Above all, we must recognize that life in the United States is too complex for families to go it alone. We must move toward greater equality and redistribute our resources more equitably in order to improve the health status of American women and their children. We must continue to organize across class, race, gender, and age lines to achieve these goals. Only through recognizing our common needs and interdependence, and by working together, can we hope to bring about these urgently needed political, economic, and social reforms.

HOMELESSNESS

Robert Wood Johnson Foundation, 1991

Homelessness is not just a poverty problem. To varying degrees with varying people, it can be simultaneously a housing problem, a disability problem, a mental health problem, a substance abuse problem, and a problem of profound social disaffiliation.

Counting the number of homeless people in the United States is complicated, in part because less than one-third of this population is chronically homeless. The majority is "episodically homeless"—homeless for only part of the year —and living with friends or relatives or even independently the rest of the time. Because researchers use a variety of methods to estimate the homeless population, these numbers range widely—from 200,000 to 2 million.

Only 1 percent to 2 percent of people living in poverty become homeless, which means that the vast majority of the poor are able to secure some type of housing for themselves and their families, despite today's much-publicized shortage of low- and moderate-income housing.

The chart on the opposite page and the following text are from a study of homeless people treated in health clinics. Although homeless people who seek medical care may not be representative of homeless people generally, this study offers a unique look at a large group of homeless people from 18 geographically dispersed cities. The gender, racial, and ethnic composition of the homeless population varied substantially among the cities.

This study found that few homeless people are old. In part, this is due to entitlement programs for people 65 and over, but it also may reflect shorter lifespans for homeless people. Blacks and Hispanics are overrepresented. Homeless children—who are mostly under age 5—are much more likely to be minority than are homeless adults.

About a third of homeless people are women. Homeless women are more likely than men to have mental disorders (35 percent *vs.* 22 percent) and are less likely to abuse alcohol.

About 40 percent of all homeless people have a significant alcohol problem, and 13 percent use drugs. Many use both. Alcohol problems are reported for homeless children at very young ages—as young as 6 to 10. About 10 percent of homeless teenagers show signs of abusing alcohol.

A quarter of homeless adults seeking treatment have some sort of injury (compared to 8 percent of the general US population seeking ambulatory treatment). A third have minor respiratory problems (compared to 5.5 percent). Overall rates of chronic disease are 37 percent (compared to 27 percent). Dental problems also are much more common (12 percent *vs.* 0.4 percent).

PEOPLE WITH CHRONIC MENTAL ILLNESSES BY RESIDENCE, 1985

In the community 59%

In inpatient settings 41%

Psychiatric facilities 4%

Nursing homes —
people with chronic
mental illness 14%

Nursing homes —
people with dementia 23%

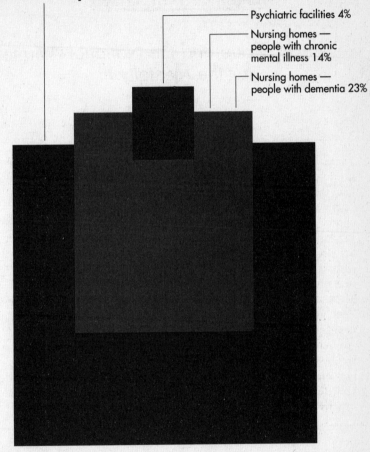

Source:

Estimates based on unpublished data from the US National Institute of Mental Health, Division of Biometry and Applied Sciences, Survey and Reports Branch.

Note:

This information on the homeless population is from demonstration projects in the Health Care for the Homeless Program, funded by The Pew Charitable Trusts and The Robert Wood Johnson Foundation.

CARE OF THE SERIOUSLY MENTALLY ILL:
Eight Current Crises

*Research Group and the National Alliance
for the Mentally Ill*

1. There are more than twice as many people with schizophrenia and manic-depressive psychosis living in public shelters and on the streets than there are in public mental hospitals.
2. There are more people with schizophrenia and manic-depressive psychosis in prisons and jails than in public mental hospitals.
3. Increasing episodes of violence by seriously mentally ill individuals are a consequence of not receiving treatment.
4. Mental health professionals have abandoned the public sector and patients with serious mental illnesses.
5. Most community mental health centers have been abysmal failures.
6. Funding of public services for individuals with serious mental illness is chaotic.
7. An undetermined portion of public funds for services to people with serious mental illnesses is literally being stolen.
8. Guidelines for serving people with mental illnesses are often made at both the federal and state level by administrators who have had no experience in this field.

The modern era in public services for people with serious mental illnesses began immediately following World War II with the realization that such illnesses were common and that state mental hospitals were on the best of days remarkably untherapeutic and on the worst of days snake pits. The response of the federal government was to create a National Institute of Mental Health, to which it gave responsibility for research on mental illnesses and for the training of increased numbers of psychiatrists, psychologists, psychiatric social workers, and psychiatric nurses.

But services for people with serious mental illnesses remained the exclusive responsibility of state government until 1963, when Congress passed President John F. Kennedy's Community Mental Health Centers (CMHC) Act. In describing what the legislation would accomplish, the President said that "reliance on the cold mercy of custodial isolation will be supplanted by the open warmth of community concern and capability."[1] Following passage of the CMHC Act, people with serious mental illnesses were made eligible for several other federal programs including Supplemental Security Income (SSI), Social Security Disability Income (SSDI), Medicaid, and Medicare. Prior to 1963, then, states had almost total fiscal responsibility for serving their mentally ill residents; after 1963, an increasing proportion of this fiscal burden shifted from the states to the federal government. Today, the federal share of the approximately $20 billion annual public cost of services to people with mental illnesses is 40 percent, or approximately $8 billion.

The CMHC Act and subsequent efforts of federal and state governments to improve services seemed reasonable at the time and clearly were motivated by the best of intentions. These efforts coincided with the introduction of antipsychotic medication, which became widely available by the late 1950s, making deinstitutionalization of people with mental illnesses feasible. In the 30-year period from 1955 to 1984, the number of patients in public mental hospitals dropped from 552,150 to 118,647, a reduction of just under 80 percent. Hundreds of thousands of mentally ill individuals who previously had been held in custodial state mental hospitals were discharged to what was supposed to be community care. The federally funded CMHCs, income assistance programs such as SSI and SSDI, and increased numbers of mental health professionals were all going to work with state governments to provide care for these individuals. That was the way it was supposed to happen.

When one surveys the current scene, it is clear that whatever was supposed to happen did not happen and that deinstitutionalization was a disaster. Despite the approximately $20 billion per year in public funds spent on services, despite almost $3 billion in federal funds spent to create community mental health centers, despite over $2 billion in federal funds and uncounted additional billions in state funds spent to train more mental health professionals, services for people with serious mental illnesses in the United States in 1990 are the shame of the nation. The road to hell truly is lined with good intentions; the gateposts on this road are painfully evident.

1. There are more than twice as many people with schizophrenia and manic-depressive psychosis living in public shelters and on the streets than there are in public mental hospitals.

Estimates of the total number of homeless individuals in the United States have ranged from 300,000 to 3 million. In probably the best study done to date, the Urban Institute in Washington, D.C., in 1988 estimated that the total number was between 567,000 and 600,000. In March 1990, the United States Bureau of the Census undertook an exhaustive count of the homeless population but that count is not yet available.

There are many causes of homelessness. Most surveys have found that between 30 and 40 percent of single homeless people are alcoholics or drug addicts; some of these people have lost their housing because of their addictions (some are also mentally ill). Another important cause of homelessness is the reduced availability of low-income housing as inner cities have become gentrified and as federal support for such housing has eroded drastically (particularly in the 1980s). There are also some homeless people who have no job skills and no family support and use shelters as places to try and get their lives together.

The most controversial segment of the homeless population is the group with serious mental illnesses such as schizophrenia and manic-depressive psychosis. The question of what percentage of homeless people this group constitutes has unfortunately become a political football, with liberals arguing that it is a small percentage (and that cuts in social programs and housing are the cause of most homelessness) while conservatives contend that mentally ill people make up a large percentage (and thus that state mental health authorities, not the failure of social programs and housing, are to blame). Many of the studies done on this question have been tainted by such political preconceptions, with widely varying results.

Increasingly, however, there is a consensus that approximately 25 to 30 percent of single homeless adults living in shelters are seriously mentally ill. Studies done in the mid-1980s in Boston,[2] Philadelphia,[3] and Washington, D.C.,[4] reported that between 36 and 39 percent of adult shelter residents had schizophrenia. With the influx of large numbers of crack users into city shelters in many urban areas the percentage of homeless persons with schizophrenia has probably decreased. A 1988 study in Los Angeles found that 28 percent of homeless people in shelters had schizophrenia, manic-depressive psychosis, or major depression;[5] this survey, however, failed to include the 15 percent of shelter residents who refused to cooperate, among whom there were certainly many with paranoid schizophrenia. Another 1988 California study of three counties reported that 30 percent of homeless people in shelters had a severe mental disorder.[6] A 1989 study of homeless people in Baltimore shelters found that 31 percent of men and 41 percent of women had schizophrenia, manic-depressive psychosis, or major depression,[7] while another 1989 study in New York reported that 17 percent of shelter residents had "a definite or probable history of psychosis" and another 8 percent "a possible history of psychosis."[8]

For homeless individuals not living in shelters but rather in parks, alleys, abandoned buildings, doorways, subway tunnels, etc., the percentage with serious mental illness appears to be even higher than 25 to 30 percent. A study of individuals living on heating grates and on the streets of New York City estimated "that 60 percent exhibit evidence of schizophrenia as manifested by disorganized behavior and chronic delusional thinking."[9] In Los Angeles, a 1988 study of homeless persons (two-thirds of whom slept in places other than shelters) found that 40 percent of them had psychotic symptoms.[10] By contrast, a study of homeless individuals living on grates and sleeping in doorways in Washington, D.C., found that only 29 percent had a history of psychiatric hospitalization as reported by the individual.[11]

Taking all available data into consideration, it would appear that approximately 30 percent of single adult homeless individuals living either in shelters or on the streets are seriously mentally ill, mostly with schizophrenia and manic-depressive psychosis. If the total number of homeless adults is conservatively estimated to be only 500,000, then the number of seriously mentally ill homeless would be approximately 150,000 individuals. By comparison, the most recent data available on patients in the nation's 286 state and county psychiatric hospitals reveals that there are just over 68,000 patients with schizophrenia and manic-depressive psychosis. *There are, then, more than twice as many people with schizophrenia and manic-depressive psychosis living in public shelters and on the streets as there are in public mental hospitals.*

Common sense says that many of the homeless people with serious mental illnesses must be the same people who were discharged from state mental hospitals, and several studies have shown that this is so. A study carried out at the Central Ohio Psychiatric Hospital in 1985 followed 132 patients for six months after their discharge and found that within that period 36 percent of the discharged patients had become homeless.[12] The truly alarming aspect of this study, however, is that these 132 patients were not the sickest people being discharged from that hospital; another 61 discharged patients "were not medically cleared by hospital staff to participate in the study because of the severity of their psychotic behavior,"[13] and it seems likely that an even higher proportion of this group became homeless. In Massachusetts, a 1983 study of 187 patients discharged from a public psychiatric hospital found that 27 percent had been homeless at least occasionally within the previous six months.[14] And in Los Angeles, a 1988 study of 53 homeless mentally ill individuals living on the streets, on beaches, or in parks reported that 79 percent of them had been previously hospitalized in state mental hospitals or on the psychiatric wards of general hospitals.[15]

Having approximately 150,000 seriously mentally ill individuals living in public shelters and on the streets in 1990 in the United States, the wealthiest nation in the world, is quite an extraordinary and unacceptable state of affairs. It was, in fact, the existence of large numbers of seriously mentally ill individuals in the nation's poorhouses in the 1820s and 1830s that led to the building of state mental hospitals as a "humane" alternative. We have, in essence, returned to where we began 170 years ago; at no time in the intervening years have there been as many seriously mentally ill individuals, most receiving no treatment, living in the community.

Staying alive on the streets or in public shelters when one's mind is working normally is extremely difficult. When the mind cannot think clearly because of schizophrenia or manic-depressive psychosis, it is a living hell.

- "I know one woman who has been raped 17 times," says an official of the Central City Hospitality House in San Francisco.[16] Infectious diseases, tuberculosis, and other untreated medical problems are endemic.
- In New York City "a homeless man, attacked by seven teenagers, was thrown over a wall and dropped about 50 feet into Riverside Park early yesterday leaving him with a fractured leg and back injuries."[17]
- In Massachusetts, a homeless man and woman were savagely beaten to death. Such vulnerable people, editorialized a newspaper, "are the natural prey of anyone looking for some loose change, a pack of cigarettes, a bottle. They are rabbits forced to live in company with dogs."[18]
- Phyllis Iannotta, age 67, had been diagnosed with paranoid schizophrenia and hospitalized. Following her discharge no follow-up or aftercare took place and she became a shopping bag lady on the streets of New York. In 1981 she was raped and stabbed to death in a parking lot on West 40th Street. In her bag were found two sweaters, a ball of yarn, an empty box

of Sloan's liniment, a vial of perfume, a can of Friskies turkey-and-giblet cat food, and a plastic spoon.[19]

There have been a few tentative steps toward solving the problem of homelessness among people with mental illness. The federal McKinney Act funds included $35 million in 1989 for mental health services for the homeless. The National Institute of Mental Health elevated the problem to "priority" status in 1989 and allocated $4.5 million for research and demonstration grants. But most care for people who are homeless and mentally ill continues to come largely on a voluntary basis from the private sector, especially the community groups, churches and synagogues that operate 90 percent of public shelters and soup kitchens. These are President Bush's 1,000 points of light, individuals who are doing their best to fill the holes left by the breakdown in public psychiatric services and by the failures of American psychiatry, psychology, and social work. The crisis of homelessness among people with mental illnesses will continue until such time as public psychiatric services are significantly improved. The private sector is doing more than its share; as *U.S. News and World Report* recently noted, "it is difficult to see . . . how the thousand points of light can put out much more wattage."[20]

2. There are more people with schizophrenia and manic-depressive psychosis in prisons and jails than in public mental hospitals.

According to the United States Department of Justice, on any given day in 1989 there were 1,042,136 individuals in the nation's prisons and jails (56,500 in federal prisons, 644,000 in state prisons, and 341,636 in local jails). Studies to ascertain how many of the prisoners have serious mental illnesses have shown varying results; a 1989 review of these studies concluded that "10 to 15 percent of prison populations . . . need the services usually associated with severe or chronic mental illness."[21] This review defined chronic mental illness as including "schizophrenia, unipolar and bipolar depression, or organic syndromes with psychotic features."

On the lower end of the scale, a study in Chicago's main jail found that only 6.4 percent of prisoners had schizophrenia, mania, or major depression.[22] A study of a prison in Maryland reported that 9.5 percent of the inmates met diagnostic criteria for schizophrenia and another 3.1 percent had a major depressive disorder.[23] In Philadelphia, 11 percent of all admissions to the city jail were said to have a diagnosis of schizophrenia.[24] In the state of Washington, 10.3 percent of prisoners were diagnosed with schizophrenia, schizotypal disorder, or manic-depressive psychosis,[21] while in Michigan's prisons, "20 percent of the state's 19,000 convicts suffered from severe mental impairment meaning delusions, hallucinations, and loss of contact with reality."[25] The Los Angeles County Jail presently holds 24,000 inmates on any given day and, according to professionals who have worked there, approximately 15 percent of them have serious mental illnesses. That means that there are approximately 3,600 seriously mentally ill individuals in that jail, which is 700 more than the largest mental hospital in the United States. The Los Angeles County Jail is, *de facto*, the largest mental hospital in this country.

Given all the data it seems reasonable to conclude that approximately 10 percent of inmates in prisons and jails, or approximately 100,000 individuals, suffer from schizophrenia or manic-depressive psychosis. For comparison, there are approximately 68,000 patients with schizophrenia and manic-depressive psychosis in the nation's public mental hospitals. *Thus, there appear to be approximately 100,000 individuals with schizophrenia and manic-depressive psychosis in prisons and jails compared with approximately 68,000 in public mental hospitals.*

There is a consensus that the percentage of inmates with serious mental illnesses in the nation's prisons and jails has "increased slowly and gradually in the last 20 years and will probably continue to increase."[21] These are, of course, the same years during which state mental hospitals were discharging patients wholesale without providing aftercare for most of them. The cause-and-effect relationship between these two trends is self-evident and was illustrated by another aspect of the previously mentioned 1985 study from Ohio. In that study, 33 individuals with schizophrenia and manic-depressive psychosis who had been discharged from the state mental hospital were located six months later. During the six months, 21 of the 33 individuals (64 percent) had been arrested and jailed.[26] Most arrests did not involve violence but were for misdemeanors such as "threatening behavior" in public and "walking in the community without clothes." Prior to their discharge from the hospital these individuals had had an average of 12.5 hospital admissions in the preceding five years and had a history of not taking their medications once they left the hospital. According to the author of the study, "the jail was an asylum of last resort, where they received little or no mental health treatment and were quickly released" to begin another cycle of streets-hospital-streets-jail.

George Wooten, age 32, was booked into the Denver County Jail in 1984 for his 100th time. He had been diagnosed with schizophrenia at age 17 and developed a fondness for sniffing paint, after which he creates "a disturbance" and the police arrest him. According to a newspaper account: "Eight years ago the officers might have taken Wooten to a community mental health center, a place that was supposed to help the chronically mentally ill. But now they don't bother . . . Police have become cynical about the whole approach. They have learned that 'two hours later [those arrested] are back on the street . . . the circle of sending the person to a mental health center doesn't work.' "[27]

Prisons and jails were not created to be mental hospitals. And yet, because of the failure of public psychiatric services, prisons and jails have become *de facto* shelters of last resort for psychiatrically ill individuals. In Buffalo, when police took mentally ill individuals to the emergency unit of the local mental health center, psychiatrists refused to admit the persons 43 percent of the time.[28] The police then charged such persons with misdemeanors and put them in jail just to get them off the streets, often for their own safety. In Oregon, a study of seriously mentally ill individuals in prisons and jails found that "in about half the cases a failed attempt at commitment had preceded the arrest."[29] The person's family had sought help for them by trying to get them admitted to a psychiatric hospital but was turned down, often because no beds were available or because the person did not meet stringent state laws for dangerousness to self or others. The person then commits a minor crime such as trespassing, shoplifting, or disorderly conduct and ends up in jail rather than in a psychiatric hospital. In many communities public officials representing mental health and corrections spend much time and effort shuttling mentally ill individuals back and forth between the two systems. As a recent reviewer summarized the situation: "With both agencies exhibiting a 'he's yours' posture, the mentally ill offender falls through a crack, if not a gaping hole, in the system of care for the mentally ill."[21]

Timothy Waldrop, 24 years old and who had been voted the friendliest boy in his high school graduating class, had been treated for schizophrenia for several years. He was arrested for armed robbery and sentenced to five years in the Georgia state prison. In prison his antipsychotic medication was stopped; "a few days later Waldrop gouged out his left eye with his fingers." Despite resuming his medication he then cut his scrotum with a razor and, while in restraints, "punctured his right eye with a fingernail leaving himself totally blind."[30]

In states like Idaho and Montana, county jails are used (sometimes for several days) to hold mentally ill individuals awaiting transportation to a mental hospital; such individuals have not been charged with any crimes.

The quality of care mentally ill inmates receive in prisons and jails varies greatly. There are a few programs that provide good psychiatric care and that have been cited as models for the rest of the country; the Contra Costa County Jail in Martinez, California, the Boulder County Jail in Boulder, Colorado, and the Multnomah County Jail in Portland, Oregon, are examples of such programs. Much more common, however, are prisons and jails where mentally ill inmates are neglected or abused. In Arizona's maximum security prison, for example, mentally ill prisoners may be "chained naked to bed posts and left there 20 hours a day for up to three days at a time," according to a 1989 report in the *Arizona Republic*. "Prison officials said the procedure is part of standard mental-health practice to keep 'self-abusive and suicidal' inmates from hurting themselves."[31]

A major problem in providing care for mentally ill inmates of prisons and jails is the inability of psychiatrists to give them medication because of stringent laws designed to protect prisoners from involuntary medication. Such laws do indeed protect non-mentally ill prisoners from the abuse of a "Clockwork Orange" system of chemical mind control. But the laws also make it difficult or impossible to medicate blatantly psychotic inmates who, because of their brain disease, have no insight into their illnesses or need for medication. In Kentucky, for example, the *Lexington Herald-Leader* described an inmate with paranoid schizophrenia who had refused to come out of his cell "for years." "He refuses to take psychotropic drugs, which probably could reduce his delusions, possibly even eliminate them. But courts almost never allow prisons or mental hospitals to force medication."[32]

3. Increasing episodes of violence by seriously mentally ill individuals are a consequence of not receiving treatment.

Mentally ill individuals are inherently no more violent than non-mentally ill persons. When they are treated, in fact, studies suggest that their arrest rate is *lower* than that of the average citizen. The wards of a well-run mental hospital are much safer on any given day than the streets of most cities.

When individuals with serious mental illnesses such as schizophrenia and manic-depressive psychosis are *not* treated, however, some of them will occasionally commit acts of violence. These acts may be in direct response to imagined threats (e.g. a belief that another person is going to kill him so he strikes first), delusional thinking (e.g. that another person is really the Devil in disguise), or auditory hallucinations (e.g. voices commanding the person to hurt another). The violent acts, in short, are usually part and parcel of the person's illness.

The mass exodus of people with serious mental illnesses from public mental hospitals in the last three decades has placed literally hundreds of thousands into the community. Many receive little or no treatment once they leave the hospital. As noted above, approximately 150,000 mentally ill individuals are living in public shelters or on the streets; another 100,000 are in prisons and jails, most of them charged with misdemeanors. Another several hundred thousand—nobody knows the precise number—are living with their families or by themselves. *The majority of all of these are receiving little or no psychiatric treatment because most public psychiatric services have broken down completely.* Occasional episodes of violence then become inevitable.

It is clear that episodes of violence by individuals with untreated serious mental illnesses are on the increase. One only has to listen to daily news reports to become aware of frequent stories about acts of violence committed by individuals identified as former mental patients. Since 1965 there have been eight separate studies documenting the rise in violent acts by untreated psychiatric patients. In one of the studies, for example, psychiatric patients in a New York City hospital in 1975 were compared with those in 1982; the latter group had had significantly more encounters with the criminal justice system and almost twice as many episodes of violence toward persons.[33]

Most such episodes need not happen if the public system of psychiatric care is operating as it should. Jorge Delgado, who walked naked into St. Patrick's Cathedral in New York in 1988 and killed an elderly man, had been hospitalized psychiatrically seven times; in the six months preceding his act of violence he had been evaluated twice by psychiatrists who found no reason to commit him involuntarily for treatment.

Lois E. Lang, 44 years old, walked into the corporate headquarters of a financial firm in New York City in November 1985 and shot to death the elderly president of the firm and a receptionist. Three months previously Ms. Lang had been arrested for at least the fifth time, diagnosed with paranoid schizophrenia, and released from the hospital after 14 days. At the time of the killings Ms. Lang was homeless and said to have a delusion that she was part-owner of the firm and was owed money.[34]

While it is not possible to predict dangerousness with a high degree of accuracy, it *is* possible to pick out those untreated mentally ill individuals who are most likely to become violent. Recent studies have shown that the four most important predictors of dangerousness in mentally ill individuals are: (1) neurological abnormalities; (2) paranoid symptoms; (3) refusal to take medications; and (4) a history of violent behavior.[35] The last factor is by far the most accurate predictor for future violence and yet *most mentally ill individuals with histories of violence are released to the community without aftercare or follow-up.*

This fact was frighteningly well-illustrated in a 1983 study carried out by Dr. Richard Lamb in Los Angeles. He followed up 85 mentally ill men who had been arrested and found incompetent to stand trial. Of the 85 men, 92 percent had been arrested on felony charges (murder, attempted murder, rape, armed robbery, assault with a deadly weapon), 68 percent had previous felony records, and 86 percent had previous psychiatric hospitalizations. Despite this record of psychiatric illness and felonies, two years after their arrest 54 of the 85 men had been released and, for 34 of them (40 percent), *no plan whatsoever had been made for aftercare or follow-up.*[36]

Such situations are deplorable, needlessly endangering both the individual who is mentally ill, the person's family members who are frequent victims, and the community at large. It is further evidence of the breakdown in public psychiatric services; when the public fully recognizes the needless dangers that this breakdown in services entails, it will demand that services for people with mental illnesses be improved.

4. Mental health professionals have abandoned the public sector and patients with serious mental illnesses.

In 1945, during Congressional hearings that led to the creation of the National Institute of Mental Health (NIMH), it was said that there were only about 3,000 psychiatrists in the United States and that many of them were not fully trained. Although half of the 3,000 were employed in the public sector—mostly in state mental hospitals caring for individuals with serious mental illnesses—it was said to be very difficult to recruit psychiatrists for rural state hospitals such as Montana State Hospital or Wyoming State Hospital, each of which had only two psychiatrists on staff. The answer, everyone agreed, was to train more psychiatrists, and the fiscal responsibility for doing so was given to NIMH.

Federally funded training for mental health professionals began in 1948 with a $1.4 million program. The money was given directly to university departments of psychiatry, psychology, and psychiatric social work to support faculty salaries and pay stipends to some students. A small program was also implemented to support psychiatric nursing. By 1969 the NIMH training funds had reached $118.7 million per year and by the early 1980s, when the program was phased down, they had totalled over $2 billion. Most states supplemented the federal training funds. Virtually every mental health professional trained in the United States since 1948 has had the majority of his or her training costs subsidized by public—federal and state—funds.

From the point of view of numbers alone, the subsidized training of mental health professionals has been a huge success. In the past 45 years, psychiatrists have increased from 3,000 to 40,000, psychologists from 4,200 to 70,000, and psychiatric social workers from 2,000 to approximately 80,000. The total increase in these three professions has been more than twentyfold, during a period in which the population of the United States increased less than twofold.

From the point of view of individuals with serious mental illnesses, however, the publicly subsidized training of mental health professionals has been an abysmal failure. The reason, quite simply, is that once psychiatrists, psychologists, and psychiatric social workers were trained, almost all of them abandoned the public sector for the monetary rewards of private practice. No payback obligation was included with the subsidized training, despite assurances from federal officials during the original 1945 Congressional hearings that a payback would be built into the program; specifically, Dr. Robert Felix, who would become the first director of NIMH, testified that "I would think that a reasonable requirement of these men [sic] would be that they would spend at least one year in public service for every year they spent in training at public or state expense."[37] However, this payback obligation was not implemented until 35 years later when federal training funds had been almost phased out.

What kinds of patients do psychiatrists, psychologists, and psychiatric social workers see in their private practices? This question was answered by a 1980 survey of mental health professionals in private practice, which found that only 6 percent of patients seen by psychiatrists and 3 percent of patients seen by psychologists had ever been hospitalized for mental illness.[38] The authors of another survey summarized it as follows: "The [psychiatrists, psychologists, and psychiatric social workers] appeared to spend much of their time treating conditions that many people would consider minor."[39]

And what has happened to individuals with serious mental illnesses who must rely on the public sector? Increasingly such individuals are seen by no psychiatrist at all. At the Wyoming State Hospital, for example, in 1987 *for almost a year there was no regular psychiatrist on the hospital staff at all.* In 1947, when there were 3,000 psychiatrists in the United States, the hospital had two full-time psychiatrists, but in 1987, with 40,000 psychiatrists in the nation (and 15 in the state of Wyoming), it had none. The Montana State Hospital, which had two full-time psychiatrists in the late 1940s, still had only two full-time psychiatrists in the late 1980s despite the fact that there were 37 elsewhere in the state. Both hospitals had to resort to private firms that hire out psychiatrists for exorbitant sums—the current rate is approximately $180,000 per year—and that are popularly referred to as "rent-a-shrink" companies. The director of one such firm noted in 1988: "Business is booming. We're getting requests all the time from rural areas."[40] Under such programs it is common for a new psychiatrist to take over the wards of a state hospital as frequently as every two weeks; the consequences for the continuity and quality of patient care are obvious.

It should be noted that many of these jobs for mental health professionals in the public sector pay decent salaries. A perusal of advertisements placed in 1990 in the newspaper of the American Psychiatric Association revealed annual salaries for public-sector psychiatrists ranging from $100,000 to $120,000, with liberal leave policy (up to six weeks vacation) and fringe benefits. A few, such as Wyoming State Hospital, even offer free housing. Despite this, most mental health professionals opt for the private sector, where monetary rewards are greater and the patients are easier to treat.

In addition to using "rent-a-shrink" companies, public-sector psychiatric facilities have filled psychiatric vacancies in the United States by hiring foreign-trained physicians. This practice became widespread in the 1970s, and it is currently estimated that approximately two-thirds of the psychiatrists in public psychiatric hospitals and clinics in the United States are foreign medical graduates. Some of these are as competent as any American medical graduate, but there is evidence from licensing examination results that many others are not.[41] The overreliance on foreign medical graduates in public mental health facilities also raises moral issues; one of the world's wealthiest nations is hiring psychiatrists from poorer countries to fill public-sector jobs that American-trained psychiatrists have abandoned. By 1986, in fact, there were more than twice as many Indian, Pakistani, and Egyptian psychiatrists in the United States as there were in India, Pakistan, and Egypt.[42] We should be grateful to foreign medical graduates for keeping American public psychiatric services from collapsing entirely, but we should also remember that they are needed because of the refusal of most American psychiatrists to work in the public sector.

The worst news of all, however, is that finding mental health professionals to treat patients with serious mental illnesses in public facilities is becoming increasingly difficult. The primary reason for this is the explosive growth in the 1980s of for-profit psychiatric hospitals, which hire away at higher salaries the few professionals remaining in the public system. These hospitals, the majority of which are owned by the Hospital Corporation of America, National Medical Enterprises, Community Psychiatric Centers, and Charter Medical Corporation, have proliferated rapidly, especially in those states that have abandoned "certificate-of-need" laws which limit the building of new hospitals.

The profit margin of these for-profit psychiatric hospitals is very high. A major reason for this is that they accept few seriously mentally ill patients. Instead, they fill their beds with substance abusers (especially alcoholics) and teenagers who are unhappy for one reason or another. In fact, these for-profit hospitals have invented a new disease—teenagism—which coincidentally lasts only as long as the family's medical insurance benefits. Through aggressive advertising these hospitals convince parents that teenage problems are best treated by psychiatric hospitalization. "If you have a child who is out of control," the advertisement reads, "send him to us." Some of these for-profit hospitals are even starting to specialize in specific teenage problems, such as Hartgrove Hospital in Chicago, which recently set up "one of the nation's first treatment programs to wean teenagers from Satanism."[43] John E. Halasz, M.D., Medical Director of Chicago's Institute for Juvenile Research, called the rapidly rising hospitalization of teenagers "a racket."[44] But it is a profitable racket and in 1989 the *Wall Street Journal* said that the four major hospital chains "plan to build at least 45 more psychiatric hospitals in the next three years."[45] The staff for these hospitals, like those built in recent years, will be drawn heavily from among the psychiatrists, psychologists, psychiatric social workers, and psychiatric nurses remaining in public-sector positions.

5. Most community mental health centers have been abysmal failures.

In 1963, Congress passed legislation setting up community mental health centers (CMHCs) with federal construction and staffing grants. The purpose of CMHCs was clearly outlined by Boisfeuillet Jones, special assistant to then Department of Health, Education and Welfare Secretary Celebrezze: "The basic purpose of the 'President's' program is to redirect the focus of treatment of the mentally ill from state mental hospitals into community mental health centers."

Since 1967 a total of 575 CMHCs have received federal construction grants ($294.7 million), and 697 CMHCs received staffing and operations grants ($2,364.6 million); the total CMHC program has thus cost $2.7 billion. CMHCs that received construction grants legally obligated themselves to provide five basic services for 20 years.

Using the federal Freedom of Information Act, the Health Research Group obtained from the National Institute of Mental Health data on CMHCs including site visit reports carried out on contract by Continuing Medical Education, Inc. A report issued in March 1990 by the Health Research Group and the National Alliance for the Mentally Ill[46] documents the magnitude of the CMHC failure:

- Some CMHCs took federal funds but "never materialized," i.e., never even began delivering services. Others simply disappeared or went out of business. Still others are being used for completely different purposes (e.g. offices for physical therapists in private practice).
- Some CMHCs were used as private hospitals or are being run illegally by for-profit corporations such as the Hospital Corporation of America.
- Some CMHCs built swimming pools and tennis courts with the construction funds, and hired lifeguards, swimming instructors, and gardeners with the staffing grants. One CMHC used federal construction funds to build both a swimming pool and a chapel, the latter presumably constructed so that seriously mentally ill individuals who were not receiving services could at least pray.
- Some CMHCs, once in operation, requested and received NIMH permission to reduce their public psychiatric beds at the same time as state and local authorities said more beds were needed.
- Many CMHCs have failed to provide "a reasonable volume of services to persons unable to pay therefor" as specified by law.
- Overall, it is estimated that approximately 140 of the 575 CMHCs, or 25 percent, are seriously out of compliance and subject to recovery of federal funds. The amount to be recovered is estimated at $50 to $100 million. Approximately another 140 CMHCs are technically out of compliance.
- Only approximately 30 CMHCs of the 575 that received construction funds (5 percent) are operating as Congress originally intended: "to redirect the focus of treatment of the mentally ill from state mental hospitals into community mental health centers."

It is important to note that a small number of federally funded CMHCs developed into excellent programs and provide quality services to individuals with serious mental illnesses. These programs further accentuate the contrast with the vast majority of CMHCs that did not develop along such lines. Among the best CMHCs identified by our survey are the following:

Aroostook MHC—Fort Fairfield, ME
Solomon MHC—Lowell, MA
Corrigan MHC—Fall River, MA
Kent County MHC—Warwick, RI
Northern Rhode Island CMHC—Woonsocket, RI
Rockland County CMHC—Pomona, NY
Shawnee Hills CMHC—Charleston, WV
Range MHC—Virginia, MN
Red Rock Comprehensive MHC—Oklahoma City, OK
Salt Lake Valley MHC—Salt Lake City, UT
San Mateo County MHC—San Mateo, CA
Spokane CMHC—Spokane, WA

Defenders of CMHCs argue that most centers are seeing large numbers of individuals with serious mental illnesses. They point to a 1988 survey carried out by the National Council of Community Mental Health Centers, the Washington lobbying office for CMHCs, which claimed that "the proportion of clients on a typical community mental health agency caseload who are seriously mentally ill averages 45 percent."[47] What they fail to point out is that in this survey "serious mental illness" was defined as including everything under the sun, such as "passive-aggressive personality disorders" which, according to the American Psychiatric Association, is a diagnosis applied to individuals who procrastinate and dawdle and are stubborn, forgetful, and intentionally inefficient. This, says the National Council of CMHCs, is "serious mental illness." A much more accurate analysis of the patients seen in CMHCs, published by the National Institute of Mental Health in 1988, showed that *only 9 percent of individuals being treated by CMHCs had either "schizophrenia" or "other psychotic disorders."*[48] By contrast, 20 percent were diagnosed as having "social maladjustment" or "no mental disorder."

Representative of many community mental health centers is the Park Center in Fort Wayne, Indiana, previously known as the Fort Wayne CMHC, which received $12.7 million in federal funds between 1977 and 1981 and which still operates predominantly with state and federal funds. Instead of providing services for individuals with schizophrenia and manic-depressive psychosis, it advertised itself in a 1989 brochure as follows:

Every year we help thousands of people face the challenges of our complex world. Most people who come to Park Center feel a need for help with a life adjustment problem. Counseling services are for those experiencing:

- *Unhappy relationships*
- *Inability to communicate effectively*
- *Anxiety*

- *Depression*
- *Indecision*
- *Procrastination*
- *Poor job performance*
- *Parenting problems*
- *Alcohol problems*

High stress levels adversely affect work and family life. Counseling services help people reduce conflicts and strengthen relationships. At Park Center, We Help You Face the World.

Individuals with serious mental illnesses do not have a "life adjustment problem" but rather a primary brain disease. They do not need "counseling" alone as much as they need medication, vocational rehabilitation, and decent housing. They do not need to "face the world" but rather to become part of the world.

Another example of one of the many CMHCs that failed abysmally in its primary function to provide services for seriously mentally ill people is the Hancock County CMHC in Ellsworth, Maine. In 1976 the Hancock County Mental Health Association received a $100,000 federal construction grant to build a free-standing, one-story CMHC to serve the residents of Hancock County. The CMHC was affiliated with the respected Community Counseling Center in Bangor, in whose catchment area it was situated. From 1977 to 1983 the Hancock County CMHC provided outpatient services, emergency services, and consultation and education, but not inpatient services or partial hospitalization.

In 1983 the Hancock County Mental Health Association essentially evicted the CMHC from the federally subsidized building and began renting the offices out for profit to private service providers such as privately operated physical therapy services. NIMH became aware of this violation of federal regulations in June 1983 during a site visit by an NIMH official. The building has been used for non-CMHC purposes continuously since 1983 in clear violation of the law. An August 1988 site visit report to NIMH noted that "none of the five essential services is being provided by the grantee either in the federally-constructed space or in any other location . . . The grantee is out of compliance."

Officials of the Community Counseling Center in Bangor tried repeatedly to bring the situation to the attention of state and federal officials. In 1989, NIMH finally referred the case to the DHHS Office of the General Counsel to initiate recovery action; no action had been taken by early 1990. The president of the Community Counseling Center wrote to the Director of NIMH as follows: "The stewardship of the taxpayers' dollars is important. No federal agency should take over six years to act on blatant violations of federal regulations. I sincerely hope that the situation in Ellsworth, Maine, is an isolated example of NIMH mismanagement and is not indicative of a widespread pattern of ineptitude and failure to ensure that buildings built with federal construction grant funds are properly used." (Letter of December 12, 1989)

The Health Research Group and the National Alliance for the Mentally Ill's CMHC report included a detailed history of the Hancock County CMHC. Following the report's release, the *Bangor Daily News* questioned the chairman of the Hancock County Mental Health Association, Robert Keteyian, who responded as follows: "Keteyian agreed that his Association was not in compliance with federal regulations, adding that his group had notified the National Institute of Mental Health in writing that it was not in compliance on numerous occasions. 'We wondered why they never responded,' he said. Placing several 'for-profit' tenants in the building along with a few nonprofit organizations, Keteyian said, was just a way to help pay the mortgage."[49]

6. Funding of public services for individuals with serious mental illness is chaotic.

One need only visit an emergency room in any large city hospital to witness the disaster of public psychiatric services for people with serious mental illnesses. In one emergency room in New York City, individuals with schizophrenia and manic-depressive psychosis "were handcuffed to the armrests of wheelchairs Friday morning as they waited for beds . . . Sometimes patients have to sleep in shifts [in the waiting area] because there is not enough room."[50] Mental health administrators in the city blame state authorities for the lack of public psychiatric beds, while the state maintains that it is the city's responsibility. What neither says publicly is that they are playing a game of shift-the-fiscal-burden; the losers in this game are inevitably individuals with serious mental illnesses.

The funding of public services for people with mental illnesses in the United States is an incredible pastiche of federal, state, and local sources with no overall coordination and with individual pieces that are often at odds with each other. Federal dollars, comprising approximately 40 percent of the total, include Medicaid, Medicare, Supplemental Security Income (SSI), Social Security Disability Insurance (SSDI), block grants, and housing programs of various kinds. State and local funds for people with serious mental illnesses come from a variety of departments including mental health, social services, housing, vocational rehabilitation, and corrections. To run a department of mental health at the state or local level one needs to be primarily an accountant to keep track of the many sources of funds and what they can be used for. This chaotic funding system has grown piecemeal over the 25 years since Medicaid and Medicare were enacted; new programs have been added incrementally, with virtually no attempt made to fit the funding pieces together into a coherent whole. The system of funding public services for people with mental illnesses in the United States is, in short, more thought-disordered than most of the individuals the system is intended to serve.

At the federal level, funding programs strongly favor hospitalization for people with mental illnesses despite an official policy of deinstitutionalization. Dr. Rohn S. Friedman has called this contradiction a "psychiatric chimera—an official policy of deinstitutionalization grafted onto an everyday practice of hospitalization."[51] Medicaid and Medicare will pay for the institutionalization of a mentally ill individual on the psychiatric ward of a general hospital or in a nursing home, but will usually not pay for maintaining the same individual in a state mental hospital. For this reason states shut down wards of state hospitals, even when the beds are clearly needed, to try to force psychiatric admissions into general hospitals or nursing homes where the federal government will cover most costs.

States publicly rationalize their action as promoting community living and a less restrictive environment for patients, but these rationalizations are often a thin veneer covering an underlying economic imperative. This was clearly demonstrated by economist William Gronfein, who published an analysis of data on deinstitutionalization from 1973 to 1975 and concluded that "Medicaid payments are very strongly associated with the amount of deinstitutionalization in the early 1970s."[52] While the states, cities, and federal governments are playing this fiscal tug-of-war, mentally ill individuals needing hospitalization get caught in the middle, handcuffed to an emergency room wheelchair while the search for a bed continues.

The consequences of chaotic funding for public psychiatric care can also be seen in nonhospital services. Older adults with serious mental illnesses who require an injection of antipsychotic medication must come to a clinic to receive it because federal Medicare will not reimburse a nurse to give the same injection at home. Individuals with serious mental illness who are able to work part-time often will not do so because employment income puts them in danger of losing their SSI income assistance and therefore Medicaid eligibility. Outreach programs to treat and rehabilitate homeless mentally ill individuals are not carried out because such programs are usually not reimbursable through federal Medicaid. There are no fiscal incentives to promote continuity of care and to prevent hospitalizations. In fact, from the state's point of view, it has been pointed out that "it is often cheaper for the patient to go to the hospital than to stay out"[51] if hospitalization costs are covered by federal Medicaid funds.

Another aspect of the chaotic funding of services for people with serious mental illnesses is the failure to implement and use service models that have proved effective. An example is the Louisville Homecare Project, carried out between 1961 and 1964, which showed that 77 percent of psychiatric admissions could be averted by using public health nurses to give medication in clients' homes.[53] The use of crisis homes in Southwest Denver was another experimental program demonstrating that hospitalization rates could be reduced dramatically.[53] Both of these programs were allowed to die because the effective mechanisms of providing service—public health nurses and crisis homes—were not reimbursable by federal Medicaid. The same is true for many model rehabilitation programs that have proven to be effective for mentally ill individuals, but which are rarely replicated because they do not fit existing federal reimbursement schemes; an example is the Fairweather Lodge, a group of mentally ill individuals who live together and operate a community business.[53]

In all of these cases states are reluctant to use a service delivery system, no matter how effective it is, if federal programs such as Medicaid will not reimburse them for it. As Dr. Charles Kiesler, a prominent researcher on mental health services, has pointed out, "Quite unintentionally, Medicaid has become the largest single mental health program in the country."[54] As early as 1978, President Carter's Commission on Mental Health concluded that "the level and type of care given to the chronically mentally disabled is frequently based on what services are fundable and not what services are needed or appropriate.''[55] This means that demonstration programs can demonstrate and model programs can model, but if their results, however praiseworthy, are contrary to the existing system of economic incentives, then such programs will be neither extended nor replicated. Demonstration programs will continue to be mere tinkerings with the status quo, demonstrating the deficiencies of the present without significantly influencing the future.

7. An undetermined portion of public funds for services to people with serious mental illnesses is literally being stolen.

Public programs serving people with serious mental illnesses are not generally thought of as likely venues for theft or other criminal activity. And yet such programs spend approximately $20 billion each year, much of it in government contracts with nonprofit corporations, with remarkably little auditing or oversight of these expenditures. It is a situation ready-made for theft, which is usually not labeled as such; rather, among mental health professionals, as in other white-collar circles, it is euphemistically called "misappropriation of public funds."

There are many forms of theft from publicly funded programs for people with mental illness. Petty theft of personal property from mentally ill patients occurs commonly in psychiatric hospitals, facilitated by the fact that other patients can be blamed and the victims themselves are often so confused that they cannot assist in pinpointing when the property was taken. Another common form of petty theft in programs for people with mental illnesses is some mental health professionals' practice of seeing private patients during the same time as they are being paid to see public patients; this has become widespread and implicitly condoned as it has become increasingly difficult to recruit mental health professionals to public-sector jobs. This is in essence the theft of time, the cost of which adds up very quickly since such professionals are comparatively well paid.

We can only guess how frequently larger "misappropriation of public funds" occurs in the delivery system for public psychiatric services. In the few instances when it has been looked for, it has often been found, sometimes glaringly obvious and undetected for years by officials who were performing virtually no oversight function. Some recent examples follow.

Timpanogos Community Mental Health Center (Provo, Utah)[56]

The Timpanogos Community Mental Health Center was established in 1967 with federal construction and staffing grants from the National Institute of Mental Health. Its function was to deliver psychiatric services to mentally ill residents of three counties in the Provo region. By 1988, it had an annual budget of approximately $8 million. In 1976, former state legislator Glen Brown was hired by the board of Timpanogos CMHC to be executive director. As such he had authority to contract for specialty services. Brown, Director of Specialty Programs and psychologist Carl V. Smith, and Business Manager Craig W. Stephens then proceeded to set up contracts under which they paid themselves for the same work more than once.

According to a 1988 investigation of the Utah Legislative Auditor General, as reported in the *Deseret News*, "In 1987 alone, for example, Smith earned $728,503.72 in total compensation, including salary, contract earnings and car and credit card allowances. Stephens earned $501,461 followed by Brown with $149,065 . . . In essence, these employees were paying themselves repeatedly to perform their regular duties." The investigation also revealed that "five employees appropriated as much as $41,000 each per year in car allowances" and that "five of the eight top center employees were given American Express credit cards for virtually unlimited use." The total amount received by Brown, Smith, and Stephens was estimated at approximately $3.6 million between 1983 and 1988.

During these same years, budget cutbacks at Timpanogos CMHC forced repeated reductions in services to people with mental illness. Waiting lists grew; patients discharged from Utah State Hospital had to wait nine weeks for an appointment at the CMHC to receive medications. The CMHC facilities also deteriorated; according to a news account, "Some tables are held up with bricks. Chairs have books stashed under them for proper balance. A lunchroom couch sags to the floor because its springs are broken."

In October 1988 the Utah Attorney General filed criminal charges consisting of 117 felony counts against Brown, Smith, and Stephens. Each pled guilty to five felony counts, is serving two years in the Utah State Prison, and will be paroled in August 1991. In addition, the court ordered that Brown make restitution of $255,000, Smith make restitution of $1,702,792, and Stephens make restitution of $1,400,994. Since 1989 Timpanogos CMHC has had a highly regarded new director and has made excellent progress in getting its programs back in order.

Tarrant County Mental Health-Mental Retardation Services (Fort Worth, Texas)[57]

Tarrant County Mental Health-Mental Retardation Services (TCMHMR), serving the Fort Worth area, is one of 35 regional public programs under the Texas Department of Mental Health and Mental Retardation. It has an annual budget of approximately $20 million, of which 50 percent is state funds, 10 percent Tarrant County funds, and the remainder federal, insurance, and fee-for-service funds. It has a staff of 680 employees and is run by a nine-member Board of Directors appointed by the Tarrant County commissioners. The Board of Directors sets agency policies and appoints the TCMHMR program's executive director, who, from 1979 until his resignation in 1989, was Loyd Kilpatrick, a former high school football coach and assistant director of a State Center for Human Development.

Services for people with mental illnesses in Tarrant County have been deplorable. Texas ranks 49th among all states in per capita funding for mental illness services, and within Texas, Tarrant County ranks 34th among the 35 regions. The new county psychiatric inpatient unit is half empty because funds are not available to staff it. Patients discharged from the state hospital at Wichita Falls often must wait several weeks to be seen for outpatient services. Supervised housing for mentally ill individuals is virtually nonexistent, and rehabilitation programs are available for only a fraction of those who need them. County officials estimate that there are between 300 and 400 mentally ill individuals among the 2,700 inmates in the county jail who are receiving no psychiatric services, and untreated mentally ill individuals are strikingly evident among the homeless population in Fort Worth.

Despite these deplorable services in a grossly underfunded public program, Executive Director Kilpatrick benefited handsomely from the program. According to a series of articles in the Fort Worth *Star-Telegram* based on outstanding investigative reporting, Kilpatrick's annual salary when he was hired in 1979 was $33,300, but by 1989 it had risen to $200,937, including retirement benefits and a leased automobile; that was more than twice the salary of the Texas governor. The chairman of the board that approved Kilpatrick's salary and benefits, Roger Williams, owns car dealerships from which TCMHMR purchased most of its vehicles, a fleet that increased from 4 vehicles when Kilpatrick was hired in 1979 to 47 vehicles when he resigned in 1989. The purchases were theoretically made using closed bids, but, according to the *Star-Telegram,* "at least two agency employees said Kilpatrick told them that sealed bids were opened early so Williams could underbid them." Bid records showed that "at least six of Williams' low bids were within $50 of the next lowest bid." The bank deposits of TCMHMR were also directed to a bank of which Williams was a director without soliciting bids for the business.

In October 1989, as the *Star-Telegram* series was being published, Loyd Kilpatrick abruptly resigned from TCMHMR "for what he called health reasons." Williams and the board thereupon gave Kilpatrick an additional $214,000 in severance pay plus "the 1989 Chevrolet Suburban that the agency was leasing for him." Texas state auditors examined TCMHMR's books and reported that the agency "may have misappropriated as much as $500,000" over 10 years, and TCMHMR was ordered to repay $200,000 to the Texas Department of Mental Health and Mental Retardation. On March 15, 1990, a grand jury indicted Kilpatrick on four counts of felony theft. In June 1990 a new executive director, said to be highly regarded, was appointed to head TCMHMR and changes were made on the board of the agency.

Harris County Mental Health-Mental Retardation Authority (Houston, Texas)[58]

Harris County Mental Health-Mental Retardation Authority (MHMRA) is responsible for public psychiatric services for 2.7 million Houston residents. Its 1988 budget was $41.8 million, of which $13.3 million came from county taxes, $14.7 million from state taxes, and the remainder from federal taxes and other sources. According to the newspapers it was headquartered in "the posh Weslayan Tower," where its monthly rent in 1990 was $9,000.

Houston ranks with Los Angeles and Miami among the cities with the worst public psychiatric services in the nation. In 1987, 6,098 patients applied for admission to the eight-bed psychiatric emergency unit at Ben Taub Hospital. Ever since the opening of the Harris County Psychiatric Center in 1988, there have been long waiting lists at both the hospital and at the six outpatient clinics staffed by the Department of Psychiatry of Baylor College of Medicine under contract to MHMRA. The large number of untreated mentally ill homeless individuals living at the Star of Hope Mission and beneath the San Jacinto River Bridge is a barometer of the gross inadequacy of Houston's public psychiatric services.

On April 5, 1990, four men were indicted in Harris County for "engaging in organized criminal activity" and allegedly sharing $700,000 in proceeds from the 1985 sale of a mental health clinic building to MHMRA for $2 million; the building had an appraised value of $1.3 million and prosecutors "would only say that the defendants kept money they allegedly overcharged the authority." Indicted were Eugene Williams, who had been the director of MHMRA for 12 years until he was fired in 1989; Dr. George L. Adams, a psychiatrist who had been a professor of psychiatry at Baylor College of Medicine until his 1988 appointment as professor of psychiatry at Dartmouth Medical School; John P. Chambers, a "psychotherapist" and president of Discovery Center, Inc.; and Joe F. Wheat, a lawyer. Bail for each of the indicted men was set at $1.4 million.

Williams had also been indicted in 1989, along with the MHMRA business manager, and "accused of stealing $800,000 in deferred income annuities"; however, a district judge threw out that indictment, "saying he found insufficient evidence that the men's annuity plans were illegal." Williams' annual salary and benefits ranged from $105,108 to $108,581 between 1985 and 1987.

Dr. Adams, as Baylor's director of community and social psychiatry programs, "helped negotiate the school's contract" with MHMRA; the contract totaled $1.76 million annually. In addition to being employed by Baylor, Dr. Adams was also employed by MHMRA on a separate contract of $33,600 per year "as a management consultant." MHMRA Director Williams, in addition to his employment by MHMRA, was employed part-time by the Department of Psychiatry at Baylor College of Medicine and was said to teach "a seminar on mental health administration." The wife of the chairperson of the MHMRA Board was also employed "as a part-time clinical assistant professor of psychiatry at Baylor" and "reportedly had worked for Adams."

John P. Chambers' organization, Discovery Center Inc., had received a $66,000 annual contract from 1984 through 1986 to provide staff for MHMRA clinics through the Baylor contract. Chambers' wife was employed by MHMRA as a social worker. Chambers was president of the land company that sold the clinic building to MHMRA for $2 million in 1985, the transaction on which the April 1990 indictment was based. Chambers was also said to be under investigation for the sale of at least two other properties to MHMRA; *in one of them a building with an appraised value of $1.5 million was purchased by Chambers and his brother for $2.1 million and sold four hours later to MHMRA for $3.3 million.*

Commenting on the land deals, Harris County Judge Jon Lindsay said in 1988: "The county got ripped off, MHMRA got ripped off, the people who need the services got ripped off." District Attorney John B. Holmes stated that MHMRA "was operated in a way that apparently made it easy to steal."

In September 1988, Eugene Williams was fired as director of MHMRA. Three months later Dr. Jan Duker, a highly respected psychologist and former state mental health commissioner, was appointed to the position and said that one of her top priorities would be "re-establishing credibility" for MHMRA.

Several replacements were also made on the MHMRA board and in early 1990 Duker moved MHMRA headquarters from the expensive leased space to a building already owned by the agency.

New York Psychotherapy and Counseling Center (Queens, NY)[59]

The New York Psychotherapy and Counseling Center (NYPCC) was incorporated as a not-for-profit agency in 1974. The purpose of the corporation was to provide outpatient psychiatric services at six clinics in Queens and Brooklyn for mentally ill residents of adult homes. Most of these residents had been previously hospitalized in state psychiatric hospitals. Approximately 95 percent of the income of NYPCC was derived from Medicaid payments for outpatient psychiatric services, usually at a rate of $53 for a 30-minute individual visit. The executive director of NYPCC was Rabbi Isidore Klein, whose son served as assistant executive director. Two psychiatrists, Jack Schnee and Harold Finn, were medical co-directors.

In December 1989, the New York State Commission on Quality of Care for the Mentally Disabled released a report entitled "Profit-Making in Not-for-Profit Corporations: A Challenge to Regulators." It claimed that "NYPCC was only nominally a not-for-profit corporation. In reality, it functioned as a profit-making corporation for its key officers rather than solely for a public purpose." The report alleged that NYPCC had used "improper Medicaid billings of $1.4 million by reporting group therapy services at their clinics as individual services for which higher reimbursement is paid, and by operation of an unlicensed clinic." The report also alleged that Rabbi Klein, Dr. Schnee, and Dr. Finn, the three senior executives, were paid "in excess of $150,000/year each, in addition to generous tax-deferred compensation, insurance, and luxury cars for personal and private use." Finally, the report alleged that Rabbi Klein, Dr. Schnee, and Dr. Finn created a limited partnership owned by themselves and their children that purchased real estate, which they then leased to NYPCC; this led to "profit-making of $720,000 over a three-year period through less-than-arm's-length property transactions with family-owned businesses, one of which realized a 4,917 percent return on a $10,000 investment."

In summarizing these findings the report noted that "there is virtually no scrutiny by State licensing and funding agencies of how money is actually spent by the not-for-profit agencies." Referring to NYPCC, the Commission noted that "although these and other irregularities in the agency's operations were called to the attention of senior state OMH (Office of Mental Health) officials in October 1988, no enforcement action has been taken by OMH either directly or by referrals to other appropriate state agencies, despite their commitment to do so, and despite repeated inquiries from the Commission in subsequent months." Finally, on December 7, 1989, the state mental health commissioner agreed to refer the Commission report to the office of the New York State attorney general's office; as of June 1990, no action had been taken.

The report on NYPCC is similar to another report the Commission released three years earlier entitled "Profit Making in Not-for-Profit Care: A Review of the Operations and Financial Practices of Brooklyn Psychosocial Rehabilitation Institute Inc."[60] In that report, Dr. Karl Easton, a psychiatrist who was the founder and medical director of Brooklyn Psychosocial Rehabilitation Institute (BPRI), was said to have "violated Federal and State tax laws." The report also stated that a treatment center run by BPRI "fraudulently billed the Medicaid program for over $1.4 million in 1985 alone." Furthermore, through a series of interlocking corporations controlled by the Easton family, "actual rents paid [since 1980] have totaled $2.7 million, which represents almost entirely profit on the landlord's initial cash investment of $150,000 and $30,000 in the properties leased to BPRI . . . The net return to the Eastons on their investment [in] the Boerum Hill Residence and adjacent apartments has ranged *from 180 to 420 percent annually since 1980.* The return on The Lafayette Center has been *from 150 to 237 percent each year since mid-1979.*" New York State subsequently revoked BPRI's operating certificate and sued it for recovery of funds which it claimed had been wrongfully diverted; as of June 1990 the case had not been settled.

These cases illustrate that it is relatively easy to steal funds from public programs for people with serious mental illnesses. The Tarrant County case came to light only after it had been investigated by newspaper reporters. The New York cases were uncovered by an independent state agency, the New York State Commission on Quality of Care. The Utah case was made public by the State Legislative Auditor General. In none of these states did the state department of mental health play any role in uncovering the misuse of funds despite the fact that it funded the largest share of these programs. There appears to be an assumption that administrators and professionals working in public programs for people with mental illnesses are dedicated individuals who do not steal. This is true for the vast majority of such individuals, but the number of exceptions will not be known until such programs are subjected to much closer fiscal scrutiny than has heretofore been the case.

8. Guidelines for serving people with mental illnesses are often made at both the federal and state level by administrators who have had no experience in this field.

The actual care of people with mental illnesses in the United States takes place in hundreds of hospitals and thousands of outpatient clinics and rehabilitation programs. Decisions about how such care should be provided, however, is often determined by guidelines established by federal and state administrators in such programs as Supplemental Security Income (SSI), Social Security Disability Income (SSDI), Medicaid, Medicare, the Community Support Program (CSP), Department of Housing and Urban Development (HUD) programs, and special grant programs such as the Stewart B. McKinney Homeless Assistance Act. These guidelines determine which services will be funded or reimbursed by the federal or state governments and which will not; since federal and state funds comprise approximately 90 percent of the funds supporting public mental illness services, the guidelines in effect determine both what care will be given and how it will be given.

One of the biggest frustrations for professionals working hands-on with mentally ill people in hospitals and clinics is trying to tailor their treatment decisions to meet federal and state guidelines. For example, for a senior citizen with schizophrenia who needs an injection every three weeks, a home visit by a nurse to give the injection is not reimbursable by Medicare, but a visit to a clinic for the injection is reimbursable. In a rural area with no public transportation, the difference between these services often is critical. Most professionals who provide direct service to mentally ill individuals have long suspected that many administrators who set the guidelines for federal and state reimbursement have had no personal experience providing direct services to people with mental illnesses and do not know what they are talking about. In most cases this turns out to be precisely the case.

At the federal level, for example, crucial decisions regarding Medicaid reimbursement for services to people with mental illnesses are made in the sprawling headquarters of the Social Security Administration in Baltimore. Since Medicaid is the single largest source of public funds for mental illness services in the United States, it might be expected that the government's theoretical think-tank on such matters, the National Institute of Mental Health (NIMH), would have expertise to contribute and input into Medicaid decisions. In fact, NIMH has virtually no input to the Medicaid funding decisions made by the Social Security Administration.

NIMH itself is virtually devoid of professionals who have had practical, hands-on experience working with seriously mentally ill individuals in the public sector beyond the brief and in some cases ephemeral exposure during their professional training, which often took place a decade or two ago. Despite having administered the $3 billion community mental health center (CMHC) program for more than 22 years, as well as the multimillion-dollar Community Support Program for the past 13 years, NIMH has almost no professional staff who can speak from experience in treating individuals with serious mental illnesses in the public sector.

To illustrate this point, information was obtained under the federal Freedom of Information Act on the training and experience of NIMH staff members in charge of guidelines and funding for the Community Support Program (CSP), which gives grants to states to develop and coordinate services for people with mental illnesses (currently $24.3 million per year), and the Protection and Advocacy Program, which funds programs protecting the rights of mentally ill people (currently $14 million per year). Of the seven professional staff persons assigned to these two programs, only one appears to have ever had any employment experience working with mentally ill individuals, and that experience consisted of administrative duties in a community mental health center half-time for eight months. The two individuals in charge of these programs have had no experience whatsoever in serving people with mental illnesses; one of them has a bachelor's degree and 21 years of experience as an administrator of psychopharmacology research grants, while the other has a master's degree in public administration, four months of experience evaluating personnel usage in a town police and fire department, and seven years of experience in various administrative capacities at NIMH.

The situation at the state level is only modestly better than at the federal level. In each state, the most important official in determining policies for state programs serving people with mental illnesses is the director of the state department of mental health. As of May 1990, only about 20 percent of such directors had ever had any clinical experience in treating people with mental illnesses. With respect to professional background, the current group of state mental health directors includes two psychiatrists, thirteen psychologists, eight social workers, two lawyers, one person with a degree in education, two people with degrees in public administration, and twenty-three people without advanced degrees but with administrative experience in state government. Only a handful of them have extensive experience working with people with mental illnesses. Deborah Allness, M.S.W, the Director of Mental Health in Wisconsin, previously ran a model treatment program; Robert Washington, Ph.D., Commissioner of Mental Health Services for the District of Columbia, previously ran a community mental health center; and Stuart Silver, M.D., Director of the Mental Hygiene Administration in Maryland, previously ran a state mental hospital. The vast majority, however, have no background or experience working with mentally ill people prior to assuming their current positions.

We do not argue that training as a mental health professional qualifies an individual to administer programs for people with mental illnesses; indeed, many mental health professionals are notoriously poor administrators. Conversely, among the most highly respected state directors of mental health have been lawyers and public administrators. We do argue that, all other things being equal, it is highly desirable for federal and state officials who are setting policies and guidelines for the treatment of people with mental illnesses to themselves have had some clinical experience working with such people. Such a background should be the rule, not the exception. This should not preclude gifted administrators with a special interest in mentally ill people from being appointed to such positions, but such administrators should then undertake to get first-hand experience working with people with mental illnesses.

In probably no other area of federal or state government—including education, corrections, social services, and transportation—has the primary responsibility for programs been turned over to administrators who have so little academic training or practical experience in the relevant field. Public programs for people with serious mental illnesses are unique in the degree to which responsibility for them has been assigned to individuals who do not know what they are talking about. Good intentions are not a sufficient qualification for important positions in this field.

NOTES

1. Kennedy JF. Special message to Congress on mental illness and mental retardation, February 6, 1963.

2. Bassuk EL, Rubin L, Lauriat A. Is homelessness a mental health problem? *American Journal of Psychiatry* 141:1546–50, 1984.

3. Arce AA, Tadlock M, Vergare MJ, *et al.* A psychiatric profile of street people admitted to an emergency shelter. *Hospital and Community Psychiatry* 34:812–17, 1983.

4. Torrey EF, Bargmann E, Wolfe SM. Washington's grate society: Schizophrenics in the shelters and on the street. Washington: Health Research Group, 1985.

5. Koegel P, Burnam MA, Farr RK. The prevalence of specific psychiatric disorders among homeless individuals in the inner city of Los Angeles. *Archives of General Psychiatry* 45:1085–92, 1988.

6. Vernoz G, Burnam MA, McGlynn EA *et al*. Review of California's program for the homeless mentally ill. Santa Monica: Rand Corporation, 1988.

7. "Survey of homeless: Mental ills and addiction." *New York Times* Sept. 10, 1989, p. 36.

8. Susser E, Struening EL, Conover S. Psychiatric problems in homeless men. *Archives of General Psychiatry* 46:845–50, 1989.

9. Cohen NL, Putnam JF, Sullivan AM. The mentally ill homeless: isolation and adaptation. *Hospital and Community Psychiatry* 35:922–24, 1984.

10. Gelberg L, Linn LS, Leake BD. Mental health, alcohol and drug use, and criminal history among homeless adults. *American Journal of Psychiatry* 145:191–96, 1988.

11. Greene MS. Data challenge ideas on D.C. street people. *Washington Post* May 21, 1989, p. 1.

12. Belcher JR. Rights versus needs of homeless mentally ill persons. *Social Work* 33:398–402, 1988.

13. Belcher JR. Defining the service needs of homeless mentally ill persons. *Hospital and Community Psychiatry* 39:1203–06, 1988.

14. Drake RE, Wallach MA, Hoffman JS. Housing instability and homelessness among after-care patients of an urban state hospital. *Hospital and Community Psychiatry* 40:46–51, 1989.

15. Lamb HR, Lamb DM. Factors contributing to homelessness among the chronically and severely mentally ill. *Hospital and Community Psychiatry* 41:301–05, 1990.

16. Cooper C. Brutal lives of homeless S.F. women. *San Francisco Examiner* December 18, 1988, p. A-1.

17. Homeless man is assaulted. *New York Times* October 6, 1986, p. B-5.

18. A ferocious crime against the helpless. *Cape Cod Times* July 22, 1984.

19. Herbert W. Lost lives of the homeless. *Washington Post* October 19, 1985, p. G-4.

20. Whitman D. Shattering myths about the homeless. *U.S. News and World Report* March 20, 1989, p. 28.

21. Jemelka R, Trupin E, Chiles JA. The mentally ill in prisons: A review. *Hospital and Community Psychiatry* 40:481–90, 1989.

22. Teplin LA. The prevalence of severe mental disorder among male urban jail detainees: Comparison with the Epidemiologic Catchment Area Program. *American Journal of Public Health* 80:663–69, 1990.

23. Swetz A, Salive ME, Stough T, *et al*. The prevalence of mental illness in a state correctional institution for men. Mimeo.

24. Acker C, Fine MJ. Families under siege: A mental health crisis. *Philadelphia Inquirer* September 10, 1989.

25. Luke P. 67% of inmates need some mental help, survey shows. *Grand Rapids Press* September 4, 1987.

26. Belcher JR. Are jails replacing the mental health asylum for the homeless mentally ill? *Community Mental Health Journal* 24:185–94, 1988.

27. Kilzer L. Jails as a 'halfway house' or long-term commitment? *Denver Post* June 3, 1984.

28. Egri G, Keitner L, Harwood TB. Not mad enough, not bad enough: Where should they go? Erie County Forensic Mental Health Service, Buffalo, 1985, mimeo.

29. McFarland BH, Faulkner LR, Bloom JD, *et al*. Chronic mental illness and the criminal justice system. *Hospital and Community Psychiatry* 40:718–24, 1989.

30. Plott M. Man who blinded self is moved from prison, *Atlanta Constitution* March 8, 1985.

31. Van Der Werf M. Nude inmates bound to "rack" for hours; practice defended. *Arizona Republic* April 27, 1989.

32. Nance K. Program for prisoners shackled by lack of funds. *Lexington Herald-Leader* June 25, 1989.

33. Karras A, Otis DB. A comparison of inpatients in an urban state hospital in 1975 and 1982. *Hospital and Community Psychiatry* 38:963–67, 1987.

34. Raab S. Deak murder suspect has been found paranoid. *New York Times* November 21, 1985, p. B-3.

35. Krakowski MI, Convit A, Jaeger J, *et al*. Neurological impairment in violent schizophrenic inpatients. *American Journal of Psychiatry* 146:849–53, 1989; Smith LD. Medication refusal and the rehospitalized mentally ill inmate. *Hospital and Community Psychiatry* 40:491–96, 1989; Hafner H. The risk of violence in psychotics. *Integrative Psychiatry* 4:138–42, 1986.

36. Lamb HR. Incompetency to stand trial: Appropriateness and outcome. *Archives of General Psychiatry* 44:754–58, 1987.

37. Torrey EF. *Nowhere to Go: The Tragic Odyssey of the Homeless Mentally Ill.* New York: Harper & Row, 1988, p. 72.

38. Taube CA, Burns BJ, Kessler L. Patients of psychiatrists and psychologists in office-based practice: 1980. *American Psychologist* 39:1435–47, 1984.

39. Knesper DJ, Pagnucco DJ. Estimated distribution of effort by providers of mental health services to U.S. adults in 1982 and 1983. *American Journal of Psychiatry* 144:883–88, 1987.

40. Worthington R. Psychiatrist shortage in rural U.S. *San Francisco Sunday Examiner and Chronicle.* November 27, 1988, p. A-1.

41. Torrey, *Nowhere to Go, op. cit.*, p. 172.

42. *Ibid.*, p. 171.

43. Psychiatrists to 'treat' Satanism. *Washington Post* September 7, 1989, p. C-6.

44. Pickney DS. Youth psychiatric hospitalization is up dramatically. *AMA News* March 10, 1989, p. 46.

45. Schiffman JR. Teenagers end up in psychiatric hospitals in alarming numbers. *Wall Street Journal* February 3, 1989, p. 1.

46. Torrey EF, Wolfe SM, Flynn LM. Fiscal misappropriations in programs for the mentally ill: A report on illegality and failure of the federal construction grant program for Community Mental Health Centers. Health Research Group and National Alliance for the Mentally Ill, March, 1990, mimeo.

47. Some facts about Community Mental Health Centers. Washington: National Council of Community Mental Health Centers, March 23, 1990. See also their original report of the survey: Services for the seriously mentally ill: A survey of community mental health agencies, 1988.

48. Windle C, Poppen PJ, Thompson JW, *et al.* Types of patients served by various providers of outpatient care in CMHCs. *American Journal of Psychiatry* 145:457–63, 1988.

49. Higgins AJ. Hancock County health center fails federal standards, Nader group charges. *Bangor Daily News* March 24, 1990.

50. Barbanel J. System to treat mental patients is overburdened. *New York Times* February 22, 1988, p. A-1.

51. Friedman RS. Resistance to alternatives to hospitalization. *Psychiatric Clinics of North America* 8:471–82, 1985.

52. Gronfein W. Incentives and interventions in mental health policy: A comparison of the Medicaid and community mental health programs. *Journal of Health and Social Behavior* 26:192–206, 1985.

53. Torrey EF. Economic barriers to widespread implementation of model programs for the seriously mentally ill. *Hospital and Community Psychiatry* 41:526–31, 1990.

54. Kiesler CA. Mental hospitals and alternative care. *American Psychologist* 37:349–60, 1982.

55. Task Panel Reports Submitted to the President's Commission on Mental Health. Vol. II. Washington, U.S. Government Printing Office, 1978, p. 369.

56. Data on the Timpanogos CMHC case was taken from "An Expenditure Review of the Timpanogos Community Mental Health Center," Report by the Utah Legislative Auditor General, April 1988; "An Investigative and Prosecution Report by the Office of the Utah Attorney General," September 18, 1989; and by news accounts of the case in the *Deseret News.*

57. Data on the Tarrant County Mental Health-Mental Retardation Services case was taken from news stories in the *Fort Worth Star-Telegram* by Carolyn Poirot, Stan Jones and Bob Mahlburg between October 1988 and March 1989, and from a letter of May 10, 1990 from Tarrant County District Attorney Tim Curry to the Board of Trustees of TCMHMR Services.

58. Data on the Harris County Mental Health-Mental Retardation Authority case was taken from news stories in the *Houston Chronicle* by Pete Slover, Stephen Johnson, Jo Ann Zuniga and R.A. Dyer and in the *Houston Post* by John Mecklin, Brenda Sapino, Robert Stanton, Katherine Kerr, and Peter Brewton between July 1988 and April 1990.

59. New York State Commission on Quality of Care for the Mentally Disabled, Profit-Making in Not-For-Profit Corporations: A Challenge to Regulators, Albany, New York, December 1989; and New York State Commission on Quality of Care for the Mentally Disabled Annual Report 1988–89, p. 16.

60. New York State Commission on Quality of Care for the Mentally Disabled, Profit-Making in Not-for-Profit Care: A Review of the Operations and Financial Practices of the Brooklyn Psychosocial Rehabilitation Institute, Inc. Albany, New York, November 1986.

HEALING THE DELTA

Frank Clancy

On a spring afternoon seven years ago, a man arrived at Dr. Anne Brooks's clinic near the Tutwiler, MS, post office with a sore back. He'd been chopping cotton in a nearby field—moving methodically up and down the rows, digging weeds with a hoe. Like most of Tallahatchie County's residents, he was black.

As a matter of principle, Brooks, a Catholic nun who trained as an osteopath, likes to suggest ways for patients to help themselves. In this case, her instinct was to recommend that the man spend the weekend in bed, putting hot towels on his back now and then. She thought for a moment, then asked if he had hot water. "No ma'am, I don't," he told her. "But I can heat the kettle." How? she asked. "I'll go outside, haul the water and chop some wood," he said, "then start a fire." Brooks told him to rest in bed, and perhaps ask a friend to rub his back.

I had gone to Tutwiler, a town of 1,176 where W.C. Handy is said to have "discovered" the blues, in the hope of learning why black Americans, in Mississippi and across the rural South, are less healthy and dying younger than their white neighbors—what physicians call excess morbidity and excess mortality. For two weeks in May and June I crisscrossed the Delta in search of doctors, nurses, and public health officials who might provide answers. I could as easily have gone to any of seven other southern states, from North Carolina to Louisiana, that make up the so-called stroke belt and have the highest infant mortality rates in the U.S. But in the Delta, where blacks constitute about 70 percent of the population and many are desperately poor, the problems are the most concentrated of any region in the country.

For more than 400 miles, from New Orleans to Memphis, US Highway 61 roughly parallels the Mississippi River and passes within 20 miles of all but one of the towns I visited. It was my life line, the road to which I constantly returned, for most of these towns are too small and too poor even to have a motel of their own. North of Vicksburg, 61 descends to the vast flatlands of the Delta, a rich alluvial plain that supports bountiful harvests of wheat, rice, and soybeans, along with the region's newest agricultural product, farm-raised catfish. And of course, there is the crop that made the Delta what it is today: cotton.

Time and again I discovered situations as complex and frustrating as Brooks's attempt to treat her patient's aching back. In the Delta, health and medicine are linked inextricably to numbing poverty, lack of education, and a social structure in which many blacks remain fundamentally powerless, unable to control their own lives. All of these forces are as entwined in local culture as the ivy that overwhelms abandoned buildings scattered across the landscape. If the pain of Brooks's patient cannot entirely be attributed to race, neither can race be absolved: White people do not chop cotton, and most white people do not live in houses without stoves and running water.

I learned, most of all, from the stories I heard. One nurse told me about a man who stood at the edge of a field waving a white flag to let a crop duster know where to spray, wearing only a T-shirt and jeans to protect him from raining poison. A physician described a patient hospitalized with massive gastrointestinal, urinary tract, liver, and skin ailments after a spring wind soaked him with herbicide he was pouring into a container.

In Mound Bayou I heard about a man who lost his manufacturing job because he missed work to get X-rays, and one doctor told me of women whose employers "don't want them to go to a doctor even if they're half-dead."

I heard of one mother who fed her infant just twice a day, when she ate, and of people forced to choose between food and heart medicine, because they didn't have money for both.

When black people in the Delta seek medical care, it's not in an integrated health care system but a haphazard patchwork assembly—one held together by too few physicians and fewer specialists. Their efforts are undermined by employers who fail to provide insurance, and Medicaid and Medicare systems that inadequately reimburse doctors and leave many patients uninsured.

"I'm not sure that the medical problems we face here in the Delta are a whole lot different from the medical problems anyplace in our country," says Brooks. "I think people are sicker longer before they get help, because of lack of money and transportation. When we finally get them in the hospital they're much worse off."

Marks

On a hot, dry morning I drive to Marks, 20 miles north of Tutwiler, where I have arranged to interview another Catholic nun, Dr. Marilyn Aiello. With giant oak trees shading well-kept wooden houses, the town at first seems relatively prosperous. As the seat of Quitman County, it sustains a decent-sized middle class. But soon I learn it is the white side of Marks that seems prosperous, for its housing is segregated, the railroad tracks as rigid a divider as the old Berlin Wall. As with legal segregation, separate does not mean equal: On the other side of the tracks are blocks of crooked wooden shacks, many built shotgun-style, with rooms stacked one behind the other. On one side of the tracks are street signs and fire hydrants, on the other, neither. Yet many black families have planted flowers in window boxes and in their front yards.

Aiello, a small, dark, gregarious woman who still retains a strong Chicago accent, traveled throughout the South before settling in Marks nine years ago. One of Marks's two doctors had died of cancer. Aiello and several other nuns moved into his office, and named it the DePorres Health Center, after a seventeenth-century Peruvian saint who worked among and healed the poor. Like Brooks in Tutwiler, the nuns integrated the clinic's waiting room.

Poverty is the most overwhelming cause of poor health among black people in the Mississippi Delta: They are ill because they don't have the resources to remain well. "Your wealthier people, with cars, they can travel to Clarksdale, to Memphis, to Oxford," says the 53-year-old Aiello. "But your poor become very sick and die. I can't tell you how many people come into the clinic who have never seen a doctor, and are seriously sick—not so much any more, because I've been here almost ten years. But in the beginning it was very commonplace. They just wouldn't go, because it was so hard for them to go."

Although she was for a time the only physician in the county, Aiello chose Marks because she found another void as deep and significant as the absence of a doctor. "The poor need people who have a sympathetic ear, who will listen to them and help identify and further their interests—an advocate," she says. "Some of the places we went to, as much as there was a medical need, there were advocates. But when we came here, there were few advocates. We felt that we could offer something beyond health care."

That something might be as simple as seeing that specialists treat her patients with respect. It can mean teaching a woman to read, or having a fellow nun, Sister Julian Betts, help a man apply for social security. With some—particularly the middle-aged men who live in sheds behind other people's homes—Betts can do little except help them get food stamps. When they are ill, she brings them to the clinic, which writes off the debt.

Despite a recent expansion of Medicaid, the government insurance program for the nonelderly poor, a number of Aiello's patients have no insurance. Adult men, for example, are rarely eligible, and the minimum-wage jobs available to poorly educated blacks, such as chopping cotton, seldom provide insurance or any other benefit. But poverty affects health in more than the obvious ways. Most poor people cannot afford medicine when they need it, and they're too poor to pay a clinic's sliding-scale fee and too proud to seek free care, even in the few places it's available. In most rural towns, healthy food is expensive and difficult to find, making it hard to control chronic diseases like hypertension and diabetes. "There aren't a lot of things poor people can change," says Sister Maryann McMahon, a nurse-practitioner who works with Aiello.

Poverty also breeds enormous stress. "They're always wondering where they're going to get money," says Betts of her clients. "If they have children, they worry about clothes, about school supplies. It's worry after worry after worry." The pressure on black men may be more severe, Aiello suggests. "They have to leave, for all intents and purposes, to find work," she says. "The only constant jobs are as farm workers, and there aren't many of those. Amtrak comes through Batesville [about 20 miles east of Marks]. It's a steady stream up north."

Aiello would like nothing better than to help heal Marks's social divisions along with its disease. A number of the town's whites donate money to support Betts's work, and among Aiello's patients, white and black, there is friendliness and respect. "We don't want to divide people," Aiello says. "We're going to go home eventually. The question is, Will we leave things better or worse?"

Tchula

Early one morning I leave for the town of Tchula, 70 miles north of Jackson. Before the sun gathers its brutal strength, the Delta has a peculiar and awesome beauty, its immense landscape dwarfing everything of human scale. A faint mist rises slowly off the highway, and white herons soar gracefully overhead.

Tchula's only physician became a minor celebrity last winter when the National Health Service Corps—which paid for Dr. Ronald Myers's education and assigned him to Belzoni, 22 miles west—tried to prevent him from opening a clinic in an abandoned restaurant on the highway. A public health official was reported to have said that Tchula, a battered town with 1,900 people and few jobs, was "too poor" to support a doctor. After Myers's battle reached *The New York Times*, television stations and Hollywood producers soon followed.

It's not hard to understand their interest in Myers, for he is a kind of black Renaissance man, an accomplished jazz pianist and ordained Baptist minister, as well as a physician. Young and fairly new to the Delta, he is a giant of a man, more than 100 pounds overweight. Though he has an ample sense of humor, he does not mince words. "Poor black Americans, in terms of their health care, get written off," he says. "When the Public Health Service says, 'We don't want you to go to Tchula, it's too poor for a doctor,' what they're saying is, 'We'll let those poor, rural black people die. We don't care.' "

He's especially bothered by the high infant mortality rates throughout the Delta. "Our country ranks 20th in the world when it comes to infant mortality," he says, "and I'm in an area that has three times the national average."

Humphreys County, just west of Tchula, has a staggering five-year average rate of 36.7 deaths per 1,000—nearly four times the state average for whites. Black infants in other counties across the state are dying, in many areas at rates of 26 per 1,000 and more. A child born in Chile or Malaysia is more likely to celebrate his first birthday than a black baby throughout much of the Delta.

Many of those dying are the children of children: Despite programs to distribute inexpensive and sometimes free birth control through health clinics, Mississippi has the highest teen pregnancy rate in the country. Fewer teenage mothers receive adequate prenatal care here, and more have low-birth-weight babies. In Tchula's county, Holmes, 25 percent of all births in 1988 were to teenagers.

There is broad agreement on one thing that must be done to lower infant mortality rates among black Americans: Black women must receive better prenatal care. Like many states, Mississippi recently expanded Medicaid for pregnant women. It also expanded WIC (Women, Infants, and Children), which supplies food to pregnant women, and has several programs aimed at reducing the teen pregnancy rate. But it faces a huge obstacle in implementing some of these programs: Most of its counties have no resident obstetrician.

Which is one reason Myers—a specialist in family practice trained to provide early-pregnancy care—gets angry when reminded that public health officials didn't want him in Tchula. "It's hard, because of the amount of poverty here," he says. "I'm not gonna make a lot of money. I collect what I can. But if it's too poor for a doctor, the government shouldn't say, 'Don't go there.' The government should say, 'Yeah, go there, we'll assist you.' "

In Tchula I see firsthand the kind of barriers that make it difficult for the Delta's poor to remain healthy. One of Myers's first patients today, a four-year-old boy, was stung on the eyelid by a wasp. His entire face is swollen, his left eye completely shut, the other a slit. Myers is worried that the stinger hit the eye and wants the boy to see an ophthalmologist, 25 miles away. His mother, Jackie, has no car. She would ordinarily have to pay $10 to $12 for a ride—a significant amount for someone earning minimum wage who has already lost a day's pay to bring her son to the doctor. I offer to take them and a friend of theirs, who has a stubborn case of pinkeye.

The two women tell me about their work in the catfish plants that Myers calls "the new plantation." It's better than welfare, they say, but it's hard work, with poison fins, pressure to work quickly, no air conditioning, and flies everywhere. "Guts be hanging out your eyes, blood be on your clothes," says Jackie. "You be smellin' like fish the rest of your life."

Tchula had been without a doctor for more than two years before Myers arrived. "It was a long time, for me," says the second woman, Harriet. "Too long." But people adjust, just as they live with the Delta's heat. She shows me a finger, swollen and infected, where a catfish fin broke off beneath the skin. She hadn't thought of showing it to Myers; it would work itself out. For the first time I realize that many black residents of the Delta never take for granted what to me had always seemed an utterly simple and available amenity—a doctor.

Mound Bayou

Mound Bayou is a town rich in history. Built on swampland by ex-slaves during Reconstruction 120 years ago, the all-black town straddles Route 61. In the 1960s, when there was a desperate need for doctors in the Delta—and the political will to defeat poverty—the federal government helped establish the Delta Health Center here, the oldest rural community health center in the country. Today several dozen such facilities are scattered across Mississippi.

At 66, Dr. Luther McCaskill is a big man with massive hands who has practiced medicine so long that he leans instinctively as he talks. When he started out 34 years ago, he was the only black doctor in Clarksdale, half an hour north on Route 61. Patients paid him, at times, with chickens or whatever else they had. A modest man, he shifts easily between the language of medicine and that of his patients ("They have enough psychology to know whether you shucking them or whether you being honest")—an important skill, since poor people often complain that doctors don't adequately explain their illnesses and treatments.

Like most physicians in the Delta, McCaskill spends much of his time helping patients manage chronic illness, especially hypertension and diabetes. As many as 4 in 10 blacks may have high blood pressure, twice the rate found among whites. They also tend to develop the disease at a younger age, are five times more likely to have severe hypertension, and have more complications, including heart and kidney disease. Across the stroke belt, west from Virginia to Louisiana and as far north as Indiana, blacks die of stroke almost twice as often as whites, and far more often than northern blacks.

While researchers have offered a variety of explanations for this abundance of hypertension (diet, stress, blacks' tendency to process salt differently), one study found that, given equal access to medical care and antihypertension medicine, blacks responded just as well as whites. The study links the disproportionate number of complications (which include stroke) to one thing: lack of access to medical care.

Things are better now, McCaskill tells me, without any real enthusiasm. Public health education, especially about high blood pressure, has taught people about the effects of diet on health. "There's a much greater awareness now," he says. "Even though they might have some indiscretions in eating salt now and then, or pork, they know it's ultimately dangerous to their health. But it's hard to get away from old habits."

Thus, physicians battle the past as well as poverty, for its influence is as pervasive as humid air before a storm. Like many black residents of the Delta, McCaskill's boss, Dr. L.C. Dorsey, grew up on a farm, the child of sharecroppers. The owner, Dorsey says, controlled access to medical care: "One of the criteria for whether you were on a 'good' plantation, with a 'good' owner, was if he gave you permission to see a doctor. I think the practice in the black community of reserving that benefit of going to the doctor for the most dire needs began then. Because before you could go, you had to go to the boss man and say, 'John is sick,' or 'His wife is sick.' It was a favor you were asking for—although you would be charged, and would pay for it at the end of the year, when a settlement was made.

"The whole process got set in place," Dorsey continues, "where people decided which member of the family was more in need of health care, as a favor. Because black males don't come. I don't think it's just being macho. Even when you make it free they will bring their wives and children, and they will come only when gasping for breath, lungs collapsed, heart giving out, or with 15 chronic diseases that have to be managed."

Although Dorsey admits her theory is untested, a recent survey found that black Americans at every economic level sought medical care less often than whites. (They also waited longer and were less satisfied with the care they received, tremendous disincentives to seeking further care.) While the authors partly attribute this discrepancy to such factors as a shortage of physicians in black communities, they think it may be due in part to "unmeasured sociocultural differences between blacks and whites."

For whatever reason, the effect can be, literally, deadly. McCaskill tells me about a disabled man he had recently treated for a severe infection. The man's mother, a retarded woman, had waited to bring him to a doctor, and his toes had fallen off. Eventually he lost both legs and died. "You see suffering so often you can't get next to it," McCaskill says. "You know you have to go on. It's pathetic when you see somebody who could've been saved, but because of neglect, because of ignorance, because of"—he stops himself. "We need so much to educate the people. The question is, how you gonna do it?"

Tunica

In a few weeks, Dr. Arlillian Savare, a 34-year-old internist, will be leaving the Aaron Henry Community Health Center, a federally subsidized clinic on Highway 61 in Tunica. She has more than a few regrets about leaving a town that was once notorious for its "Sugar Ditch," an open sewer black families lived by. Savare, who worked at the center for four years, will miss the collard greens and the fresh peas, the fish, venison, and pecans patients brought her. "I like it here," she says. "I like the people, the patients, the community. They need adequate health services. They don't deserve second-rate services just because they don't have any money."

Like Ron Myers and Anne Brooks, Savare came to fulfill an obligation to the National Health Service Corps, a government agency that paid for her medical education in return for work in a medically underserved community. For Savare, it was a sort of homecoming: As a girl she lived on a farm just 50 miles northeast of Tunica. Her parents were sharecroppers. "We had an outhouse," she remembers. "We thought it was luxury when we got a pump."

Savare is a small woman with a youthful appearance and a taste for bright lipstick. She found a reservoir of loneliness in Tunica, she says, that was in its way as deep as the need for medicine. With no one else to turn to, residents often brought her their problems. Some didn't even want advice—they just wanted to talk to someone they knew would listen.

Savare will be replaced, but other towns in Mississippi are not so fortunate. (Good fortune is relative: 45% of Tunica County's residents live below the poverty line.) The state has 58 officially designated "health manpower shortage areas," where the ratio of primary-care physicians to residents is excessively low. According to government figures, the state needed 107 physicians in 1989 to provide a minimum level of care; without them 319,000 people were left unserved. If the situation is critical now—the Reagan administration decided in the early '80s to cut scholarship money for the National Health Service Corps —it may get worse. The doctor shortage is expected to hit rural areas the hardest.

In Mississippi, the problem is not just a shortage of physicians but also poor distribution: More than half of the state's doctors practice in just eight counties. The clustering of specialists such as obstetrician/gynecologists—especially those who accept Medicaid and Medicare—is particularly uneven.

There is an undercurrent of bitterness in Tunica, the northernmost stop on my trip through the Delta. Five years ago the world heard the story of Sugar Ditch Alley, where about 200 blacks lived on an open sewer, amid rats and roaches, without running water and toilets. The Reverend Jesse Jackson called it "America's Ethiopia." In response, people from across the US sent truckloads of food, clothes, and toys, including numerous Cabbage Patch dolls to an 11-year-old girl who had wanted a black doll for Christmas. The federal government approved $3 to $4 million for subsidized apartments.

"Some things have improved," Savare says. "They did get some housing units. They did move some people off Sugar Ditch and into a trailer park. There are still families down on Sugar Ditch, though, and Sugar Ditch is still there. But nobody appears to be interested any longer.

"These people have pride," she adds. "They are not asking for a handout. They simply do not have access to jobs. If they did, some would work, and have a better standard of living. Jobs is what these folks need—bringing in industry, so the unemployment rate will go down.

"And so they don't have to stay on Sugar Ditch."

Tutwiler

More than anything else, Dr. Anne Brooks, the soft-spoken nun and osteopath, understands the relationship between the health of blacks in the Delta and the region's myriad social problems. In addition to medical care—Brooks and two nurses, both nuns, see about 600 patients a month—the Tutwiler Clinic offers counseling, literacy and general equivalency diploma classes, child care, summer programs for children, a thrift shop and field trips for senior citizens. While this array of services hints at the limits of medicine, it also underscores the importance of a physician—of a person trained to heal. Before Brooks arrived in 1983, Tutwiler had gone years without one.

Like all of the physicians I met, Brooks, now 52, expresses great respect for her patients, who confront seemingly intolerable lives with grace, humor, and dignity. "They live in situations where I would be so depressed I'd probably go hang myself," she says. "They give me much more than I give them."

Brooks is careful and meticulous, surrounding herself with charts, graphs and maps to illustrate much of what she finds important. One shows the median household income of Tallahatchie County ($9,300), while others show where her patients come from (as far as 40 miles away) and their sex (two-thirds women). She occasionally allows a simmering anger to seep through, such as when I mention Tunica's Sugar Ditch. People live like that throughout the Delta, she says. In Tutwiler, sewage empties into the bayou, which floods. "Last year it flooded five times," she says. "I've had people in the hospital because of it. There are people who won't go to their outhouses because of the snakes and the rats. You can sit in somebody's house, and rats will be on the rafters, in the kitchen. I've had people whose toes have been eaten off by rats at night. People shouldn't have to live that way. This is America. We have the technology and we have the money."

With age and experience has come patience, if not acceptance. "You learn that perhaps you can't change the whole world all at once," she says. In seven years, she has seen the health of the community improve—seen stabilizing blood pressures, and fewer strokes. Fewer people call her at home for emergencies. She attributes this improvement to better access to care: Her patients know she will treat them with or without insurance, whether or not they have money.

For now, Brooks strives to help her patients heal. "I believe there's a difference between healing and curing," she says. "Curing is getting rid of the disease: Pneumonia is finished, the antibiotic is done. But healing is the balance, the interaction with the environment. You don't kick the dog, you don't yell at your spouse, because you're well."

To keep herself well, Brooks takes Thursday afternoons off, and we will talk then, in her office. While waiting, I speak to three women who work in the clinic's outreach program.

One of them, Dorothy Dodd, tells me how she started working at the clinic. She'd been depressed after losing a job, she says, and went to see Brooks at home, just to talk. Brooks suggested she volunteer at the clinic to keep herself busy. Five years later, Dodd is an assistant to the director of outreach, helping to run the clinic's programs for children and senior citizens. In May, she testified before a government commission about the flooding of Hopson Bayou. Her mother, a diabetic, sees Brooks regularly. Her children learned to swim in the summer program. Dorothy Dodd is healthy.

She has healed.

BURNOUT IN L.A.

Frank Clancy

Like the mythical phoenix, Martin Luther King, Jr., Hospital rose from the ashes of the Watts Riot, a symbol of hope and promise to a community that had incinerated itself. Sparked by a minor incident—the arrest of a black youth on a hot summer evening in 1965—as many as 10,000 black residents of Watts and south central Los Angeles had exploded in frustration and anger. Over six days, they set fires, looted stores, beat up whites, overturned cars, exchanged gunfire with police, and stoned fire-fighters. By the time calm was restored, 34 had died and more than 1,000 had been injured.

In the wake of that violence (activists call it the Watts Rebellion), a commission was formed to determine its origins and suggest ways to avoid a recurrence. Among many grievances, the commission discovered hospitals too small and poorly equipped to serve these poor neighborhoods, eight miles south of downtown Los Angeles. It recommended the construction of a new hospital, now known as Martin Luther King, Jr./Drew Medical Center, the hub of Los Angeles' public health care system for the black community. King, 25 years later, is a source both of pride and frustration, at once the lifeblood of its community and a symbol of a promise badly broken: a hospital so overwhelmed and underfunded that it fills but a fraction of the needs its founders had hoped to address.

Los Angeles' black population suffers, in disproportionate numbers, from almost every major health problem found in the rural South, including hypertension, diabetes, cancer, stroke, kidney disease, glaucoma, cirrhosis, and tuberculosis. Here blacks share the burden of poverty with a rapidly growing Latino community.

By at least one measure, the situation has gotten worse in the past 25 years. In 1965 the commission cited the infant mortality rate in south central Los Angeles, a predominantly black area, as a sign of poor medical care—it was 50 percent higher than the citywide rate. Today that gap has nearly tripled: Los Angeles' black infant mortality rate is about 140 percent higher than its white counterpart. At 21.1 deaths per 1,000 births, it's comparable to all but the worst of Mississippi's 82 counties, and higher than that state's overall black rate (16.1).

Other statistics tell a similar story. In 1965 the commission complained that black children in south central Los Angeles were inadequately immunized. Two decades later, 75 percent of black two-year-olds in California had not been fully immunized. And although only 8% of California residents are black, they represent 25 percent of the state's pediatric AIDS cases and 42 percent of its youth homicide victims.

One of the most urgent problems—cited in 1965—is poor access to primary medical care. A recent study of hospital admissions in the area of King/Drew found inordinately high rates both for uncontrolled chronic diseases such as hypertension (six times higher than the average state rate) and treatable conditions like pneumonia. Most of those admissions could have been avoided, says study coauthor Geraldine Dallek. "There's an inadequate level of primary care in low-income minority communities. Often the only care available is at overcrowded, understaffed public hospitals and clinics."

Decades ago, Martin Luther King, Jr., Hospital was meant to be a new kind of hospital, one that combined traditional services with comprehensive primary care, community outreach, and education. "We felt we could provide care to a deprived group of citizens that would be comparable to the best medical care given anywhere in the country, in a manner that addressed both their human needs and medical needs," says Dr. Theodore Schlater, King's acting chairman of emergency medicine. "There's no doubt things are better here medically than prior to King, but I think we've fallen short of our expectations for the way we provide service."

The medical school, Drew, hoped to train "a new cadre of health care professionals for the nation," says Dr. Robert Schlegel, its chairman of pediatrics. "The philosophy was to identify the health care needs of this population and develop new ways to serve them. There was a lack of understanding of the social and economic circumstances that contribute to or cause disease."

With little money and burgeoning patient loads, King was soon forced to limit that vision. "The rug was pulled out from under those dreams," says Dr. Ezra Davidson, Jr., King's chairman of obstetrics and gynecology. "Comprehensive care was quickly narrowed, because it was clear that the resources were not going to be allocated." Thus, he says, King provides prenatal care "only in very limited kinds of ways," and has all but abandoned attempts to reach out to the Watts community. The entire public system of obstetrical care, he contends, "is so flawed and inadequate that you can't deal with outreach. There are so many disincentives that it becomes difficult to get the patient to stay in the system."

The result is deadly. Of the 3,001 black women who gave birth at King over a recent three-year period, 60 percent had received no prenatal care. One-third of those with no prenatal care bore low-birth-weight infants (less than 5.5 pounds), a rate that is far above average. Black infants died at a rate of 52.7 per 1,000 births.

Faced with a threatened loss of accreditation, the hospital last year closed three wards, even though it was, and remains, consistently full. Despite a chronic and often desperate shortage of beds, an entire wing sits empty, leaving only 350 beds in use. In the emergency room, patients lie on gurneys for as long as three days waiting for a bed. King's obstetricians discharge women early to make room for others who have just delivered; in intensive care, doctors shuffle patients to make room for newcomers. Although AIDS has disproportionately affected blacks, the hospital's AIDS clinic operates just two nights a week, staffed by a doctor and nurses volunteering their time. Because of overcrowding at King, the doctor must admit his patients to other hospitals. In King's clinics, most patients routinely wait four to six weeks for an appointment; some wait two or three months.

In the emergency room the burden is most dramatic. King treats 4,000 to 5,000 trauma patients a year, two-thirds of them victims of "intentional" injuries: gunshots, stabbings, and beatings. The U.S. Army sends its surgeons to King for experience in treating gunshot wounds; King sends its resident surgeons to nearby hospitals, where they can practice routine procedures like removing gallbladders.

"It's like a M.A.S.H. unit," says Dr. Arthur Fleming, King's chief of surgery and director of its trauma center, who was a surgeon at Walter Reed Hospital in Washington, DC, during the Vietnam War. "The casualties come in, and you've got to triage—decide who's going first, who's going second. Instead of one or two coming at intervals, there are sometimes three and four and five."

If they are not wounded, many patients reach King gravely ill. "I have to remind young doctors," says Fleming, "that when they see somebody, that person wouldn't come here unless he was really sick. We see more perforated appendixes here than probably anywhere in the world, because they didn't come in at four to six hours, when they had symptoms. They came in at four to six days, after they were dying."

King is just one piece of a public health care system that often resembles gridlock on Los Angeles' freeways. At some county hospitals, emergency-room waits of six to eight hours are routine, while other patients have waited up to three days in the E.R. At other county hospitals, women labor and even give birth in hallways. At the county's main AIDS clinic, new patients wait four months for an appointment. Elsewhere, they can wait six to eight weeks for CAT scans, an average of three months for a mammogram and two for a chest X-ray. Like King, the county's largest hospital was recently threatened with a loss of accreditation.

Like counties throughout California, Los Angeles pays the price for a state health care system in disarray. As many as 6 million Californians have no health insurance of any kind, and the state's Medicaid system (called Medi-Cal) is in crisis, with too few doctors, dentists, and hospitals willing to accept its low payments and clumsy bureaucracy. California now ranks 47th among the states in per capita Medicaid spending. "This Medi-Cal system is supposed to be freedom of choice," says Melinda Bird, a public-interest attorney in Los Angeles. "The reality is, they go to county hospitals because they are the only places they can see a doctor."

"We're at a crisis stage," says David Langness of the Hospital Council of Southern California, a trade group. "Everybody admits it. We know that unless we fix the problem the current system will collapse. We know we're not meeting the needs of Californians."

As in Mississippi, the state has tentatively begun to address the issue of black infant mortality. California recently adopted a policy to provide extensive prenatal care, including health education and nutritional guidance, to women in Medi-Cal—if they can find an obstetrician who provides these services. Though operating on a limited scale, several innovative programs were designed to take a similar approach, identifying high-risk pregnant women and providing com-prehensive care. But as of this writing, these programs are all in danger of being eliminated through budget cuts.

On the surface, Watts is an unlikely ghetto. Blocks of stucco houses, small but well-kept and occupied by working- and middle-class families, touch blocks of desperate poverty. And there are housing projects, Los Angeles-style: plain stucco buildings that resemble army barracks. Watts's most famous landmarks are the towers on 107th St., built of shells, glass, and rock by Simon Rodia, an Italian immigrant.

On one of the ghetto's busiest corners stands the Watts Health Center, a beacon of hope. Like King, it rose from the ashes, one of the first community health centers in the United States. It is an attractive stone building that sur-rounds a courtyard, with a garden at its center. It is clean and comfortable. "We have taken extreme steps not to look like, feel like, smell like a public clinic," says Dr. Clyde Oden, the president of the Watts Health Foundation. One of the largest health centers in the country, it offers a full range of medical care, including dentistry, pediatrics, optometry, physical therapy, and acupuncture. It has both X-ray facilities and a pharmacy. Under the rubric of the foundation, it offers a vast array of social and medical services, many of them creative and occasionally controversial responses to the needs of Watts: a drug treatment and education center that includes a program for addicted mothers; drug- and alco-hol-prevention services for children; in-school clinics that provide extensive medical care and counseling; a health maintenance organization; and mobile clinics that immunize children and provide primary care to the homeless.

It's not enough. "It's like bailing out a boat with a small bucket," Oden says, "and the water's coming in faster and faster. We're doing an excellent job of bailing out, but we can't make up for all that society has abdicated because of its lack of commitment, leadership, and resources."

People who work in Watts say that even a doctor on every street corner would not solve the community's health problems. After years of neglect, there is often a deep distrust of the medical profession, even when those providing the care are black.

One of the center's newest programs sends its mobile clinics to perform pregnancy tests near housing projects. If a woman tests positive, she is referred to the clinic for early prenatal care. At first, few women showed up and clinic employees canvassed the neighborhood to distribute information and talk to people. One afternoon they met a woman who was about seven months pregnant. She had not seen a doctor and had no plans to do so. She was saving money to give birth in a hospital. Because of a previous experience with Medi-Cal, she refused to believe that the clinic could help her get free or inexpensive care.

"There's a lack of trust of medical care," says Makungu Akinyela, a mental health specialist who spoke to her. "We thought just being here would be enough, that people would come out to greet us with open arms. There's something we are not doing.''

Others point to a dearth of hope—a lack of incentive to remain healthy. ''What black people do with health care has much to do with how they see themselves in America,'' says Donzella Lee, the center's director of women, adolescent and children's programs. ''Many of our kids don't see a future for themselves. If they still live in the projects, if they still see the same level of violence, if they're still unemployed, if they're still poor, why should they change?''

''The best prescription we could write to improve health care in this community is a job,'' says Oden. ''Full employment would do things to the psychological well-being of the individual, as well as the physical well-being. If you can't look forward to anything, to talk about prevention has no meaning.''

Violence, like unemployment, has taken a physical and a spiritual toll. While visiting a school in Watts, Lee says, she once asked children to name the most important thing in their lives. The answer: ''Our lives.'' Lee returned to her office and cried. ''How do you have 12-year-olds saying the most important thing is whether they live or die?'' she asks. ''They respond like they're at war.''

Those who provide health care in Watts express more than a little bitterness: They believe they've been abandoned by the people of America's wealthiest state. ''Our society has given up on our young people,'' says Oden. ''If we were committed to bailing out our inner cities the same way we're trying to protect persons who have $100,000-plus investments in S&L's, we wouldn't have a story here at all. As a society, we have turned deaf, dumb, and blind.''

While violence makes headlines, mundane and controllable diseases, such as hypertension, quietly take as great a toll. By one estimate, one-third of those hospitalized with severe high blood pressure—the people counted in the six-fold higher admission rate for uncontrolled hypertension at King—will need dialysis within one year. Blacks are 10 to 18 times likelier to suffer kidney failure related to hypertension. In Los Angeles, an average of one black person a day begins dialysis.

Such facts frustrate Dr. Clarence Grim, a professor at the Drew University School of Medicine, who has spent much of his professional life studying hypertension. ''Most patients with high blood pressure could be controlled for 10 cents to 25 cents a day, many of them for a penny a day,'' he says. ''It's almost incomprehensible that this country does not have some systems for giving free medicine to people.''

The commissioners investigating the Watts Riot—the Rebellion—25 years ago felt a similar frustration. They recommended the construction of a new hospital. King was built, then all but abandoned, left to redeem the sins of a health care system gone awry. ''Of what shall it avail our nation,'' those commissioners wrote, ''if we can place a man on the moon but cannot cure sickness in our cities?''

LEAD, RACE, AND PUBLIC HEALTH

Barbara Berney

I have been thinking about lead a lot lately. The federal Centers for Disease Control has just lowered the "level of concern"—that is, the amount of lead in children's blood that is considered hazardous—to 10 micrograms per deciliter. In the last 20 years, this threshold of concern has fallen 600 percent, from 60 micrograms per deciliter before 1970 to 40 in 1970, 30 in 1978, 25 in 1985, and now to 10.

Research published in the last five years overwhelmingly supports earlier evidence that at blood levels of 10 or 15 micrograms per deciliter (and perhaps less), lead causes decreases in IQ and interferes with attention and auditory processing. It creates learning problems and may interfere with judgment and self-control. It poisons every cell in the body and especially affects the central nervous system.

Lead poisoning makes me think about race—or, more properly, racism. Personally, I wish racism would just go away. Don't get me wrong—I don't think ending racism would be a panacea. Poverty, hypertension, heart disease, drug addiction, hatred, and even lead paint poisoning would not disappear even if racism went away. But their victims would be less predictable. And perhaps public health would develop more successful preventive interventions for these problems.

Racism and lead are intimately tied to each other. It's not that anyone put lead in paint to poison black children—or to poison anyone, for that matter. But action, inaction, and research on lead is all tied up with race. The fact that lead paint, especially deteriorated lead paint, is most often found in slum housing in black and brown communities has slowed attempts to alleviate and abate this problem.

Proving that low-level exposure to lead causes cognitive and neurobiological problems was hampered for years by the fact that lead's primary victims were and still are poor black children living in dilapidated housing. That *these* children were cognitively impaired or had trouble in school could not easily be attributed to their exposure to lead. Racism and class prejudice—and many studies—suggested that *these* children could be expected to be less than bright. Researchers hypothesized that children who were cognitively impaired ate lead-containing paint chips because they were stupid, rather than the other way around. Maybe they mouthed lead dust from their hands and toys because their mothers were bad housekeepers or bad mothers or had so many children they didn't know what to do. How could learning and behavior problems of children living in such environments be attributed to their exposure to lead rather than their "social background," critics of the lead research asked.

In order to eliminate "confounding" by race and poverty, Herbert Needleman studied lead exposure and neurobehavioral effects in thousands of white working-class school children in Somerville and Chelsea, Massachusetts. His first results were published in 1979. Then he and David Bellinger studied a cohort of upper- and upper-middle-class infants born at Boston's Brigham and Women's Hospital in the early 1980s. These studies showed the same cognitive and behavioral effects found in other studies in which the backgrounds of children were less well controlled. Once effects had been demonstrated in the white and the well-off, they were accepted as real.

Toxic Use Reduction

In the 1950s and 1960s, lead poisoning was considered a problem of poor black children living in slums who ate paint chips. The Lead Paint Poisoning Prevention Act passed by Congress in 1970 funded screening programs, which found that hundreds of thousands of children had elevated blood lead levels. In 1977, the Consumer Product Safety Commission banned the sale of lead paint. Thus began a national program to eliminate lead in the environment before it was dispersed (known as toxic use reduction).

Through the 1970s and 1980s, researchers demonstrated that lower and lower levels of exposure were harmful. At the same time, screening and national health surveys showed that exposure was much broader than previously believed. Millions of children in the general population (including large numbers of white, middle-class children) were at risk from lead exposure. The significant sources were not just peeling lead paint, but included gasoline, intact lead paint, food, and drinking water. The toxic use reduction strategy was expanded. Having begun the reduction of lead in gasoline in the mid-1970s, the Environmental Protection Agency cut the lead content of gasoline by 90 percent between 1982 and 1986. The Food and Drug Administration negotiated with food manufacturers to limit lead in food, especially for infants. That's why baby food comes in jars, not cans—there's no lead solder.

Lead is a case that demonstrates the effectiveness of toxic use reduction as a strategy. The average blood levels of American children dropped by more than 30 percent from 1976 to 1980 as a direct result of reductions of lead in gasoline. In 1980 the mean blood level of white children under 6 years old was approximately 13 micrograms per deciliter. For black children it was about 20 micrograms per deciliter. Further regulation and other actions taken over the last 10 years have reduced lead in gasoline, food, and water. Preliminary reports from the 1990 National Health and Nutrition Examination Survey show that average levels have now dropped to about 6 micrograms per deciliter. The ratio between black and white has not changed. It is estimated that some 90 percent of poor black children have blood levels exceeding 10 micrograms per deciliter, above which neurological damage occurs. In every income and geographical category, twice as many black as white children have lead levels over 15 micrograms per deciliter. The Environmental Defense Fund estimates that 3 to 4 million children under age 6 have blood lead levels above 15 micrograms per deciliter. This is thousands of times the number of children who get all the infectious childhood diseases combined.

Eliminating toxic chemicals before they are dispersed is relatively cheap and easy, as well as effective. Eliminating a toxin that is everywhere—in the soil and in the walls—is technically difficult, fabulously expensive, and a logistical and administrative nightmare. Thus, the case of lead also demonstrates the limits of toxic use reduction.

After 20 years of research, struggle, and toxic use reduction, the major source of children's exposure to lead is again leaded paint in old housing stock. The federal Department of Housing and Urban Development has just estimated that 57 million American homes have lead paint. Children under age 7 live in 10 million of them. They are overwhelmingly poor children of color. We have succeeded in removing lead from the environment of most white children.

In December 1990, the federal government announced its intention to eliminate lead paint from the nation's housing stock over the next 10 years. The cost is about $2 billion a year, $20 billion over 10 years. Over the same period, we will spend $400 billion on the savings and loan fiasco. The feds are not saying where the money for eliminating lead paint will come from. Responsibility for lead abatement will be dumped in the lap of already strapped state and local health departments. Private landlords and home owners will be expected to delead their property. Real estate values are plummeting; foreclosures and evictions are up. Without a budget and funding mechanism, the federal government's promised "strategic plan to eliminate childhood lead poisoning" will be a pipe dream, not a reality.

Racial Comparison of Health Data

Health Parameters	Black/White Comparison	Comments/Significance
Low birth weight infants (less then 2,500 grams)	Black rate 110 percent higher than white rate.	Racial discrepancy widening; low birth weight associated with large numbers of deaths, physical and mental handicaps; blacks currently experiencing rates seen in 1950s by whites.
Very low birth weight infants (less than 1,500 grams)	Black rate 2.5 times the white rate.	Physical and mental handicaps often impair survivors; racial discrepancy may be widening.
Neonatal mortality (death in first 28 days of life)	Black rate 97 percent higher than white rate.	Reflects pre-pregnancy health and prenatal, intrapartum, and neonatal care; gap may be increasing.
Post-neonatal mortality (death from day 29 to day 364)	Black rate over twice the white rate.	Reflects quality of health care for children, including prevention of controlled, treatable diseases; rate is worsening for urban blacks.
Infant mortality (death in first year of life per 1,000 live births)	Black rate twice the white rate (21.4 per 1,000).	A major indicator of health status and a measure of overall standard of living; black rate worse than that in Jamaica or Cuba.
Maternal deaths	Black rate 3.3 times the white rate; amounts to 43 percent of U.S. total.	Reflects lack of access to obstetrical care; current figures are probably an undercount; 75 percent of these deaths are preventable.
Immunization rates (black children)	48.4 percent immunized against diphtheria, pertussis, tetanus; 39.1 percent immunized against polio.	Black children still die, lose vision and hearing, and suffer brain damage from these easily preventable diseases.
Childhood tuberculosis	Black rate 4 to 5 times the rate for whites.	Funds for children's health programs being reduced despite high rates in black community.

Racial Comparison of Health Data (cont.)

Health Parameters	Black/White Comparison	Comments/Significance
Dental care	40 percent of black children under 17 years of age have never seen a dentist.	Overall, two-thirds of black children have not seen dentist in past year.
Childhood anemia	20 to 33 percent of black children are anemic.	Easily diagnosed and treated with basic child care; reflects poor nutrition; adversely affects school performance.
Toxic level leads	15 to 20 percent of black urban children may have high blood lead levels.	First loss is intellectual function; many children are either undiagnosed and untreated or mislabeled as retarded or "slow learners."
Childhood deaths (per 100,000 children)	Much higher among blacks. Age Blacks Whites 1–4 97.6 57.9 5–9 41.7 28.5 10–14 36.6 29.8	Many deaths are preventable with immunizations and early diagnosis and treatment; more of these children are being locked out of the health delivery system.
Tuberculosis among persons under 45	Black males: 17.4 times white death rate; black females: 15.6 times white death rate.	Reflects lack of access to minimal health care.
Hypertension among persons under 45	Black males: 10.2 times white death rate; black females: 13.4.	Reflects lack of access to minimal health care.
Anemia among persons under 45	Black males: 6 times white death rate; black females: 5.2.	Reflects lack of access to minimal health care.
Cancer incidence among persons under 45	Blacks: 27 percent increase; whites: 12 percent increase.	Reflects increased exposure to toxic environmental substance, poor diet, and high-risk lifestyle; gap is widening.

Category		
Cancer deaths among persons under 45	Blacks: 40 percent increase; whites: 10 percent increase.	Rates were even in 1950 when there was little treatment; black access to early diagnosis and treatment being curtailed annually.
Death rate for persons under 45	Black rate twice the white rate.	Huge numbers of person-years lost; responsible for a large portion of poverty and matriarchal families.
Diabetes	33 percent more prevalent in blacks.	Programs providing care for chronic disease are regularly cut.
	Black death rate over twice that of whites.	Largely preventable with good outpatient medical care; funding for such care is being cut.
Heart disease	Twice as common in blacks.	Programs providing care for chronic disease are being cut.
	Black death rate 1.25 times higher than white rate.	Largely preventable with good outpatient medical care; funding for such care is being cut.
Stroke	Black death rate 80 percent higher than white rate.	Largely preventable with good outpatient medical care; funding for such care is being cut.
Deaths from pneumonia and influenza	Black rate 1.5 times higher than white rate.	Preventable with access to good medical care, treatment, and timely hospitalization; access for blacks and the poor is being curtailed.
Deaths from nephritis, nephrosis, and nephrotic syndrome	Black rate 3 times the white rate.	Largely preventable with good outpatient medical care and timely hospitalization; access for blacks and the poor is being curtailed.
Excess deaths (numbers of deaths beyond those expected with equal mortality rates across racial lines)	Blacks suffer 59,000 annually; 42 percent of black deaths are "excess."	If death rates for races were equal, 4 of 10 black deaths would not occur.

Racial Comparison of Health Data (cont.)

Health Parameters	Black/White Comparison	Comments/Significance
Leading causes of death	Blacks lead in 13 of 15 categories.	Many of these deaths are preventable with known, basic cost-effective medical treatments.
Longevity	Blacks live 5 to 7 fewer years than whites.	The "gold standard" of health system performance; recent gains for blacks have slowed if not stopped.
	Black life expectancy 69.6 years.	Black life expectancy has decreased since 1984.

Reprinted with permission from W. Michael Byrd, "Race, Biology, and Health Care: Reassessing a Relationship," Journal of Health Care for the Poor and Underserved, Winter 1990:1(3), pp. 228–96.

Sources:

Cancer Facts and Figures for Minority Americans: 1986: New York: American Cancer Society, 1986; Black and White Children in America: Key Facts, Washington, DC: Children's Defense Fund, 1985; Haynes, M. A.; "The Gap in Health Status Between Black and White Americans," in Williams, R. A., ed., Textbook of Black-Related Disease, New York: McGraw-Hill, 1975; Kaunitz, A. M., "Honing in on Maternal Deaths," Contemporary Obstetrics and Gynecology, 1984:24, pp. 31–34; U.S. Bureau of the Census, Statistical Abstract of the United States, 1988, Washington, DC:U.S. Department of Commerce, 1987; and U.S. Department of Health and Human Services, Health Status of Minorities and Low-income Groups, Washington, DC:U.S. Government Printing Office, 1985.

"SIGNIFICANT GAPS IN HISPANIC ACCESS TO HEALTH CARE" GAO REPORT, 1990

Statement of Eleanor Chelimsky,
Assistant Comptroller General,
Before the House Select Committee on Aging
and the Congressional Hispanic Caucus,
September 19, 1991

In 1989, over 33 million Americans (14 percent of the population) were not covered by any type of health insurance (public or private) at any time during the year. Although lack of health insurance is a problem that cuts across every demographic category, it is especially prevalent among Hispanics. For instance, according to the Current Population Survey, 33 percent of Hispanics (over 6 million persons) were uninsured during all or part of 1989, compared with about 19 percent of blacks and about 12 percent of whites. (See Table 1.) The percentage of Hispanics not insured varies substantially across states. In addition, data from the Current Population Survey indicate that about 2.1 million undocumented aliens were living in the United States as of November 1989, with 1.6 million of these persons having been born in Mexico. We do not know the extent to which this population is included in the Current Population Survey's estimate that we are using. However, it seems reasonable to assume that these undocumented aliens are undercounted and less likely than other Hispanics to have insurance coverage.

Medicaid

In explaining the lack of access to Medicaid among Hispanics, both the literature and the experts we interviewed point to the stringent eligibility criteria in a number of states with high concentrations of Hispanics. Since eligibility criteria for Medicaid are determined, within federal guidelines, by each state, the criteria vary dramatically across states. Two of the most restrictive states are Texas and Florida, in which about three of every ten Hispanics in the United States reside.

There are two broad classes of eligibility under Medicaid: categorically needy and medically needy. Categorically needy persons are generally those who qualify for assistance under the Aid for Families With Dependent Children (AFDC) or the Supplemental Security Income programs. They are automatically eligible for Medicaid. At the option of each state, Medicaid eligibility may be

Table 1
Estimates of Types of Health Insurance Coverage by Race/Ethnicity, 1989

Type of Insurance	Percent of population covered[a]		
	White	Black	Hispanic[b]
Private	78	54	50
Medicare	14	10	6
Medicaid	6	23	15
Other public insurance	4	4	3
Uninsured	13	19	33

[a] Figures do not total 100 because persons may have more than one type of insurance coverage.

[b] Hispanic persons may be of any race.

Source:
U.S. Bureau of the Census, Current Population Survey, 1990.

extended to medically needy persons, including certain groups (for example, the aged, the blind, families with dependent children, and so on) whose income or resources are in excess of the qualification standards for the categorically needy.

Table 2 illustrates the eligibility criteria for enrolling in Medicaid through AFDC and the medically needy program in those states in which most Hispanics reside. For instance, in California, a family of three must earn less than 79.1 percent of the federal poverty-line income to qualify for Medicaid through AFDC. In contrast, a family of three in Texas must earn less than 21.9 percent of the federal poverty-line income to qualify through the same program. Thus, in 1989, a family of three that earned $6,500 (61 percent of the poverty-line income of $10,600) would have qualified for Medicaid through AFDC in California but not in Texas.

Under medically needy programs, Medicaid eligibility may be extended to persons whose incomes are in excess of the income limit applicable under the categorically needy program. However, these persons must either "spend down" or accumulate enough medical expenses to deduct from their income to meet eligibility criteria. The income criteria vary across those states where many Hispanics reside, with California having the least stringent criteria and Arizona and New Mexico not having a medically needy program at all.

The differences in eligibility criteria across states largely explain the discrepancy in Medicaid coverage across the Hispanic subgroups. For instance, as I noted previously, Mexican-Americans and Puerto Ricans both have high rates of poverty and low median incomes. However, Puerto Ricans (concentrated in New York and New Jersey) are much more likely than Mexican-Americans (with a substantial population in Texas) to meet the Medicaid eligibility criteria.

Table 2
Medicaid Eligibility Criteria for
a Family of Three in Selected States, 1989

State	AFDC eligibility		Medically needy eligibility	
	As a percent of poverty	Rank[a]	As a percent of poverty	Rank[b]
Arizona	35.0	38	c	c
California	79.1	1	106.4	1
Florida	34.2	41	45.7	26
Illinois	40.8	33	54.6	20
New Jersey	50.6	17	67.5	12
New York	64.3	7	84.6	6
New Mexico	31.5	44	c	c
Texas	21.9	49	31.8	33

[a]Rank is based on the eligibility criteria of the 50 states. Higher rank indicates less stringent criteria.

[b]Out of a total of 35 states that have a program for the medically needy.

[c]Arizona and New Mexico have no medically needy program.

Source:

National Coalition of Hispanic Health and Human Services Organizations (COSSMHO), . . . And Access for All: Medicaid and Hispanics (Washington, DC: 1990).

As a result, a higher proportion of Puerto Ricans than Mexican-Americans are eligible for Medicaid.

I should point out that, although the greatest proportion of Mexican-Americans (41.6 percent) reside in California, and although California has the least stringent eligibility criteria in the nation, nevertheless, with over 30 percent of the Mexican-American population residing in Texas, the Texas Medicaid policies play a major role in restricting health care coverage for that group.

It is also the case that making the eligibility criteria less restrictive in order to include all persons below the poverty line would still leave many working people—who earn more than the poverty-line income, but not enough to afford health insurance—without coverage. The situation in California is a perfect example of this hole in the health insurance safety net. Despite California's less restrictive criteria, 23 percent (6 million persons) of the nonelderly population of California were uninsured in 1989. Only Texas, the District of Columbia, New Mexico, and Oklahoma had higher rates of noninsurance. Being employed in low-wage jobs that do not provide health insurance has been identified as one of the factors that contribute to California's noninsurance rate. Thus, raising the Medicaid thresholds closer to the poverty line would still leave many work-ing persons uninsured.

In sum, Hispanics in general, and Mexican-Americans in particular, have difficulty gaining access to Medicaid because of the stringency in state Medicaid policies. While they suffer from similar economic disadvantages, Puerto Ricans are better able to gain access to this public health insurance program by virtue of their place of residence, thus ensuring some measure of health insurance coverage for this population. However, even states with less restrictive Medicaid policies, such as California, have difficulties providing health insurance coverage to the large proportion of people who do not meet the criteria and still cannot afford health insurance.

Nonfinancial Barriers to Medicaid Access

We discussed the issues involved in gaining access to Medicaid with Med-icaid officials in Texas, New York, and Florida. In addition to the low income-eligibility criteria in Texas and Florida noted earlier, the officials cited the complexity of the Medicaid system as a principal barrier to Medicaid access. There are numerous avenues to Medicaid enrollment that may involve such factors as family income, financial assets, family composition, age of children, and medical need. For instance, in Texas, there are nearly 10 different programs for Medicaid enrollment, each with its own criteria for eligibility (for example, pregnant women with incomes up to 133 percent of the poverty line; children born before January 2, 1982, who are eligible for AFDC; children born before October 1, 1983, with incomes between the AFDC and medically needy criteria; and so on). Officials in Texas told us that the Medicaid caseworkers engage in 4 weeks of training just to learn the eligibility criteria and how to communicate them to potential recipients.

Medicaid officials stated that they find it difficult to "market" Medicaid because of its complexity. For instance, officials in Texas said that it is difficult to enroll people in the medically needy program because people do not want to accumulate medical bills before being reimbursed. They also noted that it is difficult to effectively communicate to people that they may not be eligible for Medicaid at the present time, but that they may be eligible in the future (for example, if a woman becomes pregnant). New York state officials noted that the process of enrolling people is complicated and burdensome, and that stand-ing in line for a full day at the Medicaid office does not compete favorably with the practical alternative of receiving free care in an emergency room or a com-munity health center.

WOMEN—THE MISSING PERSONS IN THE AIDS EPIDEMIC

Kathryn Anastos and Carola Marte

Our current understanding of the public health problem posed by the acquired immunodeficiency syndrome (AIDS) in women is seriously distorted by the underrepresentation of women in official data and the misrepresentation of their disease. Through November 1989, 10,369 women in the United States were reported to have the acquired immunodeficiency syndrome—9 percent of the total number of AIDS cases.[1] In urban areas on the East and West coasts, the numbers are higher; for example, 13 percent of all people who have been diagnosed with AIDS in New York City are women. The percentage is higher still in the most recently diagnosed cases—18 percent of New York City cases since January 1988 are in women.[2]

It is unlikely, however, that these numbers accurately reflect the number of women who in fact have serious manifestations of HIV (human immunodeficiency virus) infection, for several reasons. The diagnosis of AIDS depends not only upon demonstrated infection with HIV, but also upon the clinical manifestations of the disease—that is, the ways in which those infected become sick. Because those affected first were almost exclusively men, the case definition of AIDS is centered in how the disease has manifested in men, and gynecologic conditions are not included as manifestations of HIV infection. If women's disease manifests with the same infections as it does in men, it may be recognized and reported as AIDS; if the infections, still HIV related, are different, the women are not considered to have AIDS.

For example, HIV-infected women with severe infections of their fallopian tubes (pelvic inflammatory disease or PID) are not categorized as having AIDS. This is in spite of the fact that many doctors have found that these infections are worse in HIV-infected women: treatment is more difficult and less likely to be successful.[3] This resistance to cure by ordinary therapy is the sign of a failing immune system.

Similarly, vaginal yeast infections in HIV-infected women are more severe and less likely to be cured by ordinary therapy.[4] A woman may suffer from vaginal yeast infections even before she has thrush, a yeast infection of the mouth that affects both women and men and that is officially used as one of the criteria for a pre-AIDS condition (AIDS-related complex or ARC). Does it make sense that the same infection in another orifice—an orifice not present in men—is not categorized as an AIDS-related condition?

Moreover, and most seriously, a number of published reports indicate dramatically higher rates of abnormal Pap smears and cervical cancer in HIV-infected women compared to uninfected women.[5] Cervical cancer in immune-suppressed women is known to be more severe and life-threatening than in women with healthy immune systems. It may advance with dangerous rapidity and often requires special treatment.[6] Given the many years between the time a person becomes infected with HIV and the time he or she becomes ill with full-blown AIDS—now thought to average nine years—many HIV-infected women may die from cervical cancer, a potentially treatable disease, before they die from AIDS as officially defined. Clearly, the case definitions of AIDS and ARC should be revised to include those women whose severe infections and malignancies are obvious manifestations of immune system failure induced by HIV infection.

Another major problem is that similar symptoms in both women and men are interpreted, investigated, and treated differently, because women are not expected to have AIDS. Underdiagnosis is thus a significant bias in epidemiologic data on women with AIDS. For example, one study showed that women with pneumocystis carinii pneumonia (PCP), the most common opportunistic infection in AIDS patients and a major cause of AIDS deaths, were more likely to be treated for minor respiratory ailments and not for PCP.[7] The result was life-threatening respiratory failure and a higher death rate than in men who had the same symptoms and whose PCP was recognized and treated. The potential magnitude of this problem may be seen in recent statistics showing unexplained and dramatic increases in deaths of women from a variety of respiratory and infectious diseases. For example, in New York City and Washington, D.C., there were, respectively, a 154 percent and a 225 percent increase in deaths in young women (aged 15 to 45 years) from 1981 to 1986. Idaho, in contrast, has experienced no such increase in mortality rates in women.[8] Chris Norwood of the National Women's Health Network, who compiled these statistics, has suggested that because these increased numbers of deaths in women are found in geographic areas with heavy concentrations of AIDS cases, they may in fact be uncounted HIV-related deaths.

A better understanding of the true scope of the AIDS epidemic in women requires us to reconsider all these factors. The case definition of AIDS must be changed to include gynecologic conditions. Some estimate must be made of the proportion of the observed increase in respiratory and infection-related deaths that is caused by HIV-induced immunosuppression. In addition, health care providers need to develop an increased clinical awareness of AIDS in women in order to achieve more accurate diagnoses of full-blown AIDS, even by the current case definition.

The problem of the "missing women" in the AIDS epidemic goes well beyond the epidemiology. Women have been forgotten in every aspect of AIDS medicine. Fundamental questions about the progression of this disease in women have not been asked or answered. Is cervical cancer more common in HIV-infected women? How does HIV infection affect pregnancy and childbirth? Do the different hormones in women and men affect the course of HIV infection? Do women fall prey to different opportunistic infections than men do? Do women respond differently to treatment regimens established for male patients?

Do women suffer different side effects and toxicities from AIDS medications? Do women survive a shorter time after the diagnosis of AIDS has been made? Are the causes of death in women different than in men? In particular, gynecologic disease has until recently been entirely ignored in discussions of HIV-related conditions, and current guidelines for medical management do not include recommendations for gynecologic care.[9] We have little information to indicate how often Pap smears should be done, and common symptomatic conditions such as vaginal yeast infections are not routinely discussed with patients or treated prophylactically, as are comparable oral or anal conditions.

The neglect of women with HIV disease extends to other important areas. Very few women have been included in drug trials. The original studies of AZT in 282 patients included only 13 women,[10] and many drug trials have specifically excluded women. The potential importance of gender differences in response to HIV infection is rarely addressed in current medical publications, and this lack allows only the most rudimentary understanding of AIDS in women. Physicians find little information available to help them understand HIV-related gynecologic conditions in women.

Women at Risk

In the United States, AIDS declared itself first in gay men and subsequently among intravenous drug users, who are predominantly men. This history has led to our false perception of AIDS as a disease of men. This fallacy is quickly dispelled by the observation that in large areas of the world, for example, African and Caribbean nations where the dominant mode of transmission is heterosexual contact, women and men are infected with equal frequency.[11] In addition, the increasing importance of heterosexual transmission in the United States has already produced a faster rate of increase in the numbers of women who have become sick through heterosexual transmission compared to any other group.[12] For gay men in particular, massive educational efforts have been effective in decreasing the rate of new infections.

One factor in this epidemiologic shift is the crack epidemic and its associated hypersexuality and exchange of sex for drugs. Young women and adolescent girls have multiple sexual partners in a day in exchange for a dollar or a hit, and their "clients" are frequently older men with a history of intravenous drug use. As Willard Cates of the Centers for Disease Control observed, the crack houses are for heterosexual transmission to women what the bath houses were for transmission among gay men.[13]

Of the 3,668 cases of AIDS reported in American women in the single year ending November 30, 1989, 51 percent are attributed to transmission by intravenous drug use; 32 percent are attributed to heterosexual transmission; 9 percent to transfusion; and 9 percent to "undetermined means of acquiring infection" (compared to 2 percent in this category for men).[14] The higher rate of "undetermined" risk in women is assumed to reflect heterosexual transmission in which the woman is not aware of her partner's risk-taking behaviors. The category of women at double risk—those who are both intravenous drug users and partners of infected men or men at risk—is not calculated separately for women as it routinely is for men, even though these women are at substantially increased risk for infection. This matters because it subjects them to the victim-blaming attitude held by many: Their source of infection is seen to justify their second-class treatment and care.

It is not clear how many of the estimated 1 million HIV-infected individuals in the United States are women. Among women who are HIV-infected, many are unaware that they are at risk. In a CDC study of HIV-infected blood donors, 44 percent of 34 infected women studied could not identify a risk factor associated with their source of infection, and an equal number were known to have become infected through heterosexual contact.[15] Other studies also indicate an increasing number of infected women who do not know how they acquired the infection. For example, 15 of 26 HIV-positive mothers in a South Bronx hospital and 5 of 12 mothers in a Brooklyn hospital had no history of intravenous drug use or other identifiable risk behavior.[16]

In fact, for many women, their address alone places them at risk. Although area of residence is not officially viewed as a risk factor, data on seroprevalence make clear that, in fact, it constitutes a risk because it is so strongly associated with acknowledged risk factors. Epidemiologic data collected by the Centers for Disease Control (CDC) documents that seroprevalence rates in inner-city hospitals are high even when people with known risks are not counted. Recent CDC data show that as many as 8 percent of women and 18 percent of men visiting emergency rooms in some inner-city hospitals are HIV-infected.[17] Similarly, available information about women giving birth suggests that in some inner-city areas as many as 4 to 9 percent of deliveries are to women who are HIV-infected.[18] Breakdown of New York City data by zip code area also reveals that the most socially and economically devastated inner-city areas are those with the most HIV disease, whereas contiguous affluent areas may have much less HIV disease. For example, in 1988 the Upper East Side of Manhattan below 96th Street reported an AIDS case mortality rate of 27 per 100,000 people, compared to 48 per 100,000 for East Harlem on the east side of Manhattan above 96th Street.[19]

A woman who lives in an inner-city area and follows a conventional lifestyle of marriage and raising a family, who does not use drugs and is monogamous, nonetheless runs a high risk of becoming infected because her partner has a high probability of being infected, usually because of drug use. In many cases, these women are not aware that their partner is at risk. This means again that poor black and Latina women are at unduly high risk for infection, whatever their lifestyle, because poverty and lack of resources and opportunity keep them in areas of high HIV seroprevalence.

Women as "Vectors"

Deeply ingrained societal sexism as well as racism and classism have skewed the public perception of AIDS and HIV infection in women in the United States. Since the first case of a woman with AIDS was reported in the United States in 1981 in the Bronx, women have remained a forgotten group in the AIDS epidemic. They are regarded by the public and studied by the medical profession as vectors of transmission to their children and male sexual partners rather than as people with AIDS who are themselves frequently victims of transmission from the men in their lives. Until recently, one could gain epidemiologic information concerning women and AIDS mainly from perinatal studies and, to a lesser extent, from studies of prostitutes. Women have been defined primarily in terms of childbearing activities, despite the facts that pregnancy lasts a relatively short period of time and most of the serious AIDS-related illnesses in women occur outside of pregnancy.

Both in clinical practice and public discussion, pregnant women with HIV infection are perceived as incubators of sick babies who are destined to become a burden to society, not as individuals with a life-threatening illness, nor as mothers in struggle and in pain. Mothering, which for most women is an intense and perhaps the strongest emotional bond of their lives, is seen as an irresponsible and selfish act if the woman is HIV-infected and especially if she is also poor and of color. Many doctors and other health care providers feel that it is not only their right but their responsibility to counsel and persuade an HIV-infected woman to abort her pregnancy, even in the face of clear statements by the woman that she does not want to choose an abortion.

Such providers are poorly educated about, or choose to ignore, the reasons that their HIV-infected patients may wish to carry a pregnancy to term. A woman's choice is made in the context of cultural attitudes in which bearing children may be seen as the most valuable contribution a woman can make to her family and community. Families often exert pressure to plan pregnancies or to continue pregnancies already conceived. For many women, children may be the only means of attaining a sense of identity and status. In addition, poor women may perceive as favorable the risk described to them of transmitting HIV infection to their offspring. A 20 to 40 percent chance of bearing an infected child is a 60 to 80 percent chance of bearing a healthy child. This is a risk they may be willing to take; these odds seem better than those they routinely face in other aspects of their lives.

Several studies have suggested that HIV-infected women make decisions about pregnancy for the same reasons that uninfected women do. For instance, a study of decisions about pregnancy and abortion made by women on methadone maintenance found that a woman's HIV status was not the best predictor of her decision to terminate a pregnancy.[20] These choices were more readily predicted by factors directly related to the pregnancy, such as the woman's feelings about it and whether it was planned. HIV-infected women in this study who chose to continue their pregnancies cited family pressure, religious beliefs, and the desire to have a child as important factors in making their decision—in other words, the same factors considered by women who are not infected.

Male Prerogative, Female Risk

Discussions of heterosexual HIV transmission in the United States are also frequently permeated with sexist assumptions. For example, there are a number of studies on HIV infection in prostitutes,[21] presumably because this affects heterosexual transmission to men. In contrast, there has been no discussion in the professional literature of how women's lack of empowerment affects heterosexual transmission to women. Prostitutes are frequently seen as the guilty parties in the infection of women whose husbands or steady partners are the clients and the major support of the sex industry. This shifts the responsibility away from the man who engages in risk-taking sexual encounters. How many men inform their steady partners that they are exposing them to the risk of HIV transmission? The underlying inequity between women and men, at the level of individual relationships as well as in the culture at large, contributes to much of the transmission of HIV infection, particularly to women who do not perceive that they are at risk. The prevailing ethic that it is a man's prerogative to have multiple sexual encounters without condemnation has been uncritically integrated into official attitudes and research.

Sexist and classist attitudes allow the sweeping condemnation of prostitutes as transmitters of HIV infection. Studies have clarified that intravenous drug use by prostitutes, and not the prostitution itself, places women at high risk of HIV infection.[22] The prevalence of HIV infection is low in prostitutes who don't use intravenous drugs. For example, the CDC compiled statistics from several previous studies demonstrating a seroprevalence of 3.5 to 45.3 percent in drug-using street prostitutes, whereas none of the call girls who did not use drugs were HIV-infected.[23]

Lack of empowerment is a problem for all women, and especially poorer women, in protecting themselves against HIV infection. Education is only the first step in successful prevention, and even when a woman does recognize the risk of contracting HIV infection from her sexual partner, she may not be able to protect herself adequately. A heterosexual woman is usually not an equal partner in the bedroom, and her requests that her partner use a condom may be met with refusal or even physical abuse. Many providers involved in counseling women about safe sex have had experience with patients who have been beaten because they asserted the need to use condoms. Both the woman and her health care provider must weigh the immediate risk of battering against the long-term risk of HIV infection and AIDS. Similarly, women in the sex industry often omit the use of condoms because of clients' threats or offers of higher payment to do so. It is reportedly a widespread practice among prostitutes to be more careful about condom use with their clients than with their steady partners, although the steady partners are often intravenous drug users and may represent a far greater risk to the prostitute than her clients.[24]

Sexism and the lack of empowerment it causes are having a serious impact on the AIDS epidemic. Women are unable to protect themselves adequately from infection because they are frequently unaware that they are at risk; and even when they are aware, they are unable to assert their need for protection. When women are infected with HIV, they frequently do not receive appropriate medical care because of underdiagnosis, a flawed case definition, and insufficient information about manifestations of HIV disease in women. Sexism feeds on itself with the false perception of women as vectors rather than victims of HIV transmission. When classism and racism join with sexism, as they do for inner-city women, the impact of AIDS is devastating.

NOTES

1. Centers for Disease Control, Division of HIV/AIDS, Atlanta, Georgia, personal communication, January 2, 1990.

2. New York City Department of Health, "AIDS Surveillance Update," November 10, 1989.

3. Hoegsberg, B., et al., "Human Immunodeficiency Virus in Women with Pelvic Inflammatory Disease," Fourth International Conference on AIDS, Stockholm, Sweden, 1988, abstract, p. 333; and personal communication.

4. Rhoads, J. L., et al., "Chronic Vaginal Candidiasis in Women with Human Immunodeficiency Virus Infection," *Journal of the American Medical Association*, 1987:257, pp. 3105–3107.

5. Provenchar, D., et al., "HIV Status and Positive Papanicolaou Screening: Identification of a High-Risk Population," *Gynecologic Oncology*, 1988:31, pp. 184–190; and Schrager, L. K., et al., "Cervical and Vaginal Squamous Cell Abnormalities in Women Infected with Human Immunodeficiency Virus," *Journal of Acquired Immunodeficiency Syndrome*, 1989:2, pp. 570–575.

6. Sillman, F. H., and A. Sedlis, "Anogenital Papillomavirus Infection and Neoplasia in Immunodeficient Women," *Obstetrics and Gynecology Clinics of North America*, 1987:14, pp. 537–558.

7. Verdegem, T. D., et al., "Increased Fatality from Pneumocystis Carinii Pneumonia in Women with AIDS," Fourth International Conference on AIDS, Stockholm, Sweden, 1988, abstract, p. 445.

8. Norwood, Chris, "Women and the 'Hidden' AIDS Epidemic," *Network News*, Newsletter of the National Women's Health Network, November–December 1988, pp. 1, 6.

9. See, for example, New York Statewide Professional Standards Review Council, "Criteria Manual for the Treatment of AIDS," Albany, NY: AIDS Intervention Management System, 1988.

10. Fischl, M. A., et al., "The Efficacy of Azidothymidine (AZT) in the Treatment of Patients with AIDS and AIDS-Related Complex: A Double-Blind Placebo-Controlled Trial," *New England Journal of Medicine*, 1987:317, pp. 185–191.

11. Haverkos, H. W., and R. Edelman, "The Epidemiology of Acquired Immunodeficiency Syndrome Among Heterosexuals," *Journal of the American Medical Association*, 1988:260, pp. 1922–1929; and Quinn, T. C., et al., "AIDS in Africa: An Epidemiologic Paradigm," *Science*, 1986:234, pp. 955–963.

12. Guinan, M. E., and A. Hardy, "Epidemiology of AIDS in Women in the United States: 1981–1986," *Journal of the American Medical Association*, 1987:257, pp. 2039–2042; and Centers for Disease Control, "Update: Heterosexual Transmission of Acquired Immunodeficiency Syndrome and Human Immunodeficiency Virus Infection—United States," *Morbidity and Mortality Weekly Report*, 1989:38, pp. 423–424.

13. Cates, W., quoted in M. F. Goldsmith, "Sex Tied to Drugs=STD Spread," *Journal of the American Medical Association*, 1988:260, p. 2009.

14. Centers for Disease Control, personal communication, January 2, 1990.

15. Ward, J. W., et al., "Epidemiologic Characteristics of Blood Donors with Antibody to Human Immunodeficiency Virus," *Transfusion*, 1988:28, pp. 298–301.

16. Checola, R. T., et al., "Maternal Drug Abuse and HIV Seropositivity," Fifth International Conference on AIDS, Montreal, Quebec, Canada, 1989, abstract, p. 313; and Landesman, S., et al., "Serosurvey of Human Immunodeficiency Virus Infection in Parturients," *Journal of the American Medical Association*, 1987:258, pp. 2701–2703.

17. Ernst, J. A., et al., "HIV Sero-Prevalence at the Bronx-Lebanon Hospital Center—A CDC Sentinel Hospital," Fifth International Conference on AIDS, Montreal, Quebec, Canada, 1989, abstract, p. 79.

18. Hand, I. L., et al., "Newborn Screening for HIV Seropositivity in the South Bronx," Fifth International Conference on AIDS, Montreal, Quebec, Canada, 1989, abstract, p. 120; and Novick, L. F., et al., "HIV Seroprevalence in Newborns in New York State," *Journal of the American Medical Association*, 1989:261, pp. 1745–1750.

19. *New York City Community Health Atlas* (New York: United Hospital Fund, 1988).

20. Selwyn, P. A., et al., "Prospective Study of Human Immunodeficiency Virus Infection and Pregnancy Outcomes in Intravenous Drug Users," *Journal of the American Medical Association*, 1989:261, pp. 1289–1294.

21. Cohen, J., et al., "Prostitutes and AIDS: Public Policy Issues," *AIDS and Public Policy Journal*, 1988:3, pp. 16–22; Centers for Disease Control, Survey Summaries, "Distribution of AIDS Cases by Racial/Ethnic Group and Exposure Category, June 1, 1981–July 4, 1988," *Morbidity and Mortality Weekly Report*, 1988:37 (no. SS-3), pp. 1–3; Centers for Disease Control, "Update: Heterosexual Transmission of AIDS and HIV Infection"; and Landesman, op. cit.

22. Centers for Disease Control, "Update: Heterosexual Transmission of Acquired Immunodeficiency Syndrome and Human Immunodeficiency Virus Infection."

23. Centers for Disease Control, Survey Summaries, "Distribution of AIDS Cases by Racial/Ethnic Group and Exposure Category."

24. Centers for Disease Control, "Antibody to Human Immunodeficiency Virus in Female Prostitutes," *Morbidity and Mortality Weekly Report*, 1987:36, pp. 157–161.

ABORTION: WHERE WE CAME FROM, WHERE WE'RE GOING

Ellen Bilofsky

Not quite 20 years after the Supreme Court's *Roe v. Wade* decision legalized abortion, and nearly 30 years after the beginning of the modern movement for reproductive rights, the abortion rights movement is going back to rediscover and record its history. Challenges from the anti-abortion movement have spawned some frightening judicial decisions as well as a flood of restrictive legislation touched off by the Supreme Court's Webster decision. In the face of this attack and the prospect of having to refight old battles, a spate of articles and publications have appeared reminding us of how we won this tenuous right to abortion in the first place and how we coped in the dark ages when all abortion was illegal.

Two publications from South End Press make excellent additions to this literature. *Abortion without Apology* is actually a long pamphlet that aims to teach the history of the abortion struggle to young women and serve as an organizing manual for a new generation of activists. It also has considerable value for those of us who were there when it was happening. Author Ninia Baehr emphasizes some little-known history, starting with the criminalization of abortion in the 1880s, and sets it in the context of the medical profession's attempt to gain control of women's health.

Baehr's focus, however, is the "radical history" of the abortion rights movement ("radical," as in calling for a change in the balance of power), beginning in 1959 with the "army of three": Patricia McGinnis, Lana Clarke Phelan, and Rowena Gurner. These women were organizing for women's rights and the repeal of abortion laws even before the second wave of feminism. The text, sprinkled with vintage illustrations, is largely based on interviews with these long-forgotten pioneers and others like them. Their gripping testimony about illegal abortions and the sense of empowerment they experienced in the women's self-help movement will get even jaded movement veterans angry and motivated again.

Perhaps Baehr's most important contribution is rescuing from obscurity the distinction between the liberal movement to legalize abortion and the radical movement to repeal abortion laws altogether and to put control of reproductive decisions in women's own hands. The efforts to win legal reforms of anti-abortion laws led to compromises of the more radical demands in order to achieve "winnable" gains. This process culminated in the flawed *Roe v. Wade* ruling, which granted a limited right to abortion but reasserted state and medical control over the decision to have one. Since this ruling made abortions accessible to most middle- and working-class women, the fight was essentially declared over, even while abortions were still financially and logistically denied to many poor and third-world women.

Baehr points out that we lost some of our abortion rights in the 1980s because of the way they were defined in the 1970s. The legacy of those earlier compromises is the necessity of undertaking a new struggle to preserve the narrow right to abortion. Renamed the "pro-choice" movement, it has made abortion, Baehr says, "the right that dare not speak its name." In an attempt to placate potential foes, abortion has been redefined as a necessary evil, and lost in the shuffle are all other demands for reproductive rights and control over one's sexuality, as well as the political reasons why abortion has been denied to women and the connection of abortion to other issues such as the struggles of poor women, women of color, and lesbians.

Baehr concludes *Abortion without Apology* with some "Lessons for the 1990s" about building a more inclusive coalition and broadening the demands into a true reproductive rights movement. Her last chapter is a brief organizing outline, describing her own "Abortion Rap" sessions with groups of young women. She appends a useful bibliography and list of resource groups.

Abortion Rights vs. Reproductive Freedom

From Abortion to Reproductive Freedom essentially starts where *Abortion without Apology* leaves off, with a comprehensive analysis of the current movement and an attempt to define a broader one. As the title implies, Marlene Gerber Fried (a longtime activist with the Boston-based Reproductive Rights National Network, known as R2N2), like Baehr, draws a distinction between a "pro-choice" movement for abortion rights and a movement for reproductive freedom, and her aim is to show how we can create the latter. The large number of articles in this anthology (nearly 50 in all) may be hard to digest, but its many insights are well worth absorbing. The book's great contribution is to put abortion in the context of other issues that affect women's lives. It shows the limits of a single-issue focus—even a radical one—and who is left out of such a limited movement.

In her own essay, "Transforming the Reproductive Rights Movement: The Post-Webster Agenda," Fried argues that by in effect dissolving after abortion became legal and then reconstituting itself as a "pro-choice" force, the abortion rights movement lost its guiding principle as well as its momentum. It thus gave the Right the power to set the terms of the abortion debate ("defenders" versus "destroyers" of the family) and the tactics (judicial and legislative attacks on the one hand and Operation Rescue's clinic attacks on the other). In responding to the "pro-lifers" on their own terms, the pro-choice movement has also allowed them to determine the grounds for its defense of abortion—the "necessary evil" argument. Fried sees today's mainstream pro-choice movement as an actual obstacle to broader reproductive rights goals through its narrow strategies of:

framing the issue in terms of privacy and civil rights rather than in terms of women's liberation and sexual freedom; shaping strategy and politics in accordance with the concerns of white middle-class women and ignoring the needs of other groups of women; relying on those in power to create change rather than pursuing grassroots empowerment strategies; and isolating abortion from other issues.

We have become a movement on the defensive, and, as Baehr also argues, we cannot succeed until we actively pursue our vision of what a society based on reproductive freedom would look like. Fried sees the current crisis brought on by the right-wing attacks as a chance to "get back on the offensive, and to transform our movement."

Defining the Agenda

The remainder of the articles amplify this position and begin to define a larger agenda and coalition. The editor has clearly gone to great effort to include every possible group and interest, particularly women of color. The collection includes, among others, the voices of blacks, Hispanics, Asians, lesbians, gay men, teenagers, disabled women, religious women, poor women, women with AIDS, and women in the workplace.

The book is divided, somewhat arbitrarily, into four sections. The first, which starts off with Fried's essay, is "The Politics of the Abortion Rights Movement." It focuses on analyses of the current situation, including pieces by Angela Davis and Alice Walker on racism in the movement, by Jacqui Alexander on reproductive freedom in the third world, and by Rhonda Copelon on key Supreme Court cases.

The second section, "Speaking Out for Women: Choosing Ourselves," includes a variety of personal stories. Reproductive rights activists have not forgotten the old women's liberation slogan, "the personal is political," and they know that activism grows out of our own needs and our anger. In addition to essays and poems recounting women's experiences with illegal abortion, there are articles about how women—both black and white—took control of meeting their own needs. Here are the stories of the National Black Women's Health Project, the Jane collective, and the menstrual extraction movement. Here too is Ellen Willis's essay, reprinted from the *Village Voice*, on left antiabortionists, entitled "Putting Women Back in the Abortion Debate," in which she reminds us that we need to redefine women, their bodies, and their needs as the center of the abortion debate instead of "merely the stage on which the drama of fetal life and death takes place." (Readers should note that the identification of previously published work is somewhat obscure, so that only a tiny footnote identifies the article on menstrual extraction as 12 years old.)

"Defending Abortion Rights: Confronting Threats to Access" includes a number of articles that detail the attacks from the right wing and some of the ways the pro-choice movement has fought back. There is also a balanced discussion of RU-486 by Judith Norsigian of the Boston Women's Health Book Collective that outlines both the positive and negative aspects of the widely touted "abortion pill" and the necessity of testing it in a variety of circumstances and populations.

The final section is entitled "Expanding the Agenda: Building an Inclusive Movement." It includes statements from women representing a variety of the constituencies listed earlier describing their interests in reproductive rights and the need for coalitions among these groups.

While there is plenty of room for debate and for a variety of strategies and tactics within the abortion rights movement, there is clearly need for reinvigoration—even after the brief post-Webster upsurge of activity—and for greater inclusiveness. *Abortion without Apology* and *From Abortion to Reproductive Freedom* should be required reading to help remind us where we came from and where we should be going.

THE INSURANCE GAME

New York Times, *March 1, 1992*

To the Editor:

President Bush, in his "comprehensive health plan" (front page, Feb. 3), thinks that uninsured Americans, given tax incentives, would rush out and buy insurance. I wouldn't. I'm sure I'm not the only one.

Mr. Bush's proposals reflect misunderstanding of the problems that plague health insurance. He would give the middle class a tax deduction of $3,750 to buy health insurance. This is not as ridiculous as the proposed health insurance tax credit for the poor (who don't pay enough taxes to benefit from a credit). But the deduction for the middle class would be just as ineffective in encouraging people to buy private health insurance.

I, for example, will not buy any medical insurance, even with a tax deduction because:

(1) I have never dealt with an insurance company that consistently pays its claims.

(2) I have never dealt with an insurance company that pays its claims without a barrage of paperwork. (I once had an insurance company return a copy of a doctor's bill stating that the claim could not be paid because the address of the doctor was missing. It was missing because the insurance company duplicated the bill sideways, thus cutting off the doctor's letterhead. I sent a second full copy of the bill, only to have it duplicated sideways again with the same claim of not having the doctor's address.)

(3) Insurance companies do not pay for basics like checkups.

(4) Because I live in New York, where health care costs exceed the "acceptable rates" set by insurers, even claims that are paid are not paid in full.

A tax deduction to buy private health insurance makes as little sense to me as a tax deduction to buy a broken toaster oven. I will no longer pay for private health insurance, and if I fall very ill while uninsured, I will simply get treated and then declare bankruptcy. I am not alone in my views: 35 million Americans refuse to play the insurance game.

I'm sure that Mr. Bush has never filed a claim with an insurance company, waited anxiously for a return check, suffered high blood pressure when receiving, yet again, no check and suffered financially from the insurance game. Mr. Bush refuses to listen to those who have played the insurance game and refuses to acknowledge that private medical insurance does not work.

Mr. Bush's health insurance proposal is merely a ploy to save his Presidential campaign. He is not interested in creating real solutions to the health insurance problem.

I, however, am not interested in giving any more money to private health insurance companies or voting for any Presidential candidate who does not support national health insurance.

DIANA HOLTZMAN
New York, Feb. 8, 1992

TOO LITTLE, TOO LATE: A CHILD WITH AIDS

Teresa McMillen

After six years of working as a therapist at a children's mental health clinic in New York City's East Harlem, I began to feel it was time to try something new. I never dreamed it would be working with children who have AIDS. AIDS was something that I was aware of only peripherally. It was one of many horrors in the world that I protected myself from by not thinking about. I was sure it would never touch my personal life, and that there was nothing I could do about it anyway. So when I applied for the social work position in the Comprehensive AIDS Family Care Center of Albert Einstein College of Medicine in the Bronx, it was only with the idea of exploring options. I really could not see myself working with children who were just going to die. It seemed too depressing, and I was afraid to see people suffering.

During the interview process my attitude began to change. The coordinator of social services for the center helped me see beyond the issues of hopelessness and death, but the real turning point was simply seeing the children themselves. I saw beautiful children who appeared healthy and happy, despite their HIV-positive diagnosis. I also saw for the first time in my life frightened, dying children. Suddenly my own fears and desire to avoid illness seemed unimportant. How could I turn my back on what I had seen? It seemed important to try to bring some measure of comfort and compassion to these children and their anguished parents. I had no idea at the time that I would gain from this job more than I could ever give.

One of the first families I worked with after coming to Einstein was that of an 11-year-old named Joanna. I met Joanna and her family during their second visit to the clinic in June 1990. Joanna was brought to the clinic by her mother, Ana, and her aunt Mildred. Her 6-year-old brother, Tommy, was an uncontrollable ball of energy, running in and out of rooms, up and down the halls, propelled by a force that no one could contain, although Joanna often tried. Ana was in a daze, having just found out that Joanna had tested positive for HIV infection; she barely spoke and seemed isolated from those around her. Mildred expressed her concern about how Ana, as a single mother, would manage with Joanna sick, Tommy out of control, and Ana herself eight months pregnant. The family lived in a one-bedroom, rat-infested apartment. I promised to make a referral to the city's Division of AIDS Services with requests for home care and housing.

I learned that Joanna had had a pretty normal life until her eleventh birthday, when she began to get very ill. Ana said Joanna had frequently had fevers and ear infections, but no one thought to look for HIV infection as a possibility until Joanna came down with candida esophagitis, one of the opportunistic infections associated with AIDS, in May 1990. At our first interview, Ana told me she did not believe the diagnosis. She wanted Joanna to be tested again. And, since the only possible risk factor was perinatal transmission, we asked Ana to be tested as well. When both tests came back positive, Ana had to come to terms with the severity of Joanna's illness. She had to accept her own infection as well, and face the guilt she felt at the possibility that she had infected her then new-born son, Jason. She anguished over her daughter's suffering and felt additional guilt that she herself had remained so healthy. She worried constantly that Jason would become sick and that one day only Tommy, who was HIV-negative, would be left, with no one to care for him. She was also afraid of dying.

Joanna was enrolled in a controlled treatment trial for children. The protocol involved monthly intravenous infusions of about 2½ hours each. As I spent time with the family during these monthly infusions, a connection began to develop between us. I was impressed with Joanna's maturity, intelligence, and sense of responsibility. She was a tremendous source of strength and companionship to her mother as Ana struggled to raise her children alone. Joanna had goals for her life. She was an honors student and valedictorian for her sixth grade class. She wanted to live.

Time Running Out

From the perspective of a service deliverer, caring for a child with AIDS is a difficult and frustrating task that requires the coordination and involvement of many agencies. The doctors, nurses, and social workers at Einstein contacted at least 40 different agencies in attempts to secure needed services or materials for Joanna's family. We were able to provide Joanna and her family with many important services that eased their suffering, but just as often her illness was several steps ahead of our efforts.

In July we invited Joanna to come with a group of children from the hospital to the Hole in the Wall Gang Camp in Connecticut, a camp for children with chronic illnesses. She desperately wanted to go, but already her time was running out. The day before we were to leave, she was hospitalized for severe abdominal pain at Bronx Municipal Hospital Center. (Every time Joanna needed to be hospitalized, the pediatric unit at Einstein was full. It was extremely frustrating.) This was the first warning we had that the deadly microbacterium intracellae avium infection had found Joanna. We knew then that she had less than a year to live. We all tried to bring as much comfort, compassion, and joy to Joanna's life as possible. After her bitter disappointment at missing camp, we made a referral to Starlight Foundation, which fulfills the requests of terminally ill children. They granted Joanna's wish for a TV and VCR. Joanna was unable to attend school that September. A home tutor came to Joanna every day and tried to brighten her spirits with jokes, games, or just companionship when she was too ill to study.

The Division of AIDS Services was finally able to provide a homemaker for

Ana in mid-October. She had waited for 4½ months, but it was a great relief to finally have some help. The homemaker's hours were from 8:00 am to 4:00 pm. She helped with housework and stayed with the other children when Ana had to bring Joanna to the hospital.

There were several crises when the homemaker wasn't available and Ana had to rush Joanna to the hospital. Her friends helped sometimes, but often Ana was forced to struggle alone with one child in severe pain and two others demanding her attention in a crowded hospital emergency room. It was a nightmare for her. We requested increased hours for the homemaker but were never able to get them.

Tommy was confused and disturbed by his sister's illness. As often happens in families of chronically ill children, the well children are overlooked or emotionally neglected in many ways. Tommy became the main expresser of anxiety in the family. His hyperactivity and reckless, impulsive behavior became almost unmanageable. It was impossible for Ana to follow through consistently on referrals for counseling for Tommy because the burdens of caring for Joanna were too overwhelming.

Joanna's condition deteriorated rapidly. She was in constant, often severe pain. She wasted away before our eyes, losing 40 pounds—and there was no way to stop it. One day in November, I went to meet Joanna and her mother at the emergency room of Bronx Municipal Hospital Center. Joanna had been suffering from seizures. She had numbness and tingling on her right side, her foot dragged when she walked, and her mouth contorted when she tried to talk. She was terrified by the changes in her body. I stayed with her and tried to comfort her as she cried over and over again, "Why me? Why is this happening to me?" I squeezed her hand and tried to calm her when the doctor drew her blood. She screamed each time an IV was inserted or blood was taken. Every needle stick was a torturous affront to the fragile body that she was desperately trying to keep intact. The virus was destroying her body, but to Joanna the procedures she was put through were equally terrifying and destructive.

Around Thanksgiving I went to Joanna's home. She was suffering from diarrhea and could no longer walk. Still, she was open to talking. She talked about her helplessness, her frustration at not being able to walk, her regrets about the things in life she had missed out on, her embarrassment at needing to wear diapers. I tried to comfort her by telling her that someday she would have a different kind of life. I said that sometimes our bodies just don't work right anymore. I tried to convey to her my sense that our spirit—or everything that makes us who we are, how we think, feel, and act—lives in our bodies. I expressed my belief that when our bodies get too sick or injured, God invites us to live in his house so that we can have a different, more beautiful life. I felt that Joanna understood.

In early December, Joanna had to be admitted again, this time to North Central Bronx Hospital with pneumocystis carinii pneumonia (PCP). From the time of her admission until the day of her death on January 4, the nurses from Einstein's Comprehensive AIDS Family Care Center, who were very close to Joanna, frantically worked to obtain the nursing services that would allow her to be discharged and cared for at home. Einstein's doctors also worked closely with those from North Central Bronx to coordinate her care. Numerous agencies were contacted. Only one of them could help, but not in time.

Joanna begged every day to go home. She was often alone in the hospital in the evenings and at night because the family did not have enough support and Ana had no one to take care of her other children. The nurses and social worker from Einstein visited several times a week. At Christmas, Joanna found the strength to open a number of gifts from the Children's Hope Foundation.

Anger, Frustration, and Death

The last visit I had with Joanna during which she was aware of my presence was two days before her death. Her room was filled with toys that she would never play with and could bring her no more joy. The Christmas decorations were incongruous next to the suffering in her room. Joanna was wearing an oxygen mask. She removed it only long enough to point out the IV in her ankle, which must have been even more frightening to her than the usual insertions she hated so much, and to indicate her swollen wrists. Then she panicked and put the mask back on her face.

As I drove home, I cried because I did not understand a medical system that dictates that some form of treatment must be provided even when there is no hope. Joanna's mother had struggled with and finally signed the "do not resuscitate" order weeks earlier. Why did they continue to draw blood, to put an IV in her little ankle, to take needless X-rays that were only going to tell us that she would die soon? Why couldn't Joanna be allowed to die with dignity at home? I was angry and frustrated by a home health care system that requires that a referral cross many desks and receive multiple approvals before someone actually shows up to help. I was angry at Ana's family and friends for not rallying to support her in any way they could. I was angry at myself for not knowing more about how to negotiate the health care system. No dying child should have to spend even one night alone in a hospital.

I can take you no further with Joanna than the door of her room the night she died. As Ana, her nurse from Einstein, and I waited at her bedside for her suffering to end, Joanna was blessed with unconsciousness.

Time has not eased Ana and Tommy's suffering over the loss of Joanna. Ana often feels sad. She is apathetic about life and sometimes thinks dying would be easier. Tommy is worried about everyone in his family getting sick. He is haunted by the memory of his sister. At 8 years of age, he is burdened with guilt and regret born of not treating his sister better when she was alive. The struggles of Joanna's family are not unique. I have met many courageous people like them who have taught me about life, about hope, and about what is important. They have given me strength to pass on to others in need.

Across the nation thousands of families are facing similar tragedies compounded by nonexistent, overloaded, or inadequate services. Access to services must be facilitated more quickly, and more skilled home care workers must be hired to meet the overwhelming needs of these families. One of the things I learned most clearly from Joanna's experience was that AIDS waits for no one, least of all the children.

SECTION II

THE CRISIS IN PROVIDER INSTITUTIONS: ISSUES AND AREAS FOR REFORM

INTRODUCTION

Nancy F. McKenzie

As much as the official national debate about health care reform stays within the narrow confines of financial policy, most individuals in America know that the inadequacies of the American health care system go far beyond our individual, or collective, ability to pay for health care. While lobbyists and legislators jockey for pride of place in piecemeal reform, 80 percent of Americans believe that substantial reform will be necessary to deal with our troubled national institutions.

Discussions about health care in the United States must address all the institutions that contribute to the health of individuals—whether they are service institutions that offer medical interventions, or programs traditionally designed to combat economic trends that have unleashed market forces, making one in four Americans poor sometime during 1991.

More to the heart of the matter, health care reform should be about *the convergence of poverties*: the poverty of our health care institutions, particularly those that prevent illness and provide basic care; the poverty of federal policy with respect to meaningful public health and welfare; the increased poverty of individuals. In the 1990s, the decade "of consequence" (after 12 years of the Bush/Reagan "new federalism"), this convergence *is* the health care crisis confronting the United States.

As Marianne Fahs points out in our opening article, "The Economic Consequences of Inaction," the 1980s may have been a period of economic growth for some, but it left millions poorer not only in real terms but in comparative terms as well. As the richest quarter of the population raised their standard of living between 1979 and 1987 by almost 20 percent, the poorest fifth saw theirs fall almost 10 percent. This resulted in the largest disparity in wealth in the United States since Census Bureau Records began keeping figures on wealth in 1947. From 1975 to 1987 children in poverty increased to 20 percent, more than double the rates found in the cooperating countries of the Organization for Economic Cooperation and Development (OECD).

There is a known and direct connection between poverty and serious disease (See Section I) and, as a consequence of federal inaction and direct cuts by federal agencies of "safety net" programs, transferring the burden of the poor to city and state budgets, poor individuals in the United States are today more numerous, sicker, and less institutionally connected than they have been for the last 50 years. This is as true of the elderly as it is of children in poor families. It is not surprising, then, that health provider institutions for the three-fourths of Americans who live in cities are under siege from multiply ill and poor individuals, or that "for-profit," as well as public health care providers are operating with a bunker mentality with respect to community and public health.

As McKenzie and Bilofsky point out in "Shredding the Safety Net: The Dismantling of Public Programs" (p. 140) not only were the 1980s the era of "new federalism," when states took on the role of provider that the federal government had previously, it was an era when hospital emergency rooms became the institutions of last resort, receiving, along with individuals who were sick, the destitute poor, the victims of violence, the malnourished, and the transiently or permanently homeless. As public hospitals received cuts from their state and city budgets throughout the eighties and many closed, those that remained received from all corners this invisible but virtual legion of consequences of failed health care policy. And, as Emily Friedman points out in her article "Public Hospitals" (p. 196), those public hospitals that remained open, now regarded as "vanguard" institutions, merely ended up "Doing What Everyone Wants Done but Few Others Wish to Do." They treated the sick.

The crisis in provider institutions not only involves 50 years of undernourishment of federal health care policy in the United States and the consequent further corporatization of the delivery of care (see Section 3), it involves the "new" (under Presidents Reagan and Bush) public policy with respect to labor and the workplace which has so quickened the era of early cancers, early disability, and a continuity of cynicism and callousness toward the working-class American. It involves, as Dave Kotelchuck shows in his analysis of the fire in Hamlet, North Carolina, that killed 25 individuals ("Worker Health and Safety in the 1990s," p. 133), the general evisceration of federal agencies like OSHA that have traditionally had the moral responsibility and the political clout to resist corporate attacks on occupation health and safety.

The crisis includes the lack of an environmental policy to keep our city infrastructure intact and non-toxic, and the abandonment of urban areas altogether in a battle over the role of the federal government in housing, fire, and sanitation. (See "Contagious Urban Decay and the Collapse of Public Health," p. 167.) The race and class battle between the "burbs" and the urban "ghetto" is a battle reminiscent of the 19th century where joblessness, over-crowding, malnourishment, and the exposure of city dwellers are producing new epidemics of old, treatable, infectious disease. New York City alone is three years behind in its knowledge of how to deal with the national tuberculosis epidemic.

Plaguing our health delivery institutions, those vital institutions traditionally responsible for responding to human suffering and disability, is a crisis caused by the inhumane and irrational health care delivery policy that views health care as a medical commodity and tries to calculate "disease days" through "diagnostic-related groups" (DRGs) of clinical prediction in order to cut down on hospital stays for Medicare patients. Perhaps the most obvious manifestation of this crisis is the resulting chaos seen in "gridlocked" urban hospitals, in public care facilities, in all emergency rooms (See "National Alert: Gridlock in the Emergency Department," p. 176) as the ill find fewer and fewer facilities offering routine and basic care. This situation is as much related to cuts in federal agencies as it is to the crisis of provision of services: inchoate nursing home and long-term care policy (See Cynthia Rudder's piece, "Reforming Long

Term Care," p. 181), shortages in physician involvement in basic care due to the dis-incentives of employment in HMOs and for-profit franchise clinics, as well as the low payment of federal insurance programs for early care of chronic diseases for the poor and the elderly. The crisis is compounded by wholly incoherent financing of health care delivery through third party payers—whether private insurance or federal program—who routinely drop individuals from payment protocols, or ration their care through a "spiral of exclusivity" if there is a probability that they are or might become sick sooner than some other individual. (See "Excluding More, Covering Less: The Health Insurance Industry in the U.S." in Section 3, p. 310.) Finally, the crisis in provider institutions is about a mental health policy that, in combination with housing and social services policy, has virtually eliminated care for individuals with emotional problems that might be ameliorated by group and community support.

In addition, this section addresses the era of health care rationing: the "cost/benefit" policy that has not only wreaked havoc with the health of high risk populations, but has eroded the confidence of every individual American that health care in America is, first and foremost, about care (see "And What About the Patients?," p. 190).

Ultimately, the crisis in provider institutions is evolving into a national debate over what many individuals see as not only a "two-tiered" health care system but a rigid, judgmental, and hypocritical health care system that tolerates an "apartheid-like" separation of services.

"Medical Apartheid: An American Perspective," by Durado Brooks, et al. (p. 223) compares the structures of the fragmented basic health care provision to the poor of Texas with the actual apartheid-driven structures of health care to Black South Africans. The authors find that while the former structures of delivery are not codified into law, nor offered to individuals without legal rights, they are, nonetheless, and for all intents and purposes, as obstructive of medical response, as "misinforming," as "user-unfriendly," and as destructive of health promotion and prevention as health care delivery in racially separated South Africa. This article is one of the few that address the actual quality of care that poor individuals in America receive from health care institutions.

The invisibility of the issues of health care for the poor in our national debates for health care reform is, of course, due not only to the disparities in wealth in America (and therefore in political power), but also to increasingly institutionalized disparities that disguise the actual delivery of health care: disparities in how health care is financed for the poor as opposed to moderate to well-off individual Americans (Medicaid versus private insurance); disparities in the actual structure of the institutions which deliver health care for poor Americans versus other Americans;[1] and disparities in the regulatory mechanisms for upholding individual rights within the health care system. Many states are now requesting a waiver of the federal requirement that Medicaid recipients be given a choice of provider so that the Medicaid population can be assigned to "managed care" facilities which are allowed to be owned by for-profit HMOs.

As a new administration promises financial solutions to the cost of health care coverage for every American, and progressives like Physicians for Health

Care Reform call for a Canadian-style system (for further discussion of alternative systems, see Section VI), there is *no* discussion of the discrimination inherent in the structure of the American health care delivery system—and there is incredible retrenchment on the issue of health provision for the poor, largely minority, communities. In fact, as we debate ''Managed Competition,'' it looks like there will be little change at the national level *except for changes in health services, health financing and health outcome that will adversely affect the poorest of American citizens—predominantly members of the African-American and Latino communities.*

Ultimately, the crisis in provider institutions of health care in the United States must be seen as one that calls into question the American political commitment to equality, non-discrimination, social justice, and autonomy. It is in our health institutions that the articulation of democratic values meets its truest test; how Americans treat not the ''best and brightest,'' but the sick, the disabled, the most vulnerable—each of us, sometime, somewhere, eventually.

It is of primary importance that we as a nation deal with the American health care system as it directly affects our democratic ideals and institutions, and not only at the intersection marked ''access to health care.'' Health care reform must confront the conditions of individual lives, the lack of infrastructure for health care delivery, the mean-spirited and Social Darwinian tendencies of the ''cost containment'' policies of the last decade, the consequences of the ''new federalism'' and its covert declaration that politics would and could tolerate a ''developing country'' within American shores. Finally, the nation must confront the intricacies of health care philosophy itself, a philosophy more driven by health commodification than by human need, more destructive of the human spirit than restoring of the human body.

The readings in this section are designed as a ''walk through'' our largely dysfunctional institutions of care, keeping in mind an ever-worsening economic scene, a depleted environment, and a ''deregulated'' workplace, the three major producers of illness and disability. But hopefully as we engage the other sections, we will carry with us a sense that Americans still do have a vision of a democratically organized, compassionate, and meaningful health care system, a topic we will treat in the final three sections of *Beyond Crisis.*

N O T E S

1. 50 percent of all admissions in public hospitals in 1988 were through the emergency room; in New York City in 1988 there were 27 full-time equivalent primary care physicians for 1.7 million residents of nine low-income African-American and Latino communities (1988 Public Hospital Survey, American Association of Public Hospitals; ''Building Primary Care in Low-Income Communities,'' Community Service Society, Health Unit, 1990).

THE ECONOMIC CONSEQUENCES OF INACTION

Marianne C. Fahs

The tragic and threatening consequences of the fiscal epidemic of health care cutbacks in the city of New York illustrate in miniature the profound consequences that lie ahead for the health of the nation as a whole. We are rapidly becoming a nation of big cities. Thirty years ago, less than two-thirds of the country was urban. Today, over three-fourths of our population is urban. One hundred of our 250 million live in the largest 20 metropolitan areas.[1] The challenges we face in New York are the challenges we face as an urban nation, striving to maintain a competitive edge as we look ahead to the twenty-first century.

For the past 15 years, I have been studying the relationship between economic productivity and illness. My research, and that of others in this field, shows the economic consequences of illness to our society to be vast. They include the direct medical costs of providing health care to the ill—the consequences most often cited in policy circles. But they also include the incalculable toll in human pain and suffering that disease costs American families and friends every year, and the devastating costs to our economic viability as a city, and as a nation, through significant losses in economic productivity due to disease.

The economic consequences of illness are staggering.[2] The annual loss in productivity to our national economy associated with work loss due to illness and premature death is now over *$450 billion*. This represents over 10 percent of our total economic production. Think of the tremendous boost to the economy and to our competitive world position that would result if we were able to harness this economic potential. The disturbing truth of the matter is that, according to standard preventive medicine textbooks, we *are* able to prevent over 90 percent of this economic productivity loss, using current knowledge and technology.

AIDS, "the most devastating epidemic of our century," adds an accelerating toll to our economic loss.[3] Published estimates indicate the loss in economic productivity associated with AIDS is especially high, because this disease strikes young people, often at the beginning of their most productive years. In 1991, the productive loss to our economy associated with AIDS is estimated to be over $55.6 billion.[4]

While this is a national problem, New York is especially hard hit, and shoulders a disproportionate share of this loss. With 21 percent of the nation's AIDS cases in New York State, AIDS costs the New York State economy over $12

PREVALENCE OF SERIOUS CHRONIC HEALTH CONDITIONS BY INCOME

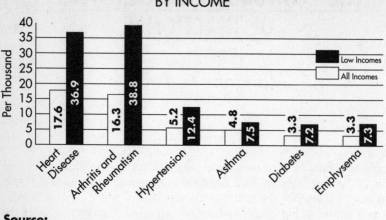

Source:

R. J. Blendon and D. E. Rogers, "Cutting Medical Care Costs," *Journal of the American Medical Association*, vol. 250, no. 14, October 14, 1983, pp. 1880–85. Copyright 1983, American Medical Association.

billion annually; $10 billion of that loss is contributed by the toll this devastating epidemic takes in New York City.[5]

We are a nation of communities. But the real cutbacks in federal support of community health programs in the 1980s, combined with the absence of federal leadership in instituting comprehensive health care reform, have resulted in a shift of responsibility to state and local governments. Cities and states have been left to fend for themselves. What constituted hard times in the 1980s, during a period of economic expansion, constitutes a real crisis in 1991. I do not use that term lightly. It is in fact both a fiscal and a moral crisis.

The 1980s was a period of economic expansion for some, but not for others. From 1979 to 1987, the standard of living of the top fifth of the population rose by 19 percent. At the same time, the living standard for the more than 40 million Americans who make up the poorest fifth of the population fell by 9 percent.[6] According to the Census Bureau, the income gap between the richest and the poorest is now wider than it has been at any time since the bureau began keeping such statistics in 1947.

During the 1980s, the poor became both poorer and more numerous.[7] The percent of the American population living below the poverty line increased from 12.3 percent in 1975 to 13.1 percent in 1988. In New York State, the percent of Americans living below the poverty line increased from 6.7 to 8.7 percent; in New York City, from 15.0 percent to 20.8 percent. The annual rate of increase is accelerating.[8]

Particularly disturbing is the record regarding children. From 1975 to 1987, the poverty rate for children in the United States increased from 16 to 20 percent.[9] Today, one out of every five children in this country lives in poverty. This is more than double the rates found in Organization for Economic Cooperation and Development (OECD) countries.[10] In New York City, the poverty rate for children is double the national average; 40 percent of the city's children live in poverty. Fully 60 percent of the city's children live in families with incomes below 200 percent of the poverty level, compared with 43 percent nationally.[11]

There is a direct relationship between poverty and the prevalence of serious disease (see chart on page 122). To quote one of the great leaders in the history of public health, Johann Peter Frank, "poverty is the chief cause of disease."[12] The federal government found that the percentage of people in the United States who consider themselves in only fair or poor health (as opposed to good, very good, or excellent health) rises precipitously as income level drops: from 4.6 percent for people with incomes over $35,000 to 21.1 percent for people with incomes below $10,000. The number of bed disability days per year is three times as high for people with incomes under $5,000 as compared to people with incomes above $25,000.[13]

What does this increase in poverty and decline in health have to do with the nation's economy? Radical reductions of funding in public health have dire consequences beyond the crippling of our ability to meet the many health needs of Americans. The short-term saving in health expenditures is, in the long run, illusionary, as the following cases illustrate.

Thwarted Promises in Our Nation's Communities

• LEAD POISONING. Lead poisoning is the most common and socially devastating disease of young children, currently damaging the intelligence and behavior of at least 3 million to 4 million children in the United States (17 percent of all children).[14] Vulnerability to lead poisoning is associated with poverty. This invisible epidemic will cost the country over $28 billion during the next 20 years.[15]

Control of this epidemic will save the US economy money. Research shows that a $34 billion investment in lead poisoning prevention programs over a 20-year period will *save* $62 billion in monetized returns, through averted health care costs, increased income associated with increased IQ, and averted special-education costs.[16]

The tragedy we face today in cities such as New York is a drastic cut in lead poisoning prevention programs. The consequences of this loss of public health leadership and vision will inevitably be borne by all of us in the form of higher taxes and further losses in productivity, as we bear the double burden of increased medical and educational costs for our affected children, and as we find our economic GNP growing more slowly than it could have, due to the disability of these individuals. The true tragedy here is that a concerted effort could virtually eliminate this disease in this country within twenty years—at substantial savings to our economy. To quote Primo Levi, "When we know how to reduce the torment, but do not do it, then we become the tormentors."[17]

• PREVENTION OF LOW BIRTH WEIGHT. In the 1980s, after years of slow decline, there was an actual increase in the percentage of infants born with low birth weight, the most significant factor in determining infant death and disability.[18] The Office of Technology (OTA) estimates that for every low birth weight birth averted by earlier and more frequent prenatal care, the US health care system saves between $14,000 and $30,000 in newborn hospitalization, rehospitalizations in the first year, and long-term health care costs associated with low birth weight.[19] The OTA reports that encouraging poor women to obtain early prenatal care through expanded public health benefits is a good investment for the nation. Further, the OTA underestimates the true savings to the economy: If the disabilities associated with low birth weight are averted, we can expect an increase in productivity.

Yet the percentage of women receiving early and regular prenatal care declined significantly in the 1980s. In 1987, more than 74,000 pregnant women received no prenatal care at all—a 50 percent increase over the 1980 rate.[20] Unfortunately, as a consequence of the proposed Fiscal Year 1992 budget cuts, all public maternity, education, and referral services would be eliminated in New York City. The 10,000 women who are currently being served by maternity and family planning services, and an estimated 18,300 newly enrolled clients in 1992, would not receive referrals to prenatal, postpartum, or well-child care.

• CHILDHOOD IMMUNIZATION. The cost-effectiveness of childhood vaccines is well established in the scientific literature. The first 20 years of measles vaccination provided a net savings to the US economy of $5.1 billion.[21] A 1983 study showed that the use of a combined measles, mumps, and rubella vaccine saved the country $60 million in direct medical costs and increased productivity.[22] Another study, in 1984, of pertussis vaccination showed a $44 million savings in medical costs for every one million children vaccinated.[23]

Despite the clearly established economic benefits, the current levels of immunization in this country are less than half of those in the United Kingdom, France, Canada, Israel, Spain, Italy, and Sweden.[24] And Dr. James Mason, head of the US Public Health Service, points out: "The current outbreak of measles is an ominous foreshadowing of what could be in store, if we don't make rapid progress in raising immunization coverage of preschoolers. . . . We could be laying the foundation for outbreaks of diphtheria, pertussis, polio, mumps, rubella, and congenital rubella syndrome."[25]

With the increase in poverty among our nation's children, and the real cutbacks in health and income-support programs of the early 1980s, preventable childhood diseases are on the rise. Unfortunately, as a consequence of the proposed Fiscal Year 1992 budget cuts, over 100,000 immunizations given annually at walk-in immunization clinics in New York City would be eliminated.

• CERVICAL CANCER AND LOW-INCOME ELDERLY WOMEN. A study conducted by the Department of Community Medicine at Mount Sinai of a cervical cancer screening program for elderly women attending a municipal hospital outpatient clinic in New York City showed that for every 100 Pap smears performed, the screening program saved the health care system over $5,000. Odd as it may seem, this study, published only three years ago, was the first economic analysis in this country of public health prevention efforts among the low-income elderly.[26] Unfortunately, the $5.4 million proposed cut in laboratory services run by the Department of Health would simply eliminate Pap smear testing from its laboratory services program.

These four examples lay bare some of the economic implications of the public health disaster we are facing in the communities of our nation. We are mortgaging our future by systematically destroying our human and economic potential. Further, with the increased suffering we are imposing on our poor, we are becoming a morally bankrupt society.

How did we arrive at such a predicament? It is not as though we haven't been trying to solve the interrelated and complex problems of health, productivity, and economic growth for some time. In the past few years, we have seen the arrival of one reform after another—all with little success. We must find new strength in the face of adversity, for the serious problems facing us are soluble. As Winston Churchill said: "Americans can always be relied on to do the right thing after they have exhausted all the other possibilities."

The Myths about the Health Care Cost Crisis

The United States, which spends 12 percent of its GNP on health care (a percentage that has been steadily increasing over time), has higher expenditures for health care than any other nation.[27] This statistic usually accompanies the handwringing over our current "health care cost crisis." Since the late 1970s, the policy response to this "crisis" has increasingly focused on reducing government expenditure on health care. The assumption is that health care expenditure increases should be fought by ever more draconian cuts to our public health care budgets. This is wrong-headed policy. Health care expenditures are not full economic costs, and, as the above examples show, cuts in government health expenditures can actually increase the full economic costs we bear.

After fifteen years of health care reform failures under Presidents Carter, Reagan, and Bush, who have all tried to follow traditional economic principles of competition and allow the "invisible hand" of the market to rule the production and distribution of health in the United States, the American public is ready for a major change. Poll after poll demonstrates that there is a crisis of confidence in the American health care system.[28] Yet today's policy responses continue to be based on economic myths that lack supporting empirical evidence.

• MYTH 1: CUTS IN HEALTH CARE EXPENDITURES ELIMINATE HEALTH CARE SERVICES ONLY. There is a fundamental principle in economics, that expenditures equal income. Health care in fact, because it is labor intensive, creates a high rate of jobs per expenditure—much higher than, say, military expenditures, which are capital intensive. Today, health care employs 37 out of every 1,000 Americans, compared with 28 out of every 1,000 10 years ago.[29] The number of health-related employees surged from 6.1 million in 1979 to 8.7 million in 1989—by 43 percent. According to Labor and Census Department estimates, by the end of the 1990s, at least 12 million Americans will work in health services, which will contain 7 of the 10 fastest growing occupations.[30] Cuts in public health budgets not only deny people needed medical care, they also deny people jobs.

• MYTH 2: HEALTH CARE SPENDING BY BUSINESS DESTROYS AMERICA'S COM-PETITIVENESS. It is an unproved myth that health care spending adversely affects America's "competitiveness."[31] According to this widely shared folklore, an automobile produced in Detroit now contains between $500 and $700 of health care costs. But as Uwe Reinhardt, professor of economics at Princeton University, argues, it is not high health care costs *per se*—in the form of insurance premiums and fringe benefits—that render American business noncompetitive at home or abroad, it is the *total* worker-compensation package—benefits *plus* cash wages—that affects business competitiveness.[32] In fact, workers have accepted tradeoffs of cash income for fringe benefits, so that total compensation packages remain competitive.[33]

• MYTH 3: HEALTH CARE SPENDING BY THE GENERAL PUBLIC DESTROYS AMERICA'S COMPETITIVENESS. It is highly unlikely that the relatively large percentage of the American GNP devoted to health care, by itself, adversely affects the nation's competitiveness. Economists are quick to point out that there is nothing magical about the current percentage of our economy spent on health care.[34] Not only is it not necessarily wrong to spend 12 percent of our economic wealth on health care, but we could even spend substantially more—say 20 percent—without adversely affecting other productive sectors of the economy.

In 1987, Americans spent a total of $194 billion on hospital care, $102 billion on physician services, and $34 billion on drugs and sundries. While these are sizable outlays, that same year Americans spent $35.6 billion on tobacco, $61 billion on alcohol, $24.2 billion on jewelry, and $26.2 billion on cosmetics.[35] Arguments that spending in health care is a misallocation of productive resources must contend with these statistics.

• MYTH 4: HEALTH CARE SPENDING BY THE GOVERNMENT DESTROYS AMERICA'S COMPETITIVENESS. The only way in which high health expenditures are likely to detract from the nation's competitiveness in the long run is if public health care spending comes at the expense of our investment in other forms of human capital (such as education) or the nation's infrastructure, both of which are largely publicly financed.[36] And this would only happen if the American taxpayers and their political representatives insist on keeping the percentage of GNP going through public budgets constant—so that more spent on public health care (about 41 percent of all health expenditures at the present time) means less spent on other public programs.[37]

Our tax burden in this country (33 percent of the GNP) remains lower than that of all the European nations in OECD, where tax-to-GNP ratios range in the mid-to-high 40 percent range.[38] We maintain the lowest tax burden despite a growing underclass of poverty-stricken children, an increase in the elderly population, and higher infant mortality rates and lower life expectancies than in almost all other OECD countries.[39]

Research shows a strong positive correlation between public health expenditures as a percent of GNP and life expectancy.[40] Countries that place a high priority on health programs have approximately two to three times lower infant mortality and child death rates than their counterparts at the same level of economic development.[41]

Further, the United States has the lowest public health to total health expenditure ratio of all 24 OECD countries; at 41 percent it is comparable only to Turkey.[42] Other countries average between 70 and 80 percent. This higher public health allocation does not adversely affect their GNP growth. For example, in comparison with Canada and Japan, our average annual GNP growth per capita between 1985 and 1988 in real dollars ranks a poor third.[43]

In New York City, the public health-care budget did not keep pace with the growth in real GNP during the 1980s, and it has been continually losing ground in real dollars. But the substantial restrictions of the proposed 1992 budget mark the first reversal in public health expenditures. There is no doubt that the impact of these shrinking resources will adversely affect the city's health. Econometric analyses have shown a quantifiable direct relationship between health expenditures and age-adjusted mortality.[44] Based on these equations, we can expect our age-adjusted mortality in New York to increase.

The Legacy of Laissez-Faire

Current federal inaction is based on the economic theory of competition, which embodies the principle of *laissez-faire*—literally, let the private market alone to do its work. The Reagan and Bush administrations have used the theoretical ideal of competition and "privatization" to sound the alarm against rising public health-care expenditures. This alarm is combined illogically with the reassurance that public program cuts and stiffer hospital and physician regulation will solve the cost problem.

Competition used this way is a wolf in sheep's clothing. The theory, as first detailed by Adam Smith in his classic *The Wealth of Nations*, predicts that the ultimate outcome of the Godlike "invisible hand" guiding the private market will be compatible with both private profitseeking and the public benefit. But even Adam Smith had moral qualms about this compatibility. According to Smith, the interest of those who live by profit "is never exactly the same as that of the public," and they "have generally an interest to deceive and even to oppress the public, and . . . accordingly have, upon many occasions, both deceived and oppressed it."[45]

Moral qualms aside, the economic and health policy literature is full of reasoned arguments and empirical proof that the special quality of health care does not meet the stringent requirements necessary before the ideals of competition can be approached.[46] For example, consumers must have time to search the market to exercise their sovereignty, yet medical care requirements are often urgent, leaving no time to shop for the best price. There must be free entry into the market, which goes absolutely against the standards of the AMA and state licensor boards. And consumers must have perfect knowledge about the quality of the product, which is extremely difficult to attain in the complex and constantly changing field of medicine.

The past decade of "competition" in health care has brought four adverse consequences:

• CONSEQUENCE 1: HIGHER COSTS. National health care spending has more than doubled from $248 billion in 1980 to over $600 billion this year—a spending increase of $1,000 per person. Adjusted for inflation, health-care expenditures have been growing at near record levels.[47]

• CONSEQUENCE 2: INCREASED REGULATION. The "market"-oriented policies of the Reagan and Bush administrations have left us with an erosion of clinical freedom. Physicians in the United States are now the most litigated-against, second-guessed, and paperwork-laden physicians in Western industrialized democracies. Rates of malpractice suits against private-practice physicians more than tripled between 1980 and 1985.[48]

• CONSEQUENCE 3: LOSS OF HEALTH INSURANCE FOR AMERICANS WHO NEED IT MOST. Because of the rising cost of health insurance premiums, insurance companies, including even Blue Cross, have responded to competition by dropping "bad risks." The horrible irony is that these are the people who need coverage most. The numbers of uninsured have increased from 30 million in 1980 to approximately 37 million in 1987, and millions more are underinsured.[49]

Further, the proportion of children in the United States without private or public health insurance increased from about 13 percent in 1977 to 18 percent in 1987.[50] Today, one-third of all poor and low-income children have no health insurance. This is a consequence of the decrease in private coverage among low-income families, and the decrease in public coverage of single-parent families.[51] Again, the tragedy is that these are children with the highest health needs; among the poor and near-poor, there is an increased incidence of respiratory infections, tuberculosis, measles, dysentery, childhood lead poisoning, and AIDS.

• CONSEQUENCE 4: DETERIORATING ADMINISTRATIVE EFFICIENCY. Because many different health insurance companies compete with each other in the United States, the proportion of health-care expenditures consumed by administration—in the form of insurance overhead, hospital administration, nursing home administration, and physicians' overhead and billing expenses—is higher than in Canada and in Britain, where there is a single-payer system. In 1983, administrative costs in the United States were 60 percent higher than in Canada and 97 percent higher than in Britain.[52] Further, between 1983 and 1987, administrative costs in the United States increased 37 percent in real dollars, whereas in Canada they declined. The proportion of health-care spending consumed by administration is now at least 117 percent higher in the United States than in Canada.[53]

Options for the Future

The economic consequences of public health inaction are severe. They include direct health expenditures, due to the costs of disease that could have been prevented, and decreases in worker productivity potential. It is an economic truism that investment in capital increases labor productivity. Our neglect of *human* capital investment will surely decrease our rate of GNP increase; health is a crucial contributor to economic growth.

Health care spending is a productive use of resources. We must educate the American public to understand what a payoff the right kind of public spending can have. If we lose the productivity of our poor and near poor, we lose a profound American dream—the dream of betterment, of the poor or working-class immigrants who work hard so that their children can go to college. The evidence is clear that the loss of access to health care during the 1980s is already robbing many Americans and their children of an opportunity for a long, healthy, and productive life. A young *uninsured* adult male now has three times the chance of dying during a hospitalization as an *insured* adult male, similar in every way except for insurance status.[54] The death of such a man can mean the end of the American dream for his young children, who must attempt the struggle toward economic improvement without the financial support of their father; it is a preventable tragedy.

In order to achieve the economic expansion we are capable of, we must adopt an active public health policy agenda, with target objectives *and* target budgets clearly spelled out. Without a federal economic and political agenda for the health of the nation, we are in danger of lurching off track each time political pressures present unexpected choices.

Our economic growth depends on our public health investments of today. Government can simply look the other way or can summon the courage to face the problem squarely.

A good investment choice is to reduce the number of Americans living in poverty. One way to approach this problem efficiently, without increasing taxes, is to decrease income disparity through a negative income tax policy. This policy would redistribute the tax burden more equitably among income brackets, with the lowest brackets getting cash returns.

Another investment choice is to form a federal community partnership to improve access to health care. The decrease in funding to community health centers has had a devastating impact on the poor served by these programs. This has been a myopic cost-cutting policy. These programs are a cost-effective use of federal health expenditures; they are targeted on high-need populations; and they have been highly successful in reducing the hospitalization rates—from 25 percent to 67 percent—of those served.[55]

How could this partnership be financed? One way is to make sure that all community health center clients are already insured when they arrive at the health center. We have the capability to achieve that at the present time, with no additional taxes. The General Accounting Office reports that *if the United States went to a single-payer system of paying for medical care*, similar to that in Canada, *the annual savings would be $75 billion*. This is more than enough to cover all the uninsured, with enough left over to cover all the deductibles, copayments and out-of-pocket costs for medical care to all others presently insured.[56] This reform offers President Bush an historic opportunity to guarantee basic health care to every American.

But to rebuild our public health infrastructure and increase the availability and accessibility of health services to our disadvantaged communities, we need both new, creative, and culturally sensitive community programs and outreach efforts, as well as new investment capital for these efforts. We can have higher taxes, or we can have *different* taxes. We might consider reviewing federal excise taxes on alcohol and cigarettes, which have been very stable since 1951.[57] Research by Michael Grossman, professor of economics at the City University of New York, shows that if we were to raise the excise tax on beer in line with the rate of inflation over the past three decades, we would cut motor-vehicle fatalities of 18- to 20-year-olds (many of which are alcohol related) by about 15 percent, saving more than 1,000 lives per year. If we were to restore the excise tax on cigarettes to its real value in 1951, 800,000 premature deaths of Americans 12 years and older would be averted.[58] These can be considered public health investment taxes. If they are used to improve services to the poor, they will have a public health multiplier effect on both national health levels and economic wealth.

We remain a nation of communities. Some of our communities are desperately ill. We cannot ignore them. The cost is too high. We must fight against ignorance, political expediency, and selfishness to uphold the ideals of community medicine, first advanced a generation ago by Dr. Kurt Deuschle, the founder of community medicine in the United States. As he has said, "In the final analysis, the diagnosis and treatment of community and social pathology, not individual pathology, must be our major concern."[59]

Our public health programs are among the most cost-effective health programs in the country. Action must come soon or health-care problems will bring this country to its knees. The most rapid and dramatic improvements in the health of the public will result not from technology-intensive medical care but from preventive measures. These are grossly underfunded at the present time; only 2.9 percent of all health dollars is spent for government public health activities. We must turn away from the narrow-minded cost-containment refrains to consider the health of our country. We need rational analysis, compassion, and an appreciation of the long-run, as well as the short-run, aspects of this complex problem.

As Joseph Califano, former secretary of the Department of Health, Education and Welfare, wrote in his autobiography: "Of course, those who govern will make mistakes. Plenty of them. But we should not fear failure. What we should fear above all is the judgment of God and the judgment of history if we, the most affluent people on earth, free to choose and act as we wish, choose not to govern justly, choose not to distribute our riches fairly and to help the most vulnerable among us, or worse yet, choose not to even try."

NOTES

1. U.S. Bureau of the Census, U.S. Census of Population; 1960 and 1970; 1980 Census of Population, vol. 1, chap. A (PC80-1-A) and Supplementary Report, Metropolitan Statistical Areas (PC80-81S1-18); Current Population Reports, Series P-26, No. 85-AL-C to 85-WY-C and Series P-25, No 1039.

2. Estimates in this discussion are derived from studies of the cost of illness by D. P. Rice, T. A. Hodgson, and A. N. Kopstein, "The economic costs of illness: A replication and update," *Health Care Financing Review*, Fall 1985, pp. 61–80. Figures for 1991 are estimated by applying the prior 17-year average annual indirect cost growth rate to 1985 cost estimates and updating the dollar values to 1991 dollars using the consumer price index.

3. J. E. Osborne, "AIDS and Public Policy," *AIDS* 3 (supplement 1), 1989, pp. S 297–300.

4. A. A. Scitovsky, "The Economic Impact of AIDS," *Health Affairs*, Fall 1988, pp. 32–45.

5. Estimates in this discussion are derived from the study by Scitovsky, "The Economic Impact of AIDS," pp. 32–45, using the proportion of total U.S. AIDS cases that are in New York State and New York City, according to data from U.S. Department of Health and Human Services, Centers for Disease Control, *HIV/AIDS Surveillance Report*, July 1991, pp. 1–18.

6. P. Passell, "Forces in Society, and Reaganism, Helped Dig Deeper Hole for Poor," *The New York Times*, July 16, 1989, p. A1.

7. Office of Policy and Financial Management, Human Resources Administration, The City of New York, unpublished data, July 1991.

8. Ibid.

9. U.S. Bureau of the Census, "Current Population Survey for New York City," Average of 1985–86 estimates of percent of population living in poverty. National data from Current Population Report, Series P-60, #158.

10. T. Smeeding, B. B. Torrey, and M. Rein, "Patterns of Income and Poverty: The Economic Status of Children and the Elderly in Eight Countries," in J. L. Palmer, T. Smeeding, and B. B. Torrey, eds., *The Vulnerable* (Washington, D.C.: The Urban Institute Press, 1988), pp. 89–119.

11. U.S. Bureau of the Census, "Current Population Survey for New York City," Average of 1985–86 estimates of percent of population living in poverty. National data from Current Population Report, Series P-60, #158.

12. H. E. Sigerist, *Medicine and Human Welfare* (College Park, Md: McGrath Publishing Co., 1970).

13. "Health Status of the Disadvantaged, Chartbook 1986." DHHS Publication No. (HRSA) HRS-P-DV86-2 (Washington, D.C.: U.S. Government Printing Office, 1986).

14. U.S. Department of Health and Human Services, Centers for Disease Control, *Strategic plan for the elimination of childhood lead poisoning*, February 1991, pp. 1–53.

15. Ibid.

16. Ibid.

17. P. Levi, *The Periodic Table*, 1st American edition (New York: Schocken Books, 1984).

18. The National Commission to Prevent Infant Mortality, *Troubling Trends: The Health of America's Next Generation*, February 1990.

19. U.S. Congress, Office of Technology Assessment, *Healthy Children: Investing in the Future*, OTA-H-345 (Washington, D.C.: U.S. Government Printing Office, 1988).

20. The National Commission to Prevent Infant Mortality, *Troubling Trends: The Health of America's Next Generation*, February 1990.

21. A. B. Bloch, W. A. Orenstein, H. C. Stetler, et al., "Health Impact of Measles Vaccination in the United States," *Pediatrics*, vol. 76, 1985, pp. 524–32.

22. C. C. White, J. P. Koplan, and W. A. Orenstein, "Benefits, risks and costs of immunization for measles, mumps and rubella," *American Journal of Public Health*, vol. 75, no. 7, 1985, pp. 739–44.

23. A. R. Hinman and J. P. Koplan, "Pertussis and Pertussis Vaccine: Reanalysis of Benefits, Risks, and Costs," *JAMA* 251, 1984, pp. 3109–13.

24. *The State of the World's Children* (New York: UNICEF, 1987).

25. J. Mason, *The Nation's Health* (newsletter of the American Public Health Association), August 1991.

26. J. S. Mandelblatt and M. C. Fahs, "The cost-effectiveness of cervical cancer screening for low-income elderly women," *Journal of the American Medical Association*, vol. 259, no. 16, 1988, pp. 2409–13.

27. Health Care Financing Administration, Division of National Cost Estimates, U.S. Department of Health and Human Services, 1989.

28. R. J. Blendon and K. Donelan, "Interpreting public opinion surveys," *Health Affairs*, vol. 10, no. 2, Summer 1991, pp. 166–69.

29. M. Freudenheim, "Job Growth in Health Care Soars," *The New York Times*, March 5, 1990.

30. Ibid. Also, K. R. Levit, H. C. Lazenby, S. W. Letsch, and C. A. Cowan, "National health care spending, 1989," *Health Affairs*, vol. 10, no. 1, Spring 1991, pp. 117–30.

31. U. E. Reinhardt, "Health care spending and American competitiveness," *Health Affairs*, vol. 8, no. 4, Winter 1989, pp. 5–21.

32. Ibid.

33. Ibid.

34. Ibid. Also, V. R. Fuchs, "The health sector's share of the gross national product," *Science*, vol. 246, 1990, pp. 534–38.

35. U. E. Reinhardt, "Health care spending and American competitiveness," *Health Affairs*, vol. 8, no. 4, Winter 1989, pp. 5–21.

36. Ibid.

37. Ibid.

38. Organization for Economic Cooperation and Development Secretariat, "Health care expenditure and other data," *Health Care Financing Review*, 1989 Annual Supplement, Baltimore, Md. U.S. Department of Health and Human Services, December 1989.

39. M. I. Roemer, R. Roemer, "Global health, national development and the role of government," *American Journal of Public Health*, vol. 80, no. 10, October 1990, pp. 1188–92.

40. Ibid.

41. S. Cereseto and H. Waitzkin, "Economic development, political-economic system, and the physical quality of life," *Journal of Public Health Policy*, Spring 1988, pp. 104–20.

42. G. J. Schieber, J-P. Poullier, "International health spending: Issues and trends," *Health Affairs*, vol. 10, no. 1, Spring 1991, pp. 106–16.

43. U.S. Department of State, Bureau of Intelligence and Research, "Economic Growth of IECD Countries, 1978–1988," Report No. IRR 205 (revised), 1989, and unpublished data.

44. J. Hadley, *More Medical Care, Better Health?* (Washington, D.C.: The Urban Institute Press, 1982).

45. R. Heilbroner, "Economic Predictions," *New Yorker*, July 8, 1991.

46. J. Hadley, J. Holahan, and W. Scanlon, "Can fee-for-service reimbursement coexist with demand creation?" *Inquiry*, vol. 16, 1979, p. 247. Also, T. Rice, "The impact of changing medicare reimbursement rates on physician-induced demand," *Medical Care*, vol. 21, 1983, p. 803. Also, L. F. Rossiter and G. R. Wilensky, "A reexamination of the use of physician services: The role of the physician-initiated demand," *Inquiry*, 1983, p. 162. Also, M. C. Fahs, "Physician response to the United Mine Workers cost sharing program: The other side of the coin," *Health Services Research*, forthcoming.

47. K. R. Levit, H. C. Lazenby, S. W. Letsch, and C. A. Cowan, "National health care spending, 1989," *Health Affairs*, vol. 10, no. 1, Spring 1991, pp. 117–30.

48. P. R. Lee and L. Etheredge, "Clinical Freedom: Two Lessons for the U.K. from U.S. Experience with Privatisation of Health Care," *The Lancet*, February 4, 1989, pp. 263–65.

49. P. J. Cunningham, A. C. Monheit, "Insuring the children: A decade of change," *Health Affairs*, vol. 9, no. 4, 1990, pp. 76–90.

50. Ibid.

51. Ibid.

52. S. Woolhandler and D. U. Himmelstein, "The Deteriorating Administrative Efficiency of the U.S. Health Care System," *The New England Journal of Medicine*, vol. 324, no. 18, 1991, pp. 1253–58.

53. Ibid.

54. J. Hadley, E. P. Steinberg, and J. Feder, "Comparison of Uninsured and Privately Insured Hospital Patients: Condition on Admission, Resource Use, and Outcome," *JAMA*, vol. 265, no. 3, 1991, pp. 374–79.

55. K. Davis, "Expanded Use of Community Health Centers: Potential Savings to Medicaid," Paper prepared for 1981 Commonwealth Fund Forum, "Medical Care for the Poor: What Can States Do in the 1980's?" Philadelphia, Pennsylvania, August 9–12, 1981. Also, U.S. General Accounting Office, Report to the Chairman, Committee on Government Operations, House of Representatives, *Canadian Health Insurance: Lessons for the United States*, GAO/HDR-91-90, June 1991.

56. U.S. General Accounting Office, Report to the Chairman, Committee on Government Operations, House of Representatives, *Canadian Health Insurance: Lessons for the United States*, GAO/HDR-91-90, June 1991.

57. M. Grossman, *Health Benefits of Increases in Alcohol and Cigarette Taxes*, National Bureau of Economic Research, Reprint No. 1414, Cambridge, Massachusetts.

58. Ibid.

59. K. W. Deuschle and F. Eberson, "Community medicine comes of age," *The Journal of Medical Education*, vol. 48, no. 12, 1968, pp. 1229–37.

WORKER HEALTH AND SAFETY
IN THE 1990S

At the beginning of the 1990s, following a decade of attack on occupational health and safety protections, the occupational safety and health movement, spearheaded by the nation's labor unions, has switched from defensive efforts to a major new initiative to reform the federal Occupational Safety and Health Act (OSHA). The Comprehensive Occupational Safety and Health Reform Act (COSHRA: HR.3160, S.1662), introduced by Senator Edward Kennedy (D-MA) and Rep. William Ford (D-MI) in the US Senate and House, respectively, is the first serious attempt by supporters of greater worker protection to eliminate some of the obvious weaknesses of the OSHAct since it took effect two decades ago in 1971.

The Fire in Hamlet, North Carolina

This legislative effort was given a tragic jump-start in September 1991 after a sudden, preventable fire at a nonunionized poultry plant in Hamlet, North Carolina, took 25 workers' lives. The incident touched a raw nerve—it reminded Americans in all walks of life how poorly this society protects the lives and safety of working men and women.

Many of the dead and injured were trapped by exit doors which had been padlocked shut or blocked shut by large, heavy objects such as trash containers. Most of the 25 victims died of smoke inhalation. Why did the company lock or block the exits? Company officials have so far refused to say, but the understanding of workers at the plant was clear: *The doors were locked to prevent workers from stealing chicken parts!* And for this, the lives of 25 human beings were taken, many of them young mothers and all precious to their families and friends.

Full time workers were paid a starting wage of only $4.90 an hour ($9,800 per year) with a top wage of just $5.50 an hour ($11,000 per year). With workers paid such meager wages, is it any wonder that they might try to supplement their income with some food from the plant?

And for these reprehensibly low wages, the company treated the workers like slaves. Workers were allowed two 15-minute breaks and half an hour for lunch each day. "Extra" bathroom breaks cost workers warning points, with permanent loss of job after five warning points. (Kotelchuck, 1991) The result: People reported frequent incidents of working in wet or soiled clothing (in a food plant, no less!). Absences, whether excused or not, also resulted in warning points or even summary loss of job. One woman reported after the fire that she had been fired when she asked for time off to care for an elderly father who broke his hip. (Kotelchuck, 1991)

After the fire, reporters found out that the plant, regulated by a federally approved state OSHA plan, had never been inspected in its entire eleven years of existence. North Carolina, administering a state plan supposedly "as effective as" federal OSHA, had fewer OSHA inspectors—35 statewide—than any other state plan. (AFL-CIO, 1991) The state's failure, which drew a temporary suspension of federal approval for its state plan—later rescinded—highlighted for many citizens the painful inadequacies of many of the nation's 23 state plans and fueled calls from across the nation for both state and federal OSHA reforms. The circumstances of the fire also echoed for many older Americans, and those knowledgeable about US labor history, the events of the Triangle Shirtwaist Fire in New York City in 1911, which killed 146 women and girls also at locked exits and sparked passage of the country's first state worker compensation laws.

The Decline in Worker Health and Safety in the 1980s

National statistics on work-related injuries and illnesses, compiled annually for OSHA by the federal Bureau of Labor Statistics (BLS) and based on management reports, show the decline in worker health and safety during the 1980s.

Between 1973, the first year BLS compiled national OSHA statistics, and 1980, the lost-time injury and illness rate climbed slowly from 3.4 to 4.0 work-related injuries and illnesses per 100 full time workers (BLS, 1991a)—that is, in 1980 4 workers per 100, or 1 in 25, suffered lost-time injuries or illnesses on the job that forced them to miss or be transferred to a lighter job for at least one full workday. This rate, already quite large, remained roughly constant during the 1980s.

Meanwhile the severity of these work-related injuries and illnesses reached record highs during this period. In 1980, the number of lost workdays per lost-workday incident was 16.3, that is, the average worker who lost workdays due to a job-related injury of illness lost a little over three weeks of work. (BLS, 1986; Kotelchuck, 1987) By 1985, this figure reached an all-time record high of 18.0 working days lost per lost-time incident, and in following years the figure rose steadily to its current (1990) record high of 20.5 days per lost-time incident. (BLS, 1991b; Kotelchuck, 1992) That is, by 1990 a person suffering a lost-time injury or illness on the job lost an *average* of about one month (four weeks) of work!

During the 1980s, the rate of job-related illnesses and their severity rose steadily. Job-related illnesses represented only 2.3 percent of all job-related incidents (injuries and illnesses) in 1980; their percentage in 1990 was more than twice as large at 4.9 percent. (BLS, 1991a) During this same period, the average number of workdays lost per illness incident increased from 19 to 32 days per incident.

Leading the rise in job-related illnesses has been the dramatic increase in incidence of repetitive trauma disorders (RTDs), such as carpal tunnel syndrome, most commonly caused by repeated bending of the wrists and elbows, pinching motions and/or extension of the fingers during work operations. In 1980 RTDs made up only 18 percent of all reported illnesses on the job, by 1989 they became the majority of all reported job illnesses, and appear still to be continuing their rapid rate of increase. (BLS, 1991a)

OSHA Enforcement

Currently, federal OSHA has only about 1,000 inspectors nationwide who cover about 3 million workplaces employing 92 million workers. (AFL-CIO, 1992a; BLS, 1991b) At the current rate, the AFL-CIO labor federation estimates that the average facility covered by OSHA can expect an inspector to visit on average about *once in 84 years*, making such visits a "once-in-a-lifetime" experience for both workers and employers. (AFL-CIO, 1992a)

Breaking this down on a statewide basis, the AFL-CIO study (1992b) finds further that it would take more than 167 years for the nine federal OSHA inspectors for Nebraska to inspect all of the state's covered workplaces, the worst state record in the nation, followed by 162 years per inspection in neighboring South Dakota and 137 in Delaware. In contrast, the *best* state inspection rate for federal OSHA is an inspection every 57 years in Idaho, still a "once-in-a-lifetime" experience, followed by once every 61 years in Wisconsin.

The enforcement picture is only slightly better in the 25 US state and territorial OSHA plans. Here again about one thousand state inspectors are responsible in most state-plan states for all private-sector and state and local public-sector workplaces. In the best staffed of these states, Nevada, Alaska, and Michigan, covered workplaces are inspected on average every 11, 12, and 13 years, respectively, far better than Idaho at 57 years, the best federal OSHA state. However, the range of inspection rates is very wide for these state-plan OSHA states as well. It comes as no surprise that the worst of the state-plan states, North Carolina, with an average of one inspection every 113 years, ranks up with the worst states under federal jurisdiction. (AFL-CIO, 1992b)

Fines for OSHA violations remain relatively small both for federal and state-plan jurisdictions. In the federal case, this effect is masked by a so-called federal "egregious case" policy under which, for multiple violations such as falsifying records or not recording serious injuries, companies may be fined separately for each violation, resulting in occasional multimillion-dollar fines. Thus total fines have risen from $11.4 million in 1986, when the new policy went into effect, to $91.7 million in 1991. (BNA, 1992a) This resulted in ten fines of $1 million or more in 1991, and may further increase as a result of the US Congress increasing maximum OSHA fines sevenfold that year. (BNA, 1992a) But the more important measure of fines is not the maximum fines, but the *average* OSHA fines, and these remain quite low. In fiscal year 1990 the average OSHA fine for a serious violation was only $273. (BNA, 1990) Similarly, repeat violations were fined only $1,098 on average, a small sum for noncompliance with initial OSHA directives. For all types of violations, OSHA assessed an average fine of $386 per violation that year. (BNA, 1990) Overall, between 1972 and 1990, the median penalty paid by an employer in an incident resulting in the death or serious injury of a worker was just $480! (AFL-CIO, 1992c) These are paltry, shameful fines.

Perhaps a better indicator of lack of governmental concern with worker health and safety are the paltry sums federal and state governments spend to deal with this problem. In the first five years of the Reagan Administration, budgets for the federal OSHA agency were slashed by an annual average of 7 percent per year in constant dollars, (Labor Research Association, 1987) and NIOSH, the federal research agency for worker health and safety, had its budget slashed almost in half in constant dollars (Greaves, 1991). Currently, according to the AFL-CIO, the "combined state and federal commitment to workplace health and safety" amounts to a paltry *$3.80 per worker per year*, less than the amount of money spent annually to protect fish and wildlife. (AFL-CIO, 1992d)

The OSHA Reform Act

One important way to compensate for the lack of federal and state OSHA inspectors is to put health and safety inspection powers into the hands of workers through the mandatory establishment of plantwide occupational safety and health committees. This would give workers the power to initiate plant inspections through these committees (currently a management prerogative), and negotiate with management about health and safety problems. If no agreement is reached on an alleged OSHA violation, workers could still request an OSHA inspection.

Other key provisions of the proposed COSHRA law include:

- *Workplace Safety and Health Programs*—Currently employers must comply with all OSHA standards and provide a workplace "free from recognized hazards," but are not required to have an overall safety and health plan for the plant or company. COSHRA requires such a plan, and it must be *written* and available for worker inspection. Also such programs must include *worker training* about plant hazards, given on company time.
- *Right to Refuse Unsafe Work*—COSHRA specifically gives workers the right to refuse unsafe work if the job threatens serious injury and if the employer *has been notified, but has not taken corrective action.*
- *Coverage Extended to Public Employees*—Currently state and local public employees, including police and firefighters, are not protected by federal OSHA. (Some are protected by state OSHA plans.) Under COSHRA, *all* public and private workers would be covered by OSHA. This includes transportation, nuclear, and longshore workers who are now covered by other, weaker health and safety laws.
- *Increased Criminal Penalties*—Currently employers can be fined up to $70,000 and face six months in jail for willful violations that result in death or serious injury. Under COSHRA, the maximum penalty for a willful violation causing death would be increased to $250,000 ($500,000 for corporations) and *up to ten years in jail.*
- *Mandatory Standards*—The proposed law *requires* OSHA to issue standards according to a fixed timetable to deal with such problems as ergonomic hazards, exposure monitoring, medical surveillance, and indoor air quality.

- *Victims Rights*—Victims of workplace accidents and their families would for the first time be given input into the OSHA enforcement process.

These are some of the provisions in the Comprehensive Occupational Safety and Health Act, introduced in Congress on August 1, 1991, just about a month before the fire in Hamlet, North Carolina. Such legislation is expected, like national health care reform, to take some years to enact, in a process involving political organizing and public education. But also like health care reform legislation, proponents of the legislation expect it to have a major effect on protecting and improving the lives of millions of Americans.

Criminal Prosecution of Dangerous Employers

While occupational health and safety activists continue their struggles to reform and strengthen federal OSHA, criminal prosecution of negligent employers continues at state and local levels.

For several years during the early 1980s, as local and state prosecutors indicted employers for crimes which OSHA refused to prosecute, federal officials attacked these efforts, arguing that the federal OSHA Act, with its weak civil and criminal penalties, preempted state and local prosecution of employers. The federal officials maintained that state and local prosecution on top of federal OSHA enforcement amounted to double jeopardy for employers. State and local prosecutors argued in turn that the federal law was essentially a civil law to prevent unsafe practices in the workplace, not a law to punish workplace criminals. Besides, they noted, OSHA doesn't enforce the few criminal provisions in the federal law—not one single employer has yet to be sent to jail during the entire two decades-long existence of OSHA, and few have even been criminally indicted.

Recently, in an important series of state and federal court decisions, this legal question has been decided: Federal OSHA does not preempt state and local prosecution of criminal actions in the workplace. In the late 1980s, and early 1990s, the highest courts in Illinois, Maine, Michigan, New York, and Texas have upheld such state health and safety prosecutions. (BNA, 1992b) In addition, in the *Chicago Magnet Wire Corporation* case heard in Illinois—where corporate executives were indicted for attacking employees by knowingly and unnecessarily exposing them to high levels of toxic workplace chemicals—the US Supreme Court refused to hear an appeal of the Illinois Supreme Court ruling upholding the state's right to prosecute. (BNA, 1992b) The US Supreme Court thereby upheld the state court's decision.

This leaves intact prosecutions and criminal convictions of employers in such notorious cases as Pymm Thermometer Company in New York City, in which two employers were fined $10,000 and sent to jail for weekends for six months for poisoning their employees with toxic mercury vapors.

Worker Training and Education Programs

Another important, positive development in worker health and safety in recent years has been the establishment and growth of worker training and education programs. Four states—Michigan, New York, Connecticut, and Maine—have created worker health and safety training funds, in most cases through a small tax (0.2 percent to 0.5 percent) on workers compensation premiums. The programs distribute anywhere from $200,000 in Maine to about $4 million in New York State in training grants to labor unions, local Committees for Occupational Safety and Health (COSH groups), hospitals, local government health and safety agencies, and private employers. Efforts are currently under way to enact similar programs in other states. These could be an important stimulus to grassroots health and safety activities by union locals and in local communities.

Health and Safety Issues for the 1990s

In addition to passing an OSHA reform law and building worker training programs, a number of important health and safety issues facing particular groups of workers need to be addressed in the 1990s. Among them are:

• *The health problems of the unemployed*—With official unemployment figures hovering between 7 and 8 percent of the US workforce, and true unemployment perhaps twice as high, working people must cope with the physical and psychological consequences of stress, such as high blood pressure and mental depression, while they seek new employment. These unemployed, with their numbers growing, are a permanent part of the US workforce. And just as the worker health and safety movement has addressed the wide range of health problems of the employed, so it must address those of the unemployed as well.

• *The health and safety problems of public employees*—Federal, state and local employees make up 15 percent of the US workforce, (US Dept. of Commerce, 1991) and are the fastest growing component of the US labor union movement, yet these employees receive little or no health and safety protection under existing federal and state OSHA laws. Their health and safety problems are serious, indeed they are equal in rate and intensity to those in the private sector (Kotelchuck and Barrett, 1991). Often their health and safety problems are unique, as in the personal security problems faced by guards and other personnel in mental institutions and prisons.

• *The health and safety problems of office and service workers*—Office workers face a growing number of hazards in their workplace, including carpal tunnel syndrome at computer typing stations, tight building syndrome, ergonomic problems associated with video display terminals, the health effects of persistent stress and various toxic chemical exposures in the workplace. Service workers are exposed to toxic cleaning and polishing compounds, asbestos dust in the bowels of large office and apartment buildings, and harmful biological agents causing AIDS, hepatitis B, and tuberculosis in hospital and nursing home facilities.

• *The health and safety problems of women and minority workers*—Women currently make up about 45 percent of the US workforce, and suffer both the ordinary health and safety problems of other workers, as well as special problems associated with pregnancy, childbirth, and frequently the lion's share of childcare. Black and Hispanic workers together make up about 18 percent of the US workforce, and these numbers are growing. They often work at the most hazardous, least desirable, lowest paying jobs due to historical patterns of racial discrimination. Health and safety activists must direct themselves to these problems. These are our brothers and sisters, and the struggle for minority workers' health and safety rights is part of the larger struggle against racial discrimination in our society.

NOTES

AFL-CIO, "North Carolina Fire Sparks a National Outcry," *AFL-CIO News* (Sept. 16, 1991) p. 1.

AFL-CIO, "OSHA Inspection Once-in-a-Lifetime Experience, Study Says," *AFL-CIO News* (May 11, 1992a) p. 1.

AFL-CIO, Dept. Occ. Safety and Health, *Death on the Job: The Toll of Neglect* (AFL-CIO, 1992b) Ch. II.

AFL-CIO, *op. cit.*, (AFL-CIO, 1992c) p. 6.

AFL-CIO, *op. cit.*, (AFL-CIO, 1992d) p. 3.

Bureau of Labor Statistics (BLS), *Survey of Occupational Injuries and Illness in 1985* (Nov. 13, 1986) Table 3.

BLS, *Bureau of Labor Statistics News* (Nov. 19, 1991a) Table 6.

BLS, *Survey of U.S. Occupational Injuries and Illness in 1990* (Nov. 19, 1991b) Table 3.

Bureau of National Affairs (BNA), *BNA Occupational Safety and Health Reporter*, Vol. 20 (1990) p. 1164.

BNA, *op. cit.*, Vol. 21 (1992) pp. 1137–39.

Greaves, Ian, "Appropriations for NIOSH," testimony before the House Appropriations Subcommittee on Labor-HHS-Education (April 28, 1991)

Kotelchuck, David, "Lost-Time Injuries More Severe," *UE News* (United Electrical Workers Union, Feb. 23, 1987) p. 15.

Kotelchuck, David, "Why Did They Lock the Doors?" *UE News* (Oct. 4, 1991) p. 15.

Kotelchuck, David, "Job Injury Rates Climb . . . And Climb . . . And Climb," *UE News* (Jan. 10, 1992) p. 15.

Kotelchuck, David, and Charles Barrett, *Occupational Injury and Illness Rates Among State and Local Public Employees (1980–1988)*, talk at APHA National Conference (1991).

Labor Research Assn., "OSHA—Who's in Charge?" *Economic Notes*, Vol. 55 (Mar.–Apr., 1987) p. 2.

US Dept. of Commerce, *Statistical Abstract of the United States: 111th edition* (USGPO, 1991) p. 401.

SHREDDING THE SAFETY NET:
The Dismantling of Public Programs

Nancy F. McKenzie and Ellen Bilofsky

Despite the promise of Ronald Reagan's budget director, David Stockman, in 1981 that they would preserve a safety net for the nation's needy, monumental and continuing cuts in what might be called the "safety net" programs—programs that guarantee a minimal standard of living in terms of food, shelter, and health care for the poor—have taken place over the last decade. And these already decimated programs are being further dismantled just when they are needed more than ever to offset the effects of the current recession.

This overview of the safety net essentially assumes that the anti-poverty programs of the 1960s and 1970s worked in keeping people poised above abject poverty. And they did. The programs did not bring people permanently out of poverty by giving them economic independence, but they did keep them from starvation and death's door. What is different now is the level of immiseration to which individuals are allowed to sink. In the last 10 years, while economic conditions for the poor have deteriorated, discretionary programs intended by Congress to target poverty and disease have been gutted.

The only major program that has held its own financially in the last 11 years has been food assistance, with a modest expansion of the Special Supplemental Food Program for Women, Infants, and Children (WIC). But, as in other entitlement programs, changing eligibility criteria have shut many people out of federal food programs, even as some specific groups were targeted for special assistance. The story of entitlements for those in need is not a seamless one, but, overall, the federal government has given with one hand and taken back with the other. Starting in the early 1980s, the progress toward eliminating hunger in this country that began in the late 1960s with WIC, food stamps, school meals, and food programs for the elderly began to be reversed by a combination of economic factors and budget cuts in discretionary programs.[1]

All safety net programs have been cut, failed to keep pace with inflation, or have lost their effectiveness in the face of the population's multiplying needs. The longer these needs remain unmet, the harder it becomes to reverse the trend (see Figure 1). And, economic and social conditions, exacerbated by this dwindling of public benefits and resources, tend to make health and health care delivery a focal concern of the poor.

Unemployment, for example, is a major correlate of ill health because it undermines a person's ability to address physical needs—either directly, through food and shelter, or indirectly through medical care. Inadequate housing is also

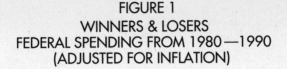

FIGURE 1
WINNERS & LOSERS
FEDERAL SPENDING FROM 1980—1990
(ADJUSTED FOR INFLATION)

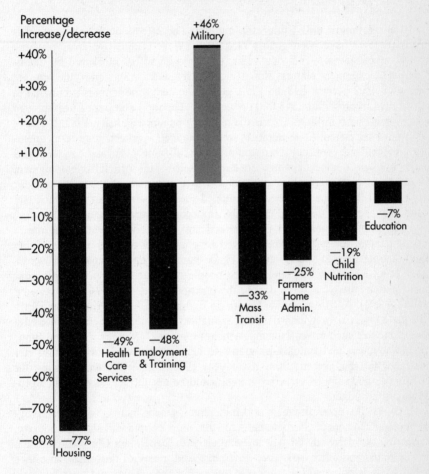

Reprinted from Jobs with Peace Campaign, Boston, MA.

Source:
OMB (Office of Management and Budget) Watch, Washington, DC.

a major factor in the destruction of health. The poor currently divert a huge proportion of their income to housing—78 percent in 1986.[2] And lack of housing is not only a cause of disease but is a major obstacle to people's attempts to regain their health by obtaining health services. When cuts in health services are added to unemployment, homelessness, and the illness consequent upon them, a line to recovery is broken. Many individuals become irretrievably lost to social and health services. And the sum of their neglect (in the devastation of individuals and their communities) is greater than its parts.

Economic Backdrop

Unemployment and Underemployment. The effects of the recession that began in 1989 have been greatly magnified by the cumulative erosion of the safety net programs—and vice versa. Unemployment (as measured by unemployment insurance claims alone) was fairly low going into the current recession—5.3 percent in June 1990. But in the next nine months it climbed to 6.8 percent, representing 543,000 new claims. The total number of unemployed is now nearly 8.6 million. This is the highest rate since January 1983, the peak of the last recession.[3] The numbers of discouraged workers, long-term unemployed, part-time workers who would prefer full-time jobs, and the length of unemployment—none of which are represented by the official unemployment figures—are also increasing. And, to add to the burden of those looking for work, 1.5 million jobs have been eliminated since the summer of 1990, and that trend is expected to continue even after the economy recovers.[4]

In addition, because of tighter federal and state unemployment insurance regulations, far fewer of the unemployed are eligible for benefits or are receiving them than in the past and fewer qualify for extended benefits beyond 26 weeks. Only about 37 percent of unemployed people received benefits in 1990, compared with as many as 75 percent of the unemployed in the 1974–75 recession[5] (see Figure 2). According to the Center on Budget and Policy Priorities (CBPP), "in the 35 years for which data are available, the nation has never entered a recession with such a weak unemployment program."[6] Moreover, federal funds for employment and training programs to help jobless workers find new employment fell 56 percent from fiscal year 1981 to 1991 (after adjusting for inflation)[7] and many of these programs would be cut further under Bush's proposed 1992 budget.

Poverty. As unemployment and underemployment increase and unemployment insurance benefits become harder to get, more people will slip into poverty, increasing the demands on Aid to Families with Dependent Children (AFDC), food stamps, and other assistance programs. And, many of those who lose jobs will also be losing health insurance coverage for themselves and their families, adding to the pool of those with limited access to health care. Currently, 50 million Americans who have some insurance cannot afford complete health care; and some 33 million Americans, 40 percent of whom are members of racial and ethnic minority groups, and over 60 percent of whom are holding down full-time jobs, lack health insurance altogether. According to the Census Bureau, 13 percent of the population—11.7 percent of whites, 20.2 percent of blacks, and 26.5 percent of Hispanics—are uninsured.[8]

There have also been great changes in what employment represents. A full-time job no longer guarantees benefits or even economic security, particularly if a family has only one wage earner, and currently one-third of those employed

FIGURE 2
PERCENTAGE OF UNEMPLOYED RECEIVING BENEFITS
1970–1990

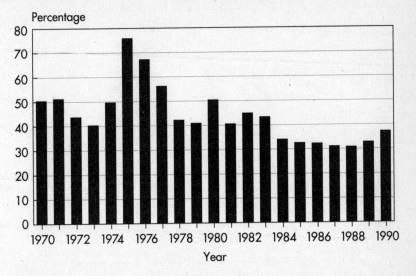

Reprinted from *A Painless Recession? The Economic Downturn and Policy Reponses.* Washington, DC: Center on Budget and Policy Priorities, 1991

Source:
Center on Budget and Policy Priorities and U.S. Department of Labor

in the United States are part-time or temporary employees. This means that they are largely cut out of job security or health and retirement benefits. The minimum wage has not kept pace with inflation, and real wages have declined across the board. According to CBPP, in 1990 average wages were at their "lowest level of purchasing power since 1964."[9] As the economy has shifted to low-paying, largely service-sector jobs (one-third of which are temporary or part-time), "half of all jobs created since 1980 fail to keep American families out of poverty."[10]

The poor were already hurting as we entered the current recession in 1989, with the US poverty rate at 12.8 percent. Although this was down from the previous high of 15.2 percent during the 1983 recession (see Figure 3), this "recovery" figure is higher than it was at any time in the 1970s and is only the starting point for the current downturn.[11] Poverty, of course, does not affect all segments of the population equally: In 1984, the average income of blacks was 57 percent that of whites.[12] Moreover, the criteria used to establish the official poverty level, as we know, creates an artificially low standard. Currently, the federal poverty level is set at an annual income of $6,280 for an individual, $8,420 for a family of two, and $12,700 for a family of four. Is it necessary to

FIGURE 3
POVERTY RATE 1970–1989

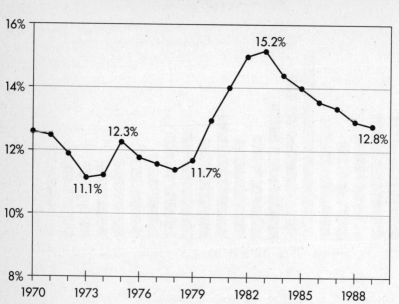

Reprinted from *A Painless Recession? The Economic Downturn and Policy Responses.* Washington DC: Center on Budget and Policy Priorities, 1991

Source:

U.S. Census Bureau

state that without additional assistance, more than 31 million Americans living on $6,280 or less per individual translates into hunger, homelessness, and sickness?

As already noted, federal and state budget cuts have taken their toll on unemployment insurance, the government's "first line of defense during a recession."[13] Moreover, two forms of cash assistance to the poor, AFDC and state or local general assistance programs, have been cut back over the last decade. A single-parent family of three living at 75 percent of the poverty level that was eligible for AFDC benefits in 42 states in 1980, would today qualify for benefits in only nine. Maximum AFDC benefits for a three-person family fell 39 percent from 1970 to 1990 (adjusting for inflation), and 18 percent from 1980 to 1990.[14]

But the cutback in benefits is not the only gauge of the jeopardy for the nation's poor. In addition, the length of time individuals, families, and communities have suffered from unemployment, housing, and multiple medical needs, as well as the degree of their current immiseration, affects the possibility of their recovery from impoverishment. According to Brown and Gershoff, government programs to aid the poor are less effective than they were 12 years ago.

"In 1979, almost one of every five families with children who had incomes below poverty was lifted above poverty by federal cash benefits programs. By 1986, that ratio had dropped to one of every nine families."[15] Whole communities have been affected by federal policy on employment, housing, and health care (see "Contagious Urban Decay and the Collapse of Public Health," on p. 167).

New Cuts. Bush's current budget proposals promise more of the same. The budget would slash $46.6 billion in benefit payments to individuals in the next five years. Although these cuts—in Medicare, veterans' benefits, school lunches, farm subsidies, and student loans—were framed as targeting mainly middle- and upper-class individuals, they will nonetheless further undermine already vulnerable populations.

Where the Cuts Are

Housing and Communities. A major factor in the current health care crisis is the loss of federal subsidies for low-income housing and housing assistance programs. Between 1980 and 1992 (if Bush's latest cuts go through), total housing and community development assistance will have fallen by 63 percent when adjusted for inflation (see Figure 4). These losses include a more than 50 percent decrease in community development block grants, the elimination of urban development grants, and a 61 percent decrease in Section 8 lower income housing subsidies. Rural programs for housing declined by 75 percent. As the table shows, these cuts have targeted those groups most likely to have multiple health needs—low-income inner-city and rural communities and the elderly, handicapped, and homeless.

Health Care. Health program funding showed large and definitive declines over the decade, with the exception of Medicare and Medicaid entitlements and specific infusions for crisis responses in 1990 and 1991. Indeed, some of the most effective and important health programs have already been eliminated.

Neighborhood health clinics, for example, were established in the 1960s and 1970s with direct grants from the federal government under the Office of Economic Opportunity. Some of them were later funded by the Public Health Service and specifically mandated to serve pregnant women as well as children. The clinics were directly responsible for the decreases in excess mortality and infant death rates that began to occur in the 1960s. At the high point of federal support there were one-third more community clinics than there are now. Many clinics still remain, but their funding is largely through Medicaid benefits, which hardly cover costs, although some receive county, city, or state funds.

These community clinic programs received a welcome boost from the National Health Service Corps. This federal program of support for physicians had three parts: medical scholarships for individuals willing to work in community clinics in underserved areas; loan forgiveness or payback of medical school costs to encourage physicians to locate in these communities; and direct payment of salaries for physicians working in community clinics. The programs were well established in the 1970s under the Emergency Health Personnel Act, but support was phased out in the late 1970s and early 1980s and, finally, ended altogether

FIGURE 4
SELECTED HUMAN SERVICES BUDGET, FISCAL YEARS 1980–1992[a]

Budget Authority	Budget Amount (in millions of dollars)		Percentage change FY 80–92	Real growth (percent) FY 80–92
	FY 1980	FY 1992		
Health				
Medicare	$32,911.0	$113,811.0	245.8	103.0
Community Health Centers	260.0	478.2	83.9	8.0
Family Planning	147.3	150.0	1.8	– 40.2
Maternal/Child Health Block Grants	424.0	553.6	30.6	– 23.4
Alcohol/Drug/Mental Health Block Grants	565.5	1,311.8	132.0	36.2
Preventive Health Block Grants	88.2	107.5	21.9	28.4
Immunizations	32.4	257.8	695.7	367.1
AIDS-CDC Funding	—	494.6	—	—
AIDS Health Services	—	261.1	—	—
Food and Drug Administration	—	779.0	—	—
Subtotal: Health	34,428.4	118,204.6	243.3	101.6
Less: Medicare	1,517.4	4,393.6	189.5	70.0
Handicapped				
Handicapped Education	1,000.5	2,731.9	173.1	60.3
Vocational Rehabilitation	982.2	2,005.1	104.1	19.8
Developmental Disabilities (HHS)	62.2	102.3	64.5	3.4
Supplemental Security Income (SSI)	6,467.6	21,080.5	225.9	91.3
Subtotal: Handicapped	8,512.5	25,919.8	204.5	78.8

Employment and Training					
Job Training (JTPA/CETA)	6,369.8	4,035.9	–	36.4	–	62.6
JTPA/CETA Block Grants	3,342.0	1,778.5	–	46.8	–	68.8
Summer Youth Employment	2,334.7	682.9	–	70.7	–	82.8
Adult Job Training Grants	–	1,088.0	–			
Youth Job Training Grants	–	1,337.6	–			
Dislocated Workers	–	527.0				
Federally Administered Programs	693.1	184.3	–	73.4	–	84.4
Job Corps	–	866.2				
Unemployment Compensation	16,440.3	26,800.0		63.0	–	4.3
Subtotal: Employment and Training	22,810.1	30,853.9		35.3	–	20.8
Community Development and Housing					
Community Development Block Grants	3,752.4	2,920.0	–	22.2	–	54.3
Urban Development Action Grants	675.0	0.0	–	100.0	–	100.0
Lower-Income Housing/Section B	23,675.5	15,862.6	–	33.0	–	60.7
Elderly/Handicapped Housing	805.9	152.8				
Public and Indian Housing	6,680.0	2,240.8	–	63.8	–	78.7
Rural Rental Assistance	393.0	611.0		55.5	–	8.7
Rural Housing Programs	4,166.2	1,774.0	–	57.4	–	75.0
Rural Development Programs	–	896.0				
HOPE, Shelter Plus Care	–	2,147.3				
Homeless Programs	–	535.7				
HOME Block Grant	–	1,000.0				
Tenant Ownership LIREEP	–	946.9				
Subtotal: Community Development & Housing	39,342.1	24,637.2	–	37.4	–	63.2

FIGURE 4
SELECTED HUMAN SERVICES BUDGET, FISCAL YEARS 1980–1992ᵃ (cont.)

Budget Authority	Budget Amount (in millions of dollars)		Percentage change	Real growth (percent)
	FY 1980	FY 1992	FY 80–92	FY 80–92
Low-Income Entitlements				
Medicaid	13,956.7	59,807.6	328.5	151.6
AFDC Benefits	8,113.3	12,135.0	98.5	16.5
Child Support Enforcement	384.5	626.0	62.8	— 4.4
Work Incentive/JOBS	357.5	1,000.0	179.7	64.2
Low-Income Energy Block Grants	1,846.5	1,025.0	— 44.5	— 67.4
Child Nutritionᵇ	(4,086.1)	(8,624.9)	111.1	23.9
WIC Supplemental Food	796.2	2,573.4	223.2	89.7
School Lunch Program	2,103.9	3,672.2	74.5	2.5
School Breakfast Program	247.0	721.9	192.3	71.6
Child Care Feeding Program	215.8	1,211.6	461.4	229.6
Summer Feeding Program	120.6	196.2	62.7	— 4.5
Commodities Procurement	445.8	226.6	— 49.2	— 70.2
Special Milk Program	156.8	23.0	— 85.3	— 91.4
Temporary Emergency Food Assistance	—	147.0	—	—
Food Stamps	9,181.6	19,650.0	114.0	25.6
Nutrition Assistance	—	1,013.0	—	—
Subtotal: Entitlements	31,840.1	95,403.6	199.6	75.9

ᵃBased on President George Bush's proposed 1992 budget, February 4, 1991.
ᵇFigures in parentheses are totals of included programs.

Source:
OMB Watch, Washington, DC, February 1991

in 1982. In 1990, the National Health Service Corps was reauthorized and given a substantial appropriation. And in 1989 some meager funds were also put back into the recruitment and education of minority health professionals.

Under Bush's current plan, funding for family planning clinics will have been reduced by 40 percent (in real dollars) between 1980 and 1992. In 1992, Bush proposes to cut grants for health professional education by 76 percent, and health services to those living in congregate housing would be eliminated altogether.[16] Alcohol, drug, and mental health programs grew by 36 percent from 1980 to 1992, but this gain was almost entirely related to drug monitoring, interdiction, and control. Bush is proposing that federal grants for advocacy for the mentally ill and mental health clinical training programs be eliminated altogether in 1992. And the President plans no additional funding for AIDS health services in 1992, which in real dollars represents a 4 percent decrease of an already grossly inadequate response to the epidemic.

The only major increase for health services in Bush's 1992 budget is for immunization. His proposal for a program to fight infant mortality in ten cities created an uproar when he announced plans to fund it in part by cutting $24 million from community health centers and $34 million from Maternal and Child Health Services Block Grants. Congress rejected this plan and instead appropriated $25 million for the campaign in fiscal year 1991. However, Bush still wishes to divert money from these programs in 1992, despite their proven effectiveness in aiding low-income communities and individuals.[17] If Bush's proposals go through, block grants for maternal and child health, as well as for preventive health, will have declined by about a fourth over the decade, although some of these losses are recouped by the expanded eligibility for maternal and child health within Medicaid programs.

Medicaid and Medicare

The only exceptions to the marked decrease in federal support are the entitlement programs, such as AFDC and Medicaid, whose funding is mandated for every eligible individual. The budget increases in these programs actually indicate trouble, however—either that more people are entitled to benefits and are enrolled or that inflation has increased the cost of the coverage. Over the last 11 years, coverage in these programs has become thinner in many states, since the states have discretion over the level of poverty at which benefits begin. There is also wide variation in the kinds of coverage or eligibility an individual receives under Medicaid. New York, for instance, which has a very progressive policy, covers almost all health care costs, while Alabama allows individuals access to Medicaid only if family income is below $1,700.

There have been constant attempts by the federal administration to control costs for both Medicaid and Medicare, but the cutbacks have not been instituted with the ferocity that they have been in other benefit programs. This has to do with the fact that the constituency for Medicaid and Medicare is not only the poor and elderly but also medical providers, who have resisted cuts in reimbursement for their programs.

Although funding for Medicaid has increased in real dollars by 152 percent between 1980 and Bush's 1992 proposals, it only covers 38 to 40 percent of the poor. Unlike Medicare, it is not indexed to inflation in most states. And, as recent analyses point out, having Medicaid is not synonymous with access to medical care when, for instance, only 25 percent of doctors in New York State participate in the program, even though New York State itself is one of the most vigorous supporters of public benefits through Medicaid.[18] Moreover, more than 60 percent of Medicaid benefits nationwide go to nursing home residents who have exhausted their resources.[19]

Besides the fact that only 40 percent of Medicaid goes to the poor, the benefits they finally receive may be altered by the way states seek to control their mandated participation in the programs offered to their residents. States can and have made large gains in balancing budgets that were drastically reduced by the withdrawal of federal funds by juggling Medicaid funds. Where benefits are mandated by federal programs, for example, states are trying to make compensatory cuts in optional benefits. Recent federal rules mandated increased benefits for maternal and children's health services to take place in July. To compensate, some states are proposing cuts in optional services such as dental, optometric, podiatric, and chiropractic care and hospice care for the terminally ill, as well as in optional coverage of people who are not poverty stricken but whose resources have been depleted by high medical bills.[20] Others are seeking federal waivers to reorganize "priorities" within Medicaid benefits to their residents. And it is now a well-established practice for states to try to cut down on Medicaid health costs by subcontracting services through increasingly mandatory prospective payment programs.

Medicare spending has increased enormously in the past 11 years, but there has been a drastic cutback in what a Medicare dollar buys in yearly health care costs. Medicare A (part one of the Medicare Trust Fund) pays for hospitals and completely covers elderly and disabled beneficiaries. Individuals must purchase Medicare B—the "major medical" part that pays for doctor care, preventive care, and some limited long-term care. Besides the monthly premiums, they must also pay out-of-pocket co-payments and deductibles. As a result, Medicare may, in fact, cover only 60 percent of beneficiaries' yearly health care costs. The Secretary of Health has the option to increase Medicare co-payments and deductibles, and this option has been exercised repeatedly over the last 11 years.

In late 1990, Bush signed legislation to cut Medicare payments to hospitals, doctors, laboratories, and suppliers of medical equipment by $32 billion over five years. Then, in February, he proposed $23 billion of additional cuts, the largest of which would be in payments to private teaching hospitals, which serve greater numbers of poor, inner-city, and sicker patients.[21] As these cuts limit access to urban teaching hospitals, more of the poor will be shunted to the nation's public hospitals, another weakening segment of the safety net.

Transferring the Burden

Reagan's "new federalism" shifted much of the burden for maintaining the safety net to the states (and Bush's 1992 budget includes additional new federalism proposals), without a concomitant shift in resources. This "transfer" has amounted to an abandonment of federal responsibility. And the states are not going to be able to pick up the slack from federal budget cuts. On the contrary, state and local budgets are being squeezed as never before by contracting revenues and cuts in federal grants. Between 1980 and 1990, federal funds as a percentage of city budgets declined by 64 percent, from an average of 17.7 percent to 6.4 percent in 1990.[22]

Moreover, most states are required by law to balance their budgets. Thus, the *New York Times* reports that "legislators in almost every state have considered cuts in health, welfare or housing programs, even as the demand for assistance rises."[23] The programs being targeted are, as already noted, some of the most basic safety net programs supporting the poorest of the poor—AFDC, Medicaid, and certain housing programs.

The Arena of Last Resort

Concern over access to health care has increased in recent years along with the dramatic increases in the numbers of the uninsured and the almost impossible burden placed on public hospitals. As this brief review tries to make clear, this is the result of an unprecedented confluence of factors, as increasing health care costs converge with the federal government's decreasing political willingness to offer a financial response and with a new level of impoverishment and immiseration that is affecting the health status of low-income communities.

It is not surprising, then, that America's public hospital system is operating at a great deficit. Members of the National Association of Public Hospitals (NAPH)—over 100 hospitals across the country—averaged 30 percent operating deficits in 1988. Occupancy rates in these hospitals are over 80 percent, and the individuals served are those most affected by the worsening economy and distorted priorities of the United States over the last 11 years. Minority communities in particular rely on a shrinking number of providers, largely in emergency rooms. In inner-city hospitals, 50 percent of all admissions are through the emergency room.[24]

When individuals already affected by poverty and homelessness develop multiple health problems, and these affect their employability or their ability to hold on to their housing, recovery becomes almost impossible. As the downward spiral of loss of employment, food, and housing is hastened by the wholesale decimation of programs that kept people from going over a physical and emotional precipice, health care delivery becomes the last stop before the final outcome—which is, of course, death. When health care delivery itself becomes impoverished, it is unable to intervene effectively. Excess deaths and early debilitation are the results.

The end stage of this downward spiral, which got its momentum from the "new federalism" of the 1980s, is that the public hospitals and emergency rooms across the nation have become the repository of those individuals who are no longer kept from disease and death by a safety net of benefits. These refuges are themselves suffering a striking depletion as a result.[25]

The "new federalism" included more than the "dismantling" and "transferring" of federal programs. It also included "cost/benefit" policies—the term for deregulating the workplace and removing the environment from federal over-sight and responsibility and for the introduction of market principles into the federal services that remained. Like the institution of DRG (diagnostic-related group) categories for in-hospital treatment under Medicare financing in 1983, these strategies affected the poor and powerless directly in myriad untold ways. The tragedy of the era is being borne now largely by the poor, by workers, by families, and by communities of color.

On the occasion of Ronald Reagan's election in 1980, progressives across America were outraged at the new "trickle down" ideology, fearing that the new order would substantially harm the poor. Few, however, no matter how long their view, foresaw how far-reaching the effects would be. Today, as we witness the substitution of shelters and streets, prisons and hospitals, for com-munities, jobs, and housing, and see death becoming the baseline of the new poverty, we are stunned by the magnitude of the devastation.

NOTES

1. Brown, J. Larry, and Gershoff, Stanley N., "The Paradox of Hunger and Economic Pros-perity in America," *Journal of Public Health Policy*, Winter 1989:10(4), pp. 425–443.

2. Ibid., p. 436.

3. Unemployment was 10.7 percent in January 1983. The worst unemployment since the 1930s was 10.8 percent in the 1981–82 recession. Uchitelle, Louis, "New Jobless Claims at 8-Year High," *New York Times*, April 4, 1991; and Hershey, Robert D., Jr., "Jobless Rate Rose to 6.8% in March, Highest Since 1986," *New York Times*, April 6, 1991.

4. Robert McFadden, "Degree and Stacks of Resumes Yield Few Jobs for Class of '91," *New York Times*, April 22, 1991.

5. Clynes, Adam, "Jobless Issue Proves Puzzle to Democrats," *New York Times*, April 28, 1991.

6. Shapiro, Isaac, and Greenstein, Robert, *A Painless Recession? The Economic Downturn and Policy Responses*, Washington, DC: Center on Budget and Policy Priorities.

7. Ibid., p. 19.

8. Bureau of the Census, U.S. Department of Commerce, *Current Population Survey: Annual Demographic File*, Washington, DC: U.S. Government Printing Office, 1988; Inter-university Con-sortium for Political and Social Research, Ann Arbor, MI, 1988; and Lewin, Tamar, "High Medical Costs Hurt Growing Numbers in U.S.," *New York Times*, April 28, 1991.

9. Shapiro and Greenstein, op. cit., p. 7.

10. Brown and Gershoff, op. cit., p. 432.

11. Shapiro and Greenstein, op. cit., p. 4; and Brown and Gershoff, op. cit. The number of officially poor in 1983 was 31.5 million. In 1989, each additional percentage point in the poverty rate represented 2.5 million people. With today's larger population, even though the poverty rate is lower, about 31 million people are still living below the poverty line.

12. National Research Council, *A Common Destiny: Blacks and American Society*, Washington, DC: National Academy Press, 1989.

13. Shapiro and Greenstein, op. cit., p. 15.

14. Ibid., p. 18.

15. Brown and Gershoff, op. cit., p. 436.

16. "FY 92 Bush Budget Proposal, Human Service Winners and Losers at a Glance," *OMB Watcher*, February 4, 1991, p. 7.

17. Pear, Robert, "Spurning Bush, Congress Provides New Money to Fight Infant Deaths," *New York Times*, March 26, 1991.

18. Kolbert, Elizabeth, "New York's Medicaid Costs Surge, But Health Care for the Poor Lags," *New York Times*, April 14, 1991.

19. Lillie-Blanton, L. "Medicare and Medicaid Program Barriers in Meeting Minority Health Care Needs," in *Access and Health Care Financing Alternatives for Minority Populations: A Chal-lenge for the 21st Century,"* Washington, DC: Office of Minority Health, 1990.

20. Pear, Robert, "States Struggle, Needs Rise: A Double Dose of Pain for the Poor," *New York Times*, April 7, 1991.

21. Pear, Robert, "President to Seek $23 Billion Savings in Medicare Costs," *New York Times*, February 3, 1991.

22. *City Fiscal Conditions. 1980–1990: A 50-City Survey*, Washington, DC: United States Conference of Mayors, January 1991, p. 3.

23. Pear, "States Struggle, Needs Rise: A Double Dose of Pain for the Poor."

24. *America's Safety Net Hospitals: The Foundation of Our Nation's Health System*, Washington, DC: National Association of Public Hospitals, January 1991.

25. See ibid., especially p. 4.

FROZEN IN ICE: FEDERAL HEALTH POLICY DURING THE REAGAN YEARS

Geraldine Dallek

Government can err, presidents do make mistakes, but the immortal Dante tells us that divine justice weighs the sins of the cold-blooded and the sins of the warm-hearted in different scales. Better the occasional faults of a government that lives in a spirit of charity than the constant omission of a government frozen in the ice of its own indifference.

—President Franklin Roosevelt
Acceptance Speech, June 1936

President Reagan came to office in 1981 with a specific health care agenda. He claimed he would cut federal programs without harming the "truly needy," transfer responsibility to the states and voluntary sector, control health care costs, and eviscerate federal regulations while giving competition free rein. After seven and a half years of the Reagan presidency, it is time to look back and assess how well he succeeded; the changes wrought because of, or despite, the Reagan agenda; and where we stand today as we look forward to the post-Reagan era.

The Reagan years have been marked by a government that cared little about the basic needs of its people, one "frozen in the ice of its own indifference." As a consequence, the nation has lost ground in its efforts to build a more decent health care system. Yet, despite the losses under Reagan, the people of the United States continue to believe in the idea of health care as a right. The goal for the post-Reagan years will be to make that idea a reality.

Federal Programs

The Poor

In the first flush of its perceived mandate to cut government fat, the Reagan administration successfully slashed health care programs for the poor. The Omnibus Budget Reconciliation Act of 1981 cut 25 percent from the budgets of most categorical health programs. It also set in place a rolling reduction of federal Medicaid matching funds—3 percent in 1982, 4 percent in 1983, and 4½ percent in 1984. Moreover, a 10 percent decrease in AFDC (Aid to Families with Dependent Children) coverage for the working poor in 1982 led some 700,000 children to lose their Medicaid coverage. States, hard pressed by the

1982 recession, responded to federal Medicaid cuts with cuts of their own. As a result, large numbers of Americans lost access to medical care.[1]

After the early Reagan years, Congress and the states lost their appetite for more Medicaid cuts. Nevertheless, today state Medicaid programs cannot adequately meet the needs of the poor for medical care. When the Washington-based Health Research Group of Public Citizens released a report in December 1987 ranking the performance of the 50 state Medicaid programs in terms of eligibility, services, and reimbursement policies,[2] no one was more surprised than advocates in California to learn that their state had one of the best Medicaid programs in the nation. After all, they had just sued the state for inadequate services. If best is inadequate, then worst (Mississippi) is dismal indeed.

State Medicaid programs ration care for the poor in subtle and not-so-subtle ways. Historically, rationing is hidden behind low reimbursement rates or utilization controls.[3] At least one state—Oregon—though, has a written policy of denying transplants to Medicaid beneficiaries and using the money saved to increase prenatal care.[4] This tradeoff makes sense from a Medicaid perspective. However, by making explicit what had been implicit, this policy brought the rationing of care to public attention as a serious ethical issue. Unlike these Medicaid recipients, privately insured children and adults are not denied life-saving operations; nor, as has happened in Oregon, are they forced to launch media campaigns—become television beggars—to raise thousands of dollars, or to leave their homes in search of a state with a more generous Medicaid program.[5]

After the 1981 budget cuts in Medicaid and categorical health programs, Reagan hit a solid brick wall of congressional and state opposition to further reductions in health programs for the poor. Remember the Medicaid "cap"— the proposed 3 percent reduction in states' federal Medicaid reimbursement— and attempts to make Medicaid co-payments mandatory? Probably not (how quickly we forget our victories), as Reagan's later efforts to slash federal health care programs arrived in Congress with small chance of survival. As Medicaid celebrated its twentieth anniversary in 1985, the program seemed to have become sacrosanct—off limits to both Gramm-Rudman and budget cuts.

Moreover, Medicaid underwent a dramatic broadening of its base when Congress, in the Omnibus Budget Reconciliation Acts of 1986 and 1987, severed the program's link with welfare. No longer is income eligibility for welfare the measure by which Medicaid coverage is granted. States now have the option of providing Medicaid to infants and pregnant women with family incomes up to 185 percent of the poverty level, as well as to children under 5, the aged, the blind, and the disabled with incomes up to 100 percent of the poverty level. Congress has not backed away from the fundamental promise of Medicaid—as an entitlement program for the poor.

Unfortunately, Medicaid's promise is meaningless for the millions of poor and near-poor who do not qualify for the program. The continuing commitment to the program and Medicaid's projected $50 billion price tag for 1988 do not buy enough health care for the nation's under-served population.

Reagan has steadfastly maintained that his policies would not harm the "truly needy." Yet, through sins of commission and omission on the part of the government, the poor among us have been harmed. The Reagan administration has watched passively as the health care fortunes of this group plummet. Today, Medicaid covers significantly less than half the nation's poor, down from 63 percent in 1975. Over 37 million citizens (17 percent) have no health insurance and little access to health care.[6] A survey by the Robert Wood Johnson Foundation documents the dramatic decline in access to care among poor and minority populations between 1982 and 1986[7]—years during which Reagan promised no harm would come to the "truly needy."

The United States does not provide for even the simplest and most fundamental health care need—prenatal care. A recent study by the General Accounting Office found that 59 percent of women on Medicaid and 67 percent of uninsured women get insufficient prenatal care.[8] Since 1979, the number of babies born to mothers who received inadequate prenatal care grew by nearly 10 percent.[9] As a result, the nation's high infant mortality rate continues to haunt us.

The number of underinsured individuals who lack adequate protection from catastrophic illness is also growing[10] and, in all likelihood, will continue to grow in the years to come. According to a survey by the Bureau of National Affairs, 27 percent of employers plan to eliminate or reduce employee health insurance coverage during 1988.[11]

Some programs and providers serving the poor—community and migrant health centers, maternal and child health programs, and WIC agencies—have done fairly well, given federal budget limits. Other major sources of care—notably inner-city and rural public and private hospitals—are in serious financial trouble, often unable to provide their patients with a minimal level of services.[12] Thus, the poor and the health care institutions on which they depend fared badly during the Reagan years.

The Elderly

No federal health program underwent a more dramatic change during the Reagan years than Medicare. PPS, DRGs, "participating physicians," and CMPs were all added to the Medicare lexicon as the federal government experimented with ways to control Medicare costs. The jury is still out on what the various changes in Medicare reimbursement will ultimately mean for the elderly and those who care for them. Although anecdotal evidence suggests that at least some elderly patients were discharged "quicker and sicker," studies have found no systematic evidence of inappropriate discharges. Moreover, given past overutilization of hospital care it is also likely that the prospective payment system resulted in less unnecessary care.

There is no question, however, that the elderly lost ground on a number of other fronts during Reagan's term of office. Twenty-five percent of the elderly population have incomes below 150 percent of the poverty level.[13] According to the Commonwealth Fund's Commission on Elderly People Living Alone, two-thirds of poor elderly Americans are not covered by Medicaid and are spending nearly a quarter of their income on health care.[14]

Although policymakers have finally recognized that lack of long-term care insurance posed a financial catastrophe for the elderly, they did little but talk about the problem. As out-of-pocket costs increased both for services covered by Medicare as well as those not covered, the administration and Congress came close to passing a catastrophic insurance program. However, the proposal, awaiting likely enactment at the time of this writing, may not give enough bang for the buck; it ignores coverage for long-term care and contains a funding mechanism based on a means test that could ultimately undermine the program's broad political support.

Perhaps the most troubling feature of Reagan's Medicare proposal, a voucher system, never got off the ground. Medicare HMOs and competitive medical plans (CMPs), however, made a shaky[15] and, in one instance, criminal debut;[16] and a new program of MIGs (no, not Soviet fighter planes, but Medicare Insured Groups) holds as many pitfalls as promises.[17]

Overall, the government seemed to have trod the Medicare waters, obsessing about expenditures and recognizing unmet need, but unable to deal effectively with either.

AIDS

Sometimes individuals and governments can make up for past mistakes. The AIDS epidemic is not one of those instances. The $1.3 billion federal budget for AIDS proposed for fiscal year 1989 cannot buy back the years lost while the federal government did precious little to address the worst epidemic of our time. An unwillingness to spend federal dollars, coupled with homophobia, stupidity, and denial, has left us with an estimated one and a half million individuals infected with the AIDS virus, continued ignorance and misconceptions about the disease, and inestimable pain and suffering. The Reagan administration's apathy and inaction during the early years of the epidemic only fanned the flames of the contagion.[18] [See "Ignoring the Epidemic: How the Reagan Administration Failed on AIDS," *Health/PAC Bulletin*, Vol. 17, No. 2.]

The Budget Deficit and Public Opinion

Along with the early indifference to the AIDS epidemic, the Reagan budget deficit will haunt us for years to come. Ronald Reagan is the biggest, freest spender we have ever had in the White House. His tax cuts and military expansion leave us with a debt that future generations will struggle to repay.

With 20 percent of total federal spending going for interest payments on the $2.2 trillion national debt, and with a budget deficit sure to exceed the Office of Management and Budget's projected $128 billion for 1988, the Reagan years have changed the way we think about new entitlement programs. Now it's strictly pay as you go, and general revenues are off limits.

Although Congress is still willing to respond, albeit inadequately, to the most dramatic of domestic needs (research and education on AIDS and support for the homeless), any new entitlement program must rest on a specific funding source if it is to have a chance of success. Thus, no matter how great the need or desire for change, the nation will find it harder than ever to enact a national health insurance program. Moreover, the budget deficit will further limit the government's spending options when the next recession comes, as it surely will.

A counterweight to the negative effect of the budget deficit is the overwhelming and widespread support expressed by the American people for a more equitable health care system. That support is found not just in liberal places like Massachusetts, where a statewide poll in April 1987 found that 89 percent of those surveyed believed that access to health care is a basic human right and 79 percent were willing to pay higher state taxes to guarantee that right. It is also found in Orange County, California, one of the most conservative, bedrock Republican communities in the nation. A September 1987 poll found that 75 percent of those surveyed supported national health insurance, and 72 percent were willing to pay higher taxes to insure that the poor get necessary care.[19]

No matter who does the polls, the results are consistent. A nationwide poll sponsored by *Hospitals* magazine found that 69 percent of the population would pay higher taxes to provide health care for the indigent,[20] while 70 percent of Californians polled in a 1988 survey regard access to health care as a right.[21] And, in the guns-and-butter debate, military spending is now on the defensive; 71 percent of the public would rather see a reduction in the nation's defense outlays than cuts in federal expenditures for health.[22]

Americans' support for an expanded health care system may not be as solid as these polls indicate. The public continues to view Medicaid at least partially as a welfare program, making it vulnerable to future cutbacks in economic hard times.[23] In addition, US citizens do not consider health care among the most important problems facing the nation, and so may not be willing to put their money where their mouth is when it comes to increased taxes. Nevertheless, the American people remain committed to providing health care for those in need, and the administration's efforts to undermine support for government involvement in the financing of health care have failed miserably.

Transfer of Federal Responsibility

The States

Along with reducing federal health care programs, the Reagan administration repeatedly proposed giving more responsibility and flexibility in administering these programs to the states. Generally, efforts to transfer responsibility—labeled the "new federalism"—failed when states realized that they were a ploy to cut federal spending.

Yet, acting on their own, states assumed increased responsibility and used it well. After 1981 and 1982, the states' flexibility in administering Medicaid was used almost exclusively to expand rather than reduce coverage. Fears over how the states would use and misuse the 1981 block grants were also unfounded.

During the Reagan years, as the aftermath of the 1981 federal budget cuts and 1982 recession became visible, over 25 states studied the problems of the uninsured, and many enacted small but significant expansions of state programs. States increased medical services for low-income pregnant women, taxed insurers to pay for uncompensated hospital care, and established high-risk pools for the "uninsurable" population. Massachusetts passed "health care for all" legislation in April 1988, and the state of Washington is soon to pilot a state-subsidized program for the uninsured working poor.

States, of course, did not operate in a monolithic fashion. Some states, most notably California, cut back on programs for the poor, especially in the early part of the decade. Others misused the new flexibility and adopted Medicaid case management programs helter skelter, without adequately protecting access to care and quality of services. But, looking back over the years, it is fair to conclude that Reagan was at least partly right in this regard. States used their new flexibility well. Within the limited confines of their budgets, they attempted to fill the void left by the federal government's inaction.

Moreover, in a number of instances when states were unwilling or incapable of addressing a major problem, Congress stepped in. A case in point is the 1986 Omnibus Budget Reconciliation Act. By acting to regulate hospitals through tough anti-dumping penalties in the Medicare Act, Congress further advanced on territory traditionally left to the states. Likewise, federal requirements that employers offer continuation and conversion insurance policies encroached on what had heretofore been an area of state authority.

The Voluntary Sector

Reagan claimed that the voluntary sector—that is, private charitable organizations—would fill in any holes left in the safety net by federal and state governments. The president was partly correct in his assessment. Although it was specious to maintain, as he did, that private money and effort could replace the federal government's role in providing care for the needy, it was nonetheless true that the voluntary sector mobilized to serve those in greatest need. Activities of organizations serving the homeless or people with AIDS are only two cases in point.

Even the more traditional charitable organizations took on new projects to meet new problems. For example, the Robert Wood Johnson Foundation moved from its seemingly knee-jerk funding of large teaching hospitals and medical schools to support innovative community organizations serving the homeless and experimental programs to insure the uninsured.

And finally—although Reagan didn't have this in mind when he spoke of the voluntary sector—health advocacy grew during the 1980s. At the national level, the Villers Foundation, the National Health Care Campaign, and Citizen Action joined already established health advocacy organizations such as the Children's Defense Fund, the Gray Panthers, and the American Association of Retired Persons to push for change at the federal and state levels.

Statewide organizations have also begun to flex their muscles. The Massachusetts Health Action Alliance was a major force in the passage of the state's new health care legislation. Health Access in California and the Health Care For All Campaign in New York have also set their sights on statewide health care coverage. And new programs for uninsured pregnant women in a number of states (Massachusetts, Minnesota, South Carolina) were enacted only after long and arduous community campaigns.

Local advocacy organizations such as Staying Alive in Boston and the Committee to Save Cook County Hospital in Chicago have survived the 1980's, maybe not stronger, but as committed as ever to saving their public hospitals. Legal services, against all odds, also made it through the Reagan years. And, finally, progressive health advocacy organizations remain a symbol for advocates who have kept the faith that this nation will have a more just, equitable health care system.

Cost Containment

Only one item on the Reagan agenda garnered widespread support—the need to control health care costs. Unfortunately, cost-containment efforts during the Reagan years largely failed. In 1981, we spent 9.4 percent of the gross national budget—$287 billion—on health care. By 1987, spending had reached half a trillion dollars ($499 billion), 11.2 percent of the GNP. In each year of the Reagan administration, health care inflation far exceeded inflation in other areas of the economy.

The most dramatic of the president's efforts to control costs was Medicare's prospective payment system. Alan Sager of Boston University calls these jerking lurches to reform our health care system "policy by spasm." In 1984, we suddenly found ourselves inundated by a plethora of new acronyms and a basically untested scheme for reimbursing hospitals in the Medicare program.

Prospective payment systems (PPSs) and diagnosis related groups (DRGs) may have kept Medicare expenditures below what they otherwise would have been. Not even this is certain, though, as early DRG payments were excessive, and outpatient and ambulatory care costs went through the roof.[24] Moreover, Medicare Part B physician payments continued to increase at a 17 percent annual rate. And hospital and physician costs show few signs of abating: a recent survey of 1,863 hospitals found that hospital charges increased 19 percent in 1986.[25] During that same year, physicians' incomes jumped 6.5 percent.[26]

Insurance rates, too, are increasing at a phenomenal rate. At the beginning of 1988, insurance companies generally raised their premiums between 12 and 25 percent.[27] As we began the decade with a "crisis" in health care costs, so will we end it. We are today spending more money than ever, yet providing care to fewer Americans.

We may have controlled payments to some providers, but we haven't controlled costs. Today, we spend approximately 6 percent of our GNP on defense and 5 percent on hospital care. Efforts during the Reagan years, planted in infertile soil, have borne little fruit. Without doubt, the vertiginous heights to which health care spending has risen since 1981 are a major failure of the Reagan administration.

Competition and Deregulation

Reaganites who came to power in 1981 believed there was only one way to control health care costs—marketplace competition. An early spokesman for this view, David Stockman, wrote that the "liberal national health care policy" was built on a number of erroneous assumptions, including beliefs that the health care sector "can be efficiently and effectively regulated by government agencies and by bureaucratic mechanisms" and that "health care is unique"—a "sort of spiritual or social or collective good." Rather, Stockman argued, health care should be treated as an economic good "so that we can bring into play those self-regulatory, economizing, efficiency-producing mechanisms that we rely on in all other sectors." Stockman offered a simple prescription for the ills afflicting our health care system: "Enfranchise consumers" through cost-sharing, provide fixed rather than open-ended federal subsidies, encourage "at-risk" for-profit enterprise, promote a competitive "retail market" for health care, and build the entire health care system on a "laissez-faire" foundation "where government specifies nothing."[28]

Certainly, the Stockman cure has not worked. A growing number of HMOs and new preferred provider organizations (PPOs) did begin to compete with each other, but without any discernible overall savings in the health care system.[29]

For-profit hospital chains were the darlings of Wall Street in the first part of the decade, only to see their fortunes plummet after 1986. Today, few would argue that the growth of for-profit health care led to greater efficiency and lower costs.[30] Hospitals did compete, but not on the basis of price. Facilities, not-for-profit and for-profit alike, continued to expand and purchase the latest, most technologically advanced and expensive equipment, resulting in gross overcapacity.[31] Predictions by the likes of Stockman that such anti-competitive behavior would lead to bankruptcy now seem simplistic. The hospitals that closed in the 1980s were generally small, undercapitalized, inner-city and rural hospitals that served the poor, not the overcapitalized giants.[32]

Moreover, to the extent that hospitals did compete for business during the 1980s, this competition had a number of negative by-products: first, private insurers were less willing to subsidize the costs of caring for the indigent; second, the amount of money spent on advertising and marketing instead of patient care was vastly expanded; and, finally, hospital-controlled inpatient services and procedures were moved to the less regulated outpatient sector to make up for lost inpatient revenues through higher outpatient profits. As one economist put it, "The competitive market is an opponent, not an ally, of cost containment. When capacity increases, advertising and marketing increase, the boundaries of the system are expanded, duplication of costly services is encouraged, and the public is pushed to consume more health care services than it needs."[33]

The unwillingness of Medicare and private insurers to continue to subsidize hospital care for the poor has had particularly negative consequences. In Los Angeles, for example, the lack of reimbursement for emergency care provided to the uninsured poor has led a number of hospitals to opt out of the city's trauma system and close or limit their emergency rooms, resulting in a crisis for the entire community.[34]

Despite the failure of Reagan's broad agenda to increase free market competition, the way health care is organized has changed. The rapid growth of prepayment and managed care has transformed the health care landscape in ways that could not have been predicted in 1981. HMOs and their brethren hold promise for curbing overutilization and perhaps controlling costs. Further, the move away from the open-ended fee-for-service reimbursement system, with its incentives to provide unnecessary services, can only be viewed as positive. Although prospective payment and capitation have their own set of problems, the existing situation was no longer tenable.

The deregulators had some successes during the Reagan years, but these were few and far between. Early in the Reagan reign, 22 categorical health programs were combined into four block grants, and over 300 pages of regulation were eliminated from the *Federal Register*. However, Congress strongly resisted other efforts to slow down the regulatory machine, making almost yearly admonitions to a reluctant Department of Health and Human Services to issue congressionally mandated regulations. The administration simply got around these mandates by shoddy enforcement of regulations that did exist.

A second major success of the anti-regulators was the final elimination of federal health planning, with the failure to reauthorize funding for the Health Planning and Development Act of 1974. Although the program was not always successful in controlling the proliferation of the high-tech medical armamentarium, its demise has resulted in an orgy of hospital and nursing home expansion in a number of states. Health planning was also a useful tool to obtain concessions from providers to serve the poor.

Despite the anti-regulation rhetoric, the administration has not been averse to using federal regulation to suit its own purposes. Its attempts at price fixing of hospitals', and, lately, physicians' fees in the Medicare program are a far cry from the laissez-faire medical care system where "government specifies nothing," envisioned by Stockman.[35] If anything, Reaganites became regulatory hypocrites with their repeated attempts to use regulations to implement their own social agenda, especially in the matters of abortion, family planning, and protection of newborns with serious birth defects.

The most ardent of free-market advocates might argue that competition was not given a fair chance during the Reagan years. They would be right. Congress, and by extension, the American people, were not willing to go the competition route. Reagan proposed a revolutionary restructuring in our health care system. Americans, generally happy with their health care (although not the costs of that care),[36] were not willing to support this revolution. It appears that the American people do not believe that medical care should be a commodity and are unwilling to eliminate many of the anti-competitive underpinnings of our health care system.[37] David Kinzer of the Harvard University School of Public Health makes this point: "If and when our nation's political establishment responds to public sentiment about universal access to medical care, it should be obvious that more law and regulation are the inescapable corollary. Where citizens' rights are involved, only government can guarantee them."[38]

Quality of Care

Although the antiregulatory, pro-marketplace approach of the Reagan agenda was rejected, its emphasis led to a new interest in quality of care. Advocates of competition argued that if consumers were to make informed and rational decisions in the medical care marketplace, they would need information on quality as well as price. This competition-driven move to inform the medical care consumer, combined with a concern that capitated systems have incentives to skimp on needed care, a hope of saving money by reducing inappropriate care, and an awareness of the recurring medical malpractice crisis, sparked a new interest at the federal level in quality of care.

During the 1980s we made some progress in figuring out how to define and measure quality. Peer review organizations (PROs) replaced their weaker brothers, professional standards review organizations (PSROs), as the government's lead agencies to monitor the quality of care for the elderly. The Health Care Finance Administration (HCFA) released data on mortality rates of Medicare patients, despite furious opposition from the hospital industry and others who argued that the data did not adequately adjust for the varying types and severity of cases handled by the different hospitals.

Although still in their infancy, research attempts to measure quality and government efforts to use information about quality of care hold promise of a more rational and safer medical care system.

The Reagan Balance Sheet

Where have seven and a half years of Reagan's efforts to transform the health care system left us? The nation's health care system provides less for the poor and elderly today than it did when Reagan became president. The truly needy have been hurt and hurt badly. To the extent that they were tried, competition, deregulation, and for-profit medicine failed to control costs. State and voluntary efforts are not viable substitutes for federal health care programs and money. And Reagan's budget deficit may well slam shut the door to an expanded, more equitable health care system.

Yet, as we look forward to the post-Reagan years, there is cause for hope. Perhaps more than ever, Americans favor expanding health care to the poor and near poor; the elderly are mobilizing to fill in the substantial gaps in insurance coverage left by Medicare; insurers are moving away from an open-ended funding system that clearly did not control costs to, we can hope, something better; health care advocacy by states and community organizations is paying off in more care to the uninsured; and the nation has finally recognized the AIDS epidemic for what it is—a plague that threatens us all.

Unfortunately, the Reagan administration has also left us without a workable plan for the future. The nation is without a clear vision of where it wants the health care system to go, and, just as important, how to get there.

Thus, with the post-Reagan years upon us, we must take cognizance of the lessons of the Reagan era. First, a health care revolution is not in our future. Policy in this country changes slowly, step by incremental step. As the American people rejected the Reagan health care revolution, so will they reject any proposal that does not build on foundations previously laid, weak as they may be. The job before us is to shore up what we have and build from there.

Second, we must face the issue of health care rationing. If we hadn't realized it before Reagan, we certainly know it now: rationing of health care exists in its most insidious and inequitable form—based on income and race. Yet, we cannot afford to provide all that medical science is capable of. As ethicist James Callahan posits in his 1987 book, *Setting Limits: Medical Goals in An Aging Society*, it is time to begin the soul-searching process of deciding how much and for whom.

A continued emphasis on quality assessment will make that search much less difficult. This is the third lesson from the Reagan years. We must find a way to control the explosive growth of expensive high-tech machines and procedures that are of questionable value. A recent RAND Corporation study showed that 32 percent of carotid endarterectomies, an extremely high-risk and very expensive procedure, were inappropriate.[39] Such findings again underscore the need to regulate the introduction of new medical and surgical procedures and technology, much as we do drugs.

We also need quality assessment to prevent underutilization of medical resources. The increase in prepayment and managed care systems during the Reagan years raises new ethical dilemmas for physicians and hospitals by allowing them to make more by doing less. We now have the worst of all worlds for quality of care—where incentives to do too much and too little exist side by side.

Fourth, we must control costs if we are to expand care. It may be that, as HCFA predicts, Americans by 1990 will spend not 11 percent but 15 percent of our GNP on health care.[40] If for that extra 4 percent and $200 billion dollars we get better care for more people, the expense will be worth it. If, however, the nation spends those extra billions only to end up with the same system we have today, the American people will have been cheated. Although many of us may disagree with how the Reagan administration proposed to control costs, one could well argue that its emphasis on the issue was well placed.

Fifth, even as we turn our attention to federal efforts to expand health care, we must continue to pursue advocacy at the state level. Fears that granting states greater flexibility in setting health care policy would prove disastrous were not realized. The states have become our laboratories for experiments on the best way to provide health care for the most people. Only a few of these experiments need to be successful for us to learn the best approaches to reforming the federal system.

Finally, it's important to remember that individuals and organizations working for a more humane and decent health care system make a difference. There would be far less care for the poor and elderly today had advocates not fought hard against the worst excesses of Reagan policy.

We have survived the Reagan years. Unfortunately, the next few years do not look promising for reshaping our health care system. Costs are out of control, the number of uninsured seems likely to grow, the graying of America will make it even harder to address the needs of the elderly, and the specter of death and disease from AIDS haunts the nation. Yet, as we look to the 1988 election and a new presidency, anything is possible. If we keep working at it, America will have one day a "government that lives in the spirit of charity" and a health care system for all.

NOTES

1. Dallek, Geraldine, "Who Cares for Health Care? The First Two Years of Reagan Administration Health Policy," *Health/PAC Bulletin*, January–February 1983: 14(1), pp. 11–14.

2. Erdman, K., and S. Wolfe, *Poor Health Care for Poor Americans: A Ranking of State Medicaid Programs*, Washington, D.C.: Public Citizen Health Research Group, 1987.

3. For example, Alabama will pay for only 12 hospital days per year, 3 outpatient hospital visits per year, 12 physician days per year, and 8 well-child screenings from birth through age 21, including only one visit during the first year of life.

4. Kolata, Gina, "Increasingly, Life and Death Issues Become Money Matters: Who Gets Bone Marrow Transplants?" *New York Times*, March 20, 1988, p. E6.

5. Egan, Timothy, "Oregon Cut in Transplant Aid Spurs Victims to Turn Actor to Avert Death," *New York Times*, May 1, 1988, p. 12.

6. Employee Benefit Research Institute, March 1987 Current Population Survey.

7. Freeman, Howard, et al., "Americans Report on Their Access to Health Care," *Health Affairs*, Spring 1987, pp. 7–18; Access to Health Care in the United States: Results of a 1986 Survey, *Robert Wood Johnson Foundation Special Report*, No. 2, 1987, p. 10.

8. *Prenatal Care: Medicaid Recipients and Uninsured Women Obtain Insufficient Care*, Washington, D.C.: General Accounting Office, 1987. *See also* "Child Health: America's Next Challenge," *Medicine & Health Perspectives*, October 19, 1987.

9. *Facts on Infant Mortality*, National Commission to Prevent Infant Mortality, 1987.

10. Farley, Pamela, "Who are the Underinsured?" *Milbank Memorial Fund Quarterly/Health & Society*, 1985: 63, pp. 476–501.

11. *1988 Employer Bargaining Objectives*, Bureau of National Affairs, 1988.

12. "Public Hospitals Struggle to Stay Afloat," *Medicine & Health Perspectives*, November 23, 1987; Richards, Bill, "Many Hospitals Feel Financial Strain as More of Their Patients Need Public Aid," *Wall Street Journal*, May 3, 1988, p. 31. *See also* Dallek, Geraldine, with E. Richard Brown, *The Quality of Medical Care for the Poor in Los Angeles County's Health and Hospital System*, June 1987.

13. *Medicare's Poor*, The Commonwealth Fund Commission on Elderly People Living Alone, 1988.

14. "Poor Elderly Uninsured, Report Says," *Medicine & Health*, 41(44), November 9, 1987, p. 2.

15. At the end of 1987, 29 of 158 HMOs serving 80,000 Medicare beneficiaries on an at-risk basis terminated their HCFA contracts. "Medicare Loses 80,000 HMO Enrollees," *Medicine & Health*, 41(44), November 9, 1987, p. 1.

16. *Medicare and HMOs: A First Look, With Disturbing Findings*, Minority Staff Report, Select Committee on Aging, U.S. Senate, April 7, 1987; Iglehart, John, "Second Thoughts About HMOs for Medicare Patients," *New England Journal of Medicine*, 316(23), June 4, 1987, pp. 1487–1492.

17. Under the MIG program, employer-based plans are paid a capitated rate to provide health care benefits to Medicare beneficiaries affiliated with the employer's retirement plan. HCFA has contracted for several MIG demonstration projects.

18. For a description of the Reagan administration's AIDS policy, see Shilts, Randy, *And the Band Played On: Politics, People, and the AIDS Epidemic*, New York: St. Martin's Press, 1987.

19. Peterson, Susan, "Poll: 75% in OC Favor National Health Insurance," *Orange County Register*, September 22, 1987.

20. "Indigent Care: Public Wants Government to Pay," *Hospitals*, October 5, 1987, p. 152.

21. Parachini, Allan, "AIDS is No. 1 Health Issue in State Poll," *Los Angeles Times*, March 29, 1988, Part V, pp. 1–2.

22. Shriver, J. (ed.), "Federal Budget Deficit," *Gallup Report 1986*, pp. 244–245, cited in Blendon, Robert, "The Public's View of the Future of Health Care," *Journal of the American Medical Association*, forthcoming.

23. While polls show significant support for health care spending for the poor, they also show very limited support for welfare. Forty-one percent of the public believes that the nation spends too much on welfare. Thus, to the extent that Medicaid is tied to the welfare system, it remains vulnerable to the anti-welfare bias and to cutbacks. See ibid.

24. Kramon, Glenn, "Outpatient Strategy Fails to Cut Health Costs," *New York Times*, March 8, 1988, pp. 1, 35.

25. "Latest Survey Shows Hospital Charges Increasing Dramatically," *Health Lawyers News Report*, February 1988: 16(2), p. 2.

26. "Physician Income Up 6.5 Percent in 1986," *Medicine & Health*, November 30, 1987, p. 2.

27. *Health Lawyers News Report*, February 1988: 16(2), p. 4.

28. Stockman, David, "Premises For a Medical Marketplace: A Neoconservative's Vision of How to Transform the Health System," *Health Affairs*, 1981: 1(1), pp. 5–18.

29. Ginzberg, Eli, "A Hard Look at Cost Containment," *New England Journal of Medicine*, 316(18), April 30, 1987, p. 1152.

30. Ibid., p. 1153; Renn, S. C., C. J. Schramm, D. M. Watt, and R. Derzon, "The Effects of Ownership and System Affiliation on the Economic Performance of Hospitals," *Inquiry*, 1985: 22, pp. 219–236.

31. Although generally we have far too many hospital beds, in a number of communities, most notably New York City, as well as in large urban public hospitals, there are too few resources to meet community needs. See Lambert, Bruce, "Hospital Shortages Hurt Patient Care in New York," *New York Times*, March 22, 1988, p. 1.

32. Richards, Bill, op. cit.

33. Ginzberg, Eli, "The Destabilization of Health Care," *New England Journal of Medicine*, 315(12), September 18, 1986, p. 760.

34. Spiegel, Claire, "Three More Hospitals in L.A. Act to Cut Emergency Care," *Los Angeles Times*, May 4, 1988, Part 2, p. 1.

35. Kinzer, David, "The Decline and Fall of Deregulation," *New England Journal of Medicine*, 318(2), January 14, 1988, p. 113.

36. Blendon, op. cit., pp. 6–7.

37. For a description of microeconomic theory applied to the economics of health care, see Newhouse, Joseph, *The Economics of Medical Care*, Reading, Mass.: Addison-Wesley, 1978.

38. Kinzer, op. cit., p. 113.

39. Chassin, Mark, et al. "Does Inappropriate Use Explain Geographic Variations in the Use of Health Care Services? A Study of Three Procedures," *Journal of the American Medical Association*, 258(18), November 13, 1987, pp. 2533–2537; "Study Finds Overuse of Surgery Intended to Prevent Strokes in the Elderly," *New York Times*, March 24, 1988, p. 13.

40. "Health Care Spending: Growing Through the Year 2000," *Medicine & Health Perspectives*, June 22, 1987.

CONTAGIOUS URBAN DECAY AND THE COLLAPSE OF PUBLIC HEALTH

Rodrick Wallace and Deborah Wallace

Rodrick Wallace and Deborah Wallace have done considerable research on the relationship between public health deterioration and the destruction of housing and communities in New York City. A version of the original study from which this excerpt is drawn was published in the Bulletin of the New York Academy of Medicine *(September–October 1990), and contains a detailed examination of the epidemic of housing fires and abandonment, population migration, and deterioration of health conditions in New York City during the 1970s and 1980s. The section of the paper presented here, most of which has not been published elsewhere, walks the reader through a hypothetical example of the process of urban decay, showing in capsule form the interrelationship between the loss of housing and the health care crisis.*

Wallace and Wallace take the widescale burnout and destruction of the South Bronx between 1974 and 1978 as their model of urban decay, but similar processes of devastation have affected inner-city areas across the country. The authors believe that much of the deterioration in the South Bronx stemmed from a policy of "planned shrinkage" on the part of the city—deliberate abandonment of the area (as well as other sections of New York) by cutting municipal services, fire services in particular, in order to displace the largely minority population and open areas for urban and industrial renewal. While many may not accept this theory of the origins of urban decay, this does not alter the usefulness of the Wallaces' analysis of its results.

The urban afflictions of homelessness, addiction, mental illness, AIDS, and sick children overwhelming our hospitals, and crime and violence overwhelming our neighborhoods and jails, are not separate and disparate problems. Rather, they are part of an interwoven pattern of urban ecological collapse and desertification whose remedy requires degrees of understanding and political will not often brought to public problems in the United States. This article examines the interplay between destruction of housing and community and the general collapse of public health. We examine how New York City's housing famine and the processes that caused it have produced several parallel, interacting public health crises that disproportionately affect communities of color and that are deeply implicated in the conditions of "medical gridlock" that now affect New York City's hospitals. What we see in New York City, through implementation of "planned shrinkage," is an apparently deliberate reversal of the great advances in public health made during the first part of this century that followed upon vast improvements of the living and working conditions of the poor.

Urban Decay and Public Health

Tuberculosis is a classic historical and, increasingly, current example of disease involving housing, overcrowding, social disintegration, and truncation of social networks. It has been suggested that onset of the epidemic of acquired immune deficiency syndrome (AIDS) accounts for recent increases in tuberculosis in New York City. Historically, however, tuberculosis is intimately related to the social conditions of the poor, conditions which have recently deteriorated badly there. But it would be difficult in any event to invoke the *deus ex machina* of AIDS to explain the patterns of irregular increase in homicide, suicide, gonorrhea, salmonellosis, drug abuse, elderly and infant mortality, low birthweight, rat infestation, and medical gridlock since the mid-1970s.[1] On the whole, another simpler and more unifying hypothesis suggests itself: *that the massive, continuing destruction and disintegration of housing and community* (*which results from a continuing failure to provide the municipal services needed to maintain urban population densities—the implementing of New York City's planned shrinkage program among black and Latino communities*) *are having serious impacts on public health and welfare and on utilization of health services.*

We are suggesting that the consequences of withdrawing municipal services from poor neighborhoods and the resulting outbreaks of contagious urban decay and forced migration that shred essential social networks and cause social disintegration have become a highly significant contributor to the decline in public health among the poor. This process of urban decay is probably also a strong ultimate cause of serious behavioral pathology, which expresses itself, among other ways, in chronically rising mental illness, substance abuse, violence, and homicide.[2]

A large literature shows that proper socialization, the prevention of psychiatric illness, and the control of socially unacceptable behavior and violent outbreaks all require strong personal, domestic, and community networks within as socially integrated a community as possible.[3] A review of the criminology literature shows how the loss of social integration and networks, from planned shrinkage or other causes, is destined to increase such behavioral patterns. These patterns themselves become convoluted with processes of urban decay that are likely to further disrupt social networks and cause further social disintegration.[4]

These processes may, we suggest, be a fundamental cause of the patterns of rising usage of the health care system that are causing medical gridlock in New York City—that is, a nexus of increasing rates of low birthweight, rising substance abuse, and associated psychiatric disorder, all compounded with the relentlessly increasing incidence of AIDS, which may itself be convoluted with the process of contagious urban decay.[5] If so, then no conceivable system of acute medical care provision can meet the health needs of a poor population for whom living and social conditions are rapidly deteriorating, thus causing a decline in general health status, and for whom, further and consequently, public health measures have failed. That is to say, a purely medical intervention paradigm will be ineffective, and compulsive fiddling only with the modalities of acute health care provision cannot solve this crisis. As the living and working conditions of New York City's black and Latino poor regress toward those of the nineteenth century, so inevitably must their health status, irrespective of purely medical interventions.

A Hypothetical Example

Let us take a walk through a hypothetical example showing the nesting of critical phenomena and variables in a single outbreak of recurrent contagious urban decay and its intertwining outcomes.

Suppose a community is subjected to reductions in municipal services or other conditions that trigger an outbreak of contagious urban decay. That is, levels of municipal services cease to be adequate to maintain urban levels of population density and to preserve badly overcrowded housing units.

First, a number of geographically scattered occupied buildings deteriorate and are abandoned by their landlords, some as the result of uncontrolled fires. After a time, buildings close to those initially abandoned are also abandoned and receive no maintenance services, so that the initial scattering of individual abandoned buildings becomes a scattering of clusters of abandoned buildings. Some of these, in turn, suffer fires or other disasters and become vacant. People begin to move out of abandoned or nearly abandoned and occupied buildings, causing deterioration in their own domestic and personal networks and in the surrounding community network.

Legitimate neighborhood economic activity begins to decline rapidly as out-migration proceeds.

Vacant and abandoned buildings now become centers of illicit activity, mainly drug related, further accelerating neighborhood decline. Fire becomes ubiquitous in the affected neighborhoods, and fire setting in vacant buildings becomes customary, driving many from still-sound nearby occupied buildings. Many of the stronger people, with the financial and emotional resources, now move completely out of the neighborhood, further seriously depleting community networks. The initial clusters of abandoned and vacant buildings now grow greatly and coalesce into a moving front of fire and abandonment.

A population concentration, bringing with it badly overcrowded housing, flees in a wave before the oncoming front of abandonment and fire. Those in the wave suffer increasingly depleted personal and domestic networks, as do those left behind. Indices of public health, including contagious disease and infant mortality, begin to show serious degradation among both the displaced population and that left behind, as social nets disintegrate for both groups.

Children, forced to move time and again, and to continually re-form their own networks of friendship, fail to learn to read. Schools increasingly seem to ''fail.'' Collapse of social networks before and behind the urban decay front triggers violent episodes within and between families and ''acting out'' by children, who are now largely unsupervised outside of the home. Gangs of unsupervised adolescents congregate on street corners, contributing to a sudden, marked rise in street crime and initiating many criminal careers.

Rising levels of criminal activity, coupled with declining levels of legitimate neighborhood economic activity, further accelerate the process of abandonment by landlords.

Those individuals with marginal mental disorders who had relied on support from personal, domestic, and community networks now begin to require increased hospitalization, often for more extended periods. Moreover, collapse of networks and decline of "quality of life" contribute to the community's disempowerment and helplessness and feed back into processes of contagious urban decay and further deterioration of mental and public health. Substance abuse and homicide become ubiquitous in the devastated neighborhood, and begin to rise among displaced refugees with truncated social networks who are now crowding into nearby neighborhoods.

As we have shown for the Bronx,[6] what had been a sharp geographic concentration of intravenous drug abuse, the principal vector for the introduction of HIV infection to the heterosexual population, now becomes broadly diffused throughout many neighborhoods. These neighborhoods suffer truncation of the social networks needed to successfully diffuse information about the control of AIDS and to reinforce limitations on high-risk behaviors. This seriously compromises subsequent attempts to control the spread of HIV.

Neighborhoods near those that burned, which received displaced refugees from devastated areas, begin to suffer severe housing overcrowding and stress on the social networks of the original residents, who themselves begin to move out from underneath the avalanche of refugees. The conditions of "susceptibility" to contagious urban decay, which underlay destruction of the first community—extreme housing overcrowding coupled with extreme poverty—now begin to exist in those nearby areas that were forced to receive displaced refugees.

The vast wave of outmigration by more affluent, largely white, middle-class residents from the now-deteriorating neighborhoods that absorbed refugees temporarily makes available their generally larger apartments to the displaced poor, lowering the percentage of badly overcrowded housing occupied by the very poor. Thus, the number of housing units susceptible to the fire/abandonment process falls below the epidemiologic threshold, and the initial outbreak of contagious urban decay begins to slow.

A large remnant elderly white population remains in the previously middle-class neighborhood now overwhelmed by displaced refugees. As the richer white population evacuates, these elderly become more and more isolated, and are often unable to make social connections with the refugees of color who move into the neighborhoods, themselves suffering, and suffering from, depleted social networks. Along with the increase of substance abuse among the displaced refugees comes an inevitable increase in victimization of this remnant elderly population, both from the general rise in community violence that comes with increased social disorganization, and from their particular targeting as "easy marks" for mugging or push-in robbery.

As fires decline in the partly devastated neighborhood, the municipality begins even further reductions of essential municipal services, causing faster outmigration of the population into adjacent, "ripening" areas, hastening renewed outbreaks of contagious urban decay.

Contagious loss of housing continues in the already devastated areas,[7] driving doubled-up residents, many of whose friends may have moved from the neighborhood, into homelessness, as middle-class outmigration from the city slows.

The now-inevitable outbreaks of disease in the newly crowded zones, particularly intensified by homicide, substance abuse, and AIDS, also contribute materially to increasing the susceptibility of these areas to contagious urban decay by encouraging another round of outmigration by those with the resources. Behavioral and mental disorders, substance abuse, violence, contagious disease, and contagious urban decay have become obscenely intertwined.

Now the health care system begins to become overburdened by the sudden increase in the rate of low-birthweight babies; by dual substance abuse and psychiatric disorder; by AIDS; and by the impossibility of finding housing for convalescent indigent patients outside of shelters for the homeless.

As homelessness proceeds and the poor begin doubling up again, housing overcrowding in poor neighborhoods begins to rise. The stage is now well set for another outbreak of contagious housing destruction in the newly overcrowded regions, and for its severe impact on community, domestic, and personal social networks. Thus, in the absence of effective interventions, a full-scale process of urban ecological collapse synergistically amplifies and replicates itself, just as the consequences of the first outbreak become unmanageable.

Housing Famine and the Collapse of Health Care

New York City's low-income housing famine is evidently the most important cause of its crisis of homelessness, although the exact mechanisms may be subtle.[8] We have suggested here a necessary parallel track to homelessness: deterioration of public health and an inevitable resulting collapse of health care provision. Thus, the concept of a housing famine provides a unifying paradigm that may help us understand, explain, and correct many otherwise disparate aspects of the accelerating New York crisis.

The dynamic nature of the failure of public health in New York City suggests that until emergency measures—including provision of adequate housing for the poor and success of programs to reestablish their social networks—can take effect, demand for acute medical care can and probably will continue to increase relentlessly and without foreseeable limit. What may be limited, however, is provision of medical care for the poor. Just as the effects of the housing famine are structured according to our social hierarchy, falling most heavily on the poor, so too may be the effects of medical care shortfall. The revenge of the poor may be to die on the doorsteps of the rich, raising, beyond certain moral niceties, questions regarding the value of real estate in a plague city.

In short, the "slow disaster" of contagious urban decay triggered by planned shrinkage has, after a relatively short delay, become a housing famine that, classically, is rapidly evolving to an interacting complex of "slow plagues," increasingly overwhelming the city's medical care system. The public health outcomes of urban burnout may, in fact, constitute yet another great disaster, as may the parallel track of collapsing public order.[9]

In any event, it is now clear that other, more rapid and more contagious, plagues are no longer inconceivable in New York City. Both medical care and public health measures are increasingly overwhelmed, while the population densities of the very poor are increasing rapidly. New York City now contains one-quarter of the AIDS cases in the United States, largely the result of factors of "social medicine" that could well apply to more rapidly spread but equally incurable diseases.

One of the principal characteristics of an event officially defined as a "disaster" is the availability of relief efforts on a very large scale. It is difficult to escape the inference that the South Bronx catastrophe has been, and remains, a continuing disaster without benefit of relief. Failure to recognize that catastrophe as a disaster may further compound the victimization of those affected. Health, behavioral, or psychological pathologies consequent on victimization may be blamed on the victims themselves. It is, of course, always ideologically useful to blame the failures of a social system or governmental structures on the victims of those failures. Indeed, blaming the victim is as American as apple pie and violence.

Victim-blaming comments and sentiments—such as Senator Daniel Moynihan's comment in 1978 to the effect that "people don't want housing in the Bronx, or they wouldn't burn it down"[10]—affect public policy. The currently popular media term "underclass" also comes to mind when thinking of those remaining in the devastated zones of New York City. However, what has been stigmatized as a particular group—an "underclass"—seems better characterized as a process producing a spectrum of symptoms and outcomes among those who have been subjected to a slow, but intense, disaster without relief. These are the effects of "planned shrinkage," a virulent and systematic program of malfeasance, misfeasance, and non-feasance conducted by agencies of government for the political purposes of a ruling oligarchy.

Recommendations

Indices of public health status and health care utilization in New York City show sharp deterioration after 1978 or, in some cases, as early as 1974, rapidly accelerating in the late 1980s. The evident Occam's razor hypothesis is that deterioration of public health and health care in New York City, possibly including psychiatric illness, substance abuse, low birthweight, and a whole spectrum of behavioral pathology, is intimately related to massive "planned shrinkage" destruction of housing, and hence of community, in poor neighborhoods caused by outbreaks of contagious urban decay. The destruction of low-income housing has, likewise, become one of the principal wellsprings behind the city's burgeoning parallel crisis of homelessness, which may have its own, separate but related, dynamic impacts on public health and health care.

The evidence strongly suggests that the impacts of the spreading and possibly recurrent epidemic of urban decay on the physical and mental health status of New Yorkers are likely to be extreme, especially given the effects of time and cuts in federal programs. It seems increasingly possible that we have only just begun to see the health and other problems that "planned shrinkage" has engendered.

Possible remedies, like apparent causes, lie in public policy:

1. Improvements in fire and other municipal services can serve as "immunization" against the recurrent cycle of contagious urban decay that continues to erode communities and displace population.
2. Communities and social networks disrupted or disorganized by New York City's planned shrinkage program must be reknit by concerted community organizing.
3. Low-income housing must be rebuilt, while preserving existing social structures, and new or rehabilitated housing must be preserved with adequate municipal services. Evidently, rehabilitation and renewal must be done in such a way as not to further destabilize existing communities, a subtle point not adequately addressed here.

Without such a closely coordinated threefold program explicitly designed to reverse social disintegration, significant public health improvement seems literally impossible, and relentlessly increasing social disintegration, public violence, homelessness, and medical gridlock appear inevitable.

New Yorkers now endure a famine of human habitat and community, triggered and sustained in large measure by government's continuing refusal to deliver the municipal services needed to maintain urban population densities. As with more conventional famines, the principal cause of mortality is likely to be disease concentrated among groups traditionally affected by famine: the poor, the very young, and the very old.[11] We have suggested mechanisms by which this might occur. However, there is likely to be ignition of another wave of "South Bronx" epidemic in New York City just as it is overwhelmed by the consequences in terms of health and homelessness of the last. There seems little time for delay of corrective measures, particularly the simplest one involving restoration of fire extinguishment and sanitation services to ghetto neighborhoods.

Relearning History

In matters of public health and welfare—particularly involving contagious phenomena well known to undergo uncontrollable explosive outbreak—a very conservative attitude appears prudent. Requiring excessive standards of scientific proof for programs to improve public health—for example, reopening of ghetto fire companies—while allowing grossly relaxed standards for implementation of ideologically driven service reduction schemes (such as the fire service cuts instituted following the recommendations of the Rand Corporation in 1969 and more recently renewed by the Koch and Dinkins administrations) has already proven fatally counterproductive on a considerable scale. Continuation of such a bizarre reversal of standards will very likely have even greater fatal impact.

Hinkle and Loring describe the decision-making process for projects which, like the provision of clean water to New York at the turn of the century, caused vast and lasting improvement of public health:

One of the traditional foci of public health administration, to prevent or reduce disease and injury in a human population, has been to change conditions in its physical environment. Historically numerous ideas for such interventions were acted upon before definitive research had determined the nature of the relationship between a particular object and a disease.[12]

We have seemingly unlearned that history: A hundred years after the beginning of the great reform movement in New York City, and more than 60 years after its success, it is yet again necessary to call for adequate fire extinguishment, adequate sanitation, and other municipal services in the ghettos of the poor as important instruments of public health. New York City, and by inference other devastated cities of America, stands in evident need of a renewal of that great reform movement, which first brought adequate public health to the poor and, indeed, to the nation.

N O T E S

1. For a detailed treatment, see Wallace, Rodrick, and Wallace, Deborah, "Origins of Public Health Collapse in New York City: The Dynamics of Planned Shrinkage, Contagious Urban Decay and Social Disintegration," *Bulletin of the New York Academy of Medicine*, September–October 1990:66(5), pp. 391–434.

2. Leighton, A. H., My *Name is Legion: Foundations for a Theory of Man in Relation to Culture*, New York: Basic Books, 1959; and Leighton, D. C., Harding, J. S., Macklin, D. B., Macmillan, A. M., and Leighton, A. H., *The Character of the Danger: Psychiatric Symptoms in Selected Communities*, New York: Basic Books, 1963; and Solomon, S., "Mobilizing Social Support Networks in Times of Disaster," in Figley, ed., *Trauma and Its Wake*, New York: Brunner/Mazel, 1986.

3. Ibid.; and Cassel, J., "Psychosocial Processes and 'Stress': Theoretical Formulation," *International Journal of Health Services*, 1974:4(3), pp. 471–482; Cohen, S., and Wills, T. A., "Stress, Social Support, and the Buffering Hypothesis," *Psychological Bulletin*, 1985:98(2), pp. 310–357; House, J. S., Landis, K. R., and Umberson, D., "Social Relationships and Health," *Science*, 1988: 241, pp. 540–544; and Hinkle, L. E., and Loring, W. C., *The Effect of the Man-Made Environment on Health and Behavior*, Washington, DC: Department of Health, Education & Welfare, 1977.

4. See Skogan, W. G., "Community Organizations and Crime," in A. J. Reiss, Jr., and M. Tonry, eds., *Communities and Crime*, Chicago: University of Chicago Press, 1986; and Skogan, W. G., *Disorder and Decline*, New York: The Free Press, 1990.

5. Wallace, R., "A Synergism of Plagues: 'Planned Shrinkage,' Contagious Housing Destruction and AIDS in the Bronx," *Environmental Research*, 1988:47(1), pp. 1–33. This is exactly parallel to the "jail gridlock" now affecting the city, arising from the same wellspring of social network disruption. Wallace, R., "Urban Desertification, Public Health and Public Order: 'Planned Shrinkage,' Violent Death, Substance Abuse and AIDS in the Bronx," *Social Science and Medicine*, 1990:31(7), pp. 801–813; and Wallace, D., "Routes of Increased Health Care Inequality in New York," *Social Science and Medicine*, 1990:31(11), pp. 1219–1227.

6. Wallace, "A Synergism of Plagues."

7. Wallace, R., "Homelessness, Contagious Housing Destruction and Municipal Service Cuts in New York City: 1. Demographics of a Housing Deficit, and 2. Dynamics of a Housing Famine," *Environment and Planning A*, 1989:21, pp. 1585–1603, and 22, pp. 5–15.

8. Ibid.

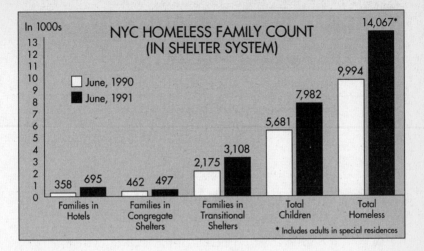

Source:

NYC Human Resources Administration, 1991

9. Wallace, "Urban Desertification, Public Health and Public Order."
10. Weisman, S. R., "Moynihan Urges Priority for Jobs in South Bronx," *New York Times*, December 20, 1978.
11. Cahill, K. M., ed., *Famine*, Maryknoll, NY: Orbis Books, 1982.
12. Hinkle and Loring, *The Effect of the Man-Made Environment on Health and Behavior*.

NATIONAL ALERT: GRIDLOCK IN THE EMERGENCY DEPARTMENT

Stephan G. Lynn

As an emergency physician from the American College of Emergency Physicians (ACEP), I'd like to bring a national perspective on what we consider today's most important crisis in health care. We are on the verge—and perhaps over the verge—of a major crisis in health care related to overcrowding in hospital emergency departments. Emergency department overcrowding occurs when admitted patients can no longer leave the department because all staffed inpatient and intensive care beds in the hospital are occupied, and no beds are available in neighboring facilities for transfer. Patients come to the emergency department requiring inpatient care, and there are no beds, no resources, no intensive care units, and no nurses available to provide that care. Those patients wait in the emergency department, sometimes for hours, sometimes for days, until a bed becomes available.

I am personally familiar with patients who have waited as long as eight days in the emergency department for an inpatient bed. There are emergency departments in New York and in other cities throughout the country in which there have been as many as 50 or 60 patients waiting for inpatient beds that were not available. In large metropolitan areas, emergency department overload can develop despite the availability of staffed beds, because additional patients are being diverted from other overcrowded facilities. When a large percentage of a community's emergency departments simultaneously adopt "ambulance diversion," "standby," or some other limited availability status, emergency departments that remain open may quickly become overwhelmed with patients. This set of circumstances can rapidly lead to emergency department "gridlock"—a particularly dangerous situation in which no emergency department in the immediate vicinity can safely accommodate additional ambulance patients. In many communities, overcrowding is severely limiting the public's right to timely emergency medical care and compromising the quality of that care. The problem in simple terms is that we have too many patients requiring access to health care and too few resources available for those patients.

As an emergency physician, this significantly limits my ability to provide quality care. Emergency departments were neither designed, planned, nor staffed to provide inpatient services, and when they are asked to provide those services, they have marginal ability to do so.

In overcrowded emergency departments today, we are able to take vital signs, we are able to give medications, we are able to monitor patients, but we cannot provide any of those things that our patients expect when they are admitted to the hospital. We cannot provide privacy, we cannot turn out the lights, we cannot turn off the noise, and we cannot provide access to telephones or visitors. It is difficult, if not impossible, for us to provide three warm meals at appropriate times. It is extremely uncomfortable for our patients to spend days sitting on an emergency department stretcher with a mattress that is two inches thick. When the emergency department is overcrowded, the quality of care suffers, and, far more important, access to care suffers as well.

When 50 percent of an emergency department's staff, space, and equipment are allocated to provide care for patients who require inpatient admission (and have no need for emergency care), what happens to the next patient who walks through the door? The role and mission of an emergency physician is to be constantly available for that next patient, whoever he or she is, whatever his or her problem is, but when most of an emergency department's resources are allocated to providing inpatient care, we are far less able to do so.

Scope of the Problem

How extensive is this problem? A few years ago, emergency department overcrowding was perceived as a problem of the East and West Coasts, with a few scattered areas in between. Unfortunately, over the last few years we have learned that this problem is substantially more extensive. The American College of Emergency Physicians conducted a survey of its chapters in 1989 to assess the extent of emergency department and hospital overcrowding nationwide. Each chapter was asked whether its members had experienced emergency department overcrowding, and to what it attributed this problem; all 54 chapters responded. ACEP chapters from 41 states (representing 94 percent of the country's population) reported overcrowding. All four non-state chapters (the District of Columbia, Puerto Rico, Ontario, and Government Services) reported overcrowding as well. Only nine state chapters reported no problem with overcrowding (Idaho, Minnesota, Nebraska, New Hampshire, New Mexico, North Dakota, Oregon, Utah, and Wyoming).[1] Similarly, the Emergency Nurses Association polled its state councilors during its 1989 Scientific Assembly, and all 50 state councilors reported overcrowding.[2]

Last winter, the entire East Coast, from Atlanta through Washington, Philadelphia, New York, Boston, and up to Toronto, was gridlocked; unfortunately, we expect that this will continue. We expect that San Diego, San Francisco, and Los Angeles will be gridlocked, but we know as well that there will be problems in Miami and Memphis. Last year Dallas and Chicago were added to the list of major urban areas that became substantially overcrowded. And when we surveyed ACEP chapters, it was extremely clear that this overcrowding is not simply an urban problem. Our chapters from West Virginia and North Carolina and Alaska told us that they had substantial overcrowding in areas that were neither urban nor poor.

The National Association of Public Hospitals (NAPH) has issued a report studying overcrowding at all of its member institutions and all the members of the Council of Teaching Hospitals. The study included replies from 277 hospitals in 43 states, among the largest and best hospitals across the country.[3] Based on the preliminary results, the private hospitals experienced the same problems of overcrowding and occupancy as did the public hospitals. Seventy-five percent of those hospitals reported increased emergency department utilization over the past three years. (In fact, in 1989 utilization rose to over 90 million visits, the largest annual actual and percentage increase that has ever occurred.) In those hospitals studied, 65 percent reported a substantial effect on quality of care as a result of overcrowding. Forty percent diverted ambulances, and approximately one-third transferred patients to other institutions during the target month (August 1988), because their hospital and secondarily their emergency department were overwhelmed with patients; there was not room for one additional patient.

Contributing Factors

What contributes to this substantial and increasing problem of emergency department overcrowding? In simple terms, there is inadequate funding and priority for emergency health care services during a period of increasing demand. There is increasing demand because more and more people are utilizing the emergency department every year for a large number of reasons. Our population is aging; we have increased drug abuse and poverty; and AIDS patients that we could never have planned for five or ten years ago are utilizing the emergency departments in our hospitals in ever-increasing numbers. And for those 37 million people we constantly hear about that are uninsured or underinsured, the emergency department has become the provider of last (and, frequently, only) resort.

At the same time that demand for services is increasing, the supply of hospital beds is diminishing. New York City in the last five years has eliminated 5,000 acute care beds. Emergency departments in California, particularly in Southern California, are closing at a rapid rate. In that state, hospitals are allowed to close their emergency departments when they become financially undesirable. There are fewer hospital beds, there are fewer emergency departments available to treat patients. There are not enough nurses; there are particularly not enough skilled nurses in emergency departments and critical care units, and it is these intensive care units that usually become the bottleneck for hospital admissions. There are not enough nursing homes. About 10 percent of the acute care bed capacity in New York City and in the state of Massachusetts in 1989 was occupied by patients who required nursing homes or home health care placement. The resources were simply not available in those states.[4]

Solutions

What will bring us to the end of this problem? The first solution is universal access to health care and universal access to health care reimbursement. The care for about one-third of all patients who come to the emergency department is uncompensated; in a national study by the American College of Emergency Physicians, 31 percent of all emergency care in this country was uncompensated.[5] The emergency department is appropriately mandated to see all patients who seek care there, but society does not provide reimbursement for that care. As a result, our hospitals, our emergency departments, and our patients are suffering.

Another factor that must be addressed is the lack of access to primary care. This is exemplified by a study done in Washington, D.C., for the District of Columbia Hospital Association, which evaluated patients characterized by three very simple factors: the patients (1) had no ability to pay, (2) came into the emergency department, and (3) were admitted.[6] Looking at those three characteristics, the study found that about one-quarter of all patients who presented to an emergency department in Washington, D.C., for admission and who had no ability to pay had an "avoidable admission"—avoidable, that is, if that patient had had access to primary care. If one other factor is added to that list—preexisting chronic disease—the percentage of "avoidable admissions" increases from 25 percent to about 45 percent. Lack of access to primary and preventive care is not only injurious, it causes a substantial number of completely avoidable hospital admissions.

Admissions through the emergency department add cost to the system in other ways, as well. The Health Care Financing Administration compared patients admitted through the emergency department and patients admitted from all other sources in the same DRG. The study showed that the length of stay and the cost to the hospital and to the health care system are substantially higher for patients with the same diagnosis who are admitted through the emergency department.[7]

Long-Term Vision

The problem of emergency department overcrowding is severe and serious today. On one Monday in September 1990 in New York City, 40 of the 55 emergency departments were on total bypass. That means that each of those 40 emergency departments already had 15 patients admitted and waiting for beds, and no inpatient beds were available. This was in the fall, not a season of traditional overcrowding, with winter still to come.

We see little hope for a solution in the short term. Major changes are not occurring to deal with either the causes of this problem—increases in infectious diseases, increases in respiratory emergencies, AIDS, drug-related health crises, and poverty—or to bring about the solutions—universal access to health care, more nurses, reweighting of DRGs for patients admitted through the emergency department, implementation of preventive health care programs, and a reorganization of health care services so that in-hospital treatment is used only for patients with acute health problems. Development of realistic and effective contingency plans may allow emergency physicians and emergency nurses and their colleagues to deal with the immediate consequences of overcrowding.[8] Such management tools, however, while crucial in the face of the immediate problem, will not produce significant long-term changes in the nature of hospital overcrowding.

Emergency departments provide the critically important safety net for our

180 THE CRISIS IN PROVIDER INSTITUTIONS: ISSUES AND AREAS FOR REFORM

nation's health care system, but our capacity to meet the needs of patients is stretched to the breaking point. Long-term resolution of the problem of hospital and emergency department overcrowding will require a substantial commitment of societal resources and vision—and, perhaps, a revolution in our national health care priorities.

NOTES

1. Lynn, Stephan G., Hockberger, Robert S., Kellermann, Arthur, Allison, E. Jackson, and Yeh, Charlotte S., *A Report from the American College of Emergency Physicians Task Force on Hospital Overcrowding and Emergency Department Overload*, Dallas, Texas, September 1989.
2. Fadale, Joanne, President-Elect, Emergency Nurses Association, report presented at the American College of Emergency Physicians Conference on Overcrowding, New York, NY, October 13, 1989.
3. Kellermann, Arthur, report presented at the American College of Emergency Physicians Conference on Overcrowding, New York, NY, October 13, 1989. The final results are published in *America's Safety Net Hospitals: The Foundation of Our Nation's Health System*, Washington, DC: National Association of Public Hospitals, 1991.
4. Greater New York Hospital Association; Massachusetts Hospital Association.
5. Statistical analysis by Mathematica, Inc., for American College of Emergency Physicians, 1986.
6. Lewin/ICF Group, "Indigent Care Project Prospective Uninsured Patient Survey," Washington, DC: District of Columbia Hospital Association, Spring 1988.
7. Melnick, G. A., Serrato, C. A., et al., "Prospective Payments to Hospitals: Should Emergency Admissions Have Higher Rates?" *Health Care Financing Review*, Spring 1989:10(3), pp. 29–39.
8. Lynn, Stephan G., and Kellermann, Arthur, "Critical Decision Making: Managing the Emergency Department in an Overcrowded Hospital," *Annals of Emergency Medicine*, March 1991.

TESTIMONY ON REFORMING LONG-TERM CARE IN NEW YORK STATE

Cynthia Rudder, Ph.D.

My name is Cynthia Rudder and I am the Director of the Nursing Home Community Coalition of New York State (NHCC), a coalition of 33 statewide consumer, civic, and professional organizations working for better nursing home care in our state.

I am pleased to be given the opportunity to discuss long-term care in New York State. Our coalition has long been struggling with these issues. We believe that it is long past time to look at ways of reforming the entire long-term care system in New York State.

Any reform of the long-term care system must include the following principles:

1. A comprehensive continuum of available long-term care services must be developed. As different parts of the continuum are developed, their context within the continuum must be considered.
2. This continuum must be based upon the needs and preferences of consumers who will use the services.
3. This continuum must be developed with the help of the consumers who will use the system.
4. Our first priority must be on making sure that alternatives and available services are in place so that consumers will have real choices and so that there will be no cracks for consumers to fall through.
5. This system must encompass the needs of all individuals needing long-term care—the elderly, the disabled, the young, people with AIDS, etc. Any system not encompassing the needs of all is bound to fail.
6. The way long-term care services are delivered and reimbursed must be reorganized to focus more on social supports and autonomy of recipients at all points on the continuum.

We must develop this continuum of long-term care services based upon the needs and preferences of all the consumers of these services. Time and effort must be put into both assessing consumer needs as well as consumer satisfaction with the available services. Ask consumers what they believe they need and want.

Our long-term care system in the past has evolved, not from the needs and desires of consumers, but from the identification, by professionals, of some specific need they believed consumers had, or as some services seemed inappropriate and/or too costly. Then, programs were often developed based upon available streams of money to pay for it. This has led to inappropriate and costly services that may not meet the need of consumers.

One example is how we tried to solve the problem of housing and caring for people with AIDS who did not need acute care, but were not sick enough for skilled nursing care. Because we had a stream of money for institutions, we decided to build special nursing homes for them even though we knew that the progression of the disease is episodic and probably will require these consumers to have to go in and out of these facilities.

Another example is our Assisted Living Program. We first produced a system of care heavily weighted toward institutionalization. We then developed a re-imbursement system for nursing homes that would encourage facilities to take only those people with the heaviest care needs. We put this in place before making sure that services were available to care for those people no longer financially attractive to the nursing homes. We then discovered large numbers of people, eligible for nursing home care, with no place to go. They were falling "between the cracks." We then decided to fill the cracks, not with an innovative way of offering supportive housing, but with an idea for which we already had an available stream of money. It was hoped that this idea would also save money, which is an overriding consideration. We then offered the Assisted Living Program, most of which will be offered in existing institutions, adult homes, as the one answer for our problem, even though it is clear that Assisted Living will probably work better in some parts of the state than in others and will work better where it is part of a continuum of services than when it is offered only in conjunction with adult homes.

How we deliver and reimburse long-term care services must be changed. Because of Medicaid reimbursement, too much of long-term care is based upon a medical model. We had to create programs that had major medical components even though we know that the major long-term care needs are social and not medical. In fact, if more attention were paid to social supports, some institutional placement would be delayed or eliminated altogether. We must find ways to pay for those social supports that help to keep consumers, both in the community and in the institutions, independent. In addition, we must reorganize our system based upon consumer autonomy and quality of life. Alert recipients of services, or if nonalert, their representatives, must be the ones who will make the decisions whether to take certain risks in long-term care placements and/or in refusing certain treatments. For example, if an alert disabled home care ventilator recipient has no informal support system to care for him/her if a home care worker does not show up, the home care professional believes that he/she must therefore be sent to a hospital or nursing home. However, the decision of what to do, whether to enter a hospital or nursing home, must remain with the consumer, not with the home care professional.

Given those major principles that we believe must help to frame our long-term care system, I would like to spend the rest of my time specifically discussing the Managed Access to Aging Services (MAAS) proposal presented by the State Office for the Aging and the public policy paper presented by Mr. Michael Dowling and Dr. Alice Lin.

MAAS Proposal

As a proposal to change one important part of the long-term care system, this proposal has much to offer. MAAS is a proposal to change one crucial part of the system: access to long-term care services for the elderly. I would like to discuss elements of MAAS.

1. The ability for the elderly to enter the long-term care system through a single point of entry would be a tremendous advantage for consumers. As most of you know, the present system is a complicated, almost incomprehensible system. The ability of one individual, on a local level, helping the elderly through the maze of options and requirements is a wonderful idea. People looking to enter the system from the community are in the worst position. They need help in understanding the options available and need help in filling out the enormous amount of paperwork. We would love to see this individual as an advocate for the elderly person entering the system. Will this individual help the consumer actually receive the service indicated?

2. Although it is unclear exactly what sets of statutory and regulatory requirements now governing access to long-term care would be eliminated and replaced with a new single set of requirements, assuming that public protections would remain in place, the change has merit if it eliminates confusing access requirements.

3. By requiring Medicaid recipients to follow developed care plans while the private sector continues to have the final say on what services they will pay for may very well lead to a two-tiered system of health care: one for the poor and one for the rich. It would be better to allow free choice to both groups of recipients. If the system works as the Office for the Aging has stated it will, with consumer choice being a prime consideration and all appropriate and available options being considered, we would expect most of the clients to follow the developed plan of care.

4. Because of the unavailability of alternative services and providers and/or the unwillingness of a provider to accept a client, consumers rarely have a choice regarding which provider to use. Thus, the consumer choice in MAAS is not a real choice. We need to build in real choices for consumers.

5. Clarification is needed on the specifics related to consumer appeals and complaints. Exactly what will they be like?

6. The idea of a single state office or agency responsible for long-term care is an interesting idea. In the past, the heads of the different agencies responsible for long-term care have not worked well together. A good example is the dual monitoring of adult homes by both the Department of Social Services and the Office of Mental Health. There have been major gaps in communication, often at the expense of the client. However, any agency that undertakes this role must be influential enough and have the strength needed to make sure that long-term care does not become a stepchild to other health care issues such as acute care. Long-term care must have the same importance in terms of policy making and supply of needed resources as other health systems.

7. Any evaluation of the MAAS system must include client satisfaction. If the proposal to only allow privately paying clients to reject the developed plan

is maintained, the evaluation must look at what percentage of the private sector use the developed plan. This should be very high if the system is working as envisioned. In addition, the potential creation of a two-tiered system of care, one for Medicaid clients and one for private pay, and the removal of any provider regulations must be carefully monitored.

Long-Term Care for the Aged and Disabled Persons in New York State: A Public Policy Framework

This is a comprehensive attempt to make sense out of the complicated and difficult issue of long-term care at a time when New York State and the country face fiscal crises and the national arena is looking at national health care.

Before I make any specific comments on this report, I would like to state one of our overall concerns. Trying to implement a new system at a time when cost containment is the driving interest is very dangerous. Programs tend never to have the promised resources they need to make the system work. When we deinstitutionalized the mentally ill population from our state's psychiatric facilities, the basic goal was to save money. As we know, promised community programs never found the needed resources. What can we do to make sure this does not happen again?

Some Specific Comments

1. We are pleased that this attempt addresses the entire class of individuals needing long-term care. As I mentioned above, only by meeting the needs of all of our citizens needing long-term care can a new structure for long-term care succeed. In addition, only by attempting to reorganize the way health care is delivered and reimbursed, can we hope to make significant change.

2. The next step must involve an equal representation of community groups and consumers with providers to begin the development of this new system. Only by including those for whom the services will be developed and for those who will use this system, will the system be successful.

3. Housing is probably the most important issue in long-term care. We must spend time on how to finance housing for the clients of long-term care.

4. Social needs must be a primary focus.

5. We must not allow the reimbursement system to drive our services. The source of funding must not define our programs. Look carefully at the incentives in our reimbursement systems. Are they driving providers into offering programs that do not meet the needs of our citizens?

6. We do not believe that co-payments by Medicaid recipients is a good idea. By their very definition, Medicaid recipients do not have money for health care. If we require them to give co-payments, they will have to choose between health care and food or rent. They will stop getting the care they need.

7. We are against any concept of filial responsibility. It can lead to many problems. Where children and parents feel comfortable and able to take and give responsibility, it will naturally happen. If children or parents are uncomfortable

or unable to take or give responsibility, many other problems can arise if they are forced to take or give responsibility.

8. We understand the need to contain costs. However, we are against the approach commonly taken to contain costs: Limit access and cut services to the consumer. Speaking to advocates in Arizona, it is clear that their system is containing costs by limiting access to people who have nowhere to go. One cost containment practice we do support is to set up a mechanism to encourage provider financial responsibility and oversight. How are providers now using public monies? What are we now paying for? Direct care or administrative costs?

PERCENT OF AGED POPULATION RESIDING IN NURSING AND RELATED CARE HOMES, BY AGE GROUP (USA, SELECTED YEARS, 1969–1985)

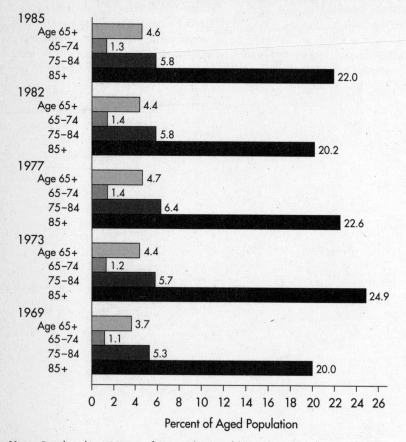

1985
- Age 65+ — 4.6
- 65–74 — 1.3
- 75–84 — 5.8
- 85+ — 22.0

1982
- Age 65+ — 4.4
- 65–74 — 1.4
- 75–84 — 5.8
- 85+ — 20.2

1977
- Age 65+ — 4.7
- 65–74 — 1.4
- 75–84 — 6.4
- 85+ — 22.6

1973
- Age 65+ — 4.4
- 65–74 — 1.2
- 75–84 — 5.7
- 85+ — 24.9

1969
- Age 65+ — 3.7
- 65–74 — 1.1
- 75–84 — 5.3
- 85+ — 20.0

Percent of Aged Population

Note: Data based on US Bureau of Census estimates of the resident population. Data for 1977 and 1982 include nursing care, personal care services, and/or supervision over activities of daily living. Adult foster care homes in Michigan and residential community care facilities in California are excluded. Data for 1973 include those care homes that do not provide nursing care.

Sources:

For 1969–1977: US Department of Commerce, Bureau of the Census. Demographic and socioeconomic aspects of aging in the United States. Washington DC, 1984 (Current Population Reports; Series P-23, No. 138).

For 1982: Data provided by A. Sirrocco, National Center for Health Statistics, and US Department of Commerce, Bureau of the Census. Projections of the population of the United States by age, sex, and race: 1983–2080. Washington DC, 1984 (Current Population Reports; Series P-25, No. 952).

For 1985: E. Hing Nursing home utilization by current residents: United States, 1985: National Health Survey. Hyattsville, MD: National Center for Health Statistics, 1989; DHHS Publ. No. (PHS) 89-1763: Table 2, p. 30 (Vital Health Stat; Series 13, No. 102).

PERCENT DISTRIBUTION OF NURSING HOMES[1] BY TYPE OF CONTROL AND BED SIZE
(USA, 1986)

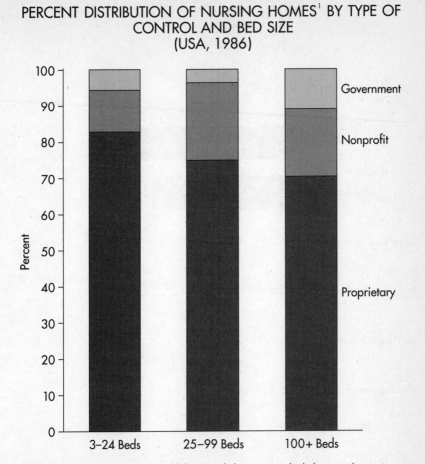

Note: 1. A nursing home is an establishment with three or more beds that provides nursing or personal care to the aged, infirm, or chronically ill.

Source:

A. Sirrocco. Nursing home characteristics: 1986 Inventory of Long-Term Care Places. Hyattsville, MD: National Center for Health Statistics, 1989; DHHS Publ. No. (PHS) 89-1828: Table 9, p. 15; Table 10, p. 16 (Vital Health Stat; Series 14, No. 33).

PERCENT DISTRIBUTION OF EXPENDITURES FOR NURSING HOME CARE, BY SOURCE OF PAYMENT (USA, 1988)

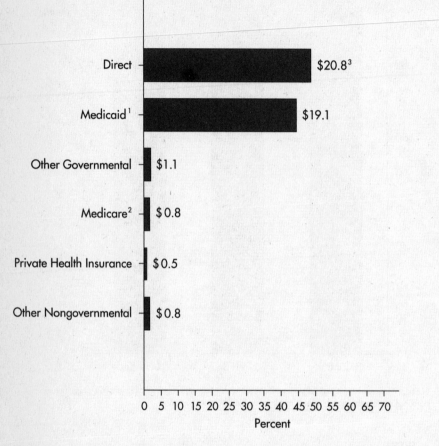

Notes:

1. Includes funds paid into Medicare trust funds by states under "buy-in" agreements to cover premiums for public assistance recipients and for persons who are medically indigent.

2. Represents total expenditures from trust funds for benefits. Trust fund income includes premium payments paid by or on behalf of enrollees.

3. Dollar amounts are in billions of dollars.

Source:

Department of Health and Human Services. Health Care Financing Administration. HHS News. May 3, 1990.

NATIONAL EXPENDITURES FOR HOME CARE, BY SOURCE OF SPENDING (USA, 1988)

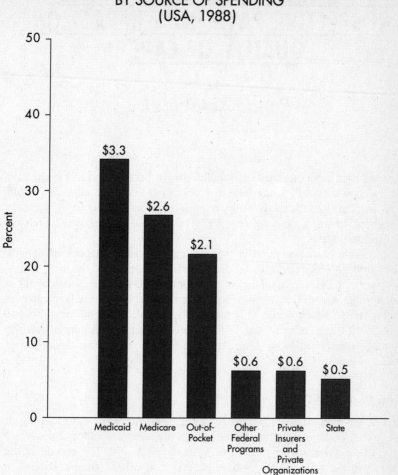

Note: Numbers on top of the bars are actual expenditures in billions of dollars.

Source:

The Pepper Commission. A call for action. Washington, DC: US Government Printing Office, 1990: Table 3–1, p. 93.

AND WHAT ABOUT THE PATIENTS? PROSPECTIVE PAYMENT'S IMPACT ON QUALITY OF CARE

Ronda Kotelchuck

Three years after implementation of Medicare's prospective payment system, no one really knows what PPS has done to the quality of care for some 29 million older Americans. Are the quality-of-care problems now coming to light the tip of an iceberg, or just a floating ice cube? as one Rand Corporation researcher posed the question.

Considerable obstacles stand in the way of answering the question. That's because, unlike widely available hospital cost and utilization data, there is neither a universal definition of quality of care nor a data collection system to allow its monitoring. Are the problems encountered under PPS actually greater or fewer than those which occurred before its inception? At the moment no one can say. Until quite recently, the Federal Government, which administers the system, has utterly failed to take responsibility for answering these critical questions.

Quality Concerns

PPS raises three major concerns regarding the quality of American health care. The first is the danger that the enormous pressure to achieve cost savings under the new system may lead to undertreating patients. The second is the inadequacy of the system's key instrument, diagnosis-related groups (DRGs), to account for the severity of a patient's illness, prompting hospitals to avoid or dump these patients. The third is whether certain types of care formerly provided in the hospital will be available to patients in alternate care settings such as nursing homes.

By paying a flat price per case instead of hospital cost, PPS is the first hospital payment system to force hospitals to reduce costs if they are to survive or prosper. These economies include reductions in length of stay (LOS) and the decreased use of ancillary testing, pharmaceuticals, medical supplies, and therapies—usually leveraged through the hospital's physicians. The system has prompted some dramatic reductions in these areas. In 1984, the first full year of PPS, Medicare length of stay fell by 9 percent—three times the decrease of any previous year. In 1985 it dropped an additional 8 percent. Simply put, quality of care may be threatened for the first time by PPS's incentive to provide too few, as opposed to too many, services.

The new system has also prompted hospitals to cut their workforce, which currently accounts for over 60 percent of their total costs. In fact, in the year following PPS's implementation, the hospital workforce fell 3.5 percent. It was the first such drop in post-war history. In 1985 there was a 5 percent reduction. Nursing staffs, which comprise the vast majority of all hospital personnel, are particularly vulnerable. The California Hospital Association reported a 9 percent cut in full-time nurses and a 37 percent drop in part-time nurses in 1983. As one examines these numbers it is important to keep in mind that, aside from physician competence, nursing care is the single most important determinant of the quality of inpatient care.

DRGs, the 471 categories of illness used as the basis for reimbursing hospitals for patient care, are seriously deficient in a number of ways which may compromise the quality of that care. Most seriously, they do not reflect severity of illness. Because DRGs limit themselves to only five pieces of data to categorize a patient and establish the rate at which the hospital will be reimbursed, they fail to account for the additional costs of treating patients with multiple conditions or very advanced disease. Patients with these conditions pose serious financial liabilities, often prompting hospitals to transfer or avoid them altogether. DRGs do not recognize the use of different treatment modalities, some of which may be costlier, but more beneficial. In addition, DRGs will not reimburse hospitals for treating more than a single condition, even though this may be best or, in certain cases, crucial for the patient's recovery.

Finally, PPS incentives to shorten a patient's length of stay and reduce treatment costs are forcing a major shift of subacute care services from hospitals to nursing facilities and patients' homes. Medicare discharges to skilled nursing facilities increased 40 percent and discharges to home health care rose 30 percent in the year following PPS's inception. As these shifts occur, patients are in danger of falling into a "no care zone" as the demand for aftercare services outstrips supply. Not only are aftercare providers unequipped to deal with these more intensely ill patients, but Medicare coverage for these services is extremely limited. As a result, many patients simply cannot obtain the care that was previously provided and paid for in the hospital.

The types of quality problems that may arise from these cost-cutting incentives include: inappropriately refusing to admit patients; inappropriately transferring patients to other hospitals; underusing the necessary services; substituting quality materials, devices and supplies with inferior ones; and prematurely discharging patients. These problems are compounded by public confusion about Medicare coverage and patients' rights and appeal options under PPS, a confusion which leaves patients helpless to challenge decisions affecting their care.

The Primitive Art of Assessing Quality

As noted previously, the extent of these problems cannot be measured because we lack not only a widely accepted definition of quality, but also the relevant data and a system for measuring it. HCFA (the agency that administers Medicare) should take responsibility for overcoming this deficiency. Instead, the

Health Care Financing Administration exploits the absence of information to dismiss reported quality-of-care problems as few, isolated, and anecdotal.

In addition to showing no embarrassment over its irresponsibility, HCFA has been seriously negligent in complying with Congressionally mandated reporting on the impact of PPS. At least eight such reports and studies required over the last two and a half years are overdue. The first report, due in December 1984, was released in draft form a year later, but only in response to a subpoena from the Senate Special Committee on Aging chaired by Senator John Heinz (R-Pa.). HCFA's report addressed hospital cost and utilization issues, but not quality concerns. Its second report is now a year late.

HCFA also failed to issue an impact report due two years ago on skilled nursing facilities. Although the agency had completed an impact report on home health care, it opted for an oral briefing rather than to publish its findings. In the briefing, HCFA officials denied that a significant increase in discharges to home health care had taken place, blatantly contradicting their own internal data. Their failure to report on the impact of PPS has spawned considerable speculation that they are incompetent, hiding something, deliberately snubbing Congress, or all of the above.

Meanwhile, a host of outside studies conducted by such groups as the Commission on Professional and Hospital Activities and the Rand Corporation are underway and expected to provide some answers.

What obstacles prevent the government from assessing PPS's impact on the delivery of care? The most vital quality-of-care information cannot be measured in the hospital, but is reflected in a patient's health status outcome following discharge from the hospital to the home or long-term care setting. Unfortunately, current data collection and review systems stop at the hospital door, and studies which attempt to overcome these limitations tend to be laborious, costly and one-shot at best.

If it really wanted to, HCFA could help solve this problem. Data systems exist which can help assess patients' health status outside the hospital. For example, physician and outpatient claims, paid under Medicare Part B (which reimburses physician services), constitute a potentially important data source. Claims data, available from skilled nursing facilities and home health agencies, and post-discharge death data, which is available from Social Security files, could also be used. Clearly, all of these data sources could be merged to yield ongoing, easily usable information on the most important measure of quality: health status outcome. It should be underscored that the obstacle is neither technical expertise nor resources, but political will.

What the Professionals Say

Lack of scientific data has forced those concerned with the system's impact on quality to seek out other sources of information, including professional opinion polls and Congressional hearings. Both have been pivotal in shaping current public perceptions that PPS has caused the quality of American health care to falter.

According to many professional association polls, physicians strongly believe that the quality of care has deteriorated under PPS. Sixty-six percent of hospital medical directors responding to a 1986 AMA survey indicated that the quality of care had suffered and 43 percent noted pressure under PPS to discharge patients early. Forty percent acknowledged that they were in fact discharging Medicare patients earlier under PPS. The terrible irony is that nearly all of these respondents indicated that earlier discharges worsened patients' health.

Among hospital administrators, 54 percent said they expected quality of care to diminish as a result of PPS (in contrast to only 20 percent of consumers polled), according to a survey by the National Research Corporation. While fears were greatest among administrators of small hospitals, 65 percent of these respondents also said they expected their hospitals to profit under PPS.

Many of these surveys are admittedly unscientific. They have low response rates and respondents are likely to be among the most dissatisfied, especially physicians who are traditionally hostile to regulatory forces that restrict their independence. The poll results are nonetheless important because they voice concerns from those people with front-line responsibility for quality of care.

The Heinz Committee

More than any other group, the Senate Special Committee on Aging, known as the Heinz Committee, has raised the quality-of-care issue under PPS to the level of a grave public concern. At Senator Heinz's request, the General Accounting Office (GAO) conducted the first study of premature discharges. Surveying six communities, the GAO found patients being discharged "sicker and quicker," home health agencies facing heavier caseloads of more intensely ill patients, and an inadequate supply of nursing home beds to meet the burgeoning need. As expected, PPS's defenders, in particular HCFA, once again dismissed these findings as unscientific.

The Committee's three well-publicized hearings on the quality impact of the PPS system were held in late 1985. One after another, patients, physicians, relatives, hospital and nursing home administrators, and advocacy groups testified to the worst imaginable abuses under the PPS system, with special ire reserved for HCFA. One 65-year-old-woman told of her mother's death 14 hours after being prematurely discharged to a nursing home. "I feel like all of this is what killed my mother. It is just like murder to me," she said, referring to the system which thrust her frail, dying parent out of the hospital. For lack of any other, these hearings became the sole public forum where patients, advocates for the elderly, providers of all types, and researchers could bring their experiences, findings, and concerns.

Patients' Rights Gone Wrong

Among the many concerns raised by the Heinz hearings was the great frustration over PPS's baffling and virtually dysfunctional system of patient appeal rights, rights intended to safeguard the quality of patients' care. Thanks largely to these hearings, gains have been made in the patient appeal process. But until recently, patients seeking to appeal abuses under PPS would have to have been both healthy and clever enough to outwit a system that was nearly the perfect Catch-22.

Under this Byzantine system, patients could challenge a premature discharge only if they were notified in writing of the hospital's intention to release them, or to charge them if they refused to go. This "notice of noncoverage" was the only source of information about appeal rights and procedures that hospitals were required to provide. Worse yet, they were not required to issue these notices unless they intended to bill the patient. This allowed hospitals to inform patients of their discharge verbally, preventing them from ever seeing the notice of their appeal rights.

It was a gap that invited misinformation and abuse. Most patients simply accepted what they were told and left the hospital, too intimidated to challenge such statements as, "Your DRG is up," "Your Medicare days are up," or "Your benefits are expiring." Patients simply didn't know that their Medicare eligibility and benefits remain unchanged under PPS, or that only physicians— not hospitals—can discharge them, and then only when deemed medically appropriate.

Also unavailable to patients was clear information about Medicare's coverage of different levels of aftercare and their impact on patients' discharge rights. For instance, a patient, when no longer acutely ill, may not be discharged if he or she is in need of skilled nursing care and none is available outside the hospital. Until placement can be found, Medicare will continue to pay the hospital as if that patient were acutely ill. This is not the case, however, for patients requiring lower levels of care, such as intermediate care, home health care, or home support services. By Medicare standards, discharging patients who require home or intermediate care is acceptable, regardless of whether such care is available. Thus, gaps in Medicare coverage itself seriously weaken the quality and coordination of care and compound the confusion over when it is appropriate to discharge the patient.

Finally, patients who successfully cleared these hurdles to challenge their discharge encountered yet another contradiction: They were given two calendar days notification before being charged. If they appealed, a determination was required within three working days. Thus, in order to exercise appeal rights, a patient had to risk paying for at least one day of care—or several days—if the process spanned a weekend. If the patient was dissatisfied with the review determination, he or she could seek administrative and then judicial appeal. However, the risk of personal financial liability ruled out doing this while remaining in the hospital.

Stung by criticism, HCFA moved to address this major flaw in the appeal system. Effective March 24, 1986, hospitals must distribute to every Medicare patient upon admission a notice entitled, "An Important Message from Medicare." In language agreed upon by five major provider and patient advocacy groups, the document spells out the circumstances under which a patient may be discharged, along with the appeal rights and procedures available.

In addition, Congress has recently removed the financial risk of patient appeals by postponing the time when hospitals can charge patients until after the appeals have actually been determined. While hardly adequate to protect the quality of patient care, these reforms offer significant improvements.

UNDERSTANDING THE DRG APPEALS PROCESS

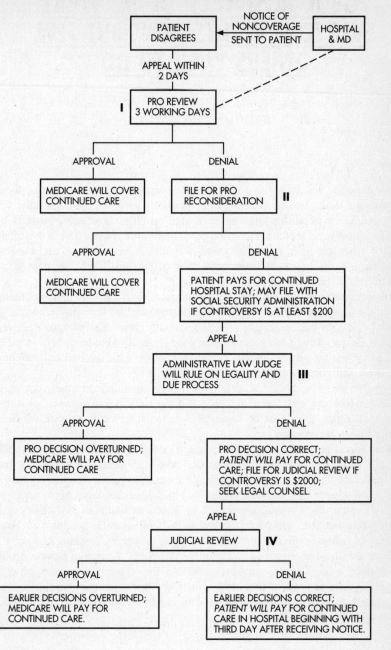

Source:
Massachusetts Executive Office of Elder Affairs

PUBLIC HOSPITALS: DOING WHAT EVERYONE WANTS DONE BUT FEW OTHERS WISH TO DO

Emily Friedman

American public hospitals—that is, institutions owned by federal, state, or local governments in the United States—today present a series of contradictions.

Among urban public hospitals are several of the oldest health care institutions on the continent, yet that heritage often earns them little respect. Public hospitals in many cities are filled to capacity and suffering severe financial and clinical problems as a result; but in rural areas, lack of business threatens many government health care institutions.

Residencies in public teaching hospitals are often eagerly sought; yet many physicians who trained in such residencies hesitate to refer their patients to these hospitals. Several public hospitals—Cook County Hospital, Chicago; Bellevue Hospital Center, New York City; Boston City Hospital—are legendary in medical history; but the physical plants of the Boston and Chicago hospitals (among others) are sadly deteriorated.

The demise of the public hospital was widely predicted after the passage of Medicare/Medicaid legislation in 1965. But the anticipated wave of closings never took place, and most of those who called for closure or sale of these hospitals have fallen silent.

The federal government issued a postage stamp in 1986 in honor of public hospitals (originally proposed to note Bellevue's 250th anniversary), but has been reluctant to offer financial support to them. Yet public hospitals survive. Some 1600 general hospitals are owned by cities, counties, city-county arrangements, hospital districts and authorities, or states; as many as 300 others also exist. Public facilities represent more than half of all rural hospitals, a large minority of urban hospitals, and the majority of university teaching hospitals.

They are, in some ways, an anachronism—a public force in a private health care market, a huge government presence in a free-enterprise economy. Yet it is probably true of most of them that if they did not exist, they would have to be invented; for they do a job—several jobs, in fact—that everyone wants done, but no one else wishes to do.

". . . the Infirm, the Aged . . ."

The public hospital tradition is intertwined with that of the almshouse—the British practice, imported to North America, of establishing a specific institution for those who were viewed as the failures of society. As public hospital historian Harry Dowling, M.D., notes, after Henry VIII closed many religious institutions in England in the 1530s, "Local officials found themselves responsible for the aged, chronically ill, and permanently disabled; homeless women before and during childbirth; foundlings and orphans; the insane, feebled-minded, and alcoholics; and persons with medical and surgical illnesses who today would be placed in a general hospital" (Dowling HF: *City Hospitals*. Cambridge, Mass.: Harvard University Press, 1982).

At a time when "respectable" people received care at home, those who could not were social outcasts, even if their only crimes were illness and poverty. The almshouse was also a workhouse, where able-bodied pauper and recovering patient alike were expected to work off at least part of what they owed society for shelter, food, and what medical care had been afforded them.

That tradition, too, followed the emigrants to colonial America. Almshouses were founded early on—in Henricopolis, Virginia, in 1612; in New Amsterdam (New York) in 1658; and in Boston in 1665, for example.

But these early institutions would not become hospitals. They did care for the sick; but this task was not viewed differently from any other in the almshouse. Nor were the ill differentiated at first from healthy paupers or other "undeserving" residents. It was in these early days that one attitude took root that continues to haunt public hospitals: the idea that because the inmates (as they were often called) were not socially worthy, the conditions in which they were given food, shelter, and medical care need not be equal to conditions elsewhere.

Indeed, in puritan America, it was appropriate that almshouse conditions be less than kind, so as to encourage the inmates to reform and go back into productive lives in society as soon as possible. This attitude extended, illogically, to the aged, infirm, and chronically ill who constituted a significant part of the almshouse population. Why one came to the almshouse was, in fact, much less important than the fact that one did.

As a result, writes University of Pennsylvania historian Charles Rosenberg, Ph.D.: "Admission to an almshouse ward—even for unavoidable illness or injury—was a confession of failure" (Rosenberg C. From Almshouse to Hospital: The Shaping of Philadelphia General Hospital. *Milbank Fund Mem Q* 1982;60[1]:108–154).

The first almshouse that would evolve into a public hospital was founded in Philadelphia in 1731 or 1732. It provided medical care for inmates who were already there, and also admitted patients whose sole reason for seeking refuge there was illness. On Jan 21, 1736, a French seaman and merchant named Jean Louis died in his adopted city, New Orleans; he willed his estate to establishment of a hospital there for the poor, which was done on March 10 of that year. This institution would become Charity Hospital.

Later in 1736, the Bellevue Infirmary was founded "on top of the first almshouse in New York, located at the present site of City Hall," reports Marty Davis, spokesman for the New York City Health and Hospitals Corporation. Its charge: to house "the infirm, the aged, the unruly, and the maniac."

The founding of Charity and Bellevue at almost precisely the same time has led to a lively debate between the two as to which is the oldest continuously operating hospital in the United States. (Philadelphia General closed in 1977.) Bellevue's claim is based on the fact that New York became a state in 1776, whereas Louisiana did not become one until 1812. Charity's advocates point out that as neither New York nor Louisiana was a state at the time the hospitals were founded, the determining factor should be the age of the institution.

Bellevue has temporarily won the battle, having been selected as the site for the introduction of the ''Public Hospitals'' 22-cent stamp in 1986. It must be added, however, that the stamp had been the brainchild of the late Sen. Jacob Javits of New York, and the ceremony might well have been held at Bellevue in any case.

Other almshouse-hospitals followed: in Baltimore in 1776, Washington, DC, in 1806, Cleveland in 1837, Seattle in 1877, Los Angeles in 1878. Boston City Hospital was founded as a freestanding institution in 1864, as was Cook County Hospital in 1866 in Chicago. Smaller communities were also erecting alms-houses.

David Rothman, Ph.D., director of the Center for the Study of Society and Medicine at the Columbia University College of Physicians and Surgeons, notes that ''between 1820 and 1840, some 60 towns in Massachusetts constructed new almshouses, and many others rehabilitated existing ones. By 1840, the state had 180 almshouses.'' In New York, he says, ''By 1833, all but four of the state's 55 counties had erected a poorhouse.'' The same was true in many states.

Rothman adds: ''The essential function of the almshouse, until the 1830s, was to serve as the great catch-all: it housed those who were unattached to family or other social support and who had no call on private charity. The 'worthy poor' were connected—to family, friends, or church. The 'unworthy poor' were unconnected.''

As a result, these institutions had a highly heterogeneous population to deal with—able-bodied paupers (although these were probably few in number and became even more scarce as time went on), unwed pregnant women, the frail elderly, unwanted or disabled orphans, alcoholics, victims of contagious disease, the severely mentally ill. As the nineteenth century proceeded, another group appeared: immigrants, especially ethnic minorities, who were also ''uncon-nected.''

After Massachusetts General Hospital was founded in 1821, for example, its services were soon sought by large numbers of immigrants (Boston City Hospital would not be founded for another 43 years). Dowling notes the resistance of the hospital's board of trustees to caring for Irish patients, because, the board claimed: ''Admission of such patients creates in the minds of our citizens a prejudice against the Hospital, making them unwilling to enter it. It thus tends directly to lower the general standing and character of its inmates'' (Dowling, City Hospitals).

In time, Boston City Hospital would provide a solution to such problems, although Massachusetts General dropped its restrictions on certain ethnic groups before the city hospital was built. In general, long after the private hospital appeared, the almshouse-hospital was still expected to care for the unworthy or unconnected patient.

Rosenberg points out that until World War I, "the proportion of men to women in urban public hospitals was as high as two or three to one. The reason is that these patients were unconnected workers—a large proportion of them immigrants. Also, it was a much bigger disgrace for a woman to be a patient in a public hospital than for a man to be there."

Later—and it remains the case—black and other nonwhite Americans would also be cared for, to a disproportionate degree, in public hospitals.

Emergence From the Almshouse

Gradually, the public hospital began to emerge from the overall context of the almshouse. Several factors contributed to the change, of which two were paramount.

First, social reformers started to separate out the various populations that had been grouped in the institution. Rothman says, "What sparked this was the coming of a persuasion in the early nineteenth century that if the perfect institutional routine could be devised, it would solve the problem at hand." Thus more specialized institutional environments were needed. He adds, "The idea was that a well-ordered, well-disciplined prison or mental hospital instills in the patient habits of order, thus effecting a cure."

As a result, he says, "Children went to 'orphan asylums.' The mentally ill went to mental asylums. Petty criminals often ended up in jails."

Furthermore, he says, "Some of this cult of asylum did spill over onto the almshouse; there was some notion that the almshouse could rehabilitate its inmates. But the almshouse never became an honored institution in pre-Civil War America, the way that prisons and mental hospitals did. They became the glory of the new republic; de Tocqueville came to America, in fact, to study our prisons."

The almshouse did not join the institutional honor roll; but as the people housed there for social reasons were drawn off, the medical and quasimedical populations remained. In some cases, these people had already been separated out from the others, by means of differently colored uniforms, distinct wards, and, more and more, separate infirmaries whose sole purpose was to provide medical care, whether acute, long-term, or psychiatric.

A second factor leading to the development of the public hospital as an entity in itself was another deeply rooted almshouse tradition: medical education. Patients avoided the almshouse unless they were in extremis; but physicians eager to teach and learn were drawn to it.

The history of medicine was written in part within the forbidding walls of Philadelphia General Hospital, where Benjamin Rush and later Samuel D. Gross taught; of Cook County Hospital, where Christian Fenger became a legend; of Boston City Hospital, where David Williams Cheever was a member of the original attending staff; and many other public institutions. This legacy of excellence has continued, in some hospitals. Ronald Anderson, M.D., director of Parkland Memorial Hospital, Dallas, points with pride to the fact that two Nobel laureates see patients at Parkland. Bellevue physicians Andre Cournand, M.D., and Dickinson Richards, M.D., garnered the Nobel Prize for medicine in 1956 for their contributions to the development of cardiac catheterization. More recently, Olga Jonasson, M.D., a surgeon at Cook County (also professor of surgery, University of Illinois, Chicago), headed the national Task Force on Organ Transplantation.

Given that they were the only places where physicians and students had access to patients who could be required to participate in teaching (and where was born the unfortunate phrase, "clinical material," to describe them), it is not surprising that medical education came early to the almshouses. The most stigmatized of institutions became the teaching grounds of the most prestigious of physicians.

However, medical education in public hospitals prior to the twentieth century was mostly a passive experience for the students. Large clinics held in amphitheaters consisted of lectures and demonstrations by faculty members who only rarely allowed a student to enter the pit and actually examine the patient.

Sometimes there were "ward walks" as well, in which an attending physician and students would tour patient areas. One story, apocryphal or not, tells of a patient at Cook County in the late 1800s who observed such a group walking through and then turned to a fellow patient to say, "Ole, we ought to be a hell of a lot better. The professor has just walked by."

Nevertheless, as the years wore on, more and more students attended lectures and demonstrations and watched autopsies and physical examinations as part of an increasingly formal education process. Residents became a fixture at the teaching hospitals and would remain so for more than a century; in many hospitals, they became the unquestioned rulers. A tension that still exists today became apparent: "House officers tended to believe that administrators were not really interested in making people well, but only in getting involved in politics, pinching pennies, and slavishly following a rigid set of rules. Administrators, on the other hand, felt that house officers, in their zeal to learn and practice, were willing to flout every rule to the point of destroying the hospital" (Dowling, *City Hospitals*).

For both social and technical reasons, physicians had an incentive to improve and refine the public hospital and separate it from the almshouse by the mid-nineteenth century. Attending physicians and residents alike played a key role in upgrading what were often appalling conditions—poor food (some patients developed scurvy during their stays), inadequate nursing (which, until Florence Nightingale's ideas were promulgated widely, was often provided by other inmates), understaffing, unproductive political appointees in key jobs, insufficient plants and equipment. Physicians, often in partnership with crusading "society ladies," helped ameliorate some of the worst problems.

Rise of Private Hospitals

After the Civil War, the revolution in medicine changed the status of the hospital—no matter what its ownership—from the site of care of last resort to the best place to receive care. Private hospitals started to come into being at the same time that public hospitals were achieving identities separate from the almshouses.

Why did the public hospitals survive? Why were they not abandoned in favor of private facilities?

There were many reasons: a public hospital infrastructure in many cities; the social and clinical unattractiveness of many public hospital patients; the fact that private patients would be less willing to participate in teaching activities (given that they usually had a choice, unlike public hospital patients); and the desire of governments to retain the power, prestige, and patronage that accompanied public hospitals.

The increasing effectiveness of medicine was also a factor. If society accepted the idea of segregating the undeserving and/or unconnected poor, it still had to grapple with the question of whether they should be denied the benefits of health care. (This was an interesting ethical question, given that it was largely the almshouse poor whose bodies had been used to learn much of what was making medicine more effective.)

As Rothman says, the public hospital provided a perfect solution: "The municipal hospital performed the function of keeping everyone's conscience clear in terms of health care for the lower classes. Once hospital care was understood to be socially desirable, and, indeed, very important, could society really say that those without funds should go without it? The answer was, 'No. We have a municipal hospital as our grand act of charity.'"

Most of the context of the contemporary urban public hospital, then, had been established by the late nineteenth century. The nature of the teaching relationship changed, of course, especially after the release of the Flexner Report in 1910 and the coming of stricter standards for medical education and medical care itself.

The growth of private university hospitals, and private hospitals affiliated with medical schools, created a competition for resources and faculty in which many public hospitals came out second best. But many did not; and the ever-present residents continued to serve as a force for high quality of medical care, if they were not always as effective in achieving high-quality overall conditions in the hospitals.

The final element influencing the development of the public hospital has been its public ownership. Government in the United States has a curious love-hate relationship with itself, which is reflected in the ambivalence it shows toward the institutions for which it has responsibility. Nowhere is this more evident than in the public hospital. This is not to say that politicians have ignored public hospitals; indeed, figures such as Mayor James Michael Curley of Boston and Gov. Huey Long of Louisiana were vocal proponents of the institutions they sponsored.

But they and others tolerated corruption, patronage hiring, underfunding, lax accounting and management practices, and the erection of cumbersome, sometimes impossible procedures that made the operation of the institutions a nightmare. In many cases, these practices were not only tolerated, but encouraged. This hobble was in evidence soon after the first public hospitals were built, and its scars are deep in many cities.

Politicians, for obvious reasons, also liked to build huge institutions. In 1910, Cook County Hospital had 1350 beds; by 1960, it had 3260. In 1910, Boston

City Hospital had 1061 beds; by 1950, it had 2376. Similar figures could be cited for other cities. Given the hospital administration axiom that no facility larger than 500 beds is manageable, these behemoths would have been a problem even if they had not often been labyrinthine mazes constructed in stages on the bones of eighteenth- and nineteenth-century plants.

Nevertheless, the end of World War II saw the public general hospital still very much in evidence. It was often a prestigious teaching facility if located in a city—and most of the 100 largest cities had at least one such institution. The passage in 1946 of the so-called Hill-Burton legislation, which made federal funds available for hospital construction, spurred rural areas to build hospitals, the majority of them publicly owned—often by hospital districts, which became popular in the late 1940s, especially in the West.

Not only did public hospitals survive in the postwar period; they multiplied. In 1946, there were 785 general short-term hospitals owned by states and localities; in 1955, there were 1120. By 1960, there were 1260; by 1965, 1453.

Decline of Sanitariums

At the same time, one class of public hospitals was headed in the other direction. Of all the contagious scourges that had swept the populace in the eighteenth and nineteenth centuries, tuberculosis had proved one of the most intractable, and public sanitariums had become a fixture in most states. Changes in treatment had a fatal effect on these institutions from World War II on: in 1946, there were 412 nonfederal tuberculosis and respiratory disease hospitals; in 1955, there were 347. From then on, their doom was speedy: in 1960, there were 238; in 1965, 178; in 1970, 101; in 1975, 36; in 1980, 11; and in 1985, 7.

A staple of nineteenth-century society has passed from the scene. An event that many predicted would cause most public hospitals, at least in the cities, to suffer a similar fate took place in July 1965: Congress passed Public Law 89-97, creating Medicaid and Medicare.

Time had dimmed the remembrance of the heterogeneous constituency of the public hospital; it had been forgotten that although most of the patients shared the state of poverty, it was about all they did share. The chronically ill, the person suffering from both medical and psychiatric problems, the homeless, the alcoholic, and those compromised in other ways were all still largely the responsibility of the public hospital. But in the flush 1960s, they were all grouped together as simply the poor and sick. And Medicaid and Medicare were configured to underwrite the care of the majority of the poor and the sick at any hospital, public or not (even if in the long run, that did not prove to be the case).

It was widely predicted that, given a choice, the public hospital patient would abandon that institution for more comfortable private hospital care. Many of them did. Medicare patients, particularly, fanned out among many institutions. Many patients in need of long-term care found a welcome in the burgeoning nursing home and intermediate care facility industries. And many of the poor tested private waters as well.

Most urban public hospitals faced a decline in inpatient utilization, and they reacted by reducing the number of beds they operated. Boston City Hospital's 2376 beds in 1950 had dropped to 859 by 1970; Cook County Hospital's 3260 beds in 1950 were down to 2263 in 1970. District of Columbia General Hospital lost 433 beds between 1950 and 1970; Baltimore City Hospitals went from 1810 beds to 857 in the same period. Los Angeles County Hospital (later Los Angeles County-University of Southern California Medical Center) had 3439 beds in 1950 and 2105 beds in 1970; San Francisco General Hospital went from 1101 beds in 1950 to 822 in 1970.

Alan Sager, Ph.D., an associate professor at the Boston University School of Public Health, reports that between 1950 and 1980, the number of urban public hospital beds declined by 38.3 percent, while private urban hospital beds increased by 60.6 percent. Some entire institutions closed as well. But no massive rush of closings materialized.

Why not? There is no one answer. But one major factor was that, as Rothman says, "Voluntary hospitals remain uncomfortable with large numbers of any down-and-out group, whether or not they are insured: the Skid Row alcoholic, the Skid Row AIDS patient, many other marginal patients. It is not at all clear that the public hospital's mission of serving the undesirable was necessarily obviated by Medicare and Medicaid."

Furthermore, although Medicaid and Medicare started out paying hospitals fairly well, Medicaid payments soon declined, in some states precipitously. Furthermore, Medicaid never covered the entire poverty population. At its height in 1977, it sponsored 92 percent of those living below the federal poverty line, according to the Health Care Financing Administration; other analysts argue that it never came that close. Today, Medicaid covers between 38 percent and 42 percent of the poverty population.

Finally, the role of the urban public hospital (whether university-owned or university-affiliated) in medical education remained central, some 200 years after Benjamin Rush first made rounds at the Philadelphia almshouse. In 1976, a national commission on public-general hospitals was convened by the Hospital Research and Educational Trust, an affiliate of the American Hospital Association. With support from the Robert Wood Johnson and W. K. Kellogg foundations, it conducted an in-depth study of government hospitals. It reported on its findings in 1978.

Among the highlights of the report: in 1976, more than ten years after the enactment of Medicaid and Medicare, there were 1905 public general hospitals in the United States. In addition to those located in the 100 largest cities; 357 were located in other metropolitan areas; 45 were university-owned; and 1413 were rural. Of the 100 largest cities, 76 still had public facilities: 49 had 1, 21 had 2, 5 had 3 or 4, and New York City had 15.

Perhaps most striking, the occupancy rates in these hospitals were far higher than might have been expected: 69.9 percent in all public facilities, 76.5 percent in university facilities, 73.7 percent in urban facilities in the 100 largest cities, 72.4 percent for other metropolitan facilities, and 65 percent in rural facilities.

The same year, average occupancy for all US hospitals was 76 percent; for private nonprofit acute general and related hospitals, it was 77.1 percent; for investor-owned acute facilities, it was 64.8 percent. In 1978, public hospitals in the aggregate accounted for 45.3 percent of all ambulatory hospital visits in the country, and nearly half of such visits in the 100 largest cities. They trained nearly 40 percent of all medical and dental residents and 20 percent of other health care professionals who trained in hospitals. Public facilities represented 48.5 percent (1413) of the 2912 rural hospitals in the United States, and 67 percent (99048) of the 147387 rural hospital beds. Reports of the death of the public hospital had been greatly exaggerated. It had not triumphed, perhaps, and there had been casualties, but it had survived.

In 1732, the Philadelphia almshouse opened its ambivalent doors to the homeless outcasts of a judgmental society. Four years later, the almshouse that would become Bellevue did the same. In 1864, Boston City Hospital was completed. It seemed somehow fitting, then, that as urban homelessness made a tragic comeback in the 1980s, some of these landmark institutions would come full circle.

In the early 1980s, Boston City Hospital opened a shelter for the homeless in a public long-term care facility. Bellevue Hospital Center moved into a modern tower in 1975, but many of the buildings on its campus had by then earned historic landmark status. Recently some of those buildings were reopened, also as shelters for homeless people. These new outcasts now sleep amidst the ghosts of brethren who have sought similar refuge within those walls for 250 years.

DEMISE OF PHILADELPHIA GENERAL AN INSTRUCTIVE CASE: OTHER CITIES TREAT PUBLIC HOSPITAL ILLS DIFFERENTLY

Emily Friedman

Despite the remarkable staying power of public hospitals, not all have survived. The pattern of closure, however, is complex, especially in cities. Alan Sager, Ph.D., associate professor, Boston University, conducted a survey of hospital closings in 52 large U.S. cities between 1937 and 1980. Defining a closure as "cessation of acute inpatient services in a hospital within the city boundaries," he found "only three public hospital closures or relocations outside the city between 1937 and 1950." From 1950 to 1959, there were six; from 1960 to 1969, there were three. From 1970 to 1980, however, there were ten.

"There was a burst of closings between 1978 and 1982, probably due to recession and economic problems," Sager reports; four more hospitals were shuttered between 1980 and 1983 for a total of 14 in the five-year period. However, there have been no closings among the hospitals in his sample since 1983. Sager ascribes this apparent deceleration to "a perception that the need for public hospital care has grown with the increasing number of uninsured patients," of whom the current Census Bureau estimate is 37 million or more. Also, he says, "I think local government has become more sophisticated, and when it desires to contain its obligation to the uninsured, it finds methods more politically palatable than closure."

Elliott C. Roberts, chief executive officer of Charity Hospital in New Orleans, has overseen public hospitals in New York City, Detroit, and Chicago, as well as in New Orleans, and he resists generalizing about closures: "Each situation is unique."

Dennis Andrulis, Ph.D., director of research and policy of the National Association of Public Hospitals (NAPH), adds, "It is difficult to say if there has been a trend in the closing, sale, or lease of urban public hospitals. It's an idiosyncratic process, dependent on a number of political factors. A politician might use his or her own clout to put forth a proposal that would adversely affect a public hospital; but that doesn't happen too often. What does happen is that from time to time, a critical point is reached in terms of the capital cycle of a facility. There may be periodic attempts or proposals to change the ownership of a public hospital, but it happens most when there is need for either renovation or replacement."

The Philadelphia Story

Of all public hospital closings in the past 20 years—if not of all those in the modern era—none has been studied, discussed, or debated as much as the 1977 closure and subsequent demolition of the oldest hospital of any kind in the United States, Philadelphia General Hospital (PGH). Its closing appears to be more controversial in hindsight than it was at the time; as Charles Rosenberg, Ph.D., a historian at the University of Pennsylvania, has observed, "It succumbed with surprisingly little public protest" (Rosenberg, *From Almshouse to Hospital*).

The core issue, in fact, was not whether the hospital should have been closed; by 1976, when the decision to close it was announced, PGH was a largely empty, deteriorating hulk. Ernest Zeger, executive director of the public Philadelphia Nursing Home, who served as general director of PGH during the closing process, recalls, "In 1976, there were as many as 1800 beds that were not being used on any given day. Its facilities were antiquated, and with Medicaid and Medicare, the patients were not coming to the hospital for acute care. We were down to around 250 acute patients, and 400 'disposition patients'—those who did not need acute care but placement of whom in other settings was not possible."

Philadelphia General Hospital still had approximately 160000 outpatient visits a year, however. The question is how, in 30 years, one of the most prestigious teaching hospitals in the country, where obtaining a residency was a major accomplishment, could fall on such hard times.

For long-time observers of the Philadelphia scene, there is little mystery about it. "Prior to the end of World War II," says Robert M. Sigmond, scholar in residence at Temple University and former president of Philadelphia's Albert Einstein Medical Center, "PGH was an extremely fine medical institution. Physicians seeking to become specialists by an informal process were delighted to be associated with it. When residency requirements changed, specialty boards sought full-time directors of programs, however, and residency programs began to shift. The public hospital model was no longer seen as the preferred model. So good liberal thinking began to favor affiliation of public hospitals with medical schools."

Enter Philadelphia politics, particularly the 1951 city election, in which power was seized from the old Republican machine by a reform-minded, if elitist, Democratic administration headed by new mayor Richardson Dilworth. Walter Lear, M.D., president of the Institute of Social Medicine and Community Health, who served as acting executive director of PGH in 1967–68, recalls, "The basic philosophy of the new administration was couched in terms of 'public-private partnership,' as we now use the term. It was expressed in a variety of major city activities. The administration assumed that the city's medical schools, of which there were five (University of Pennsylvania, Temple, Thomas Jefferson, Hahnemann, and what was then Women's Medical College), had the talent and credibility to take over leadership of the city health department," which included PGH and an infectious disease hospital that was closed in the 1950s.

In 1958, the Dilworth administration pushed through an affiliation plan that involved all five medical schools in the operation of PGH. The goal, according to health policy analyst Paul Socolar, was "a reorganized PGH under private, expert management, freed from the patronage system" (Socolar P: The closing of Philadelphia General Hospital. Presented at the 1986 Meeting of the American Public Health Association). What the city got was something less.

"No one was really responsible for programs at PGH," Sigmond recalls. "Each medical school had its own special interest. In medicine, for example, there were five services—each an adjunct of the overall service at the medical schools and the hospitals they owned. No one was focusing on the institution as a whole." Lear adds, "The medical schools were primarily interested in their goals, which were good teaching programs; as long as they could count on a quantity of medical service activity to meet the requirements of residency training, they were satisfied. They didn't really care what was happening to the hospital otherwise. I don't mean to depict the medical schools as consciously and deliberately trying to kill PGH; they just did not have any real interest in its survival. They pursued those activities that they considered appropriate to meet their goals as academic medical institutions."

Interinstitutional rivalries and tensions led to problems in division of responsibility, and later to virtual warfare. Eventually all the schools but the University of Pennsylvania either withdrew from the arrangement or were forced out. At the very end, Hahnemann was the only medical school involved, and then only briefly, according to Lear.

The lack of medical school loyalty to PGH as an entity might have been balanced by the city, but the municipal government "was less than vigilant," according to Socolar. Dilworth was succeeded by James Tate, who was more of a practitioner of patronage politics. As PGH was no longer available for patronage jobs because of the medical school affiliations, the city did not focus on the hospital or its problems. In fact, in 1969, after the passage of Medicaid and Medicare and a concomitant loss of some patient volume, Tate offered "to turn the hospital over to the University of Pennsylvania altogether," Socolar reports, but the offer was rejected.

Other nails were driven into PGH's coffin during the 1960s. Sigmond reports that although federal health dollars were available almost for the asking for urban health initiatives, "PGH, to the best of my recollection, did not respond at all." As a result, he says, "The energies that were mobilized in Philadelphia in terms of community health and leadership among the poor went in other directions. There were no Great Society initiatives at PGH, although there were at other hospitals—Einstein, University, Hahnemann, and Temple."

So patients eligible for care under those initiatives were drawn away from PGH. Meanwhile, the hospital's 1920s physical plant was beginning to fall apart. Finally, changes in medical education during the 1960s brought an end to PGH's long-time irreplaceable role as the center of teaching in the city. Private hospitals were now heavily involved in teaching activities, and privately insured patients as well as the indigent were the focus of educational activities. Also, with more payment available, low-income patients were being treated at many hospitals, including those owned by the medical schools.

By the late 1960s, only the University of Pennsylvania still conducted extensive teaching activities at PGH. Socolar and other critics charge that the university took advantage of the situation; its own hospital being within a stone's throw of PGH made it easy to "skim" paying patients and refer them to the university hospital, he says. Certain teaching programs were transferred to the private facility in their entirety, including pediatrics, obstetrics, and neurosurgery.

Although the accusations against the medical school may well be overdrawn, there are indications that it was not overly concerned about the ongoing decline of PGH. That may not have been its responsibility; the hospital, after all, was owned and subsidized by the city, and the primary guardian of the hospital should have been the city. As Sigmond observes, "The medical school wasn't the villain; there was no massive plot. It was just a case of clinical department heads acting like typical clinical department heads of that era. The problem was really the failure of the city to create a mechanism to protect the mission of the institution."

In 1971, a master plan to build a new 600-bed acute care facility was announced, and $945000 in planning funds was approved in the November election that year. But that election also saw former police commissioner Frank Rizzo chosen as mayor, and that spelled the end of PGH. Rizzo said as early as December 1971 that PGH should be closed, Lear reports, and that was that.

Although the formal closing was announced in 1976 and completed in 1977, PGH's last years were spent in a dismal environment of declining patient volume, disinterest on the part of the city and most of the medical community, and continued deterioration of the physical plant. Rizzo attributed the decision to close PGH to its crumbling physical plant and the unavailability of capital to rebuild it. However, the real reason was rooted in decisions made by an administration 20 years gone. As Rosenberg observes, "The city's saying that PGH had to be closed because it was a poor-quality hospital was equivalent to pleading for mercy as an orphan after you've killed your parents."

The actual closing was more controversial on technical grounds than on philosophical ones. Mark Levitan, now president of Albert Einstein Medical Center, was executive director of the Hospital of the University of Pennsylvania from 1974 to 1983, and he recalls fearing that his hospital "would be inundated with patients." Once PGH was gone, he says, "The only effect was in obstetrics, where our caseload increased by 500 or 600 deliveries. Otherwise there was no evidence that our hospital or, to my knowledge, any other hospital saw much of an impact." Levitan recalls, "What we took issue with was not the closing, but the process."

Zeger contests this view, pointing out that the city established six outpatient family care centers, each affiliated with a backup hospital, and operated outpatient services at PGH for a year to ensure that patients would be enrolled in one of these centers. "I think the program worked very well," he says.

The city also converted a former state tuberculosis hospital into the Philadelphia Nursing Home in order to provide care for the 400 or so chronically ill and otherwise hard-to-place "disposition patients" who were left at PGH at the end. One woman patient was described at the time as having lived in the hospital for decades. The nursing home continues to provide services, operating at 90 percent occupancy, soon to be 95 to 98 percent, Zeger reports.

Nevertheless, there seems to have been widespread confusion about the closing, chiefly because there seems to have been widespread ignorance about how many patients the hospital was treating, who they were, where they would go —and what patients were supposed to do once PGH closed. Although there was an information campaign, its design was curious for a program seeking to inform low-income, socially marginal individuals. For example, one technique used— placing ads in the *Philadelphia Inquirer*—was likely not the best way to go about it.

Questions Remain

Two questions remain, after all these years. One is, why was there relatively little opposition to the closing? In other cities, there have been demonstrations, sit-ins, and near-riots when public hospitals were closed or threatened with closing. But not in Philadelphia. For one thing, says Sigmond, "Historically, PGH's constituency was more a medical-political one than a social one. I don't think low-income people were ever well-organized in this town, politically or otherwise."

Lear adds that the hospital's civil service physicians, "the principal advocates of PGH," had largely been deprived of power and voice over the years. As for the union representing hospital employees, he says, its leaders were convinced early on that the hospital would be closed, no matter what, and thus "devoted their energies to fighting for other jobs for their members, rather than fighting for the survival of the hospital." At the end, according to Lear, PGH "did not have a really loyal constituency that had any power."

The other question is, what was the effect of the closing? This is the focus of continued debate, even today, simply because there are no data. The Fellowship Commission of Philadelphia conducted a three-year study that was released in 1979 and concluded that "services were generally 'available' for most former users," although it could not account for "the fact that aggregate use rates at other facilities failed to increase enough to compensate for the absence of the public services" (Isaacs M, et al: *The Urban Public Hospital: Options for the 1980s.* Washington, DC, Alpha Center, 1982). However, there have been so many changes in urban hospital utilization that this does not necessarily mean compromised access to inpatient care. Also, the acute care census at PGH was quite low at the time of the closing; it would be difficult to track absorption of a few hundred patients in a city with so many hospitals.

On the other hand, Lear quotes from a press release issued in connection with the commission report: "Tens of thousands of financially needy and/or medically underserved Philadelphians did not have their health care needs met by the combined health services of public and private facilities before the closing of PGH, and their needs are still not being met today." No study has tracked individual patients; the Fellowship Commission sought to examine medical records, but the request was refused on grounds of confidentiality, according to Lear. Although the debate will continue, as the years pass, it becomes less and less likely that anyone will know whether access to acute inpatient care was affected by the closing.

Access to other forms of care is another matter, according to Zeger, who cites possible problems for patients with "combinations of medical problems and mental disability, for whom there is no longer a viable institution." These patients, he says, fall into a crack between the hospital and the nursing home. He also expresses concern about the homeless, because there is no "institution of last resort" for them.

Levitan says that although "a 1700-bed nursing home," which is what PGH had become, is not needed in the city, "a 300- or 400-bed acute public hospital would be useful, to provide for patients who have no other recourse. If an institution is there, it's easier to glean support for it. The government can walk away from a responsibility to the private providers, which is essentially the case in Philadelphia. It is appropriate for charitable institutions to provide charity care, but it gets to the point when it's an insurmountable problem."

To Sigmond, "This city would be better off if PGH were still here. I do not believe in two-track medicine; I would work to enable private services to be provided to patients from the institution's service area. But there was a great tradition here, which represented the commitment of the city to health care in a way that a public health department does not. This is not to say that a city that has never had a public hospital, like Pittsburgh, should start one. But when there exists the tradition of the oldest public hospital in the United States—with a fine reputation—it is criminal to destroy it."

Other Cities, Other Scenarios

There are happier stories of closings. It is interesting that although some were accompanied by far more acrimony than the one in Philadelphia, their long-term results appear more positive.

New York City's public hospital system has closed several facilities in recent years, sometimes despite great community opposition, but it seems to have worked out. Jo Ivey Boufford, M.D., president of the New York City Health and Hospitals Corporation, reports on the closing of five public hospitals—Delafield, Morrisania, Sydenham, Cumberland, and Greenpoint. "By and large," she says, "each was a case in which the facility had become physically obsolete." In addition, she points out, a replacement or equivalent facility was usually made available. The new, almost luxurious Woodhull Hospital was opened just as Greenpoint and Cumberland closed; the new (and later expanded) Harlem Hospital Center helped ease the closing of Sydenham.

Furthermore, she says, the city opened neighborhood family care centers to provide comprehensive outpatient services to patients of the closed hospitals. The idea appears to have worked better in New York than it did in Philadelphia. Boufford adds, "Constituencies in New York are very vocal and active. Any medically underserved community will be very concerned about loss of resources. The dialogue that has ensued around hospital closings thus has been successful—and patients are using the new facilities." There are no hard data, she says, but occupancy and utilization figures would indicate that the replacement facilities have gained acceptance. Also, in a city with 15 public hospitals, the loss of one is different from the closure of the only such facility in town.

There are other examples. Homer G. Phillips Hospital in St. Louis was closed in 1979 quite suddenly, leaving the pathetic picture of an older man standing on the steps of the closed facility, seeking his wife, who had been a patient there the day before. The closure caused enough political problems for the mayor that some observers cited it as a reason for his defeat in the 1980 elections. His successor pledged to compensate for the hospital's loss, and the area now has a public regional medical center that combines elements from closed city and county facilities—although it has financial problems of its own.

Other urban public hospitals have been transferred to private ownership, leased, or sold. What becomes evident is that there is no pattern, no one set of indicators, no overall point of no return. When you've seen one urban public hospital closing, as the joke goes, you've seen one urban public hospital closing. Despite the fears set off by the closure of Philadelphia General, relatively few city or county hospitals have been shuttered without replacement in the ten years since the demise of PGH. Those that have closed were usually "dead on their feet," to use Robert Sigmond's description of PGH at the end.

In fact, it seems that the best way to close an urban public hospital is to starve it first. As Bruce Vladeck, Ph.D., president of the United Hospital Fund of New York, has observed, "A full hospital never closes."

Closings Outside Cities

Rural public hospital closings have been less well documented than those in urban areas. Until recently, the closing of a hospital was seen as a sign of administrative failure, and was thus best completed out of sight. This is more easily done in rural areas than in media-minded cities.

A study by the American Hospital Association found that 22 state and local government rural general hospitals closed between 1980 and 1985, as did 24 public rural specialty hospitals. The closed general hospitals represented 1.7 percent of all rural general hospitals—a lower rate of closure than occurred in urban areas during the same period.

The authors of the study conclude that "rural hospitals may have a high degree of community support, may be one of the largest employers in the community, and may be viewed as an important element in attracting new individuals and industries to the area" (Mullner R, McNeil D: Rural and Urban Hospital Closures. *Health Aff* 1986;5[fall]:131–141). Furthermore, the authors conclude, many rural hospitals (public or private) are the only ones in the counties where they are located; therefore, every effort is made to retain them. Of the 85 rural hospitals of all types that closed between 1980 and 1985, the authors found, only 6 were in counties that were left with no hospital after the closure.

MEDICAID AND MANAGED CARE: TESTIMONY SUBMITTED TO THE HOUSE SUBCOMMITTEE ON HEALTH AND THE ENVIRONMENT

Michele Melden

Editor's Note: This is an edited version of testimony submitted by the National Health Law Program on September 14, 1990, in response to a request by the House of Representatives Subcommittee on Health and the Environment.

Over the past decade, the National Health Law Program (NHeLP) has monitored extensively the effect of health maintenance organizations (HMOs) and other managed care programs on Medicaid recipients. Based on this experience, the Subcommittee asked NHeLP to address the Bush Administration's stated intent to repeal two essential protections for Medicaid recipients enrolled in managed care plans: the current requirements that Medicaid recipients' enrollment in managed care be voluntary and that Medicaid recipients be enrolled alongside nonpoor, non-Medicaid recipients. If the Administration is successful in repealing these protections, the result would be mandatory Medicaid-only managed care programs.

Based on our experience, we urge this Subcommittee to reject any attempts to expand the use of managed care and to reject the proposal to abandon the two existing protections that are vital to our clients. Enrollment should be voluntary, and Medicaid recipients should be enrolled alongside non-poor, non-Medicaid recipients.

Introduction

Managed health care can be defined in many ways, one of which is a system that provides access to a range of needed services that are coordinated and monitored by a specific, appropriate health care manager. However, most forms of managed health care also contemplate use of capitation, a reimbursement method by which prepayment is made to cover a given patient's or patient group's health care needs. Capitation is used as an incentive to discourage overutilization of unnecessary services. Therefore, managed care coupled with capitation is principally a device used to control costs.

In states' implementation of managed care for Medicaid recipients, many problems have resulted in programs using capitation. This testimony will address itself principally to the relationship between capitation as an incentive to control overutilization and the special problems for Medicaid recipients that result from this incentive mechanism.

Because capitation poses significant risks to Medicaid recipients, protecting their freedom to choose between managed care and fee-for-service care, and instituting requirements that Medicaid recipients be enrolled alongside nonpoor, non-Medicaid recipients are essential to offset and compensate for these risks. In addition, a number of other safeguards should be added in order to rectify the problems posed by existing Medicaid managed care programs.

The Effects of Capitation

Capitation is a mechanism for paying an organization a set amount in advance to provide for the anticipated health care needs of a given group of patients. As used in managed care programs, capitation is supposed to institute incentives against overutilization of unnecessary services. The belief is that additional controls on utilization will result in greater efficiencies. In fact, proponents believe that the incentives to save will even improve care, because providers will be encouraged to devote more resources to preventive and primary care and to coordinating care.

Capitation must be contrasted to "fee-for-service" care. Under "fee-for-service" care, physicians are paid each time they provide care. Typically, an outside third party, such as an insurance company, pays for this care and assumes the risk of paying for care provided to a given patient group. Under this system, the physician is not placed at any financial risk; only the payor is at risk. In contrast, under capitation, the managed care plan responsible for providing the care is paid in advance to provide care to a given patient group. Therefore, the provider is placed at financial risk for the amount of care required. The provider thus doubles up as both a type of "insurer" and a provider. The extent to which the provider is placed at financial risk will affect the amount of care provided.

Many managed care plans translate their financial risks into risks imposed on the physicians as well. According to a recent study in the *New England Journal of Medicine*, the vast majority of HMOs impose financial incentives on physicians to control costs. These include the following: (1) the HMO withholds income, and if the physician or the group comes out with a deficit, the HMO retains the funds; (2) financial penalties are imposed on physicians for deficits that exceed the withheld amounts; (3) physicians are required to pay directly for laboratory and specialty referrals; and (4) bonuses are offered to physicians who spend less than the group average.[1] These incentive mechanisms are often reinforced with rigorous peer review for overutilization.

One scholar, Bruce Spitz, who has studied these systems, has criticized this use of physicians as "small insurance companies," because it places the physician in an "adversarial and pernicious" relationship with the patient.[2] Indeed, a recent study appearing in the *New England Journal of Medicine* documented that financial disincentives to serve will result in less service.[3]

In theory, the pressures posed by capitation are only supposed to encourage more "efficient" practice. However, the extent to which the capitated levels are inadequate to meet a patient group's needs will tip the balance toward "underservice."

The Medicaid Experience

Experience throughout the states has demonstrated that use of capitated managed care for Medicaid recipients has not resulted in more efficient or better care. Instead, these programs often have institutionalized incentives to "underserve" a population already suffering grossly inadequate access. Indeed, we must determine whether, in the cases in which "savings" are realized, these savings have resulted in worsened care to the already underserved. If so, there is no justification for shifting the limited dollars that states allocate for Medicaid recipients to the additional layers of bureaucracy, administration, and profit-taking involved in using managed care systems.

Underfinancing

Experience has shown that the use of capitation as an incentive to control overutilization compromises the quality of care that Medicaid recipients receive. The principal reason is that the capitated rates used in Medicaid managed care programs are based on a presumption that less must be spent on managed care than is spent in states' Medicaid fee-for-service systems.[4] In most states, the capitated rates are set at 90–95 percent of the Medicaid program's fee-for-service rates.[5] However, most states' Medicaid fee-for-service rates are highly underfinanced.[6] This underfinancing is directly related to a shortage of physicians willing to accept the Medicaid rates, and the resulting shortage of physicians willing to treat Medicaid recipients.[7]

Requiring that managed care programs save costs so that they justify themselves in relation to the existing underfinanced Medicaid system will result in continued underfinancing. This underfinancing, in turn, aggravates the managed care programs' incentives to underserve, creating the danger that managed care will replicate Medicaid's currently inadequate provider participation. The principal difference between managed care and fee-for-service care, however, is that managed care programs will be taking funds and *not* providing care, while fee-for-service physicians are not paid when they reject inadequate Medicaid rates.

Inability to Meet Medicaid Clients' Needs

We should be particularly concerned about putting people covered by Medicaid at risk through underservice. Most Medicaid recipients are low-income women and children, and disabled individuals. Since both of these groups have high health care needs, they are placed at high risk by inadequate access. For example, low-income pregnant women are at least twice as likely as higher-income pregnant women to have a child die within the first year of birth. This high infant mortality rate is due primarily to inadequate prenatal care. In addition, the maternal mortality rate for black and other non-white women is four times as high as for white women, and low-income children are two times as likely to suffer long-term disability at birth, in major part because of a higher risk of low birth weight. These statistics show that any disincentives to providing this population with health care, and any barriers to the population's receiving care, could result in more infant and maternal deaths, as well as more disabilities.

The purported ability of managed care plans to save costs may not apply to a population with high health care needs. Considerable evidence demonstrates that managed care programs that serve the non-Medicaid population engage in "skimming"—*i.e.*, they market to and enroll a disproportionately healthy group of people.[8] In fact, studies demonstrate that when people become unhealthy they are more likely to become dissatisfied with a managed care plan and disenroll.[9]

Indeed, studies of Medicaid managed care programs have shown that these plans were unable to meet the special needs of high-risk pregnant women and children, or of patients with chronic needs.[10] According to a 1989 study of the Medicaid demonstration projects, the amount and timeliness of prenatal care were inadequate at all sites.[11] Most women did not receive any prenatal care until their second trimester of pregnancy; and the average number of prenatal visits at all sites was less than 8—far fewer than the 12 prenatal visits recommended by the American College of Obstetrics and Gynecology. In addition, immunizations for children were inadequate at all sites. These findings were consistent with a 1987 study of Medicaid managed care plans in 30 states, which found that capitation levels for maternity care were seriously underfinanced throughout the programs.[12]

These studies also are consistent with reports from advocates across the country. For example, in analyzing the state of Ohio's 1989 quarterly reports on the Dayton Area Health Plan, a mandatory Medicaid managed care program for AFDC recipients, the Legal Aid Society of Dayton found that only 12 percent of eligible children were provided with mandatory EPSDT services, and the referral rates were one-third or less of the national rates reported for referable conditions. According to Bruce Spitz, who studied these figures, these rates are "scandalously low."[13]

Studies and reports show that many of these programs not only failed to provide early and continuous prenatal and pediatric care, but also failed to meet the needs of patients with chronic health conditions.[14] These inadequacies may be due to lack of experience with patients who have high health care needs, rapid implementation of the programs, and the fact that these recipients' special needs make them particularly vulnerable to incentives to control overutilization. For example, the Santa Barbara Health Initiative, in California, has enrolled a large population of disabled individuals, many of whom must rely on specialized orthopedic care to meet their primary needs. However, the program limits disabled enrollees' access to specialty providers to a hospital clinic that employs only medical school residents who rotate through the clinic one day a week. This prevents any continuous care, which is essential to meeting the health care needs of disabled recipients with chronic conditions.

Other managed care programs rely similarly on medical school residents in hospital clinics to deliver care. For example, in Philadelphia, the providers listed on many recipients' cards are the doctors who supervise at the teaching hospitals' clinics. However, recipients must wait a minimum of four weeks to see the named provider, and therefore most obtain their care from the medical students instead. Again, this results in a lack of continuity, as well as inadequate quality of care.

Inappropriate Delays and Denials

Most managed care programs use "gatekeepers" to control utilization. A "gatekeeper" is usually a primary care physician who determines whether a patient should see a specialist or obtain particular services, such as laboratory testing. In theory, managed care systems are supposed to encourage physicians to provide preventive and primary care in order to avoid the high costs of inappropriate specialty or emergency care.

In adopting the use of a gatekeeper system, it is presumed that the cost of care is too high because of overuse of specialty care. Either the patient is seeking or the provider is providing specialty care inappropriately. Whether this presumption applies to Medicaid recipients is questionable.

A great deal of research and documentation demonstrates that, for the most part, Medicaid recipients are unable to find physicians willing to accept Medicaid, because the rates are abysmally low.[15] The Medicaid rates are typically set in relation to states' budgetary constraints, and therefore are greatly discounted below the private-pay rate. In the competition between Medicaid and private-pay patients, Medicaid patients have come out the clear losers. Therefore, because of inadequate access to preventive and primary care, presumptions about Medicaid clients' overutilization are not valid. Instead, Medicaid recipients have been forced to rely on emergency services, which are much more costly, especially once recipients' health has declined substantially because of inadequate access in the fee-for-service system.

Medicaid managed care programs have not, however, fulfilled their promise of providing expanded preventive and primary care, which are necessary to offset the need for emergency care. Indeed, strict use of "gatekeepers" has resulted in a pattern of inappropriate delays and denials to basic preventive and primary care. Reports from advocates nationwide reflect this pattern.

For example, an advocate in Pennsylvania reported that a woman receiving treatment for breast cancer was inappropriately denied approval for surgery after already being admitted to the hospital for preoperative procedures. The problem was straightened out only after a legal services attorney intervened.

Another advocate in Utah reported that a client requiring dental surgery for a cleft palate, and for whom the preliminary surgical treatment had been performed, was abruptly terminated from services when the managed care plan inappropriately denied payment based on a procedural error caused by the participating provider's confusion over how to obtain prior approval.

During the Santa Barbara Health Initiative's first few years of operation, some women waited for over two years for gynecological examinations. One family served by the Santa Barbara Health Initiative that has received approval for their daughter to see a pediatric orthopedist has waited nine months for the program to identify a particular specialist for approval—and they are still waiting.

Unfortunately, managed care plans' incentives against overutilization are not counterbalanced by incentives that reward coordinated and follow-up services. Furthermore, states are not taking sufficient steps to monitor the quality of care provided, or to detect patterns of underservice.

It is also ironic that to the extent that Medicaid recipients have been limited to receiving expensive emergency room services in the fee-for-service system, managed care plans have successfully blocked even this limited access, while failing to fulfill their promise to provide preventive, primary care. For example, a report prepared by the emergency pediatric department at Children's Hospital of Philadelphia studied the follow-up care given to children denied approval for emergency care by HealthPass, a Pennsylvania Medicaid managed care program.[16] The report offered several examples of inappropriate denials. One such case was a two-month-old infant who was turned away, only to return a few hours later with respiratory arrest; another example was a child who arrived with a fever of 104 degrees Fahrenheit, and, upon being rejected for coverage by the managed care plan, suffered a seizure before leaving the building. The child required an endotracheal intubation. After Children's Hospital had completed this six-month study, it decided to treat all children who presented themselves to the emergency room, whether or not HealthPass approved the care, unless the child could be assured of seeing a primary care physician immediately.

HealthPass, like many other Medicaid managed care programs, had adopted a system whereby emergency care was not approved unless the patient was suffering from a ''life-threatening'' emergency. Such a determination is difficult to make unless a physician actually performs a physical examination. However, as in many Medicaid managed care programs, the HMO would not approve even the physical examination unless the patient already was determined to be suffering from a ''life-threatening'' emergency. Nonmedical personnel at the HMO often made these decisions, relying solely on information communicated by an emergency room clerk.

Inappropriate emergency room denials are rampant across Medicaid managed care plans throughout the country. For example, a Chicago advocate reported a client whose child came to an emergency room covered with burns. The HMO refused coverage and, instead, called in the child for an appointment. When the HMO physician did not show up for the scheduled appointment, the parents returned to another local hospital emergency room that accepted the child despite the HMO's stated refusal to cover services.

Advocates have also reported inappropriate denials for other services that tend to be expensive, such as drug and alcohol treatment. For example, in Pennsylvania, HealthPass was consistently denying approval for drug and alcohol treatment for pregnant women or women with children. Some of these same recipients were lucky enough to get admitted to programs outside of the HMO, but had to establish their residence outside of the geographic area mandatorily covered by the HMO. However, the process of disenrollment took a minimum of two months, serving as a substantial disincentive to recipients eligible for these needed services.

Institutional Barriers

In reality, many managed care programs, including Medicaid managed care programs, do not rely principally on the "gatekeeper" or primary care physician to deny care in order to control utilization, but rather rely on institutional barriers, which function equally well, if not better, to limit access. These include long telephone waiting periods to make appointments, delays in making specialty referrals, and limited as well as lengthy internal review procedures for denials. These barriers are particularly dangerous to Medicaid recipients because of their high health care needs.

Moreover, low-income individuals have more trouble overcoming these barriers due to conditions related to poverty and the lack of disposable income. A person unable to afford a telephone cannot sit for long periods of time on the telephone to schedule appointments. Recipients may not be able to reach HMOs or follow up referrals to specialty care because providers are located in areas difficult to reach by public transportation. Without disposable income, recipients cannot afford second opinions in order to challenge denials.

Indeed, a study by the Rand Corporation found that, in comparing the health outcomes of lower-income people inside and outside of HMOs, lower-income people in HMOs experienced significantly worsened health results than lower-income people using fee-for-service care, including more hospital days and greater risks of dying.[17] In addition, lower-income people in HMOs experienced significantly worsened health results than middle-income people in HMOs. The report postulated that the worsened health results were related to the combination of HMOs' predisposition to underserve with the following barriers used to delay and deny care: (1) telephone-based queueing systems for scheduling appointments; (2) restrictions on the use of accident and emergency departments; and (3) greater difficulties in arranging transportation.[18]

These institutional barriers also translate into bureaucratic mazes that can pose the most significant barriers to access when combined with Medicaid's own bureaucracy. As one advocate in Pennsylvania noted, most of the problems faced by Medicaid clients result from either recipients' or providers' confusion about how to verify eligibility and obtain approval. Therefore, it is not uncommon to find that recipients have been inappropriately disenrolled, or have not been enrolled in a timely manner, or have been denied coverage inappropriately because providers are confused about how to obtain prior authorization. On the surface, most of these problems relate to "paperwork," but in reality they reflect a pattern behind which the most flimsy excuses are proffered to justify the HMOs' refusal to cover appropriate services. This pattern is consistent with the incentives that favor underutilization, which are aggravated by underfinancing.

The Question of Expanding Access

One argument offered in favor of managed care is that it expands access to recipients who otherwise could not find providers at all. However, nationwide experience has shown that when states institute managed care plans they do not

expand access, but rather the same providers who served the Medicaid population continue to do so.[19]

In a study of the demonstration projects, only one had utilized an existing
HMO that was serving a non-Medicaid population.[20] The remaining six projects
had failed to attract new physicians to Medicaid and, instead, had relied on
traditional Medicaid providers—*i.e.*, hospitals, physicians, and neighborhood
health centers. The report concluded that expanding use of managed care will
not improve access to a broader array of mainstream physicians. Therefore, the
danger of relegating Medicaid recipients to the bottom tier of available medical
care remains.

Is This a Wise Use of Limited Medicaid Dollars?

We must analyze closely the health risks faced by Medicaid clients when
the state passes on the financial risks of providing care to high-need patients at
inadequate capitation levels. In the last two years, the managed care industry
has lost $900 million per year.[21] The vast majority of HMOs that lost money in
the last five years were "individual practice associations" (IPAs);[22] the majority
of HMOs serving Medicaid recipients are IPAs.[23] At the same time, the extent
to which HMOs have been able to operate without a loss may be related in
large part to the fact that they serve a predominantly healthy population group
—far healthier than most Medicaid recipients.

Some scholars have pointed out that managed care rates for Medicaid recipients must be based on the Medicaid population's unique needs, and not on the
HMOs' experience with disproportionately healthy populations.[24] If the rates are
not adequate, the danger is that Medicaid clients will be at increased risk of
underservice. However, if managed care is viewed as a cost savings mechanism,
then it will be politically infeasible to set adequate rates.

As a result of the inadequate access to the managed care programs, states
may have to spend more, because recipients will be forced to rely on emergency
room care after their health has declined substantially. Therefore, in order for
states to realize cost savings on this population in the long term, they should be
prepared to spend more on preventive and primary care than they do presently.
This means that they must not base capitation levels on the existing Medicaid
fee-for-service experience.

States also must factor in additional administrative costs that will be incurred
both by the managed care plans and the states. The states must be able to address
the varied enrollment systems and institute procedures for reviewing the plans'
utilization controls. A report reviewing Milwaukee's managed care plan pointed
out that the state's savings were offset by the administrative costs involved in
monitoring HMO quality and utilization controls.[25] Indeed, the report was highly
critical of Wisconsin's failure to spend the amounts necessary to gather usable
data to monitor utilization and detect inadequate care.

It is not clear that the cost savings justify additional administrative costs. In
a study of four demonstration sites, no clear pattern was established that utilization changes were directly translatable into program savings.[26] According to

a 1985 report on Citicare, a Kentucky managed care program used to serve Medicaid recipients, the program allotted 14.2 percent of its revenues to profit and to administrative costs, while the Medicaid agency had spent only 4.4 percent on administrative costs.[27] One Washington Medicaid managed care program paid an administrative agency over $360,000 to run a system expected to generate $65,000 in savings.[28] Whatever "efficiencies" are derived through capitation do not justify this cost-shifting. In fact, one of the reasons that California's Expanded Choice proposal was not adopted in San Diego was that the state concluded that the extra costs involved in prepaying the HMO, and thereby forfeiting the interest that could be earned by paying retrospectively for care, would not offset the cost savings.

The Importance of Quality Safeguards

The present administration's stated plan to relax freedom of choice and mixed enrollment protections threatens to compromise Medicaid enrollees' already fragile position within managed care plans. Mandatory enrollment will turn the Medicaid population into a captive base for the profit-taking motives of the managed care plans. Without the freedom to choose between managed care plans and fee-for-service physicians, Medicaid recipients will not be able to express their dissatisfaction by disenrolling, and the plans will not be forced to compete for their enrollment.

This lack of accountability will be aggravated further by a relaxation of the requirement that managed care plans serving Medicaid recipients also enroll at least 25 percent non-Medicaid and non-Medicare recipients.[29] Without mixed enrollment requirements, the plans will not be forced to compete for middle-income clientele. This is likely to result in all kinds of unscrupulous practices, as evidenced by the California experience in the 1970s, when many entities arrived on the scene merely for profit-taking, seeking to exploit "the margin between capitation payments and expenses for services rendered."[30]

Congress is aware that increased vigilance has been necessary to ensure that Medicaid managed care enrollees are not underserved. For example, in 1987, Congress passed a number of changes to the HMO Act that increased civil penalties against managed care plans that fail substantially to provide medically necessary services and items required under Medicaid.[31] However, reliance on civil penalties to respond only to the most egregious violations is insufficient to balance recipients' need to "vote with their feet." Forcing these managed care programs to remain competitive in relation to both the Medicaid and the non-Medicaid population is a much better and more efficient safety valve to safeguard the quality of care that recipients receive.

In addition, Congress should be wary of any attempts to bring about a rapid expansion in the use of managed care programs. Recent Medicaid experience has shown that expanding managed care will not result in new providers participating in Medicaid, but, instead, in the conversion of already participating providers into groups that accept the prepayment amounts. Rapid expansion of the use of managed care systems often creates a significant danger that the so-called "Medicaid mills" will be converted into managed care plans, likely to provide inadequate care and engage in corrupt and unscrupulous practices. Therefore, implementation must be planned carefully. Indeed, according to some studies, at least two years are required for each new plan to make sure that the confusion regarding enrollment and cost controls is minimized.[32]

Conclusion

By capping amounts that states will pay to serve Medicaid clients, states are in effect rationing the care to be provided. However, through the use of managed care plans and capitation, states are delegating responsibility for these rationing decisions to the providers accepting the financial risks involved with capitation. Unfortunately, the incentives against overuse have not been accompanied by incentives to follow protocols that promote primary, preventive, and coordinated care. Just at the time when coverage obligations are expanding toward more comprehensive care for pregnant women, infants, and children, expanded use of managed care programs threatens to undercut these needed improvements.

A number of studies have improved our knowledge of how to bring down unconscionably high maternal and infant death and disability rates.[33] High-risk mothers and children require early, stable, and continuous enrollment, adequate reimbursement, mechanisms for providing follow-up services so that care remains continuous, and health education. This care is likely to cost more than states have been prepared to spend in the past, although the costs of caring for low-birth-weight and disabled infants may be substantially reduced. Nonetheless, the fact is that adequate information is not available on the exact amount that the states must spend to do a good job in this area because states have not yet spent at necessary levels. Therefore, any methods by which capitation levels are measured against past Medicaid experience will be faulty.

If any expanded use of managed care plans is contemplated, we urge that states be required to make enrollment voluntary, and that managed care plans be required to enroll Medicaid recipients alongside nonpoor, non-Medicaid recipients. States should not be permitted to base the capitated rates on already inadequate Medicaid fee-for-service rates. In addition, they should be required to proceed *gradually* in order to ensure that the managed care plans with which states contract can prove that they are solid financially and can deliver care responsibly, and to determine whether the cost savings justify additional administrative costs, incurred by both the plans and the states.

N O T E S

1. Hillman, *Special Report: Financial Incentives for Physicians in HMOs*, 317 NEW ENG J. MED. 1743 (Dec. 31, 1987).

2. Spitz & Abramson, *Competition, Capitation, and Case Management*, 65 MILBANK Q. 348, 360 (1987).

3. Hillman, Pauley, Kerstein, *How Do Financial Incentives Affect Physicians' Clinical Decisions and the Financial Performance of Health Maintenance Organizations?*, 321 NEW ENG J. MED. 86 (July 31, 1989).

4. Spitz & Abramson, *supra* note 2, at 355–57; Anderson & Fox, *Lessons Learned from Medicaid Managed Care Approaches*, HEALTH AFF. 71, 80 (Spring 1987).

5. Spitz & Abramson, *supra* note 2, at 355–57.

6. *Id.*

7. *See* Perkins, *Increasing Provider Participation in the Medicaid Program: Is There a Doctor in the House?*, 26 HOUS. L. REV. 77 (1989).

8. Anderson & Fox, *supra* note 4, at 81; Strumwasser, Pasanjpe, Ronis, McGinnis, Kee, & Hall, *The Triple Option Choice: Self-Selection Bias in Traditional Coverage, HMOs, and PPOs*, 26 INQUIRY 432 (Winter 1989).

9. DesHarnais, *Enrollment In and Disenrollment From Health Maintenance Organizations by Medicaid Recipients*, 6 HEALTH CARE FINANCING REV. 39 (Spring 1985) (showing higher than average utilization during three months following disenrollment).

10. *See* Freund, Rossiter, Fox, Meyer, Hurley, Carey, & Paul, *Evaluation of the Medicaid Competition Demonstrations*, 11 HEALTH CARE FINANCING REV. 81 (Winter 1989) [hereinafter Freund & Rossiter]; Anderson & Fox, *supra* note 4, at 80.

11. Freund & Rossiter, *supra* note 10, at 94.

12. Rosenbaum, Hughes, Butler, & Howard, *Incantations in the Dark: Medicaid Managed Care and Maternity Care*, 66 MILBANK Q. 661, 685 (1989) [hereinafter Rosenbaum & Hughes].

13. Bruce Spitz's letter analyzing these figures is available from NHeLP.

14. *See* Anderson & Fox, *supra* note 4, at 80.

15. *See* Perkins, *supra* note 7, at 77.

16. Shaw, Selbst, & Gill, Indigent Children Who are Denied Care in the Emergency Department (July 31, 1989) (paper prepared by the Children's Hospital of Philadelphia) (available from NHeLP).

17. Ware, Rogers, Davies, Goldberg, Brook, Keeler, Sherbourne, Camp, & Newhouse, *Comparison of Health Outcomes at a Health Maintenance Organization with those of Fee-for-Service Care*, LANCET 1017 (May 3, 1986).

18. *Id.* at 1021.

19. Anderson & Fox, *supra* note 4, at 83; Freund & Rossiter, *supra* note 10, at 95.

20. Anderson & Fox, *supra* note 4, at 83.

21. Wogensen, *The HMO Squeeze*, THE NEW PHYSICIAN 12, 13 (Apr. 1990).

22. *Id.* at 13–14.

23. Intergovernmental Health Policy Project, Cost-Containment in Public Programs (Mar. 1990).

24. Freund & Rossiter, *supra* note 10, at 91; Anderson & Fox, *supra* note 4, at 80–81.

25. Rowland & Lyons, *Mandatory HMO Care for Milwaukee's Poor.* HEALTH AFF. 87 (Spring 1987).

26. *See* Freund & Neuschler, *Overview of Medicaid Capitation and Case-Management Initiatives*, HEALTH CARE FINANCING REV. 81, 89 (1986 Annual Supplement).

27. National Health Law Program, An Advocate's Guide to Medicaid Case Management Systems 80, n.539 (1989).

28. *Id.* at 80.

29. The 25-percent non-Medicaid and non-Medicare population also should not include other poor enrollees. A federal court recently struck down the Health Care Financing Administration's approval for Ohio to include general assistance recipients in this 25-percent population. Oglesby v. Berry, No. C-3-89-125 (W. D. Ohio, Nov. 17, 1989) (consent decree) (Clearinghouse No. 45,472).

30. D'Onofrio & Mullen, *Consumer Problems with Prepaid Health Plans in California*, 92 PUB. HEALTH REP. 121, 124 (Apr. 1977).

31. *See* Medicare Catastrophic Coverage Act of 1988, Pub. L. No. 100-360, § 411(k)(12), 102 Stat. 683, 797 (1988).

32. Freund, *The Private Delivery of Medicaid Services: Lessons from Administrators, Providers and Policy Makers*, 9 J. OF AMBULATORY CARE MGMT. 54 (1986).

33. *See* Rosenbaum & Hughes, *supra* note 12, at 661.

MEDICAL APARTHEID: AN AMERICAN PERSPECTIVE

Durado D. Brooks, M.D.;
David R. Smith, M.D.;
Ron J. Anderson, M.D.

The suppressive policies and practices of apartheid in South Africa have directly contributed to preventable morbidity and mortality in black Africans. Due to socioeconomic segregation ("functional apartheid"), America's citizens of color also suffer excess death and disability. Health status measurements in the United States confirm the failure of the current fragmented health care system to recognize or respond to the unmet need or the barriers that exist. Predictably, the changes needed to improve the health status of black South Africans are similar to those that are necessary to remedy the situation in the United States. Community-Oriented Primary Care is a health service provision model that holds promise as a comprehensive community-based strategy that can begin to address some of the shortcomings of the current medical care systems of both nations.

(JAMA. 1991;266:2746–2749)

The Republic of South Africa has been the target of international protests, boycotts, and derision based on the treatment accorded their black majority population. Many of the most strident demands for change have come from the United States. While it is clear that the South African system must be dramatically restructured, it should also be noted that the plight of America's black and brown citizens is in dire need of attention. This is particularly evident in the area of health care.

Most Western nations treat health care as a public good, similar to education for the young. The United States and the Republic of South Africa share the dubious distinction of being the only industrialized countries that continue to view health care as a privilege. This failure to ensure access to basic health care services for all citizens results in substantial economic and human losses for these countries.

The medical care system of present-day South Africa has been recently described by Nightingale et al.[1] The segregated nature of this system is not surprising, but the similarities to health care provision in the United States are startling. The health care systems of both nations are characterized by inadequate (or totally absent) care for large segments of their population, gross inequities

in the allocation of health care resources, and poorly coordinated and economically inefficient bureaucracies.

While apartheid in South Africa is strictly along racial lines, the segregation
in our country occurs primarily as a function of socioeconomic status. However,
since ethnic minorities comprise a disproportionate share of our country's poor,
these groups remain the primary victims of oppression. African Americans and
Americans of Hispanic descent are more likely to be uninsured and less likely
to have access to health care than the non-Hispanic white population.[2] Among
hospitalized patients, lack of insurance has been correlated with significantly
fewer expensive diagnostic studies and an increased risk of in-hospital death.[3]

Despite dissimilarity in the structure and process of apartheid between the
United States and South Africa, the manifestations are the same. The wide disparity in socioeconomic status, preventable disease incidence, and life expectancy between white citizens and people of color in both nations bear witness
to the myriad inequities of the current social and health care systems.

Systems of Care

Nightingale et al[1] describe a South African medical system in which a large
number of narrowly focused agencies have been established to address different
aspects of health care. The result is a multiplicity of competing authorities that
add layers of bureaucratic lethargy and costs, and prevent the efficient provision
of health care services. This is analogous to the factionalism present in most
metropolitan areas of the United States. In Dallas County, Texas, a variety of
city, county, and private agencies provide limited services on varying days at
inconsistent locations. Areas of overlap and, more important, major gaps in
services abound. Well babies may be seen at one location, but immunizations
must be obtained at a different site, while ill children must travel to different
clinics or the county hospital. Sites for comprehensive health care services are
almost nonexistent. Collaborative attempts to create such comprehensive networks are often met with resistance due to the self-interests of involved agencies,
without regard for the needs of the service population.

Through the apartheid laws, the South African government has rigidly divided the nation's population into racially defined groups (white, Asian, colored,
and black). On this scale, socioeconomic level and standard of living decline
dramatically as cutaneous melanin level rises. Dr. Nightingale places much of
the blame for the poor health status of South Africa's blacks on the living
conditions, which relegate the black population to periurban "townships" and
rural "homelands." Defined as "separate and rigidly segregated communities,"
these areas are typified by miserable housing, poor sanitation, and inadequate
or nonexistent health care. Who can read this description and fail to recognize
the haunting similarity to America's inner cities, the *colonias* of south Texas,
or our Native American reservations?

Financial and nonfinancial barriers to health care have been built into and
reinforced in America's metropolitan areas. Long ago, medicine abandoned urban neighborhoods and completed a process of involution. Primary care and
other medical services were pulled from the community, and coalesced at in-

accessible "medical centers." These barriers have created and propagated growing segments of our populace that can be aptly described as *Les Miserables*—people constantly searching for ways to get over, around, or through these very real barriers.

South African hospitals that serve the disenfranchised majority population are overcrowded and overwhelmed by the sheer numbers of people needing assistance. Many of these institutions face the additional burdens of outdated equipment and facilities, limited staff, and grossly inadequate budgets.[4]

In many areas of the United States, public hospitals constitute the only health care alternative for the impoverished. Parkland Memorial Hospital in Dallas, Texas, is the primary provider of medical services for the economically disadvantaged of Dallas County. This 940-bed facility has been recognized as one of America's premier medical institutions.[5] Despite this national reputation for excellence, Parkland fights a daily battle for continued economic viability. Like similar public institutions throughout the nation, our service population is overwhelmingly poor and minority. Many of the inequities described in the South African medical system are mirrored in the medical environment in Dallas and in the indigent health care arena across the United States.

Parkland's occupancy rate generally exceeds functional capacity, requiring diversion of ambulances away from our emergency department. Due to the volume of patients needing Parkland's care, medical admissions were diverted to other facilities for a total of 93 days in 1990. Fortunately, diversion of trauma patients has not yet been necessary. However, the 30 percent increase in trauma volume last year (due largely to drug- and gang-related violence) is threatening to overwhelm this system and thereby diminish resources dedicated to the care of victims of automobile accidents, industrial mishaps, and other trauma.

In addition to the nearly 150000 patients treated in the emergency department each year, Parkland's outpatient clinics see 1500 scheduled patients every day. While patients with appointments are seen in a timely fashion, an additional 300 patients a day are processed through our walk-in ambulatory care clinic. Waiting times for the ambulatory care clinic average seven to eight hours. Due to the lack of accessible primary care services for Dallas' poor, this is the only available site of treatment for many patients. Although many view this as "free care," the burden imposed on the working poor by the loss of a day's wages makes this anything but free. In addition, the long waits cause approximately one of every nine of these nonscheduled patients to leave prior to receiving care. These patients often return later in a more advanced stage of their illness, necessitating more intensive (and expensive) treatment, or hospitalization. Public hospitals across our nation serve a similar "safety net" function, straining their already limited resources.

Conditions are more tenuous for the residents of rural areas in South Africa and the United States. Medical facilities are primitive or nonexistent for South Africa's homelands, and a similar situation is developing in our nation. More than 20 percent of Texas' 254 counties have no acute care hospital, and 119 counties do not have hospital obstetrical or newborn services.[6] While only 8 percent of US births occur in Texas, we account for fully one third of all out-of-hospital births nationally (and these births are disproportionately among minority women). This may contribute to infant mortality rates in some rural counties that are seven times greater than the national average.[6]

While the options for care in rural America are diminishing for many, barriers to service for the poor have always been severe (particularly for the poor of color). Without a rural equivalent of public safety net hospitals and their house-staff providers, even those minority patients with Medicaid coverage often cannot find a private physician to provide their care. Recently, in Denton County, Texas (a wealthy county with 33 obstetrician-gynecologists), a patient who had Medicaid coverage was unable to find a physician willing to accept her for pregnancy care (Klein D. "Children at Risk." New York, NY: Public Television, WNET; aired on PBS, November 1, 1991).

Preventable Disease

A number of other parallels between the health care systems of South Africa and metropolitan areas in the United States are evident. These regions share strikingly high rates of black infant mortality, and a greater prevalence of diseases such as tuberculosis, pneumonia, and measles. These diseases have been all but eliminated among South Africa's white minority population through improved education, nutrition, sanitation, and immunization programs. Similarly, US blacks die at much higher rates than whites from preventable diseases. Blacks and Hispanics suffer disproportionately higher complications from diabetes and hypertension, and African-American men in Harlem have a shorter life span than men in many impoverished Third World nations.[7-9]

Precise quantitative comparisons of morbidity and mortality rates in the United States and the Republic of South Africa are difficult due to woeful inadequacies in South African data. This is particularly true for data regarding their black population.[10] However, available information exemplifies the shared health care problems of the non-white populations of both nations.

Infant mortality has been viewed as a sensitive indicator of the health status of a population, reflecting adequacy of medical care and social systems. Adverse social circumstances have been strongly associated with increased levels of infant mortality.[11] Despite its position as one of the world's wealthiest nations, the infant mortality rate in the United States remains distressingly high compared with that of other industrialized nations. The US rate of 10 infants lost for each 100000 births (twentieth in the world)[12] is a national disgrace.

Even in states such as Texas that have achieved infant mortality rates lower than the national average, there remain danger zones. Analogous to "drowning in a river only 3 feet deep," there are communities in the very shadow of America's finest medical institutions where infant mortality rates rival those of Third World nations.

Accurate figures for black infant mortality for the entire Republic of South Africa are not available, and existing records demonstrate tremendous geographical variation. Black infant mortality rates as high as 282 per 1000 births have been documented in rural homelands,[13] and a national mortality rate for black infants is estimated to be between 94 and 124 deaths per 1000 live births.[14] This is in stark comparison with the nationwide average of 13.5 deaths per 1000 births among white South Africans.[15] Data from selected urban areas in South Africa demonstrate the potential benefits of improving access to health care services (even substandard services). While the ratio of black-to-white infant deaths remains approximately 3:1, black infant death rates as low as 27 per 1000 births have been achieved.[16,14] This rate is actually superior to current black infant mortality rates of up to 38 per 1000 births in some large standard statistical communities of Dallas County (Bacchi, D. Unpublished data, 1990).

Hypertension is prevalent in the black and white populations of both nations. Complications of hypertension such as end-stage renal disease (ESRD) can be prevented through early detection and adequate treatment. Studies of patients with ESRD in two urban areas of South Africa found hypertension to be responsible for 32 percent and 33 percent of kidney failure among blacks, but only 10 percent of the disease in whites.[17,18] In a similar fashion, 42.5 percent of black patients with ESRD in the United States have hypertension as the primary cause of their renal disease, while hypertension accounts for only 17.4 percent of ESRD in the US white population.[19] Other investigators have calculated the risk of ESRD from hypertension in Jefferson City, Alabama, to be nearly 18 times higher in blacks than in whites.[20]

Measles is yet another preventable disease that takes a heavy toll on the impoverished of both nations. Non-white children in South Africa continue to experience significant morbidity and mortality from this disease, while it has been largely eliminated among the white minority.[21,22] Poverty-related factors such as overcrowding, poor sanitation, and malnutrition are clearly related to the spread of this disease, but the failure to ensure immunization of infants and children is the primary reason for the persistence of this scourge.

Along with Los Angeles, California, Dallas will long be remembered in our nation's conscience as the center of America's 1990 measles epidemic. Although the disease occurred primarily in ethnic minorities and the poor, the entire Dallas community was affected. The financial costs of more than 2500 cases of measles and the tragedy of young lives lost to this totally preventable disease will haunt us for years to come. The failure to provide a $3 immunization in some cases resulted in thousands of dollars in hospital expenses, while 12 young people paid the ultimate price—death.

Opportunities for Change

Testimony to the similarity of health care issues in the United States and the Republic of South Africa is also provided by perusal of recent medical literature. Access to care, health care financing, national health insurance, and related topics are frequently recurring themes in the major journals of both nations. It is encouraging to find many of South Africa's physicians and medical institutions at the forefront of the anti-apartheid movement. Organizations including the Progressive Primary Health Care Network and the National Medical and Dental Association have worked aggressively against apartheid and toward a health care plan for post-apartheid South Africa.[1,23] In addition, the Medical Association of South Africa (the country's largest physician organization) has called for the abolition of apartheid and the establishment of a social and health care system free of racial and economic discrimination.[24]

The changes proposed to improve the health status of black South Africans are similar to those that are necessary to remedy the situation of the impoverished of Dallas and throughout the United States. The fragmented, categorical system that currently attempts to serve underprivileged citizens should be replaced. This system is inefficient—it creates barriers for patients, resulting in costly delays and duplication of effort. What is needed is ready access to comprehensive primary care services, lack of which has been clearly correlated with morbidity and excess deaths.[7,25,26] Community education and health promotion activities are desperately needed. Any meaningful long-term solution must also include measures to increase the number of minorities pursuing careers in health-related fields.

Dallas County is making strong efforts to improve the deplorable local situation through Parkland Hospital's Division of Community-Oriented Primary Care (COPC). In this model of care, the health status and needs of a defined community are assessed, and a health care plan is designed and implemented based on these identified needs. The COPC approach combines epidemiology, individual patient care, and general public health concerns. The COPC model has been favorably reviewed by the Institute of Medicine.[21] These concepts have been applied in a number of settings in the United States with varying degrees of success.[27,28] Ironically, the basic philosophy and structure of COPC originated in South Africa more than 40 years ago. Working with the native community in Polela, South Africa, Sidney L. Kark, M.D., and his associates organized one of the first successful COPC models.[29] Many of the current efforts in COPC have their genesis in the work of Dr. Kark.

With the support of Dallas' citizens and local government, Parkland Hospital's division of COPC is establishing a network of health centers conveniently located in economically deprived neighborhoods. Emphasizing preventive medicine and promoting healthy lifestyles, these centers provide a full spectrum of health care services at accessible locations. Providers are on call 24 hours a day, available to answer questions from worried parents, refill prescriptions, and decrease costly, unnecessary emergency department visits. Care is also provided in nontraditional settings, reaching those in need in homeless shelters, churches, and schools. Evening and weekend office hours ensure access for the working poor (for whom losing a day's wages due to a visit to a physician may have catastrophic consequences). The system is designed to give these disenfranchised citizens something they have never had—a family physician.

Community education programs are an integral part of COPC. These programs are designed to make at-risk populations aware of early signs of disease, the importance of routine preventive care, and the benefits of reducing risk factors for many diseases. The community is empowered by such knowledge, and citizens are encouraged to take a much more active role in their own health care.

The physicians, nurses, and other health care providers of COPC are of diverse ethnic and societal backgrounds, matched with the populations that they serve. In addition to providing medical care, these providers are encouraged to take an active role in community affairs, and serve as role models for the communities' youth.

The effectiveness of this program is measured by an assessment of baseline health attributes of the target population, and the formation of specific health outcome goals and objectives. Attainment of these objectives will benefit the entire community, and provide direct benefit to health center staff through an incentive program based on these outcomes (a unique aspect of Parkland's COPC model).

The value of such comprehensive care was demonstrated during Dallas' recent measles epidemic. Certain standard statistical communities served by COPC in collaboration with the Dallas County Health Department experienced 60 percent fewer measles cases than projected for these high-risk areas (Dallas County Health Department, unpublished data, 1990).

This process of assessing the health status, risk factors, and beliefs of a community, then designing interventions based on this profile is undergoing a much needed resurgence in South Africa. Projects such as the Mamre Community Health Project[30] and a recently initiated door-to-door study of cardiovascular risk factors among urban blacks[31] are using techniques pioneered by Dr. Kark 40 years ago.

Societal Implications

Programs like COPC can change the face of indigent health care provision in South Africa and the United States and we should encourage the development of more such innovations. However, it must be realized that health care does not exist in a vacuum. Nightingale observes that "health specific effects are superimposed on the more general consequences of apartheid," and elsewhere states, "even if apartheid policies ended tomorrow, their effects on health would persist for years."[1] Society must appreciate the interrelatedness of health, decent housing, education, and economic opportunity. Recent work has shown that, in addition to commonly recognized hazards (diabetes, hypertension, lack of accessible care), poverty functions as an independent risk factor for premature death in African Americans.[32] Poverty and lack of health insurance have also been postulated to be the greatest impediments to health care for Hispanics.[9]

It must be emphasized that there are clear differences in the discriminatory policies in force in South Africa and those functioning in the United States. The Republic of South Africa is a nation in which all social, economic, and political institutions have developed within an all-pervasive racist ideology. Apartheid in South Africa is a legally sanctioned (and in many instances, legally required) policy. Laws such as the Group Areas Act and the various land acts proscribe where one may live and work and who may own property. The recent repeal of these laws will no doubt lead to a gradual improvement in the economic station of some South African blacks; however, this improvement will be years in the making. Meanwhile, apartheid laws and policies continue to disallow any meaningful political participation by the black majority, and severely limit the influence of the Asian and colored populations.

Conversely, in the United States, most legal obstacles to non-white progress have been dismantled over the past 40 years, and legislation has been advanced to ensure equal protection under the law for all citizens. This has allowed significant gains in many aspects of life for America's ethnic minorities. Unfortunately, the removal of legal barriers alone is not sufficient to reverse the devastating effects that centuries of discriminatory policies have had on income and educational attainment. Due to these historical inequities, the majority of America's black and brown populations continue to lag far behind the white majority with regard to economic achievement and stability. Though legally sanctioned discrimination based on race has declined, educational and economic realities have imposed and maintained de facto apartheid for a substantial portion of America's minority citizenry.

Conclusion

It is clear that South Africa's system of apartheid has entered a terminal phase. As the persecuted majority prepares to reclaim the land of their ancestors, plans for a postapartheid South Africa are under way. Similarly, our nation must anticipate and prepare for its future.

Those who view America's impoverished and disenfranchised populations solely as a burden on society are failing to recognize economic realities. Over the next 10 years, blacks, Hispanics, and other minorities will make up a large share of the expansion of the US labor force, while white males will constitute only 15 percent of new entrants to the job market.[33] America cannot maintain its lead position in the international marketplace with a poorly educated, unhealthy work force. It therefore serves the self-interest of today's affluent and middle-class citizens to provide adequate health care and opportunities for educational and economic advancement for our nation's underclass. We must deal with hopelessness and helplessness and the conditions that spawn unhealthy behaviors through policies that encourage inclusiveness and social justice. Only through such empowering processes can we hope to eliminate this functional apartheid from America's medical and social system.

N O T E S

1. Nightingale EO, Hannibal MA, Geiger J, Hartmann L, Lawrence R, Spurlock J. Apartheid medicine: health and human rights in South Africa. *JAMA*. 1990;264:2097–2107.

2. Trevino FM, Moyer ME, Valdez RB, Stroup-Benham AS. Health insurance coverage and utilization of health services by Mexican Americans, mainland Puerto Ricans, and Cuban Americans. *JAMA*. 1991;265:233–237.

3. Hadley J, Steinberg EP, Feder J. Comparison of uninsured and privately insured hospital patients. *JAMA*. 1991;265:374–379.

4. Abkiewicz SR, Ahmed AS, Alli MA, et al. Conditions at Baragwanath Hospital. *S Afr Med. J.* 1987;72:361.

5. Dietrich HJ, Biddle VH. *The Best in Medicine: How and Where to Find the Best Health Care Available.* New York, NY: Harmony Books; 1990:18.

6. Texas Hospital Association. *Women and Children First: A Plan for Improving Texas Maternal and Child Health Outcomes in the 1990s.* Austin, Tex: Texas Hospital Association;1991:14.

7. Schwartz E, Kofie VY, Rivo M, Tuckson RV. Black/white comparisons of deaths preventable by medical intervention: United States and the District of Columbia, 1980–1986. *Int J Epidemiol.* 1990;19:591–598.

8. McCord C, Freeman HP. Excess mortality in Harlem. *N Engl J Med.* 1990;322:173–177.

9. Council on Scientific Affairs. American Medical Association. Hispanic health in the United States. *JAMA.* 1991;265:248–252.

10. Botha JL, Bradshaw D. African vital statistics: a black hole? *S Afr Med J.* 1985;67:977–981.

11. Molteno CD, Kibel MA. Postneonatal mortality in the Matroosberg Divisional Council Area of the Cape Western Health Region. *S Afr Med J.* 1989;75:575–578.

12. Children's Defense Fund. *The State of America's Children.* Washington, DC: Children's Defense Fund; 1991:60.

13. Knutzen V, Bourne D. The reproductive efficiency of the Xhosa. *S Afr Med J.* 1977;51:392–394.

14. Yach D. Infant mortality rates in urban areas of South Africa, 1981 1985. *S Afr Med J.* 1988;73:232–234.

15. Rip MR, Bourne DE. The spatial distribution of infant mortality rates in South Africa, 1982. *S Afr Med J.* 1988;73:224–226.

16. Wyndham CH. Mortality rates of black infants in Soweto compared with other regions of South Africa. *S Afr Med J.* 1986;70:281–282.

17. Seedat YK, Naicker S, Rawat R, Parson I. Racial differences in the causes of end-stage renal failure in Natal. *S Afr Med J.* 1984;65:956–958.

18. Gold CH, Isaacson C, Levin J. The pathological basis of end-stage renal disease in blacks. *S Afr Med J.* 1982;61:263–265.

19. Eggers PW, Connerton R, McMullan M. The Medicare experience with end-stage renal disease: trends in incidence, prevalence, and survival. *Health Care Financing Rev.* Spring 1984; 5(3):69–88.

20. Rostand SG, Kirk KA, Rutsky EA, Pate BA. Racial differences in the incidence of treatment for end-stage renal disease. *N Engl J Med.* 1982;306:1276–1279.

21. Bourne BE, Rip MR, Woods D. Characteristics of infant mortality in the RSA, 1929–1983. *S Afr Med J.* 1988;73:230–232.

22. Kettles AN. Differences in trends of measles notifications by age and race in the western Cape, 1982–1986. *S Afr Med J.* 1987;72:317–320.

23. Mji D, Vallabhjee KN. Health in post-apartheid South Africa. *S Afr Med J.* 1990;78:122–123.

24. Policy statement on discrimination in medical practice. *S Afr Med J.* 1989;75:560. Editorial.

25. Dana MR, Tielsch JM, Enger C, Joyce E, Santoli JM, Taylor HR. Visual impairment in a rural Appalachian community. *JAMA.* 1990;264:2400–2405.

26. Council on Ethical and Judicial Affairs, American Medical Association. Black-white disparities in health care. *JAMA.* 1989;263:2344–2346.

27. Connor E, Mullan F, eds. *Community Oriented Primary Care: New Directions for Health Services Delivery.* Washington, DC: Institute of Medicine, National Academy Press; 1983.

28. Nutting PA, Wood M, Conner EM. Community-oriented primary care in the United States. *JAMA.* 1985;253:1763–1766.

29. Kark SL. *The Practice of Community-Oriented Primary Health Care.* New York, NY: Appleton-Century-Crofts; 1981.

30. Klopper JML, Tibbit L. The Mamre Community Health Project. *S Afr Med J.* 1988;74:319–320.

31. Heart disease study launched in western Cape. *S Afr Med J.* 1990;77:12.

32. Otten MW, Teutsch SM, Williamson DF, Marks JS. The effect of known risk factors on the excess mortality of black adults in the United States. *JAMA.* 1990;263:845–850.

33. *Workforce 2000, Work and Workers for the 21st Century: Executive Summary.* Washington, DC: Hudson Institute Inc: 1989:89–95.

POINT OF RETURN
Bill Landis

Walking down Avenue C toward the needle exchange run by the Lower East Side AIDS Strategy Group every Wednesday and Saturday between 11 A.M. and 2 P.M., I flashed on an ugly memory from 1984's Operation Pressure Point. Me and a black streetwalker had been picked up for copping. We were handcuffed in the back of an unmarked police car, which was speeding uncontrollably after its next mark—a lone junkie who managed to avoid getting busted by tearing into a tenement. I was frightened. I wished I'd run too.

There is something about this area that strikes a palpable fear if you've ever messed with hard narcotics. You're doing something wrong and everybody knows it. All eyes are on you. Your mere presence pisses everyone off, even the dealer taking your money.

AIDS activists have been there, never once apologizing for people's personality traits. Faced with death, people who've had trouble confronting what they're about, be it queers or needle freaks, were given the choice of accepting themselves as human beings or dying silently by themselves.

Prior to the needle program, the works buy was obligatory for junkies who could afford it. The works salesman is the Ratso Rizzo of the drug trade, oblivious to whom he or she hurts for $3. Oft-times enraged but cautious junkies have to discard used sets complete with blood marks.

Needle exchange eliminates these risks. All ethnicities turned up the day I was there: white- and blue-collar workers, stone Jersey junkies, cabbies, guys on bikes, homeless people. The bond of masochism and junkie self-loathing cuts through every stratum of society. But the activists treated no one condescendingly. The overwhelming feeling was love, for one another and for the people they were reaching out to.

People received a diabetic set for each one they returned. A client with none was given two. Old sets were dropped into plastic containers. Bleach, water, alcohol swabs, cookers, and condoms were distributed in Ziploc bags. And though most clients were hardcore junkies who cannot handle the vile psychodrama a trip to welfare lays on the needy, the activists offered bilingual health referral cards and contact with social workers.

A most demanding Freewheelin' Franklin with an old suit jacket covering multiple tracks and abscesses screamed for a dozen sets even though he had none to return. "THE POINT IS PREVENTION? ISN'T IT? ISN'T IT?" But there was also a young Latino couple with two babies in strollers. Most people were cool and grateful to get, every face stamped with that look of anxiety and shame. Inevitably, works salesmen showed up, too, returning dozens of sets. At least they'd have clean goods to sell. Like can collectors, they're now motivated to return needles found on the street and in playgrounds, eliminating another hazard.

Until a few weeks ago, when the program's needles became exempt from the drug laws, the cops hassled the program repeatedly, and even today relations with the police seem uneasy. But despite some warnings to restrict their activities to Avenue C, volunteers began canvassing the neighborhood at around 11:30. As they started toward East Broadway, a bunch of young Latino guys who looked like good-natured Saturday-afternoon beer drinkers politely asked for supplies.

The contingent continued to a needle park. It's dominated by Methadonian needle freaks from a nearby clinic—in the age of AIDS, shooting up isn't enough to get you kicked off a program. These nickel-and-dime pagans did it all—their Meth, pills, dope, shitty nickels of coke. Their affiliation with the welfare system made them better off financially than the average street junkie, with a state dole, health care, and counseling if they're in the mood, and the more coherent and better dressed of them returned enormous numbers of used needles. A white dude who had been HIV-positive since '86 spoke of multiple operations for pancreatic abscesses. An innocuous little old man, a former Talmudic student, said he has been HIV-positive since '83. A streetwalker in a coke spasm splayed her new condoms all over the sidewalk.

Nearby was the Manhattan Bridge, under which live the people of Shantytown. Men and women had constructed living spaces of discarded planks. Remnants provided wall to wall carpeting. Generators had been obtained. Nothing was wasted. Like any family, they tipped off some activists not to wear jewelry so that a dope-sick brother or sister wouldn't get an itch and do something wrong. Totally outside the welfare system, some with jobs, they were steadfast about their responsibilities. Every dirty needle was religiously returned, all instructions were followed, and everyone was grateful to receive bleach, water, swabs, cookers—things that the squatter's life wouldn't normally allow.

A white hooker came out with her works practically in her arm, so earnest was her desire not to pass anything along. A genteel if very stoned black dude was giving back his booty for the last week—30 works. While he dumped them in the bucket, one fell on an activist's bare foot encased in a sandal. A beat passed. "The point on that's gone," he screamed. He was more terrified than her. "Take it easy, just be more careful," she gently but firmly told him, and reassured him that he was getting a boxful of sets.

If David Dinkins wants to see a New York mosaic, he should check out the needle exchange. This is the least racist subculture in the city—there are so many fucking things to fight about that the color of the skin is the least concern. Everyone has a right to live, *including* junkies.

MEDICINE: A BEDSIDE VIEW

Dawn McGuire, M.D.

The medicine that today's house officers dreamed about, which they went to college and medical school and deep into debt for, no longer exists. Our young physicians are bemused and beleaguered, and they feel they have been betrayed.[1]

It is curious that the voices usually absent from discourses on medical ethics are those of the sick and their immediate caregivers, the house officers and ward physicians responsible for day-to-day care. It should not surprise, really, for our discourse is not powerful. We are each strained and vulnerable, and for the most part we are transient as well; for the sick will heal in some fashion or die, and the house officer will complete training and move on. So our status is low, we for whom this drama matters most, and the mandarins, medical and legal, find it easy to speak for us, "objectively."

I welcome, though with trepidation, the opportunity to speak for myself, a house officer, one intimate with the actual care of the very ill in their time of crisis; with trepidation, for it is a difficult and somewhat painful task, since much of what I shall say concerns conditions against which I defend myself with a sort of desperate vigor. I begin, then, with a story by Kafka, whose "fiction" can both disarm and ready one for truth.

According to Kafka, the Great Wall of China was built to protect the Empire from the People of the North. Dutifully, the wall builders laid brick on brick, night and day, wherever they were directed. So there arose many odd, discontinuous fragments of wall over the countryside. These were a pious people, and they trusted that a master plan was indeed being executed by their small labors (though some wondered, quietly, how a wall built in fragments could protect).

None actually knew the extent of the wall, how near it was to completion, nor if it would "work" for the purposes planned. There was rumored to be an Office of the Command; but no one knew where it was nor who commanded. In fact, despite their dedication, no builder knew the wall as well as did the People of the North, the barbarians it was designed to keep out. They rode on their dirty ponies up and down the thousand hills, and they saw and knew everything.

Those of us who spend our days and nights on hospital wards defend and maintain the health care empire. Far from the office of the command, we can only dimly perceive its unwieldy 400-billion-dollar dimensions. So we must look to the "barbarians" for clarity, and this extraordinary anthology includes the most erudite among them. Here we find the critics and visionaries with whose help we may piece together, with discomfiting ease, the picture of an empire at war with itself. A graceless, antique empire, it is probably indefensible in its present form. The structure is feeble; the "cracks" between which people fall are fissures. Its walls are arbitrary, and the excluded become its enemies. Even its pious defenders are demoralized: by the end of a residency, too often the love of medicine and the affection for the sick have been so exploited that young physicians, like the workers on the Great Wall, are, in Kafka's words, "quite exhausted and [have] lost all faith in themselves, in the wall, in the world."

Kafka's tale ends abruptly. His narrator falls silent when he realizes that it is mortal whim, and not vision, behind such walls. The narrator is a politic and pious man. If I risk impiety in pursuing my remarks, it is not recklessly, but out of regard for my trade, and in fear of its disintegration. So I will describe the country of my experience, where I take care of sick people; it is 1989, the age of HMOs and DRGs, of "provider units" and "capitation units"; the age of the "medicolegal document"; the age of AIDS.

It is, first, a country morally imperiled, and those of us who care for patients cannot but do so in bad faith. This country and South Africa stand alone among industrial powers in having no national system of health care. Here, we have elected the commercialization of medicine rather than its socialization. The only aspect of our health policy which resembles a system is the systematic exclusion of millions. It is the fittest who benefit, not the frail, and not the vulnerable. So my work entails filtering the white noise of a moral disquietude. I live and work in the richest state in the richest country in the world, and here one quarter of the children have no medical care. The ironies are not artfully concealed; the attention is just aimed elsewhere. To expect that the commercialization of medicine will protect the public health requires the kind of optimism that builds broken walls: the smug optimism of the unscathed.

In brief, these are the gaps and discontinuities as seen from a great height; but, like a chaotic coastline, the crazy contour repeats itself on smaller and smaller scales. So I would next describe the hospital, where on entering one acquires a peculiar sort of vision: a tunnel vision which manages to cheapen life, while making a cruel expense of "keeping alive"—some, that is. If the standard is the surgeon's knife, or transplanting the untransplantable, or "salvaging" the unsalvageable, then we deserve praise. Cut and cure is better than ever; but *care* is mediocre, when you can get it. Long after the terribly ill, inexorably dying person has uttered her last meaningful word, she is "salvaged." Too often this is not discussed with patients or their families beforehand. Then families are confronted when they are most vulnerable with a painful decision and little realistic guidance: "Do you want us to do everything for your mother?" So the fist crashes on the heart with all the *don't die* wrath of a child. The next breath is forced by machine, the person chemically paralyzed so as not to resist. This is what "doing everything" looks like here.

The 600-gram *abortus* which manages to stir and is therefore "viable" is salvaged: months in intensive care, surviving but with scarred lungs and a damaged brain; sick, unwanted, "difficult to place"; one quarter of a million dollars spent. Yet tens of thousands of wanted children are born without benefit of prenatal care for lack of funded programs. But salvage we must, for we are "obligated"; by whom or by what it is unclear, and it should be clear what obligates us to such cruelty and wastefulness.

I am not a seasoned doctor. I am not dispassionate. Contradiction nags me, suffering grieves me, waste offends me. But nagged, aggrieved, offended, impatient, I am no less a disciplined doctor. I do my job, and this is the context in which I work; this is what I see.

I see a devastating disease, the dimensions of which mock the facile claim that medicine is science and not politics. The phenomenon AIDS has exposed the social diseases which killed long before HIV: denial of health care to millions; the use of drugs to regulate a passive underclass; the easy tolerance of violence toward gay and lesbian people; the intractable racism with its myriad masks and intentions. AIDS is revealing ourselves to ourselves. The afflicted are mostly the oppressed, but, once afflicted, all become marginal, and the easy targets of bigotry. In San Francisco, gay men painstakingly acquired a modest political power before the epidemic. They organized quickly, and have been able to exercise some control at least over the medical community's response. There are AIDS wards, hospices, support for partners; there is some *care* for these men. Yet it is also true that they are well-educated, middle-class, mostly white, comfortable with power, male-identified, and male. They could be doctors, scientists, senators. They "fit" power. Nonetheless, their vigilance to some extent protects all those affected. It would not happen, as in New York, that Jorge, a Puerto Rican gay man, would spend thirty hours in an emergency room, vomiting, incontinent, febrile to 105 degrees, to be sent away without care. This reflects the lifeboat politics of a city disorganized and stressed beyond tolerance. In New York City, AIDS is mostly in the underclass, and it kills faster there. The forces which shape the medical response to this disease are first, second, and third *political*. The political agenda shapes our science and it shapes our service.

Is this the vocation to which I was called? It is, and it isn't. *Ars toto requirit hominem*: the art takes all you've got to give. That part is certainly the same. I recall what compelled me to medicine: the sense of deep privilege and just good fortune that I could learn the mysteries and heal the wounds. And where I could not cure, I could nonetheless assist my patients toward their own "good" death. What is true is that while I can shock to life a dying heart, I have left many broken ones unattended. My training, technically impeccable, doesn't reach this far, and even mediocrity in this regard is above the accepted standard. Daily I deal clumsily with the most important moments in my patients' lives. The scenes which should be played before a hushed house I attend, barely, half in, half out of a psychological doorway. It may be my thirtieth working hour, or even my thirty-sixth. My beeper is bleating. My neck is in spasm, and I feel nothing except the drive to be horizontal. The light from my private life is so remote as to be doppler-shifted. I make just over minimum wage for a week that can exceed one hundred hours. My debt from training has the next decade mortgaged. Yet, despite the structural limitations, and my own, I *am* the intimate companion of *this* sick person. It is we two who meet and probe one another, sense each others' strengths and frailties, who trust one another or not. This particularity, this relationship, however disguised and tyrannized, is the level on which it makes sense to speak of healing. It is unique; it cannot be reproduced; it is not a science.

But I am trained in science, not in healing. I "treat" patients. And of the patients I have treated, I have probably helped only a third; to another third, I have at least kept my oath and done no harm. As for the rest, I have certainly added to their suffering, especially the oldest, the most frail, those with no advocate to speak out when they are silenced by disease. To these, I have "done everything," as my job obliges. And there is something darkly depleting about having so little to offer the sick.

So there is a wounding to this work. The relationship between the wounded healer and the art of healing is a very ancient one. Even Galen, father of our science, tells us he was cured of a mortal illness by Aesculapius in a dream.[2] Native healers from the Four Corners to the Sub-Sahara still must undergo a "shamanic illness" in their training, from which they recover, often after years, and become healers, or else succumb. And so do we, for three to seven years, live sleep-deprived, hypervigilant, anxious, isolated, and often secretly terribly sad. We should perhaps celebrate, then, our initiation illness, through which we may learn to use our power gracefully. However, unlike the training shaman, we do little in the way of meditation on our journey. We remain only crudely aware of our own affliction, and the most defended are the most rewarded here. The passage is endured, merely; we are reduced, but not refined. The experiences, unprocessed, weigh on us like lead. That it could be otherwise seems as improbable as alchemy.

I think patients must often sense the wounds of their doctors. But we are so protective of our role, and so defended against our vulnerabilities, that we thwart their care toward us. The expected comportment is that of studied concern, unflappable authority, taut patience. Their concern for us is inappropriate, we say. It breeches boundaries. But don't we doctors, with our hidden sores, know this: that it is part of being healed, to heal?

Where are the teachers, our guides for this passage? The list of scientists I admire is long; but when I consider healing, I see not Osler, Virchow; not even Lewis Thomas, nor Victor Sidel. I see a fat, pale baker from a story by Raymond Carver.[3]

"A Small, Good Thing" is a quietly remarkable parable of healing; not that it tries to define healing, nor to dissect the healing relationship. Its aims are simple, its vision local. The story just shows the "close work" of healing; and so restores it to its mystery and simplicity, its particularity, its breathtaking exactness.

A boy is hit by a car on his birthday. The physician, wishing to reassure— himself? the helpless parents?—insists that the boy is not "really" in a coma. He is a *nice* man, but his caring is brief, embarrassed, inept. He is not "good" at helplessness, except to conceal it. Hungry as the young parents are for nurturance, his best is to send them elsewhere for it. *Feel free to go out for a bite. It would do you good.*

When the boy dies, the physician is truly sorry. *A hidden occlusion,* he explains vaguely. *A one-in-a-million circumstance.* He embraces the couple, then hurries them to the parking lot. *He seemed full of some goodness she didn't understand.*

Throughout the hospital vigil, the couple had been getting bizarre phone calls. A man's voice would ask: *Your Scotty, I got him ready for you. Have you forgotten about Scotty?* On the night the child dies, his mother remembers the cake she had ordered for his birthday. She remembers the strange, sour baker —it had been *he*, then, calling about the cake!

She is so angry she feels crazy. Her husband drives her to the bakery in the dark of night. It is a petty, sinister little man who reluctantly opens his door to them. He is snide and contentious at first: the sixteen-dollar cake is stale. And then he hears her: *He's dead, you bastard.* The baker stops his work. He takes off his apron. He pulls up three chairs and makes a space at the table. He allows the impact of what he has done to impress upon him fully: he has added to their unspeakable suffering. He opens himself to their grief. And then he speaks, disarmed, from his heart:

Listen to me. I'm just a baker. I don't claim to be anything else. Maybe once, maybe years ago, I was a different kind of human being. I've forgotten, I don't know for sure. That don't excuse my doing what I did, I know. But I'm deeply sorry. I'm sorry for your son, and sorry for my part in this. . . . Please, let me ask you if you can find it in your hearts to forgive me?

Then the baker feeds them. They, who are more empty than they've ever been, eat fresh sweet rolls from his oven. He tells them, *There's all the rolls in the world here. Eating is a small, good thing in a time like this.*

As the three sit together in the early light, the baker also shares himself. *They nodded when the baker began to speak of loneliness, and of the sense of doubt and limitation that had come to him in his middle years. He told them what it was like to be childless all these years.* Such a gifted healer, this baker. He gives exactly what he has, and it suffices, exactly. He permits these suffering people to extend themselves, through their grief, to him, and their emptiness relents. *They listened to him. They ate what they could. They talked on into the early morning. And they did not think of leaving.*

Imagine the baker's first speech delivered by the physician. *I'm just a doctor.* . . . What he did say was, sadly, true: *I'm so very sorry, I can't tell you.* How empty we sound when, failing cure, we distrust ourselves, and reject whatever small, good thing that might be ours to offer. Full of some opaque, private goodness, we do not ask forgiveness, and we do not forgive ourselves.[4] I think it must be in the setting of forgiveness that healing becomes possible, for any of us.

But small, good things won't be coming from doctors in doorways, half-asleep. The standards must be articulated, the structure of care and training changed to accommodate the standards. To say there isn't time, or money, or the physician labor force to make *care for all* a meaningful concept, is to say there isn't the political will. The conditions we have accepted, which our values have determined, are as arbitrary as they are resistant to change; and can, none-theless, be changed.

This work belongs to all of us, for we are healers, all. And it remains, despite this painful stage, the best work I can imagine.

NOTES

1. J.E. Hardison. "The House Officer's Changing World," *New England Journal of Medicine* 1986; 314: 1713–5.

2. Galen, "On His Own Books," from Arthur J. Brock, *Greek Medicine*, J.M. Dent and Sons, London, 1929. p. 177.

3. Raymond Carver, "A Small, Good Thing," from *Cathedral*, Alfred A. Knopf, Inc., 1983.

4. Cf. David Hilfiker. Facing Our Mistakes, *New England Journal of Medicine* 1984; 310:118–22.

WASHINGTON COULD HELP US FIGHT AIDS

Kathryn Anastos

Two weeks ago I stood alone at the bedside of one of my patients, a man for whom I held great fondness and who had previously expressed ambivalence about living. We locked eyes as I asked him if he wanted to live, and he answered with an unequivocal "yes." I arranged transfer to intensive care, where three days later he died. The morning after his death, I stood at the bedside of another man with AIDS with his weeping mother and brother, and watched as his body shuddered with his last breaths, ending his mother's long vigil.

Two months prior I had watched as another patient, the mother of six young children, slowly relinquished her cognizance of her surroundings, including her sense that she was failing her children by dying before they were grown. She died a few days later. And shortly before that I had been called to the home of another woman, also with young children, to pronounce her dead so that her family could be spared the shame of having the police come to the home.

I am a primary-care physician—that is, my patients are mostly those who seek care early enough that they can walk into my clinic. They know that they have one doctor (me) and that if they become acutely ill I or a covering physician am available to them at any time. I am responsible for all the medical care they need, and when they are sick enough to be hospitalized, I continue to be their physician, often until their death.

Because I work in the South Bronx, most of my patients are not accustomed to this kind of care, a standard that I and most middle-class Americans expect, even take for granted. I am proud to be a part of an institution, Bronx Lebanon Hospital Center, that is committed to providing this standard of care to the South Bronx.

It is from this perspective that I am angered by the U.S. health care system and failure of the public health response to the AIDS epidemic. By June 30, 1992, 230,179 Americans with AIDS—more than 24,000 women, 200,000 men and nearly 4,000 children—had been reported to the Centers for Disease Control. Seventy-five percent of women, 72 percent of children and 42 percent of men with AIDS are African American or Latino and live in inner cities. This is a heavy burden to carry in communities already struggling with poverty, homelessness, racism and drug use.

Recently our nation was gripped by the debate over whether we as a society should invest hundreds of millions of dollars yearly to test all health-care workers for HIV. Such an initiative could at best have prevented a handful of new cases each decade.

Those of us who work or live in communities ravaged by HIV have not seen even a fraction of such resources devoted to prevention efforts in our neighborhoods, where hundreds or thousands of new cases could be prevented. What we have witnessed instead are multiple examples of social neglect.

We have yet to see adequate sex and HIV-prevention education for teenagers and adults; or public health messages that are explicit in their recommendations for preventing sexual transmission of HIV; or accessible health care for our communities; or serious consideration of needle exchange. Is it sound policy to consider spending millions to prevent a few middle-class cases of AIDS while thousands of new cases occur in low-income communities?

I was taught that to be an effective physician means to be an advocate for my patients, and that to advocate for them I must look at life and its choices through their eyes. It is the greatest source of satisfaction in my work, and also the greatest source of pain. As I try to view life through their eyes, as I picture myself dying in that hospital bed and leaving behind my own young children, I see a society that does not provide pre-natal care to pregnant women, nor immunizations for children. People making such choices must not be able to imagine themselves in my patients' circumstances. For if we all saw each other as equal human beings, how would we possibly choose to allocate our resources the way we do?

SECTION III

THE CHANGING MEDICAL/INDUSTRIAL COMPLEX: THE BOTTOM LINE VS. THE PUBLIC AGENDA

INTRODUCTION

Hal Strelnick

For many years the health system in the United States was described as a "non-system," certainly not a "health" system working toward maximizing the health of its people. At best we have a "medical care" system that both medicalizes social problems and applies as much technological diagnosis and treatment as insurance permits. Public health, primary care, health promotion, and disease prevention have been poor cousins to the dominant modes of private practice medicine and high-tech hospital care, so much so that public health advocates have called for an "ounce of prevention"—the commitment of one-sixteenth of health spending to prevention. Other nations spend substantially more.

Inflation double that in the rest of the economy has plagued health care costs almost continuously since World War II, resulting in a steady increase in its portion of the gross national product. In 1990 one dollar in eight went into the health system, a total of $666 billion. This aspect of the health system follows a traditional marketplace model; i.e., increased purchasing power through expanding health insurance to more and more people drives up prices. During the postwar period this expansion was propelled by growing private health insurance and Blue Cross/Blue Shield coverage through employment benefits, first won by labor unions during the war. In the 1960s the expansion was infused directly with public dollars with the enactment of Medicare and Medicaid. (The "tax expenditures" given to employers and their employees for health insurance benefits that are not taxed as income continue to exceed the dollars directly spent about two-to-one.) Because of this inflation many are worse off now than before; the elderly now pay more out of pocket for health care than *before* Medicare was enacted!

Health resources like hospitals, clinics, physicians, dentists, and other health professionals have also followed market forces that fill their beds and appointment books with paying (i.e., insured) patients. Doctors and hospitals have abandoned poor rural and inner city communities and flocked to the suburbs and Sunbelt. Despite token public programs to buck these trends, young doctors have pursued high-paying careers in surgical and medical subspecialties and the "life-style" specialties like ophthalmology and anesthesiology with banker's hours, resulting in surpluses of specialists and shortages of generalists. Of course, recent studies published in the *Journal of the American Medical Association* have shown that for the same medical problems, generalists generate fewer costs than specialists *without* compromising quality. Public health facilities have always been designed to protect those abandoned by the private market and have over time served a smaller, narrower, and more powerless segment of the population.

In other ways the health system defies traditional market forces. For example, the more competition between hospitals in a given city, the *higher* the costs in that city because hospitals do not compete on price but on appearance, service, prestige, and reputation. Many have noted that health insurance insulates the consumer from costs. Insurers have used mechanisms such as deductibles and co-payments to curb utilization and encourage wiser shopping. However, except for seeing their physician or filling a prescription, most consumers have little to say on the costs generated by diagnostic tests, medications, other treatments, or hospitalizations, all decisions made by their doctor. "Defensive medicine," the practice of exhaustive diagnostic testing to protect against malpractice suits, only drives these costs higher.

In the 1980s, despite the incremental expansion of Medicaid for children and pregnant women, the uninsured population grew. Classic economics would suggest that prices would stabilize with decreased demand, especially with the widespread efforts to contain and control costs using prepayment (e.g., HMOs, IPAs, etc.), micromanagement (e.g., utilization review, preadmission reviews, second opinions, etc.), and disincentives (e.g., greater co-payments, deductibles, and exclusions). Cost inflation continued unabated because of a phenomenon called *intensification* that describes the growing complexity of clinical care with more personnel and technology employed for any measurable unit of clinical care, such as hospital admission or a physician visit. For an episode of pneumonia, for example, a pulmonologist may order a new, expensive antibiotic rather than penicillin, several tests to exclude other possible diagnoses, and respiratory therapy. The old-fashioned nearly extinct family doctor might have given the same patient an injection of penicillin and followed the illness at home. The former has become the US standard of care—it is more expensive . . . and more profitable for all the providers involved.

In 1970 Health/PAC, borrowing from President Eisenhower's farewell warnings a decade earlier about the "military-industrial complex," coined the phrase "medical-industrial complex" that appeared thereafter in *Fortune* and soon in the vernacular. Eisenhower's Iron Triangle of the Pentagon, military contractors, and key congressional committees was simple compared to the complex then described between the medical establishment, the insurance industry, and federal health bureaucrats. This complex has grown infinitely more complex with the interests of the pharmaceutical and medical technology manufacturers, state and local governments, academic medicine and researchers, for-profit hospital and clinic chains, malpractice insurers and attorneys, entrepreneurial non-profits and professionals, health benefit managers, employers, and an alphabet soup of acronyms for new partnerships and regulators. The bottom line, however, remains the bottom line: profitability.

In the accompanying Table 1 (p. 247) the US health system is described in a matrix of functions and sectors, divided between the public sector levels of federal, state, and local government and the private sector of for- and non-profit (voluntary) enterprises. The non-profit sector can further be subdivided into religious or sectarian organizations and nonsectarian or secular institutions. The

Table 1
The US Health System by Function and Sector

FUNCTION	FEDERAL	STATE	LOCAL	NON-PROFIT*	FOR-PROFIT**
Capital & Construction	Hill-Burton grants & loans	Public capital bonds	Public capital bonds	Tax-exempt bonds, subsidized loans	Stocks & bonds, market-rate loans
Manufacturing (supplies & pharmaceuticals)	Rare vaccines				Medical & hospital supplies, drug & sundries, biotechnology
R&D (information)	AHCPR, NIMH, NIH, CDC, OTA, NIOSH grants, contracts	Health Research Council, grants, universities	Departments of health, universities	Universities, institutes, foundations, AMA, ADA	Industrial R & D, consultants & contract research
Education/Training	grants, indirect & direct medical education (Medicare)	Universities, academic medical centers, grants	Academic medical centers, universities & community colleges	Academic medical centers, universities, colleges, hospital schools of nursing, AAMC	Private technical schools
Financial Aid	Loans, scholarships, subsidies	Loans, scholarships, subsidies	Public subsidies	Foundations	Guaranteed student loans
Regulation	FDA, OSHA, FTC, CPSC, NTSC	Health departments	Health departments, zoning	Institutional planning	Business coalitions, consultants
Licensure, Accreditation & Certification	Some laboratories	Health/education departments, clinicians, hospitals, nursing homes	Vendors	JCAHO, LCME, RRC, ABMS, professional boards	
Reimbursement/ Insurance	HCFA (Medicaid, Medicare)	Medicaid, bad debt & charity pools	Medicaid, medically indigent	Blue Cross/Blue Shield, some HMOs	Private insurance, for-profit HMOs

Table 1 (cont.)
The US Health System by Function and Sector

FUNCTION	FEDERAL	STATE	LOCAL	NON-PROFIT*	FOR-PROFIT**
Clinical Services: Hospitals	VA, IHS, PHS, military	Mental health, chronic care	Public hospitals, chronic care	Voluntary hospitals	Proprietary hospitals, hospital corporations
Primary Care	NHSC, CHCs, MHCs	CHC funding	Public health clinics	CHCs, some HMOs	Private practice, PPOs, IPAs emergicenters, HMOs
Long Term Care	NIA, Medicare/caid funds, VA	Chronic care, nursing homes	Chronic care, nursing homes	Home care, VNS, some nursing homes	Proprietary nursing homes, home care
Mental Health	NIMH, NIDA, NIAAA, CMHCs, OSAP grants	Psychiatric hospitals & clinics, drug & alcohol program funding	Mental health clinics, drug & alcohol programs	CMHCs, voluntary social agencies, drug & alcohol treatment programs	Proprietary psychiatric hospitals, drug & alcohol treatment facilities, private practice
Health Promotion Disease Prevention	CHCs, MHCs, Surgeon General	Grants	Health departments	AHA, Am Cancer Society, etc.	Employee wellness programs
Health Planning	Grants	SHPDAs	HSAs	Institutional planning	Business coalitions, consultants
Public Health	EPA, CDC, PHS, NTSC	Health departments	Health departments	Public interest groups	Waste management
Special Populations	Refugees, military, veterans, dialysis, elderly,	Mentally ill & retarded, developmentally delayed	Medically indigent	Homeless outreach	Well-insured

* **NON-PROFIT** may be further divided between religious or sectarian and non-secarian institutions
** **FOR-PROFIT** may be further divided into corporate and entrepreneurial or individual ownership

for-profit sector may also be subdivided by ownership with both publicly and privately held corporations and individually or entrepreneurially owned businesses and practices. The vast majority of medical and mental health care is provided in this last sector in the private practices of individuals and groups (partnerships) of professionals. Most hospital care is provided in voluntary, not-for-profit hospitals by private practitioners, although the mix of public, voluntary, and for-profit hospitals varies greatly by region and city.

The functions identified in the table are not exhaustive (e.g., among areas not included are occupational and environmental health and malpractice and risk management). Among those areas identified are those directly related to finance (capital and insurance/reimbursement), the preparation of the workforce (education/training and financial aid), clinical services, public health and regulation, and responsibilities for special populations.

What the matrix demonstrates most clearly are that certain functions are distributed among all sectors (e.g., clinical services), while others are concentrated in one or two sectors (e.g., manufacturing in the for-profit sector or licensure in state governments and the non-profit professional organizations that have developed to preserve professional autonomy and avoid direct state regulation). Research takes place mainly in the public and voluntary sectors, while its fruits are produced and profits generated only by for-profit enterprises. However, as information itself becomes a profitable commodity, for-profit vendors of publicly gathered data (e.g., census data) have proliferated, what Vicente Navarro of Johns Hopkins would call "the conversion of public sector services into private commodities."

Similarly, education takes place almost exclusively in the public and voluntary sectors, while the prepared workforce is employed more broadly with professionals capable of becoming individual entrepreneurs in private practice. Academic medical centers, what Health/PAC has called "medical empires," dominate the health system ideologically, establishing the professional standards of practice through research, training, and education, but are themselves rarely for-profit and provide only a small fraction of all clinical care. Foundations play a similar modest but important ideological role, framing the questions asked about the health system and often systematically excluding from consideration important alternatives.

One view of the history of the health system is the struggle between these sectors for control and exclusion. Expansion and contraction of the three levels of the public sector are not even and do not always counterbalance expansions and contractions of the private sector, dependent as they are on tax revenues. In the 1980s the New Federalism tried to limit federal commitments, and state and local governments had to compensate. Special populations that have not been welcome in the private sector (e.g., refugees, veterans, the mentally ill, and the retarded, etc.) and expensive categories of service (e.g., dialysis, burn units, trauma centers, etc.) have traditionally become the responsibility of a specific level of government, often for historical reasons long forgotten. The public sector has joined with the voluntary sector in undertaking the unprofitable but necessary maintenance of the physical, technical, and human infrastructure of the health system and protecting the most vulnerable from the harshness of the wide open marketplace.

The most striking concentration of function in the US system has been in the production of goods; everything from manufacturing pharmaceuticals and over-the-counter nostrums to crafting fiberoptic endoscopes, multimillion-dollar Positron Emission Tomography scanners, and genetically engineered artificial organs is done in the private, for-profit sector. This means that private investors and entrepreneurs, not doctors or patients or elected representatives, are deciding what technologies to bring to market, based upon their estimate of the market's size and profitability. Concentrating production in the for-profit sector has left the US health system with countless "me too" drugs and too many so-called "orphan" drugs and technologies. The so-called "me too" drugs that have proliferated to compete for "market share" of the huge profits available treating arthritis and high blood pressure offer no demonstrable improvement over existing therapies. "Orphan" drugs and technologies have been shown effective in research but without prospects for large or profitable markets have failed to attract a corporate sponsor to move them through the regulatory process. For example, lithium carbonate, a simple salt that could not be patented, was orphaned for years, even though it was the only effective treatment known for manic-depression.

Historically, the 50 states have retained responsibility for public health with federal intervention beginning under the rubric of regulating interstate commerce when quarantine was the major intervention available and expanding during the New Deal under the "general welfare" clause of the US Constitution. Legislation has followed the "categorical imperative" with programs targeting specific diseases, age groups, or institutions or providing specific services, to address visible crises rather than planning and building toward a comprehensive health system. As a consequence of this history, the federal health bureaucracy is scattered among many different departments and agencies, including the Departments of Health and Human Services, Agriculture (WIC), Treasury (tax expenditures), Labor (OSHA), Transportation, Education, and the Environmental Protection Agency, Federal Trade Commission, Agency for International Development, National Academy of Science and National Science Foundation (see Table 2, p. 251).

The static matrix presented in Table 1 (p. 247) cannot portray the myriad of complex interactions between the various sectors that constitute the real US health system. A recent example may serve to better illustrate the interplay between public and private; federal, state, and local governments; and the body politic that is the *real* US health system.

The nation's childhood immunization system is a patchwork of public and private sector efforts that includes private physicians, and local, state, and federal governments. Half of all vaccines are administered in the private sector and half in the public sector. Only 45 percent of indemnity insurers cover immunizations, forcing pediatricians and other providers to pass on costs to parents or refer patients to already overtaxed public clinics. Since 1963, the federal government through the Centers for Disease Control (CDC) has provided grants to states and some large county and city health departments to assist in purchasing ad-

Table 2

The Health Industry and the State: The Federal Bureaucracy at a Glance
Secretary, Department of Health & Human Services

Office of the Assistant Sec'ty of Health

Office of:
- Management
- Disease Prevention & Health Promotion
- Smoking & Health
- Adolescent Pregnancy Program
- Health Research, Statistics, & Technology
- HMOs
- International Health

AHCPR

ADAMHA
NIAAA
NIDA
NIMH

CDC
NIOSH
NCHS

FDA
Nat. Center for Toxicology Research

HRSA
Bureau of Hlth Planning & Development
Bureau of Hlth Professions
Bureau of Community Health Services (NHSC) & Bureau of Medical Services (PHS & IHS)

NIH
NIA
NIAID
NIAMDD
NCI
NICHHD
NIEHS
NEI
NIDS
NHLBI
NINCDS
Div. of Research Resources

Health Care Finance Admin.
Office of Special Programs (EPS, DT)
Office of Research, Demonstrations, & Statistics

Office of Human Development Services
Administration of Aging (IV)
Admin. for Child, Youth, & Families
Office of Policy Development
Office of Program Coordination & Review (Title XX)

Dept of the Treasury
Internal Revenue Service

Consumer product Safety Commission

Dept. of Education
Office of Comprehensive School Health

EPA

FTC

AID
National Academy of Science
Institute of Medicine (IOM)

Community Service Admin. (OEO)
National Science Foundation

Dept. of Labor
OSHA
Mine S & HA

Dept. Of Transprotation
Auto Safety

USDA
WIC
food stamps

Congress
Office of Technology Assessment

equate supplies of vaccine and in supplementing their immunization efforts. Federal grants currently cover *half* of the total public sector need; state and local governments try to meet the remainder. According to the National Vaccine Advisory Committee's 1991 Measles White Paper, "there is no formal national coordination of the federal role in vaccine delivery."

Between 1966 and 1974 the CDC spent $180 million dollars on childhood immunizations and saved an estimated $1.3 billion in medical and long-term care costs. According to the House Select Committee on Children, Youth, and Families, one dollar spent on immunization saves $10 in health care costs, compared to $3.38 saved when spent on prenatal care, $3 when spent on WIC nutrition supplements, or $4.75 when spent on Head Start. Dollar for dollar, immunizations are the *best* ounce of prevention.

Yet, the 1980s began with the Reagan administration proposing a 25 percent cut in funds for childhood immunizations; most of his subsequent budgets also proposed cuts that were rejected by Congress. Federal spending increased during the 1980s, from $31 million in 1981 to $158.3 million in fiscal year 1990, but this did not keep pace with the dramatic inflation in the cost of vaccines. In 1983 there was a nationwide shortage of vaccines, aggravated by publicity about adverse events associated with the pertussis vaccine and the liability insurance crisis. The manufacture of each vaccine was then monopolized by a different drug company. Inflation for DPT (diphtheria-pertussis-tetanus) was 99.5 percent from 1983 to 1984 and for polio vaccine 36 percent in 1986 alone. Complete immunization that cost $47 in 1986 cost $91 in 1990. In constant service dollars federal support fell below 1981 levels; two million fewer children were served in 1986 than in 1981. To address the manufacturers' "production slow-down," Congress created a national stockpile of vaccines and limited the manufacturers' liability through the National Childhood Vaccine Injury Act of 1986.

In 1976 we faced a similar crisis with increases in measles, rubella, and pertussis (whooping cough). In 1977 the Childhood Immunization Initiative was begun, and the complete elimination of measles set as a national goal. In 1982 the US had only 1,742 cases of measles, one-tenth the cases of 1979, and fewer still in 1983. Since that time a major measles epidemic has broken out across the nation's cities, including Los Angeles, Chicago, Dallas, and New York with more than 25,000 cases and 64 deaths in 1990, higher than any year since 1971. A combination of vaccine shortages and expense, reductions in federal support, and cases among unimmunized infants and toddlers have fueled an epidemic that persists in 1992. However, the major CDC initiative has been a mix of priorities. The mandatory distribution of three information booklets on the basic vaccines (DPT, MMR, and polio) to *every* parent of an immunized child (Childhood Vaccine Injury Act of 1986) was passed primarily to reduce the vaccine producers' liability. Parents must sign to indicate that they have received and read the brochures. This has created a paperwork nightmare for providers. A $4.44 per MMR dose excise tax pays for a compensation program for vaccine-related injuries. Rather than an all-out war to eliminate measles, the Bush administration proposed (and then abandoned) linking AFDC and Medicaid benefits to up-to-date immunizations and sponsored six model programs nationwide.

Is this mixed public-private system working? In 1988 fourteen other nations immunized their one-year-old infants for polio better than the US. Our immunization rates for children from one to four years are all declining; they peaked for DPT (67.3 percent) and polio (78.7 percent) in 1971, for measles (65.9 percent) in 1976, and for mumps (59.5 percent) and rubella (64 percent) in 1983. From the early 1970s to 1985 the gap in immunization rates between whites and non-whites has *widened* for every vaccine!

This brief review of our immunization system highlights the problems of our complex, mixed public-private system. Despite its impressive cost-effectiveness, only a minority of private health insurance covers immunizations, leaving the gap to be covered by parents or public clinics. The cost of the basic vaccine package has increased from both profiteering and technical improvements in comprehensiveness and timeliness. Near monopolies of the production of vaccines produced a crisis when product liability suits were proliferating, vaccine costs skyrocketing, and supplies plummeting. The industry sought and received the protection of Congress, which became the insurer of last resort through its excise tax-supported compensation program. The executive branch of the federal government abandoned its financial commitment and leadership role to the states just when a major *preventable* epidemic was breaking out nationally. (Readers may see many parallels here in the federal response to AIDS.)

In the articles that follow similar relations and interactions will be examined in greater detail. David Whiteis and Jack Salmon review the relationship between the public and private sectors that leads to an impoverished public sector. Regina Neal details how an academic health center, Columbia Presbyterian Medical Center in New York City, has responded to its changing community environment, showing the role that the academic medical center plays between the private sector and public need. And Louanne Kennedy details how the difference between for-profit, voluntary, and public hospitals are eroding under marketplace incentives for efficiency.

With the Donald Light piece, we get a review of the newest approaches of the health insurance industry to reduce its risks, and with the Kotelchuck piece a discussion of the wisdom of states' moves to cut cost by embracing "Medicaid Managed Care" for their citizens. "A Staff Report of the Senate Special Committee on Aging" examines the extraordinary profits and practices of the pharmaceutical industry and Eric Holtzman and Hal Strelnick examine the medical supply and biotechnology industry, major components of the "medical industrial complex" along with the profit enhancing strategies of the "franchise" walk-in clinics for women's health.

As health care delivery changes so do the roles of its providers—physicians, nurses, and health care workers. The last articles by John McKinlay and John Stoeckle, Pat Moccia and Susan Reverby, and Sumner Rosen speak to these changes and to the changes in power and labor among physicians, to the issues of race and class in medical education, to the gender relations of care giving and about the battles for strong workers unions in the "medical industrial complex." This section ends with the "voice" of Harry Krulevitch, M.D. who speaks directly to the conflict between the need to care and the institutional demands of profit.

TOTAL US GROSS DOMESTIC PRODUCT AND PERCENT OF EXPENDITURES FOR HEALTH, EDUCATION AND DEFENSE 1970, 1975, 1980–1988

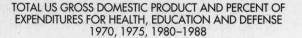

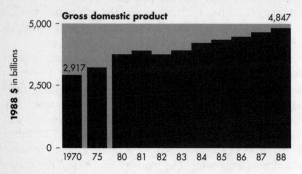

Note: Data in this chart are inflation-adjusted to 1988 dollars.

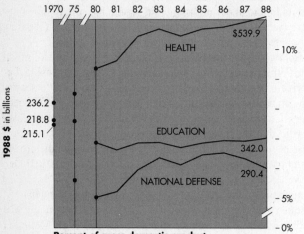

Note: Data in this chart are inflation-adjusted to 1988 dollars.

Robert Wood Johnson Foundation, 1991

Sources:

1970–1987 GDP data: Organization for Economic Cooperation and Development. *National Accounts 1960–1987.* Volume I, Main Aggregates. Paris, France, 1989. Pp. 32–33.

1988 GDP data: Unpublished data from the US Council of Economic Advisors.

Health data: Unpublished data from the US Health Care Financing Administration.

1970–1987 education data: US Department of Education, National Center for Education Statistics. *Digest of Education Statistics: 1989.* Washington DC. NCES Pub. No. 89-643, 1989. Table 25, p. 29.

1988 education data: Unpublished preliminary data from the same source.

Defense data: US Office of Management and Budget. *Historical Tables: Budget of the United States Government: Fiscal Year 1990.* Washington DC, 1989. Table 3.1, pp. 42–44.

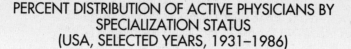

PERCENT DISTRIBUTION OF ACTIVE PHYSICIANS BY SPECIALIZATION STATUS
(USA, SELECTED YEARS, 1931–1986)

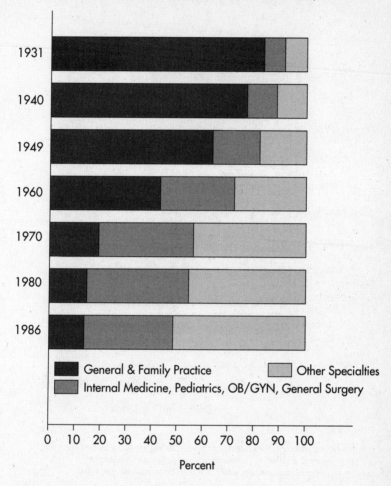

Percent

Note:
In the years 1931, 1940, 1949, and 1960, general and family practice also includes physicians who report being part-time specialists, physicians not reporting any specialty, and those reporting specialties "not recognized" by the American Medical Association; pediatrics also includes pediatric allergy and pediatric cardiology. In the year 1940, surgery includes other surgical specialties except orthopedic surgery. In the years 1970 and 1980 the categories "unspecified," "not classified," and "address unknown" are excluded. In 1986, the figures include approximately 90% of the physicians who are not classified according to activity status by the AMA and whose addresses are unknown; pediatrics includes pediatric allergy and pediatric cardiology.

Sources:
For 1931–1960: US Department of Health, Education, and Welfare. Health manpower source book. Manpower supply and educational statistics for selected health occupations, 1968. Washington DC, 1969; DHEW Publ. No. (PHS) 263: Table 41, p. 42.

AVERAGE NET INCOME OF PHYSICIANS,[1]
BY SPECIALTY, IN CONSTANT 1988 DOLLARS[2]
(USA, 1973, 1988)

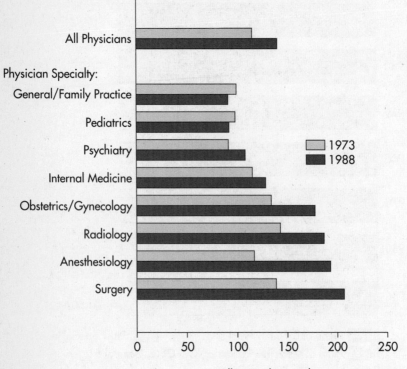

Dollars in Thousands

Notes:
1. Net income includes all earnings from medical practice after expenses but before taxes including fringe benefits and deferred compensation plans. Based on reports by a sample of nonfederal physicians predominantly in patient care, excluding resident staff.
2. Calculated using GNP Implicit Price Deflator to reflect 1988 constant dollars.

Sources:

For 1973: US Department of Commerce, Bureau of the Census. Statistical abstract of the United States, 1989. Washington DC, 1989: Table 751, p. 464.

Reynolds RA, Ohsfeldt RL, eds. Socioeconomic characteristics of medical practice 1984. Chicago: American Medical Association, 1984: Table 39, p. 110.

For 1988: US Department of Commerce, Bureau of the Census. Statistical abstract of the United States, 1990: Washington DC, 1990: Table 775, p. 480.

Gonzalez ML, ed. Socioeconomic characteristics of medical practice 1990/1991. Milwaukee, WI: American Medical Association, 1991: Table 58, p. 154.

THE PROPRIETARIZATION OF HEALTH CARE AND THE UNDERDEVELOPMENT OF THE PUBLIC SECTOR

David G. Whiteis and J. Warren Salmon

Introduction

Two major and interconnected issues confronting health care delivery in the United States today are hospital failure and the rapid encroachment by the for-profit sector. The operational influence on the entire delivery system can be seen by analyzing the dramatic growth of investor-owned hospital chains during the early years of this decade. The *Modern Health Care* survey shows a 15.0 percent increase in total beds owned, leased, or managed by investor-owned multi-hospital chains between 1982 and 1983 (1, p. 66), and a 15.1 percent increase between 1983 and 1984 (2, p. 76). During the latter time period, profits of the investor-owned chains responding to the survey rose 28.5 percent from $693.5 million to $89.1 million (2, p. 76), continuing a trend that had shown a 37.7 percent increase (from $530.5 million to $730.7 million) between 1982 and 1983 (1, p. 66). Alongside these corporate profit figures, however, have been huge losses by public hospital systems, which recorded a $360 million deficit for 1984, 57.2 percent greater than the $229 million deficit they suffered in 1983 (2, p. 76).

A closer examination of U.S. hospitals in the 1980s reveals a significant amount of financial crisis among those not blessed with ongoing capital reserves from the stock and bond markets, and well-paying privately-insured patients. The American Hospital Association (AHA) reported that 156 community hospitals closed between 1980 and 1984, with the greatest single concentration of closings (28.9 percent) being in large metropolitan areas with populations over 1.5 million (3, p. 15). The great majority of failed hospitals during this time (84.5 percent) were *not* members of multi-hospital systems (3, p. 17). Preliminary results from a study in progress at the University of Illinois at Chicago indicate that a similar pattern exists for hospital closures during the period 1985–87 (4). These findings reveal that, even in the current era of cost-cutting, retrenchment, and increased financial pressure, some hospitals continue to thrive while others are in jeopardy.

The relationship between the rampant growth of the proprietary sector (accompanied by an increasing corporatization of "not-for-profit" hospitals mimicking their for-profit counterparts), the deepening crisis in the public health sector, and the implications for the medical profession have been noted extensively (5). Corporate strategizing has encouraged such cost-saving techniques as "cream-skimming" of middle-class clienteles on the part of many hospitals, leaving smaller voluntary and public hospitals more financially vulnerable and at a higher risk (6). The AHA's portrait of "the typical closed community hospital" between 1980 and 1984 is instructive in this regard (3, p. 1):

> Under 199 beds in size, investor-owned [but not, as noted above, owned by a large national chain] or nongovernment, not-for-profit; the provider of a small number of facilities and services . . . a non-teaching hospital; located in a metropolitan area; in existence for approximately 35 years; not a member of a multi-hospital system; and not the only community hospital in the county in which it was located.

Recent federal policy has encouraged and exacerbated the financial pressures on hospitals already most at risk. The American Hospital Association reports that annual unreimbursed care more than doubled to $5.7 billion between 1980 and 1984 (7). In the face of this pressure, many hospitals are increasingly unable, or unwilling, to care for the medically indigent. Management pressure has increased on emergency room officials to restrict access to Public Aid patients, resulting in well-documented and drastic increases in the "dumping" of patients on already-overburdened public institutions (8, 9).

This consolidation of health capital into concentrated markets and the incessant push toward a for-profit health care industry at the expense of public medicine represents a condition of development and underdevelopment (10). As such it reflects the economic system of capitalism as a whole. As Navarro points out (11, p. 41):

> We cannot understand the maldistribution of resources in the health sector without analyzing the distribution of economic and political power in these societies, i.e., the question of who controls what and whom, or, as it is usually phrased in political economy, who controls the means of production and reproduction?

In the wake of this push toward corporate consolidation, those left behind —the working poor, the unemployed, racial minorities, many elderly women and children—are gradually being denied access to the vital resources needed to participate actively in their own health and the health of their communities. As we will show, the structure of the health care industry, its long history of technology-intensive intervention, and the current trends toward for-profit care with removal of services to those left behind in the wake of the corporate siphoning of public resources, are all of a piece. They are signs and symptoms of the larger illness, the underdevelopment of public resources under corporate development. To quote Navarro again, "the way to break with the underdevelopment of health is to break with the sickness of underdevelopment" (11, p. 33).

Scientific Medicine, Technology, and Corporate Self-Interest

The long history of the alliance between the medical establishment—including medical education, research and development, and the establishment of medical professionals as an elite within society—and the corporate sector has been well-documented (12–14). Seen in this context, it is obviously no accident that the course of medical research in the United States has been largely dictated by an emphasis on disease-focused, individual-based, physician-centered intervention. Social, economic, and environmental origins of disease have been largely ignored by modern biomedicine, despite increasing epidemiological evidence linking disease and illness to poverty, occupation, unemployment, and political powerlessness.

The history of U.S. medicine throughout the twentieth century has been characterized by the joining of spectacular technological advances with a hospital-dominated system to promote both research and the technology it has spurred. By original intent the medical training system has focused upon in-hospital, postgraduate education at university-affiliated (and often corporately endowed) teaching institutions, thus providing a ready labor supply to fill hospital beds. Since the implementation of Hill-Burton in 1946, many of these beds have been constructed with massive federal subsidies, further cementing the alliance between corporate medicine and federal policy.

This alliance has been strengthened through reimbursement mechanisms, as well. The fee-for-service payment system, buttressed strongly by the introduction of Blue Cross and Blue Shield in the late 1930s, was finally solidified by the introduction of Medicare and Medicaid in the mid-1960s. Such a payment structure encouraged dependent care-seeking behaviors and disease-focused, technological interventions propelled by the profit motive (15), as befitted an industry under ever-increasing corporate influence. A rational investigation of more thorough preventive care and more effective, community-based models to meet human health needs, focusing as it necessarily would on social and environmental causes of illness, continued to be downplayed. Such an alternative focus may have given the United States an entirely different urban health care system.

The interconnection of the medical industry with the larger economic system is clear: the emphasis on a "technological fix" to fix human health problems created ready "markets" for an entire array of medical services and products, ranging from hospital equipment and construction, pharmaceutical and medical supplies to consultants, lawyers, financial advisors, and most recently, computer systems and software. Large-scale corporate suppliers quickly realized that the medical industry had several desirable features: a large and available market of people who have traditionally considered health a priority in their lives; access to a ready labor market and a large supply of valuable technology through close associations with medical facilities and schools; and state and federal programs to financially bolster the health care industry (16). With these recommending characteristics, it is no wonder that the health care "market" soon attracted corporate suppliers who established their power and gained a monopoly over a burgeoning range of goods and services for which technological interventions created increasing demand. Not to be ignored is the fact that this medical model of care was the result of findings gathered over years of scientific research conducted largely under corporate sponsorship, either directly or through major universities (14).

A major step in furthering corporate inroads in health care delivery came with the Health Maintenance Organization (HMO) strategy of the Nixon administration. Designed to increase private sector involvement in health care, it did not accomplish the hoped-for results for several reasons: consumer and professional misgivings about HMOs, the mid-70s recession, chaos inflicted on the federal bureaucracy by Watergate and its aftermath, and, ironically, insufficient funding of HMOs because of Nixon administration cutbacks and impoundments. However, propelling forces toward proprietarization were set in place for the investor-owned hospital firms and health maintenance organizations (17).

As health care costs skyrocketed through the 1970s, largely spurred by the upward spiral of new capital investment and the resultant expenditures as more sophisticated equipment and methods became *de rigueur* for hospitals competing for their market share, business purchasers found that employee health benefit costs were cutting into their profit levels. The corporate class, encouraged by its policy organizations' studies and recommendations, expanded its own health-related activities to provide preventive programs for employees and began to muscle health providers and insurers on cost containment. The motivation was stated explicitly: to encourage employees to "enjoy healthy lifestyles while affording the employer the ability to stabilize costs," in the words of one corporate position paper (18, p. 18).

Large business purchasers also sought to influence public policy through lobbying by the US Chamber of Commerce and the Washington Business Group on Health (19) and through formation of local business health care coalitions. An overall thrust began toward health care as an investment in human capital, rather than as a human need for everyone in society. Worker productivity, reduced absenteeism, higher morale, and lower health benefit outlays were seen as advantageous to labor and management alike since, as another corporate policy paper put it, "they are footing much of the bill" (20, p. 1).

More insidious has been the Reagan administration emphasis on "marketplace competition" and its resultant pressure on all providers, including private "not-for-profit" hospitals that formerly shared community responsibility for caring for the indigent, to ". . . either get out of the starting block first or do a better job than the pioneers and end up dominating the market . . ," as recommended by *Modern Healthcare* (21, p. 2). To do this, the hospital industry has been pressured by third party payers, HMOs, and local business coalitions to reduce excess bed capacity and length of stay, amidst a shrinking hospital sector resulting from federal reimbursement cuts and the adoption of Medicare's diagnostic-related groups (DRGs). Avoiding the estimated 35–40 million Americans without health insurance or other means to contribute to hospital profits has become in some cases an organizational survival strategy.

The effect of growing corporatization of health care goes far beyond strategies to affect financial security. An ever-growing fixation on a bottom-line approach can be seen throughout the literature in exhortations to find, as *Hospitals*, the journal of the American Hospital Association, recommended as far back as 1978, "a method for capacity reduction that gives priority to corporate consolidations and unilateral closure of entire hospitals which is . . . likely to result in the greatest cost savings" (22, p. 63). Tinged with fear of financial disaster and a preoccupation with "trying to capture as much of the health care market as possible" (20, p. 2), hospital strategies have evolved that perceive even the "legitimate concerns and interests" of those fearing the repercussions of closure as "obstacles to effective action" to be "addressed and resolved from a balanced perspective" (22, p. 66). This "balance" between human need and economic interest may be ultimately defined, of course, by local business coalition participants in the debate.

In several cities, entire neighborhood areas are losing most or all of their hospital services (23, 24). This has resulted in diminution or complete elimination of emergency and outpatient services and a loss of economic enterprises "that employ a large number of people that contribute to the economic well-being of their communities . . . and the quality of life in the community" (22, p. 66). Thus, patients are denied access, health worker jobs are lost, and neighborhoods disintegrate even further.

The relationship between this community deterioration and the further withdrawal of health services is a dialectical one. Since the mid-1970s, data have shown a growing phenomenon of economic crisis and hospital closure among institutions serving the poor and minority populations of major US cities (25). Obscured as these figures have been in analyses of the alleged "health" of the industry, they nonetheless paint a very different picture when viewed in the light of the historical perspective given here. They must also be examined along with the trends they portend—trends toward an increasing stratification between the availability of health care for the affluent and the dismantling of the delivery system that has traditionally served the underserved segments of the population.

Attention must also be given to the overall phenomenon of increased disinvestment in public goods as a necessity of the current economic crisis, both in the United States and abroad. The global move toward privatization, in health care as in other services, is characteristic of an overall historic direction to remove many state-guaranteed or provided services from the general population. This contextual development has given rise to the emerging multi-tiered health care system in the United States. The system is thus an outcome of larger historical processes which, we maintain, result from increasing corporate power and economic consolidation. It signifies an accompanying decrease in the provision of health, human services, and economic support to "unproductive" segments of the population and to their communities.

Privatization and Capitalism: Let the Buyer Be Well

As we have seen, corporatization and proprietarization trends in health care, and the submission to corporate class restructuring, did not begin with the current economic crisis. Nor did they originate the commodification of health needs to be purchased by those who have the means to afford care for the benefit of those who sell it. However, it is clear that closures of urban hospitals and the present restructuring of the health sector are part of a larger move toward removal of public goods and services from certain population segments: the "unproductive" poor working class, aged, and disabled.

Placed in the context of the late twentieth-century capitalist development, this dismantling of health care institutions to exclude the "unproductive" population comes at a time when there is a rerouting throughout the international economic order of substantial amounts of formerly public monies into private accumulation, in an effort to shore up sagging profit levels. Navarro outlines the situation confronting the major industrial countries (26, p. 108):

(1) Extremely high levels of unemployment; (2) unprecedented levels of inflation; (3) an economic slump [indicated by continual declines in the GNP of the major Organization for Economic Cooperation and Development (OECD) countries during the past year and a half]; (4) a dramatic decline . . . of world trade with substantial balance of payments deficits in most OECD countries; and (5) an alarming growth of public debt in most of the western core states.

Navarro goes on to analyze this crisis as being largely precipitated by strengthening working-class movements in Western capitalist nations: the challenge of newer economic powers ranging from West Germany and Japan to Taiwan, Korea, and Brazil, among others; the emergence of anti-imperialist and anti-colonialist movements in peripheral countries, which make it more difficult for continued exploitation there; and the rise, through greater areas of the world, of socialist forces offering alternatives to world capitalism (26, p. 109). These factors have all precipitated serious curtailment of public spending to cut collective consumption throughout the United States, the United Kingdom, West Germany, and France.

More specifically, in the United States we have seen a dramatic drive to privatize a wide range of formerly public goods. The criminal justice system shows signs of an incipient corporate encroachment: Corrections Corp., a for-profit prison management firm, cofounded by Kentucky Fried Chicken mogul Jack Massey (who was also instrumental in beginning Hospital Corporation of America), is being considered by the Tennessee legislature as manager for that state's penal system (27). Likewise, corporate inroads on public education (28) and both the storage and dissemination of a wide range of information and knowledge (29) are being noted. *The Nation* has reported that corporate predictions for the growth of the information industry show as much as 90 percent of all communications facilities in the United States under the control of 15 large companies by 1995 (29, p. 710).

This prediction is strikingly similar to some that have been made about the consolidation of health care. Ellwood has estimated that by the mid-1990s "there will be ten giant national firms providing 50 percent of the medical care in this country" (30, p. 1). In 1985, four companies—Hospital Corporation of America, American Medical International, Humana, and National Medical Enterprises—owned or managed 12 percent of all U.S. hospitals (30).

In recent years, this unlimited expansion has slowed somewhat. Pressures brought on by overenthusiastic corporate expansion have forced the corporate giants to retrench, slow down their acquisition schemes, and slough off some of their less profitable hospitals. Overall profits fell 47.1 percent between 1985 and 1986 (31), and by a far smaller 4.8 percent between 1986 and 1987 (32).

However, such strategies as diversification into ambulatory and long-term care continue to reap enormous benefits for large-scale health entrepreneurs. Profits for corporate chains which cleared $105 million in 1987, Humana ($192 million) and NME ($81 million) continue at a healthy pace (33). More significantly, the success of corporate medicine has hastened the adoption, throughout the health care system, of a business approach toward the production and distribution of what was formerly considered a public good. This process of corporatization has transformed the nature of U.S. health care delivery in the late twentieth century, and is itself a part of a larger effort on the part of the corporate class to divert formerly public resources into profit-making enterprises.

Hospital Failure and the Disinvestment in the Public Goods

The stark contrast between recent corporate growth and the underdevelopment of public sector health care for the uninsured and poor has already been noted. Especially revealing are studies by McLafferty in New York City, which show a strong positive correlation between closure and the percentage of minority population in a hospital's service area, especially for voluntary and municipal hospitals (25). Proprietary hospitals were found less vulnerable to neighborhood change and socioethnic composition because many serve populations primarily from areas outside their specific neighborhoods, do not provide outpatient or emergency care for the uninsured, and draw most of their patients from physician referrals, which do not necessarily reflect the immediate area's demographic makeup (25). It should be noted here that proprietary hospitals in McLafferty's study were not owned or managed by large corporate chains but rather by smaller, local concerns. It is possible to expect that this contrast between proprietary and the public and voluntary institutions will become even greater as large-scale proprietarization takes place and local hospitals become managed by investor-owned firms with little or no local involvement. Thus, the increasingly corporate approach toward bottom-line business portends an exacerbation of urban hospital closures.

Numerous other studies and surveys have identified additional causes and predisposing factors that put hospitals at high risk of closure. A survey in 1982, conducted by the American Hospital Association, found five primary reasons: 1) financial (26.8 percent of all closures), 2) replacement by a new facility (23.4 percent), 3) low occupancy (14.3 percent), 4) an outdated facility (13.4 percent), and 5) lack of medical staff (10 percent) (34). As noted above, hospital size is also an important variable. AHA data and evidence from ongoing investigations show that no closure has occurred among community hospitals with 500 or more beds between 1980 and 1987, while the great majority of closures have been suffered by hospitals with under 199 beds (3, p. 4; 15).

The success of multi-hospital, for-profit chains and the accompanying high-risk status of smaller community "not-for-profit" and public hospitals must be seen in the context of overall social policy redirection (35). The trend toward emphasizing private development over the redistribution of public goods did not begin, as some liberal theorists would have us believe, with the Reagan administration. The number of persons covered by Medicaid, for instance, declined by 1.5 million even before Reagan took office (between 1977 and 1979) (36, p. 13).

Cutbacks under Reagan have surely exacerbated this, creating new barriers to equity in the receipt of health services. Since 1980, with deep federal cuts in social welfare programs, Medicaid rolls have been reduced more drastically than ever before. In 1981, Medicaid cuts were proposed or enacted in 28 states, and 6 dropped Medicaid entirely for families with unemployed parents; in 1982, federal cuts in Aid to Families with Dependent Children (AFDC) resulted in loss of coverage for approximately 661,000 children and 181,000 adults. The end result has been that less than half of the country's poor are now covered by Medicaid. In some states, such as Mississippi and Texas, as many as 75 percent of all indigents are excluded (36, p. 13).

These cuts, along with the Medicare DRG reimbursement strategy, have had a devastating effect on urban hospitals with older facilities, serving large numbers of minority and elderly patients. Such hospitals, already at high risk of closure, often have less capital to invest in high-technology equipment and thus lose out in attracting or maintaining medical specialty services. While private for-profit institutions perceive the uninsured and poor as pariahs, often refusing them care outright, certain voluntary and municipal hospitals have patient loads with increasing numbers of the uninsured and poor. More and more voluntary institutions are following the example of their proprietary counterparts by denying admission to unprofitable patients. A survey of 23 large urban public hospitals in 1983 revealed that they received an average of 13 percent of their revenues from private insurers. Grady Memorial in Atlanta received 8 percent, Chicago's Cook County Hospital received 7 percent, D. C. General only 3 percent, and Bellevue in New York received none (37, p. 594). These figures may even have decreased by now.

Reductions in Medicaid reimbursement have a dual effect; filling public hospital beds with more patients needing intense, complex care, for which the hospital will not be sufficiently reimbursed; and denying hospital care to an ever-growing number who find themselves without the "safety-net" of Medicaid. These people are increasingly refused care by other than public hospitals, which now continue to treat patients only at a financial loss (7–9).

Meanwhile, economically strapped inner city hospitals with patient loads consisting almost entirely of publicly funded patients depend on these revenues to keep operating. As public, as well as private, reimbursement becomes more restricted, these institutions—the most dependent upon recipients of public monies to remain in operation—lose proportionately more patients than other hospitals (24). Thus the clarion cry of competitionists, concerned about revenue loss from unfilled beds, has become elimination of "excess capacity" in for-profit and "not-for-profit" hospitals alike (22), meaning more closures of marginal hospitals, many of which are located in city neighborhoods and small towns of most need.

The growing ranks of the uninsured and underinsured, as well as Medicaid recipients and some Medicare beneficiaries without private supplemental insurance, are facing the erosion of the delivery system upon which they previously relied. Alternative sources of care will continue to become more limited in the absence of a new infusion of funds, such as in a national health program or even state health insurance schemes. Meanwhile, the corporate sector rushes to take advantage of current technological and policy developments to further consolidate its hold on the entire spectrum of health care delivery.

Expansion and Diversification: Surgicenters, Emergicenters, Franchising, and Academic Medicine

As corporate hospital profits grew, the logic of capitalist expansion demanded that these firms move into other related areas of care. Proprietary chain ventures into the insurance business had promise, during the early 1980s, to capture patients from "not-for-profit" institutions. These diversifications sought to engage national contracts from corporate purchasers for their nationwide system operations (38). In practice, this strategy was overambitious (39); the chains have largely withdrawn from the insurance business, although close corporate ties still exist, such as those between Hospital Corporation of America and the Equitable Life Insurance Company (40).

Other ventures have proven far more lucrative. Major investor-owned nursing home companies increased their number of beds by 17.1 percent to 153,655 in 1984. Industry experts predict that by the end of the decade, the majority of chain-operated beds will be controlled by 10 to 20 firms (3, p. 126).

Predictably, corporate inroads into other areas of health care are giving patients fewer places of "last resort" when hospitals will not accept them. The nursing home industry is solidly corporate-owned; the option of transfer for patients whose hospital care is uncovered under Medicare's prospective payment system (PPS) will be less certain for the poor unless Medicare, which does not pay for nursing home services, shifts funds to catastrophic or long-term care coverage. Observers predict a growing push on the part of for-profit nursing homes to attain a greater percentage of privately insured patients, even to the point at which "if payments to nursing homes are cut too much, nursing homes will stop accepting Medicare and Medicaid patients" (41, p. 132).

This problem will likely be exacerbated by increased growth and competitive pressure from the corporate multi-national chains. Observers predict an eventual takeover of nursing home companies by the corporate health giants (41) as "more 'ma and pa' operations . . . [are] falling by the wayside" in the face of drastic increases in beds owned and constructed by corporate multi-institutional chains (42, p. 137–138).

The rapid proliferation of freestanding health care centers and home health care agencies can be seen as symptomatic of the tendency of U.S. medicine to focus on intervention-oriented, disease-specific techniques, instead of a preventive approach to address the larger social and environmental origins of disease. Home health care agencies posted the greatest growth in the non-hospital arena between 1983 and 1984, with an 80 percent increase; other leaders included urgent care centers (a 65 percent jump); primary care centers (27 percent); and durable medical equipment dealers (72 percent) (43, p. 144), furthering the strategic corporate link between technology and medicine. Again, predictions show the freestanding centers, currently suffering some financial difficulties, being used more and more as feeders into already existing corporate-owned hospitals, and eventually also becoming absorbed by the multi-system chains (44).

Corporate control has also extended into the proliferating surgicenter industry, taking advantage of new technology and also of regulations that exempt outpatient care from the payment restrictions of PPS. Although independent centers continue to outnumber chain-owned facilities, corporate-owned surgicenters are growing in strength and number, and conduct a disproportionate share of the procedures performed (45, pp. 148, 150). As in the hospital business, a few powerful entities are becoming dominant. Especially notable is the geographic distribution of the facilities, which appear to be following the migratory pattern of U.S. economic development. The Sun Belt hosts the preponderance of freestanding surgicenters: the largest are Medical Care International (Houston), AMI (Beverly Hills), Surgical Care Affiliates (Nashville), and Alternacare (Los Angeles) (45).

Similar growth has been experienced in other areas of health service. The number of retail store dental centers rose 160 percent between 1980 and 1982, although non-traditional settings still provide a small percentage of dental services nationwide—2 to 5 percent (46, p. 160). The leading retailer in housing dental clinics is Sears, Roebuck & Company, which operated 43 dental facilities in 19 states in 1985 (47, p. 152). This growth is described by industry spokespersons as "explosive" and is expected to continue "as part of a trend affecting all professions" (46, pp. 160, 163). Privatization of health care to for-profit auspices has pervaded all aspects of health care delivery. Ambulance service, for example, was once a local government service. It is now under private contract in over 55 percent of the nation's towns and cities; another 15 areas are reportedly ready to switch. The proprietary trade association, American Ambulance Association in Sacramento, California, represents 800 companies whose revenues total more than $1.5 billion (48).

Eye care, foot care, weight loss, dermatology, and liposuction and other cosmetic surgery are other profitable areas of commodified health needs fit for corporate production, found increasingly in freestanding centers. It should be noted that this for-profit surge in the ambulatory arena maintains its opposite in the underdevelopment of public health clinics and other community-based agencies. Such out-of-hospital ventures to insured persons with disposable incomes siphon away more patients and income, reinforcing a survival mentality among local public and "not-for-profit" institutions. Closures and cutbacks have been spreading through federally-funded community health centers and local public health departments across the nation.

Finally, there is evidence that academic medical centers, the health care venue of last resort for many poor and uninsured patients, are being targeted for corporate takeover. Teaching hospitals, like public hospitals, rely disproportionately on Medicare and Medicaid, and they also bear a great burden of bad debt, giving more "free care" than non-teaching hospitals (49). Several teaching institutions, beginning with the University of Florida Hospital in 1982, have entered into contractual arrangements with corporate chains to construct new facilities or manage existing ones (49). It should be noted that specific details of these contractual arrangements differ from case to case, and not all observers think that this constitutes a major trend at present. However, given the history of corporate involvement in U.S. medical care from the earliest days to the present, these nascent trends bear careful examination. Berliner and Burlage (50) point out that ownership or leasing of a major academic medical facility can be an important component of corporate marketing and public relations strategy. This strengthened emphasis on marketing of health care as a commodity is a vital component of overall corporatization and proprietarization trends, and portends an intensification of corporate strategies to consolidate and seize formerly public goods for corporate profit.

Health as a Commodity: Individualization, Segmentation, and Nonholistic Health

The concept of health as an individual concern, disassociated from the political, economic, social, and environmental contexts in which we live, certainly did not begin with present corporatization trends. Isolated, intervention-oriented, high-technology services for separate conditions in different offices, all for different individual bodies, is a nonholistic approach to the human body and the wellbeing of the person, analogous to the preferred capitalist perspective of society as consisting of isolated individuals, joined together only by market forces and competing self-interests. Such a push toward procedural interventions in a profit-driven health system only serves to increase this fragmentation and limit health achievements.

This individualization of the concepts of health and illness, and the isolation of these concepts from an overall picture of today's social reality, has been further imbedded in our consciousness by the models of medical intervention favoring the profit drives of major corporations. Americans are being told that large-scale, more efficient corporate-run health organizations promise an improved state for health care delivery. Thus, people are distracted from conceptualizing the larger social context in which human health is primarily decided (16).

As inner city and remote rural hospitals close and retrench in the face of massive disinvestment, and as under-supported public hospitals and strapped teaching institutions struggle more with the burden of taking on the public responsibility for health, many communities are left behind with little or no access to care. These people are at high risk for major diseases. They are also the uninsured, lacking sufficient public goods such as housing, education, nutrition, social support, and employment. The emphasis on a "technological fix" to a whole array of political, cultural, and personal conditions leading to chronic degenerative illness further alienates people from their day-to-day health necessities. The class nature of this condition for poor and working people is apparent.

Meanwhile, the more affluent are enticed to consider their health a consumer good to be provided like a movie or a hamburger; entertainment, nourishment, even pre-packaged beauty and social acceptance can be obtained from health spas and fitness centers. Faddish, often pseudo-scientific health products, lines of cosmetics, and diet and vitamin regimens proliferate throughout the private sector. Such methods of individual health groping may do little to alleviate problems created by high-stress, competitive, and overly consumptive lifestyles in which the upper-middle class is compelled to participate to climb the corporate ladder of success. Ultimately it may be shown that the emergent corporate health care model is unhealthy for the more affluent, as its attendant underdevelopment is for the poor. The collective nature of society and the class nature of illness is obscured in the face of the myth that an individual's own behavior is the sole source of his or her illness or well-being.

In summary, for-profit health care in the United States and the resultant corporatization of the "not-for-profit" firms is removing health care from those Americans most in need. The exclusion of this population from necessary services appears to be related to a systematic attempt to curtail public consumption of health and other formerly public resources. The implications of this corporate transformation portend further breakdown of family and community caring networks, which may harm all "consumers" of health care, not only the poor. Seen in the light of current efforts on the part of international capital to shore up profits by diverting public goods into private control, urban slums exist as the United States' domestic Third World. In this perspective, development and underdevelopment are again seen to go hand-in-hand.

N O T E S

1. Johnson, D. E. Multi-unit providers: Survey plots 457 chains' growth. *Modern Healthcare* 14(5): 65–84, 1984.

2. Johnson, D. E. Investor-owned chains continue expansion, 1985 survey shows. *Modern Healthcare* 15(2): 75–90, 1985.

3. Mullner, R., McNeil, D., and Andes, S. National trends in hospital closure 1980–1984. American Hospital Association, Office of Policy Analysis Publication no. 59, pp. 1–32, Chicago, 1985.

4. Mullner, R., Rydman, R., Whiteis, D., and Rich, R. "U.S. Hospital Closures 1980–87: An

Epidemiologic Case Control Study." Center for Health Services Research, University of Illinois School of Public Health, Chicago. Unpublished manuscript, 1988.

5. Rhein, R. W. Hospitals in trouble: Crisis for doctors. *Medical World News* 21: 58–68, 1980.

6. Relman, A. S. The new medical-industrial complex. *New Engl. J. Med.* 303: 963–970, 1980.

7. Reinhold, R. Treating an outbreak of patient dumping in Texas. *New York Times*, May 25, 1980, p. 4.

8. Chicago's private hospitals deny care to the poor. *All-Chicago City News.* July 23, 1983, p. 6.

9. Schiff, R. L., et al. Transfers to a public hospital: A prospective study of 467 patients. *New Engl. J. Med.* 314(9): 552–559, 1986.

10. Dowd, D. F. *The Twisted Dream: Capitalist Development in the United States Since 1776.* Winthrop Publishers, Cambridge, Mass., 1974.

11. Navarro, V. *Medicine Under Capitalism.* Prodist, New York, 1976.

12. Starr, P. *The Social Transformation of American Medicine.* Basic Books, New York, 1982.

13. Brown, E. R. He who pays the piper: Foundations, the medical profession, and medical educational reform. *Int. J. Health Serv.* 10(1): 71–88, 1980.

14. Markowitz, G. E., and Rosen, D. N. Doctors in crisis: A study of the use of medical education reform to establish modern professional elitism in medicine. *Am. Q.* 25(1): 83–107, 1973.

15. Salmon, J. W. The competitive health strategy: Fighting for your health. *Health and Medicine* 1(2): 21–30, 1982.

16. McKinlay, J. B. (ed.). *Issues in the Political Economy of Health Care.* Tavistock Publications, New York, 1984.

17. Salmon, J. W. *Corporate Attempts to Reorganize the American Health Care System.* Doctoral dissertation, Cornell University, 1978 (unpublished).

18. *Highlight of an Effective Employee Benefit Management System.* Position paper, BPI, Inc., Westmont, Ill., 1980.

19. *The Formation of a Medicine and Business Coalition.* American Medical Association, Office of Corporation Liaison, Medical Practice and Professional Relations Group, 1981.

20. *Health Care Horizons '77.* Touche Ross & Co., New York, 1977.

21. John, D. E. Chains integrate health care services into local networks. *Modern Healthcare* 15(12): 2, 1985.

22. Gottlieb, S. R. Reducing excess capacity is a tough but necessary job. *Hospitals* 52: 63–68, 1978.

23. *The Killing of Philadelphia General Hospital.* Health Information and Action Group, Philadelphia, 1976.

24. Sager, A. Why urban voluntary hospitals close. *Health Services Research* 18(3): 450–475, 1983.

25. McLafferty, S. Neighborhood characteristics and hospital closure. *Soc. Sci. and Med.* 16: 1667–1674, 1982.

26. Navarro, V. The crisis of the international capitalist order and its implications on the welfare state. In *Issues in the Political Economy of Health Care*, edited by J. B. McKinlay, Methuen/Tavistock Publications, New York, 1984.

27. Montgomery, J. Corrections Corp. seeks lease to run Tennessee's prisons. *The Wall Street Journal*, September 13, 1985, p. 8.

28. Kraft, S. Corporations enter the classroom: Private companies fill the gap left by dwindling government funding. *Valley Advocate*, Springfield, Mass., January 1, 1986, pp. 1–6.

29. Shiller, H. Information: A shrinking resource. *The Nation*, December 28, 1985/January 4, 1986, pp. 708–710.

30. Hull, J. B. Medical turmoil: Four hospital chains facing lower profits, adopt new strategies. *The Wall Street Journal*, October 10, 1985, p. 1.

31. Bell, C. W. Hospital systems report 47.1% drop in profits last year. *Modern Healthcare* 17(12): 37–90, 1987.

32. Multi-unit providers survey. *Modern Healthcare*, June 3, 1988.

33. *Forbes 500 Annual Directory* 41(9), April 25, 1988.

34. Hernandez, S. R., and Kaluzny, A. D. Hospital closure: A review of current and proposed research. *Health Serv. Res.* 18(3): 419–436, 1983.

35. Weiss, K. Corporate medicine: What's the bottom line for physicians and patients? *New Physician* 9: 1–25, 1982.

36. *Health Care Financing Program Statistics/The Medicare Medicaid Data Book* 13, p. 111. Health Care Financing Administration, 1981.

37. Dallek, G. The loss of hospitals serving the poor. *Health Serv. Res.* 18(3): 593–597, 1983.

38. Koenig, R. Humana earnings increased by 15% in fourth period. *The Wall Street Journal*, October 9, 1985, p. 2.

39. M. D. behavior seen as cause of losses. *American Medical News*, May 1, 1986, p. 2.

40. Kenkel, P. J. Managed-care growth continued in 1987 despite companies' poor operating results. *Modern Healthcare*, June 3, 1988, pp. 20–38.

41. Punch, L. Investor-owned chains lead increase in beds. *Modern Healthcare* 15(2): 126–136, 1985.

42. Punch, L. Chains expand their operations, expecting prospective pay boom. *Modern Healthcare* 14(5): 131–140, 1984.

43. Wallace, C. Ambulatory care facilities multiply. *Modern Healthcare* 15(2): 142–146, 1985.

44. Punch, L. Freestanding units lose money, but that doesn't stunt growth. *Modern Healthcare* 14(5): 150–153, 1984.

45. Henderson, J. Surgery centers double: Consultant. *Modern Healthcare* 15(12): 148–150.

46. Gondela, E. Franchise, retail dental operations record major gains. *Modern Healthcare* 14(5): 160–163, 1984.

47. Gondela, E. More clinics opening, but growth rate falls. *Modern Healthcare* 15(12): 152–154, 1985.

48. Hollie, P. G. Ambulances go private. *New York Times*, May 25, 1986, Section 3, p. 1.

49. Reading, A. Involvement of proprietary chains in academic health centers. *New Engl. J. Med.* 313(3): 194–197, 1985.

50. Berliner, H. S., and Burlage, R. K. Proprietary hospital chains and academic medical centers. *Int. J. Health Serv.* 17(1): 27–45, 1987.

CORPORATIZATION AND THE SOCIAL TRANSFORMATION OF DOCTORING

John B. McKinlay and John D. Stoeckle

We are witnessing a transformation of the health care systems of developed countries that is without parallel in modern times (1, 2). This dramatic change has implications for patients and, without exception, affects the entire division of labor in health care. What are some of these changes and how are they manifesting themselves with respect to doctoring?

The Changes

Over the last few years especially, many multi-national corporations, with highly diverse activities, have become involved in all facets of the generally profitable business of medical care from medical manufacturing and the ownership of treatment institutions to the financing as purchase of services in PPOs and HMOs (3, 4). Conglomerates like General Electric, AT&T, and IBM, among many others, now have large medical manufacturing enterprises within their corporate divisions. Aerospace companies are involved in everything from computerized medical information systems to life support systems. Even tobacco companies and transportation enterprises have moved into the medical care arena. In addition to this industrial or manufacturing capital, even larger financial capital institutions (e.g., commercial banks, life insurance companies, mutual and pension funds and diversified financial organizations) are also stepping up their involvement in medical care and experiencing phenomenal success (5, 6).

Besides corporate investments in health care, corporate mergers of treatment organizations and industrial corporations are also taking place. Privately owned hospital chains, controlled by larger corporations, evidence continuing rapid growth. Much of this growth comes from buying up local, municipal and voluntary community hospitals, many of which were going under as a result of cutbacks in government programs and regulations on hospital use and payment. By 1990, about 30 percent of general hospital beds will be managed by investor hospital chains (5, 7–9). Because the purpose of an investor owned organization is to make money, there is understandable concern over the willingness of such organizations to provide care to the 35 million people who lack adequate insurance coverage and who are not eligible for public programs (10–15).

Responses

Regulations

Confronted with an ever deepening fiscal crisis, the state continues to cast around for regulatory solutions—one of the latest of which is DRGs for Medicare patients which reimburse hospitals by diagnosis with rates determined by government. If the actual cost of treatment is less than the allowable payment, then the hospital makes a profit; if treatment costs are more, then the hospital faces a loss, even bankruptcy, especially since an average of 40 percent of hospital revenues come from Medicare patients. This probably ineffective measure follows many well-documented policy failures (e.g., PSROs) and its consequences for the health professions are profound. These regulatory efforts, corporate mergers, investor-owned hospital chains, federally mandated cost containment measures, among many other changes, are transforming the shape, content and even the moral basis of health care (16–19). How are these institutional changes affecting the everyday work of the doctor?

New Management

By all accounts, hospitals are being managed by a new breed of physician administrators (20–22) whom Alford aptly terms "corporate rationalizers" (23). While some have medical qualifications, most are trained in the field of hospital administration, which emphasizes, among other things, rationalization, productivity, and cost efficiency. Doctors used to occupy a privileged position at the top of the medical hierarchy. Displaced by administrators, doctors have slipped down to the position of middle management where their prerogatives are also challenged or encroached upon by other health workers. Clearly, managerial imperatives often compete or conflict with physicians' usual mode of practice. Increasingly, it seems, administrators, while permitting medical staff to retain ever narrower control of technical aspects of care, are organizing the necessary coordination for collaborative work, the work schedules of staff, the recruitment of patients to the practice, the contacts with third party purchasers and determining the fiscal rewards.

Some argue that many administrators are medically qualified, so they act so as to protect the traditional professional prerogatives. This view confuses the usual distinction between status and role. As many hospital and HMO doctors will attest, when a physician is a full-time administrator, he is understandably concerned to protect the bottom line, not the prerogatives of the profession. When these interests diverge, as they increasingly must, it becomes clear where the physician/administrator's divided loyalty really resides. One recent survey of doctors shows that a majority do not believe that their medical directors represent the interests of the medical staff. As a result, the AMA has concluded that "as hospital employees . . . medical directors may align their loyalty more with hospitals than with medical staff interests" (24). To counteract these trends, it has been seriously suggested that "physicians should be trained in organization theory . . . to act as liaisons among all those with an interest in medicine, including patients, health care providers, insurers, politicians, economists, and administrators.''

Specialization-Deskilling

Specialization in medicine, while deepening knowledge in a particular area, is also circumscribing the work that doctors may legitimately perform. Specialization can—with task delegation—reduce hospitals' dependence on its highly trained medical staff. Other health workers (e.g., Physician Assistants and Nurse Practitioners) with less training, more narrowly skilled, and obviously cheaper can be hired. Doctors, while believing that specialization is invariably a good thing, are being ''deskilled''—a term employed by Braverman to describe the transfer of skills from highly trained personnel to more narrowly qualified specialists (25). Many new health occupations (PAs, NPs, CNs) have emerged over the last several decades to assume some of the work which doctors used to perform. Not only is work deskilled but it is increasingly conducted without M.D.s control as other professional groups and workers seek their own autonomy. These processes receive support from administrators constantly searching for cheaper labor, quite apart from the controlled trials which revealed that ''allied health professionals'' can, in many circumstances, do the same work just as effectively and efficiently for those patients who must use them. Preference for the term ''allied health professional'' rather than ''physician extender'' or ''physician assistant'' reflects the promotion of this occupational division of labor.

Just over a decade ago, Victor Fuchs (26) viewed the physician as ''captain of the team.'' Around that time, doctors (usually males) were the unquestioned masters and other health workers (usually female), especially nurses, worked ''under the doctor'' to carry out his orders. That subordination is disappearing. Nowadays, physicians are required to work alongside other professionals on the ''health care team.'' The ideology of *team work* is a leveler in the hierarchical division of healthcare labor. Other health workers—for example, physiotherapists, pharmacists, medical social workers, inhalation therapists, podiatrists, and even nurses in general—may have more knowledge of specific fields than physicians, who are increasingly required to defer to other workers, now providing some of the technical and humane tasks of doctoring. While some M.D.s continue to resist these trends, and have publicly complained about ''the progressive exclusion of doctors from nursing affairs'' (27–29); still others have accommodated to the changing scene captured in the title of a recent article: ''At This Hospital, the 'Captain of the Ship' is Dead'' (27).

Commentators have identified the ''gatekeeping'' function performed by doctors (to determine and legitimate access to generally scarce resources: e.g., certain medications and highly specialized personnel) as a special characteristic that distinguishes them from other health occupations and reinforces their central position in the division of labor. But even this gatekeeping function appears to be changing. For example, in some 21 states, nurses are now able to prescribe a wide range of medications. Despite opposition from doctors, pharmacists in Florida may now prescribe drugs for many minor ailments (30). Physician organization and resistance has been unable to curtail the introduction and growth of midwifery in some areas of the country.

Specialization has also weakened the political position of doctors because they now tend to affiliate only with disparate professional societies relevant to their own field of practice, rather than the generic and increasingly distant AMA. AMA membership continues to decline annually and there are estimates that less than half of all doctors now belong. Fragmentation of the profession through sub-specialty societies severely curtails the influence of the AMA representing all the profession. One recalls the power of the AMA only a decade ago when it successfully delayed and then shaped Medicare and Medicaid legislation. In contrast, the AMA is now losing significant battles in the courts over issues which affect the position and status of doctors. Antitrust rulings (permitting doctors to advertise), and decisions prohibiting any charges over and above the federally determined DRG rates, are major examples. In Chicago this year (1987) a federal judge issued an injunction ordering the AMA to immediately end its professional boycott of chiropractors on the grounds that it violated the Sherman Act with "systematic, long-term wrongdoing and the longer-term intent to destroy a licensed profession" (31). Responding to recent proposals to introduce a flat, all inclusive payment for doctors' services associated with each type of hospital case, Dr. Coury (Chairman of the AMA's Board of Trustees) claims doctors are becoming "indentured servants of the government" (32).

Doctor Oversupply

The growing oversupply of doctors in developed countries reinforces these trends in medical work and professional power by intensifying intraprofessional competition and devaluing their position in the job market. During the 1970s, the supply of physicians increased 36 percent, while the population grew only 8 percent. U.S. medical schools continue to pump 17,000 physicians into the system annually. One report projected an oversupply of 70,000 physicians in the United States by 1990 and an excess of 150,000 by 2000. The ratio of doctors to the general population is expected to reach one in 300 by 1990 (33, 34). This level of intensity, obviously much higher in the Northeast and West Coast, renders fee for service solo practice economically less feasible. Again, the changes that are occurring are captured in the title of a recent article "Doctor, the Patient Will See You Now" (33). There are reliable reports that doctors are unemployed in a number of countries and increasingly underemployed in quite a few others (34). Doctors have apparently received unemployment payments in Scandinavian countries, Canada and Australia. Official recognition of physician oversupply exists in Belgium, which is restricting specialty training, and the Netherlands, which is reducing both medical school intake and specialty training (35).

The oversupply of doctors is thought to be a major reason for the recent shift to a salaried medical staff, which has been so dramatic as to be termed "the salary revolution" (36). There are estimates that over a half of all U.S. doctors are now in salaried arrangements, either part- or full-time (36). By the year 2000 it is projected that the proportion of doctors in solo or independent fee for service practice will have declined to about one quarter (36–40). Young medical graduates are especially affected by the trends described and often prepared to accept a limited job (and role) for a guaranteed fixed income (without heavy initial investment in setting up a practice and obtaining liability protection from astronomical malpractice insurance premiums) with the promise of certain perks (regular hours, paid vacation, retirement plan, etc.). The division of labor in health care is increasingly stratified by age and gender, with females and younger doctors disproportionately in salaried positions. Forty-seven percent of physicians under thirty-six years of age were salaried in 1985, while only 19.4 percent of their colleagues over 55 were employees. The percentage increase for this youngest category of physicians between 1983 and 1985 was significantly larger than for the other age groups, increasing 5.3 percentage points. Female physicians were nearly twice as likely to be employees as their male colleagues. Only 23.5 percent of males were salaried in 1985 versus 45.5 percent of females. Again, the percentage increase for female employee physicians was larger than for males over the years 1983–85. While self-employed physicians consistently earned nearly $38,000 more per year than salaried physicians ($118,600 versus $80,400 respectively for 1985), self-employed doctors worked an average of one and a half weeks more in 1985 (47.4 weeks versus 45.9), spent an average of six more hours per week on patient care activities (52.6 hours per week versus 46.6) and saw an average of 19 more patients per week (122.6 visits per week versus 103.9) (42). One survey of over 2,000 hospitals found that the trend to a salaried medical staff was most marked in areas with high ratios of doctors to population. Physician oversupply and their associated economic vulnerability may force doctors to accept lower incomes and the increasingly alienating work conditions practicing in HMOs, clinics and hospitals of "today's corporate health factors," just as nineteenth century craftsmen accepted the factory floor forced on them by their move to the industrial plant (43).

Anecdotal reports from older doctors indicate that medicine today is not like "the good old days" (44). The malpractice crisis, DRGs, the likelihood of fixed fees, and shrinking incomes (projected at a 30 percent decline over the next decade) all combine to remove whatever "fun" there was in medical practice. Some wonder aloud whether they would choose medicine if, with the benefit of hindsight, they had to do it all over again (45). While doctors used to want their children to follow in their footsteps, many report that they would not recommend medicine today. Recent graduates have doubts of other kinds. They fear their debts will force them into specialties on the basis of anticipated earnings, rather than intrinsic interest (46). College advisors may dissuade the highly talented students they counsel from choosing medicine because its job market looks so bleak. The number of medical school applicants dropped 4.8 percent in 1986 and is expected to decline 9 percent more in 1987, according to the AMA and the Association of American Medical Colleges. First-time enrollments in medical schools in 1986 were down for the fifth straight year. Although it is difficult to identify a single factor responsible for these declines, it appears students fear a glutted market, concern over an average debt of $33,499 (117.2 percent increase since 1980), alarm over soaring malpractice insurance rates and a perception that the practice of medicine is becoming less individualistic, with more government regulation and more doctors working in "managed care" systems that have corporate-like structures (47). These professional concerns are expressed in the urban academic medical centers (where physicians with international reputations presumably enjoy a privileged status) as well as local community hospitals throughout the country.

Unionization—A Harbinger of a Trend?

There are reports from across the United States that physicians are rebelling against the continuing challenges to their authority and attempts to cut their incomes by Health Maintenance Organizations (HMOs) and other corporate-like means of organizing the profitable production of medical care (34, 48, 49). One recent manifestation of doctors' frustration with the profound changes already described is increased interest in unionization. Several unions have been or are being formed in different areas of the country to represent doctors working as full-time employees of state and local government, and in HMOs. The largest is the Union of American Physicians and Dentists, based in Oakland, California, with a membership of around 43,000 in 17 states. Some unions (e.g., the Group Health Association in Washington, D.C.) have even staged strikes. The HMO organizational structure and that of other similar prepaid health-care plans appear to generate disgruntlement among its salaried physician employees who were socialized to expect considerably more status and professional autonomy than the HMO permits. There are now 625 of these medical factories in the United States serving some 25.8 million people, up from 260 with 9.1 million subscribers in 1980. There are legal obstacles to physician unionization because antitrust laws prohibit independent businessmen, including doctors in private practice, from organizing to fix prices. Recognizing this, Minnesota Medical Society recently passed a resolution asking the AMA to seek government permission to form a union. National attention has recently focused on a struggle in Minneapolis where salaried physician employees of the Physician's Health Plan of Minnesota (the largest HMO in the state) are organizing to unionize (50). According to Dr. Paul Ellwood (a leading health services researcher who first coined the term "health maintenance organization") the Minneapolis dispute portends "a critical turning point. . . . There are very few places where it's gone as far as it has here, but it's moving in that general direction everywhere" (50).

For understandable reasons, many physicians and the lay public recoil at the thought of and disparage unionized doctors. Only a decade ago unionization among physicians was unthinkable, the movement commonly considered to be working class. Aaron Nathensen, an ophthalmologist with the Minneapolis Physician's Health Plan, expresses a widely held view as follows: "When I entered the practice 15 years ago, unionization was thought of as totally unprofessional, unmedical and unAmerican. But there's a growing feeling that we're losing control—losing control of patients, losing control of the health industry" (50).

Theories of Change

Some of the forces transforming medical care and the work of doctors have been described. How does one *explain* what is occurring? *Why* is it happening?

Probably the best account of the stage by stage transformation of the labor process under capitalism is provided by Karl Marx. Although not concerned with health care (51) his thesis is applicable. During the precapitalist period, small-scale independent craftsmen (solo practitioners) operated domestic workshops, sold their products on the free market, and controlled the production of goods. Over time, capitalists steered many of these skilled workers into their factories (hospitals) where they were able to continue traditional crafts semiautonomously in exchange for wages. Eventually, the owners of production (investors) began to rationalize the production process in their factories by encouraging specialization, allocating certain tasks to cheaper workers, and enlisting managers to coordinate the increasingly complex division of labor which developed. Rationalization was completed during the final stage when production was largely performed by engineering systems and machines, with the assistance of unskilled human machine minders (52). The worker's autonomy and control over work and the workplace diminished, while the rate of exploitation increased with each successive stage in the transformation of production.

Weber's account of the same process (bureaucratization) is strikingly similar (53). According to Weber, bureaucracy is characterized by: 1) a hierarchical organization, 2) a strict chain of command from top to bottom; 3) an elaborate division of labor; 4) assigning specialized tasks to qualified individuals; 5) detailed rules and regulations governing work; 6) personnel are hired based on competence, specialized training and qualifications (as opposed to family ties, political power, or tradition); 7) a life-time career from officials is expected (54). He described how workers were increasingly "separated from ownership of the means of production or administration." Bureaucratic workers became specialists performing circumscribed duties within a hierarchical structure subject to the authority of superiors and to established rules and procedures. According to Weber, bureaucratic employees are "subject to strict and systematic discipline and control in the conduct of the office" they occupy. For Weber, the bureaucratic form of work was present not only in the area of manufacturing but also in churches, schools, and government organizations. It is noteworthy that he also included hospitals: ". . . this type of bureaucracy is found in private clinics, as well as in endowed hospitals or the hospitals maintained by religious orders." While Weber viewed bureaucracy as the most rational and efficient mode of organizing work, he also saw the accompanying degradation of working life as inevitable (27, 54).

It is argued that the process outlined by Marx and Weber with respect to a different group of workers, during a different historical era, is directly applicable to the changing situation of doctors today, now that the "industrial revolution has finally caught up with medicine" (George Rosen). Whereas, generally speaking, most other workers have been quickly and easily corporatized, physicians have been able to postpone or minimize this process in their own case. Now, primarily as a result of the bureaucratization that has been forced on medical practice, physicians are being severely reduced in function and their formally self-interested activities subordinated to the requirements of the highly profitable production of medical care.

While Marx offers a most complete and theoretically well-grounded explanation of the social transformation of work (including doctoring), other commentators have described threats to professional autonomy. C. Wright Mills (55) warned of a "managerial demiurge" suffusing all the professions, including doctoring. In 1951, he wrote:

> Most professionals are now salaried employees; much professional work has become divided and standardized and fitted into the new hierarchical organizations of educated skill and service; intensive and narrow specialization has replaced self cultivation and wide knowledge; assistants and sub-professionals perform routine, although often intricate, tasks, while successful professional men become more and more the managerial type. So decisive have such shifts been, in some areas, that it is as if rationality itself had been expropriated from the individual and been located as a new form of brain power in the ingenuous bureaucracy itself (55, p. 112).

Describing "The Physicians' Changing Hospital Role" over 20 years ago, Wilson (56) saw the growth of specialization in medicine producing diminished perceptions of doctors' expertise and a routinization of charisma. This theme was developed by Myerhoff and Larson (57) when they argued that doctors were losing their charisma and becoming culture heroes: a major difference between the charismatic and culture hero is that the former is a force for social change, while the latter is the embodiment of tradition. The culture hero appears to serve as an agent of social control (58).

During the 1970s, Haug (59, 60) detected a trend towards deprofessionalization which had its origin in the changing relations between professionals and consumers. The unquestioned trust which a client has in a professional is often thought to distinguish professionals from other "ordinary" workers. According to Hughes (61) relations with professionals are embodied in the motto *credat emptor*, "let the taker believe in us," rather than *caveat emptor*, "let the buyer beware," which exists in most other areas of commerce. According to Haug, (59, 60) consumers' unquestioning trust in professionals is diminishing as the knowledge gap between the medical profession and the consumer diminishes. She regarded the modern consumer as better educated and more likely to comprehend medical subjects, which results in a narrowing of the knowledge gap. She also viewed the computerization of knowledge as making it more accessible to all. New specialized occupations have arisen around new bodies of knowledge and skills that physicians themselves are, understandably, no longer competent to employ. These and related trends have, in her view, deprofessionalized medicine, a consequence of which is to reduce physicians to mere specialists dependent on rational, well-informed consumers who approach their service with the same skepticism (caveat emptor) that they bring to other commodity purchases. As a result of deprofessionalization, doctors are becoming just another health occupation.

Margarli Larson (62) provides a penetrating systematic description of the progressive loss of autonomy and control over work among professionals. She distinguishes three areas in which the loss of autonomy (or alienation) is occurring: economic, organizational, and technical. According to her formulation, doctors experience *economic* alienation when they become salaried employees of hospitals or when, in common with most other workers, they must place hospital interests above their own. *Organizational* alienation occurs when cost-conscious hospital administrators, or managers, create systems and procedures to increase doctors' productivity and efficiency, and coordinate their work with others in the division of medical labor. *Technical* alienation refers to the process of curtailing or removing the actual decisions involved in diagnosing and treating patients. From what has been described above, it appears that doctors are experiencing loss of autonomy on all three of these dimensions, albeit at different rates depending on where they work and what specialty they practice.

Is the Profession Still Dominant?

During the late 1960s, Freidson developed a view of professionalism (articulated in two influential books published in 1970, *Profession of Medicine* and *Professional Dominance*) which asserted that the medical profession (doctors) dominated other health care occupations in the division of labor. Nearly two decades after his original work and while conceding profound organizational changes and a transitional status (63, 64), he still views the medical profession as:

> Dominant in a division of labor in which other occupations were obligated to work under the supervision of physicians and take orders from, with its exclusive license to practice medicine, prescribe controlled drugs, admit patients to hospitals, and perform other critical gatekeeping functions, the medical profession is portrayed as having a monopoly over the provision of health services (64, p. 13).

Attention is focused here on Freidson's view of professional dominance solely because it remains the dominant view of professionalism. However, it is increasingly subject to challenge (1, 48, 52, 62, 65, 66). In one of his more recent contributions (64), Freidson tests the adequacy of alternative explanations of the changing position of doctors (especially deprofessionalization and proletarianization) against the "standard" of his own view of professional dominance.

While perhaps an adequate description of the situation of doctors back in the 1960s, much water has passed under the bridge since that time. Indeed, Freidson seems to overlook the period that has elapsed since his original important contributions. Defending his position in 1985 (64), he refers to the position that he "asserted not long ago" (1970). A great deal of change has occurred over the intervening 15 years however, some of which has been described above. There is nothing wrong with modifying, refining or evolving a position on the basis of intervening change, or new data and experience (67).

Quite apart from the fact that it is now necessarily somewhat dated, Freidson's description and approach has additional limitations:

1. Grounded in the social constructionist perspective (68), it *raises more questions than it is able to answer*. Its ability to accommodate the macrostructural changes that have occurred in health care has been described elsewhere (48).

2. The professional dominance perspective is a *description of an earlier state of affairs*—a snapshot of the position of doctors back in the 1960s—*not an explanation or theory* which sustains close scrutiny today. Practicing physicians familiar with Freidson's work view it as a fairly accurate account of an earlier and much preferred golden age (69). Freidson bases his work in the past (1960's) and attempts to explain the present. The thesis of corporatization, or proletarianization, looks towards the future and argues, on the basis of what is presently occurring and has already occurred in other sectors of the economy, that this is also likely to happen to doctors in the future.

3. Freidson (64, 70) bemoans the absence of evidence to support the rival theories of deprofessionalization and proletarianization. One should note that apart from the observational work reported in *Doctoring Together* (1975), Freidson has *never gathered or reported primary data to support his own viewpoint* (only secondary sources are ever used). Moreover, it is extraordinarily difficult to obtain information from, say, the AMA, or to gain access to medical institutions. The evidence for professional dominance is no stronger, or weaker, than that used to advance the rival theories of deprofessionalization and proletarianization. The point is we are all groping under the same light, which is often kept deliberately dim. Moreover, it is very difficult, if not inappropriate, to apply traditional positivistic techniques to the study of change of the order captured by the notion of proletarianization. Imagine asking yeoman farmers and artisans in Elizabethan England, through questionnaires and interviews, if they appreciated the long-term consequences of the enclosure movement! Quite the same limitation is present in the modern study of the historically changing relation of doctors to the means of medical care production.

4. Freidson (64) has often depicted competing theorists as political visionaries—their work being "too grand and sweeping to have much more than a rhetorical and possibly political value"—". . . proletarianization is not a concept as much as a slogan," and "it would be a mistake to regard such literature (proletarianization) as evidence of actual change instead of desire for change" (64). One should note that concern over the changing situation of doctors and the worrisome direction of health care is also coming from conservative circles—from Harry Schwarz, in the *New York Times* (30), who writes that, "MDs are getting a raw deal" to Arnold Relman, editor of *The New England Journal of Medicine* (18), who warns of the danger of the medical industrial complex—a work that bears a resemblance to earlier work on the medical industrial complex in *Monthly Review* in 1978 (71).

Toward Proletarianization

The healthy debate over the changing position of doctors within the rapidly changing health care system is likely to continue for some time. Along with others in Britain (72, 73), Australia (74), Canada (52, 64, 72, 75, 76), Scandinavia (77), and the U.S. (24, 33, 43, 66, 76) we have elaborated one viewpoint (proletarianization), and have presented as much data as can be easily mustered. Although Freidson views it as "equivocation," several clarifying caveats have been deliberately introduced in an attempt to minimize misunderstandings associated with the notion of proletarianization. The theory of proletarianization seeks to explain *the process by which an occupational category is divested of control over certain prerogatives relating to the location, content, and essentiality of its task activities, thereby subordinating it to the broader requirements of production under advanced capitalism.* That is admittedly and necessarily a general definition. However, in order to provide operational specificity, and to facilitate the collection of the evidence which everyone desires, seven specific professional prerogatives which are lost or curtailed through the process of proletarianization are identified as follows: 1) *The criteria for entrance* (e.g., the credentialing system and membership requirements; 2) *The content of training* (e.g., the scope and content of the medical curriculum); 3) *Autonomy regarding the terms and content of work* (e.g., the ways in which what must be done is accomplished); 4) *The objects of labor* (e.g., commodities produced or the clients served); 5) *The tools of labor* (e.g., machinery, biotechnology, chemical apparatus); 6) *The means of labor* (e.g., hospital buildings, clinic facilities, lab services); and 7) *The amount and rate of remuneration for labor* (e.g., wage and salary levels, fee schedules) (34).

Which of these prerogatives is lost, or curtailed, through proletarianization, is associated with the relative power of any occupation and is a function of the degree of unity or cohesiveness within an occupational group, the stage of production associated with the sector in which the occupation is located, and the extent to which the tasks of the occupation can be technologized.

Table 1 lists these important prerogatives and contrasts the situation in the United States of small-scale fee-for-service doctors in the past (say, around the turn of the twentieth century) with the situation of bureaucratically employed doctors today. Every single prerogative listed has changed, many occurring over the last decade. The net effect of the erosion of these prerogatives is the reduction of the members of a professional group to some common level in the service of the broader interests of capital accumulation. One of the difficulties for the proponents of proletarianization is that the process is very difficult to recognize. Indeed, it is occurring at such a level and so slowly in some cases that it may only be amenable to historical analysis some time in the future. It would be a mistake to view this as a cop-out.

With regard to doctors who are increasingly subject to it, the process is masked both by their false consciousness concerning the significance of their everyday activities and also by an elitist conception of their role, so that even if recognized, doctors are quite reluctant to admit it.

While experiencing, on a daily basis, what has been described above, many physicians do not comprehend the historical magnitude of the process we have been describing. To capture the level of our analysis of what is occurring, it may be useful to parallel it with early industrial developments in cottage industry based Elizabethan England or, closer to home, changes in American agriculture—in both of which situations industrialization and corporatization slowly shunted aside small-scale production, eroding the market situation of independent workers. A major effect of the enclosure movement in England was to slowly drive many small growers and grazers off the land into the cities where factories were developing and where they would become wage earners. These factories, in turn, eventually penetrated the countryside, destroying the yeoman-based agriculture and cottage industry in much the same way that large-scale agricultural interests in the United States have been squeezing out small farmers.

It is our argument then that the industrial revolution has fully caught up with medicine. We are beginning to see the same phenomena in this sphere of work. From the preceding description, it is clear that we view the theory of proletarianization as a useful explanation of a process under development, *not* a state that has been or is just about to be achieved. The process described will most likely continue for a considerable period of time. An earlier article, on the social transformation of doctoring, was entitled, "Toward the Proletarianization of Physicians," not "The Proletarianized Physician" (34). The term "proletarianization" denoted a *process*. Use of the preposition "toward" was intended to indicate that the process was still continuing. Roemer (78) has recently offered a critique of the notion of proletarianization. He raises serious points and no doubt the thesis could benefit from some fine tuning (79). No one can have the final word on this subject, especially when we are attempting to explain a trend of which we are in the midst. Only time will tell who is most correct in assessing the historical trends discussed. Perhaps, this work should be put aside until the turn of the century. If what occurs in the next 17 years is anything like the dramatic transformation we have witnessed over the last 17 years (since 1970), doctoring then will bear little resemblance to that which is being discussed today.

NOTES

1. Starr, P. *The Social Transformation of American Medicine*. Basic Books, New York, 1982.
2. Light, D. W. Corporate medicine for profit. *Scien. Am.* 255: 38–54, 1986.
3. McKinlay, J. B. (ed.). *Issues in The Political Economy of Health Care*. Tavistock Publications, London, 1984.
4. Institute of Medicine. *For-Profit Enterprise in Health Care*. National Academy Press, Washington, D.C., 1986.
5. Salmon, J. W. Organizing medical care for profit. In: *Issues in the Political Economy of Health Care*, edited by John B. McKinlay, pp. 143–186. Tavistock, New York, 1984.
6. Navarro, J. *Crisis, Health, Medicine*. Tavistock Publishers, London, 1986.
7. Salmon, J. W. Profit and health care: Trends in corporatization and proprietization. *Int. J. Health Serv.* 15(3): 1985.
8. Kennedy, L. The proprietarization of voluntary hospitals. *Bull. NY Acad. Med.* 61: 81–89, 1985.
9. Eisenberg, C. It is still a privilege to be a doctor. *New Engl. J. Med.* April 1986, p. 1114.
10. Robert Wood Johnson Foundation. *Updated Report on Access to Health Care for the American People*. Princeton, N.J., 1983.

11. U.S. Bureau of the Census. Economic characteristics of households in the United States: Fourth quarter 1983. In *Current Population Reports*, p. 70–84. Government Printing Office, Washington, D.C., 1985.

12. Farley, P. J. Who are the underinsured? *Milbank Mem. Fund Q.* 63: 476–503, 1985.

13. Iglehart, J. K. Medical care of the poor—a growing problem. *New Engl. J. Med.* 313: 59–63, 1985.

14. Sloan, F. A., Valvona, J., and Mullner, R. Identifying the issues: A statistical profile. In *Uncompensated Hospital Care: Rights and Responsibilities*, edited by F. A. Sloan, J. F. Blumstein, and J. M. Perrins, pp. 16–53. Johns Hopkins University Press, Baltimore, 1986.

15. Himmelstein, D. U., Woolhandler, S., Harnly, M., et al. Patient transfers: Medical practice as social triage. *Am. J. Pub. Health* 74: 494–496, 1984.

16. Daniels, N. Why saying no to patients in the United States is so hard. *New Engl. J. Med.* May 22: 1380–1383, 1986.

17. Cunningham, R. M., Jr. Entrepreneurialism in medicine. *New Engl. J. Med.* 309: 1313–1314, 1983.

18. Relman, A. S. The new medical industrial complex. *New Engl. J. Med.* 303: 963–970, 1980.

19. Relman, A. S. The future of medical practice. *Health Affairs* 2: 5–19, 1983.

20. Eisenberg, L., and Virchow, R. L. K. Where are you now that we need you? *Am. J. Med.* 77: 524–532, 1984.

21. Freedman, S. A. Megacorporate health care: A choice for the future. *New Engl. J. Med.* 312: 579–582, 1985.

22. Himmelstein, D. U., and Woolhandler, S. Cost without benefit: Administrative waste in U.S. health care. *New Engl. J. Med.* 314: 441–445, 1986.

23. Alford, R. *Health Care Politics: Ideological and Interest Group Barriers to Reform.* University of Chicago Press, Chicago, 1975.

24. American Medical Association. Effects of competition in medicine. *JAMA* 249: 1864–1868, 1983.

25. Braverman, H. *Labor and Monopoly Capital.* Monthly Review Press, New York, 1974.

26. Fuchs, V. *Who Shall Live?* Basic Books, New York, 1975.

27. Blackwood, S. A. At this hospital 'the captain of the ship' is dead. *RN* 42: 77–80, 1979.

28. Garvey, J. L., and Rottet, S. Expanding the hospital nursing role: An administrative account. *J. Nurs. Admin.* 12: 30–34, 1982.

29. Alspach, J., et al. Joint physician-nurse committee ensures safe transfer of tasks. *Hospitals* 56: 54–55, 1982.

30. Florida says pharmacists may prescribe drugs. *New York Times*, April 12, 1986.

31. AMA ordered to end chiropractic boycott. *Boston Globe*, August 29, 1987.

32. Plan would alter doctors' payment under Medicare. *New York Times*, November 14, 1984.

33. Friedman, E. Doctor, the patient will see you now. *Hospitals* 55: 117–118, 1981.

34. McKinlay, J. B., and Arches, J. Towards the proletarianization of physicians. *Int. J. Health Serv.* 15(2), 1985.

35. Berube, B. Italian health care: Who's minding the clinic? *Can. Med. Assoc. J.* 130: 1625–1627, 1984.

36. Anderson, A. *Health Care in the 1990's: Trends and Strategies.* American College of Hospital Administrators, Chicago, 1987.

37. Freshnock, L. J. *Physician and Public Attitudes on Health Care Issues.* AMA, Chicago, 1984.

38. Glandon, G. L., and Werner, J. L. Physicians' practice experience during the decade of the 1970's. *JAMA* 244: 2514–2518, 1980.

39. Taylor, H. *Medical Practice in the 1990's: Physicians Look at Their Changing Profession.* H. J. Kaiser Family Foundation, Menlo Park, California, 1981.

40. Iglehart, J. K. The future supply of physicians. *New Engl. J. Med.* 314: 850–854, 1986.

41. Schroeder, S. A. Western European responses to physician oversupply. *JAMA* 252: 373–384, 1984.

42. Socioeconomic Monitoring System Survey. Center for Health Policy Research. American Medical Association, Chicago, 1986.

43. Berrien, R. What future for primary care private practice? *New Engl. J. Med.* 316: 6, 334–337, 1987.

44. Friedman, E. Declaration of interdependence. *Hospitals* 57: 73–80, 1983.

45. Freidson, E. Review essay: Health factories, the new industrial sociology, 1967.

46. McCarty, D. J. Why are today's medical students choosing high-technology specialties over internal medicine? *New Engl. J. Med.* 317: 567–568, 1987.

47. *New York Times*, August 30, 1987.

48. McKinlay, J. B. The business of good doctoring or doctoring as good business: Reflections on Freidson's view of the medical game. *Int. J. Health Serv.* 8: 459–488, 1977.

49. Marcus, S. Unions for physicians. *New Engl. J. Med.* 311: 1508–1511, 1984.

50. Doctor's dilemma: Unionizing. *New York Times*, July 13, 1987.

51. Marx, K. *Capital*, Vol. I. Random House, New York, 1977.

52. Wahn, M. The Decline of Medical Dominance in Hospitals. University of Manitoba, Winnipeg (Canada), unpublished manuscript (1985).

53. Weber, M. *Economy and Society*, Bedminster Press, New York, 1968.

54. Gerth, H., and Mills, W. C. *From Max Weber*. Oxford University Press, New York, 1968.

55. Mills, C. W. *White Collar*. Oxford University Press, New York, 1953.

56. Wilson, R. The physician's changing hospital role. In *Medical Care*, edited by W. R. Scott and E. H. Volkart, pp. 408–420. Wiley and Sons, New York, 1966.

57. Myerhoff, B. G., and Larson, W. R. The doctor as cultural hero: The routinization of charisma. *Hum. Org.* 17, 1958.

58. Zola, I. K. Medicine as an institution of social control. *The Soc. Rev.* 20(4): 487–504, 1972.

59. Haug, M. Deprofessionalization: An alternate hypothesis for the future. In *Professionalization and Social Change*, edited by P. Halmos, pp. 195–211. Sociological Review Monographs (20), Keele, 1973.

60. Haug, M. The erosion of professional authority: A cross-cultural inquiry in the case of the physician. *Milbank Mem. Fund Q.* 54: 83–106, 1976.

61. Hughes, E. C. *The Sociological Eye*. Aldine, New York, 1971.

62. Larson, M. S. Proletarianization and educated labor. *Theory and Soc.* 9: 131–175, 1980.

63. Freidson, E. The medical profession in transition. In *Applications of Social Science to Clinical Medicine*, edited by L. H. Aiken and D. Mechanic, pp. 63–79. Rutgers University Press, New Brunswick, N.J., 1986.

64. Freidson, E. The reorganization of the medical profession. *Med. Care Rev.* 42: 11–33, 1985.

65. Coburn, D., Torrance, G. M., and Kaufert, J. M. Medical dominance in Canada in historical perspective: The rise and fall of medicine? *Int. J. Health Serv.* 13: 407–432, 1983.

66. Oppenheimer, M. The proletarianization of the professional. In *Professionalization and Social Change*, edited by P. J. Halmos, pp. 213–227. Sociological Review Monograph 20, Keele, 1978.

67. McKinlay, J. B. On the professional regulation of change. *Soc. Rev. Monog.* 20: 61–84, 1973.

68. Bucher, R., and Stelling, J. Characteristics of professional organizations. *J. Health Soc. Behav.* 10: 3–15, 1969.

69. Burnham, J. C. American medicine's golden age: What happened to it? *Science* 215: 1474–1479, 1982.

70. Freidson, E. The future of professionalization. In *Health and the Division of Labour*, edited by M. Stacey, et al., pp. 140–144, Croom Helm, London, 1977.

71. McKinlay, J. B. On the medical-industrial complex. *Monthly Rev.* 30(75), 1978.

72. Armstrong, D. The decline of medical hegemony: A review of government reports during the NHS. *Soc. Sci. and Med.* 10: 157–163, 1976.

73. Parry, N., and Parry, J. Professionals and unionism: Aspects of class conflict in the national health service. *Soc. Rev.* 25: 823–841, 1977.

74. Willis, E. *Medical Dominance: The Division of Labor in Australian Health Care*. Allen and Unwin, Sydney, Australia, 1983.

75. Esland, G. Professionalism. In *The Politics of Work and Occupations*, edited by G. Esland, pp. 213–250. University of Toronto Press, Toronto, 1980.

76. Crichton, A. The shift from entrepreneurial to political power in the Canadian health system. *Soc. Sci. and Med.* 10: 59–66, 1976.

77. Riska, Elianne. *Power, Politics and Health: Forces Changing American Medicine*. Societies Scientiarum Fennica, Commentationes Scientiarum Socidium 27, 1985.

78. Roemer, M. Proletarianization of physicians or organization of health services. *Int. J. Health Serv.* 16(3): 469–471, 1986.

79. McKinlay, J. B., and Arches, J. Historical changes in doctoring: A reply to Milton Roemer. *Int. J. Health Serv.* 15(3), 1986.

THE EMPIRES STRIKE BACK

Regina Neal

Broken Promises: Columbia-Presbyterian Medical Center

Columbia-Presbyterian Medical Center is a huge complex overlooking the Hudson River in northern Manhattan. Its influence spreads into the surrounding communities beyond the immediate Washington Heights neighborhood. During the summer of 1989, the clinical staff of Presbyterian Hospital, the teaching hospital for the center's medical school, was informed of a three-phase plan to reduce ambulatory care services in the outpatient department, Vanderbilt Clinic. The first phase of the plan, which was already being implemented, involved referring all patients without health insurance who live outside the medical center's immediate area to other hospitals. Selected specialty clinics would then be "consolidated"—that is, closed. With this tactic, Columbia-Presbyterian would shift an estimated 39,000 mainly primary care visits from these uninsured patients—many of whom have a long history of using this clinic—to other providers and cut an additional 14,000 specialty visits, while still being able to claim that it was providing primary care for its own community.

Phase two of the plan, which, according to recent newspaper reports, is still being contemplated,[1] calls for a 50 percent reduction in the number of specialty clinic sessions, resulting in the elimination of 142,000 specialty visits annually. The third phase of the plan, while not spelled out in detail in the Columbia-Presbyterian document, can be assumed to be the elimination of all outpatient services at Vanderbilt Clinic—a reduction of some 360,000 visits annually.

These events are the most recent development in a long struggle between the New York State Department of Health and Columbia-Presbyterian—a struggle heightened by the existence of a well-organized and articulate community in the area around the medical center. They are also the direct consequence of a health care policy in New York State that pays lip service to the importance of primary care and relies largely on the academic medical centers to provide it. The lever used to gain the cooperation of these centers has been stipulations attached to the approval of their major capital projects. However, the state has been unwilling to confront the ensuing conflict between the medical centers' established mission of teaching and research and the imposed obligation to serve the needs of local communities. Moreover, during the nearly decade-long tenure of Health Commissioner Dr. David Axelrod, the chronic underfunding of ambulatory care by the state through Medicaid funding has made it impossible for the medical centers—or any other provider, for that matter—to be responsive to and responsible for their communities.

In 1983, faced with $5 billion worth of hospital construction plans and with more hospital beds than were needed, New York State imposed a moratorium on approving requests for expansion and renovation of hospital facilities. State regulators announced that in return for approving construction, they would require the major institutions to serve the needy, and Governor Mario Cuomo and Dr. Axelrod announced that expansion and renovation plans addressing the needs of the poor would be given the most favorable reviews.[2]

At the time, Columbia-Presbyterian had submitted a certificate of need (CON) for a $500 million project to renovate the hospital at the medical center's main site at 168th Street in Manhattan and to build a "community hospital" of 300 beds at the northern tip of Manhattan. The medical center's original intention was only to rebuild the hospital at the main site; however, the New York State Department of Health pressured the hospital to fill in the gap for health services that had been created in the Washington Heights and Inwood neighborhoods of northern Manhattan by the closing of five community hospitals in the area over the previous ten years.

The medical center initially resisted, but in the end it agreed and submitted a plan for both rebuilding the main hospital site and constructing a new community hospital. The new "community" hospital met the letter of Axelrod's demand, but hardly the spirit. It was to have a small emergency room and no outpatient clinics and would be located in an area remote from the greatest need. Clearly, it was oriented more toward the affluent Riverdale community across the river. The CON also included plans to establish an ambulatory care network that would create primary care resources at a variety of locations in the Washington Heights and Inwood communities. The state, convinced that Columbia-Presbyterian's response was adequate and that it indicated the willingness to take responsibility for the needs of the community, praised the plan, as did New York City's Health Systems Agency (HSA). Four months after the moratorium on expansion and renovations was lifted in December 1983, Columbia-Presbyterian's plans were approved.

The Community Fights Back

However, the moratorium gave the Washington Heights and Inwood community a chance to review the proposed project plans as described in the CON. The review left the residents far less optimistic about the adequacy of the proposed system to provide for the needs of the community. Determined to have their views represented, a group of community residents formed the North Manhattan Health Action Group (NMHAG) in September 1983. The group set as its initial goal an assessment of the health needs and health resources in the community and evaluation of the adequacy of the plans proposed by Columbia-Presbyterian.

The review was considered essential by the community of approximately 180,000 residents, whose health needs are great. The area depicted in NMHAG's report is made up of a large number of relatively young families, many of them recent immigrants from the Dominican Republic.[3] As described by a variety of economic indicators, the community is poorer than Manhattan and New York City as a whole, and its health status is much worse. Of particular note is the high proportion of pregnant women—a large number of whom are teenagers—who receive late or no prenatal care, a clear indicator of the lack of primary care resources and financial access to health care in the area.

NMHAG found serious problems with Columbia-Presbyterian's proposal. The primary care resources to be developed were inadequate, and community physicians, including those who would work at the ambulatory care sites, would not be able to admit patients to either hospital site. At the time of the NMHAG survey, only 4 of 175 physicians in the area had admitting privileges at Presbyterian Hospital. Despite the community's reservations, the New York City HSA and the New York State Department of Health approved the CON.

Determined to have their concerns heard and reflected in changes to the plan, NMHAG mounted a year-long, highly organized "bottom-up" campaign that mobilized the community. Their efforts resulted in an unprecedented arrangement in which Axelrod required Columbia-Presbyterian to work with NMHAG to "resolve the issues and to produce a model for primary health care in the community."[4] NMHAG and representatives of Columbia-Presbyterian signed an agreement in October 1985.

The agreement specified the size, general location, and scope of services that were to be provided at each of five ambulatory care network sites that were to be established in 1986. It also reflected an agreement on the scope of the physician shortage in the area and on ways to alleviate it. The primary care physicians in the ambulatory care network would "have the ability to admit and follow their patients in the Hospital," and Columbia-Presbyterian also agreed to a steering committee for the ambulatory care network that would have community participants as full members.[5] The future seemed to hold promise.

Broken Promises

Fulfillment of the promise was slow in coming. Not until October 1987, a year after all of the sites in the ambulatory care network were to have been operating, was the first site, a geriatric center in the Fort Washington Houses complex, opened. A second site opened in 1988, and the third in January 1989. But none of these sites were located in the areas of greatest need within the community.

There is disagreement on what caused the extensive delays in establishing the promised sites in the network. The community charges foot dragging on the part of Columbia-Presbyterian—a sign of the familiar reluctance of the medical center to be responsive to the needs of the community. The medical center claims otherwise. During this same period, however, Columbia-Presbyterian hardly slacked off on its other priorities. It was able to establish three medical office complexes for doctors on staff at the center in Riverdale, on the Upper East Side, and in Chinatown. And by late 1989, Columbia-Presbyterian had also managed to rebuild the main hospital site (now called the Milstein Pavilion) and build the new hospital, known as the Allen Pavilion.

Clearly, the community has not gotten what it had hoped for and what it was promised when it signed the agreement with Columbia-Presbyterian in the fall of 1985. Only three of the original five ambulatory care network sites have been opened, and the remaining two are those to be located in the areas of greatest need. The three clinics that are operating are at full capacity, and there are long waits for first visits for new patients, attesting to the need for these services. The ambulatory care network steering committee, of which NMHAG is a member, is currently evaluating the need to expand evening and Saturday hours at the clinics. There are no signs of any serious attempt on the part of Columbia-Presbyterian, in its role as a teaching hospital, to address the shortage of physicians in the community, however, nor has there been more than a marginal improvement in the ability of community physicians to admit and follow patients at the Columbia-Presbyterian hospitals.

During the summer of 1989, it became clear that the community's access to health care from the medical center was only going to get worse and not better. A year earlier, Columbia-Presbyterian had begun to make public a serious financial deficit that it attributed to its outpatient services. Chiefly responsible were the increasing volume of ambulatory services provided to uninsured patients both within and outside the Columbia-Presbyterian community and the inadequacy of the reimbursement for ambulatory services under Medicaid. This strategy ironically laid the groundwork for Columbia-Presbyterian to propose radical cutbacks in ambulatory care services, which began with the closing of its outpatient pharmacy in March 1989, even as it promised to expand primary care to the community.

The latest actions by Columbia-Presbyterian and the results for the community suggest another example of how costly and difficult it is to badger large academic medical centers to do what they do not want to do: take responsibility for meeting community needs. And it would also seem to justify the community's widely held perception that narrow self-interest and deception are the primary forces that move the medical empires. Yet, while Columbia-Presbyterian's actions are extremely distressing, considered in the context of the current fiscal realities of providing ambulatory care in New York State, they are less than surprising. For ten years, the state Department of Health, headed by Dr. Axelrod, has produced an endless supply of talk on the priority that primary care must be given by all providers in New York State. For the same ten years, however, reimbursement of ambulatory care clinic services under Medicaid has been frozen at $60 per visit; private physician's rates have been frozen since the mid-1970's and now average $11 per visit. These rates are now driving even the so-called Medicaid mills out of business. Add to this the mounting numbers of uninsured individuals who have increasing needs for health care services, and the result is the crisis we face today.

In the age of high-technology medicine, primary care is the stepchild. New York State's current primary care policy has failed utterly. This failure stems not only from the lack of adequate mechanisms to finance services. It is also a result of ignoring the fact that academic medical centers' established missions of teaching and research are not naturally compatible with a mission of primary care service to the community. So, while the concept of forced responsibility has driven the state's policy, judging by the outcome, virtually no energy has been put into developing other community-based alternatives for the provision of primary care—let alone into financing such alternatives. The result has been the continuing shrinkage of primary care services in the communities with large and growing needs for these services and with the fewest alternatives, and a further erosion of trust on the part of these communities for the institutions that have promised to meet their needs.

Given this context, Columbia-Presbyterian's actions can be seen as a direct response to disincentives to providing primary care that have been established by New York State. One has to wonder how many other providers are also dumping ambulatory care patients and shrinking services in response to the same disincentives. The only thing that may make Columbia-Presbyterian different is that it went public.

Ignoring the Community's Needs: St. Luke's-Roosevelt Hospital Center

In the past 20 years, the New York City communities of Harlem and northern Manhattan have witnessed the closing of seven community hospitals: Jewish Memorial, St. Elizabeth's, Cabrini, Delafield, Wadsworth, Logan, and Sydenham. During this same period, these areas have also suffered a rapid decline in the number of physicians in private practice. More recently, Presbyterian Hospital began a phased reduction of ambulatory care (see "Broken Promises," p. 285), and in March 1989 both Presbyterian Hospital and Mt. Sinai Hospital (which lies on the border of East Harlem) abandoned outpatient pharmacies that together provided 758,000 visits in 1987.[6]

Already hurt by these reductions, the communities of Central and West Harlem now face yet another retrenchment in services in the form of the plans for modernization of St. Luke's-Roosevelt Hospital Center. Although the community supports modernization of the existing facilities, it strongly opposes the part of the plan that calls for consolidating the inpatient obstetric, neonatal, and pediatric services now offered at the St. Luke's Hospital site at 114th Street on the Upper West Side with those at the Roosevelt Hospital site, located approximately three miles south at Columbus Circle in midtown Manhattan. There is no direct public transportation link to Roosevelt for many of the people now served by St. Luke's, so in urban terms, this facility would be geographically inaccessible to those most in need of the relocated services. Poor people are typically less mobile, and this would be particularly true for women who are pregnant or in labor or who might be traveling with sick children. Moreover, the population now served by St. Luke's Hospital is at substantial risk of giving birth to babies who need emergency and ongoing treatment because they are premature, low birth weight, or born with HIV disease or addicted to drugs. With neonatal intensive care located at the Roosevelt site, the public health consequences of parents having limited access to their infants over a period of many months become severe.

Roosevelt Hospital is located in one of the most rapidly and intensively gentrifying areas in midtown Manhattan. Columbus Circle is the site of the former New York Coliseum building, which is targeted for major residential and commercial development. The area is becoming increasingly residential, with land to the west slotted for a massive housing development by Donald Trump, while the Times Square area to the south is in the process of a major publicly sponsored redevelopment plan that will render the commercial nature of the theater district considerably more upscale. These market changes are obviously a part of the impetus for this part of the St. Luke's-Roosevelt modernization plan. Clearly, the medical center wants to cast its lot with the growing gentry located in the area of its downtown site.

By contrast, St. Luke's Hospital, on the southern border of Harlem, is in a community with a much larger, younger, and poorer population. Household size in the St. Luke's hospital area is larger by 66 percent, and the median income, at $14,149 in 1985, was 52 percent lower than that in the Roosevelt Hospital area. The two communities differ in their racial and ethnic composition as well, with the St. Luke's area 59 percent black and the Roosevelt area 71 percent white.[7]

The consolidation of these inpatient services to the Roosevelt Hospital site is part of a $467 million modernization plan first proposed in 1986.[8] The New York State Department of Health approved the plan in December 1986, with the recommendation of the New York City Health Systems Agency (HSA), the local planning agency charged with making presumably disinterested recommendations to the state on community health needs and allocation of resources. Although protests organized by a coalition of community organizations against the dislocation of services failed to halt the plan, they did lead the Department of Health to attach a number of conditions to its approval of the medical center's certificate of need (CON). Among them, the state required that demand for obstetric, neonatal, and pediatric services be monitored over time and that decisions about the need for and location of these services be reevaluated before any consolidation took place.

The New York State Department of Health clearly held out the promise that if the needs for these services changed, the decision would be modified. Yet, Raymond Sweeney, director of the Office of Health Systems Management (the branch of the state health department that covers hospitals), acted to foreclose the possibility that the decision could be altered by creating bureaucratic obstacles to any change. "If a determination is made that additional services are needed at the St. Luke's site," he wrote in a letter to the president of St. Luke's-Roosevelt in March 1987, "it is recognized that a proposal would constitute a separate certificate of need application, subject to affordability and financial feasibility reviews." In other words, to make any alterations in the plan would mean having to fulfill the CON requirements for an entirely new project, substantially delaying the plans and creating financing problems. This could bring the entire modernization project to a halt and ultimately cause it to fail.

Sweeney's letter goes on to suggest expanded outpatient and emergency services "as an alternative to inpatient care at the St. Luke's Division" and urges "accelerated and ongoing education efforts [to show that] the new configuration of the services is, in fact, not detrimental or negative, relative to the respective communities.'' While the alternatives Sweeney proposes are undoubtedly crucial, his suggestion is essentially a diversionary tactic—an attempt to divert attention away from the threatened services and focus on another needed—but currently nonexistent—set of services.

The Community's Needs

In the ensuing three years, the northern Manhattan and Harlem communities have experienced the same scourge of illness and poverty that has engulfed other New York City neighborhoods: increasing infant mortality rates; growing numbers of women who receive late or no prenatal care; and rising numbers of newly reported cases of tuberculosis, syphilis, measles, and AIDS. Although these problems can be found throughout the city, poor communities have among the highest rates for all these health indicators as well as a small and rapidly shrinking pool of resources to deal with them.

In response to the continuing concern expressed by the community coalition, the state Department of Health provided funds to the Health Action Resource Center to organize the West Side/West Harlem Community Planning Coalition for an independent study of maternal and child health needs in the community. The resulting ''Report and Recommendations on Maternal and Child Health Needs'' compellingly documents the pressing health needs of the community and the probable effects of withdrawing obstetric and neonatal services. It recommends that these services be maintained at both the St. Luke's and the Roosevelt sites and also that prenatal care for substance-using women and ambulatory care for women and children with HIV illness be enhanced. The West Side/West Harlem Community Planning Coalition presented the report to Dr. David Axelrod, New York State Commissioner of Health, in April 1989, along with a demand that the decision to move services out of the Harlem community be reconsidered.

Rather than squarely confronting the problem, Axelrod instead turned it back to the HSA, charging it to conduct yet another study and make yet another set of recommendations. The new HSA study, ''Assessment of Maternal and Child Health Needs in Upper Manhattan,'' reads like a brief for maintaining obstetric and neonatal services at St. Luke's for the mostly poor residents of Central and West Harlem.

Of greatest significance are the findings that 77 percent of obstetric patients and 89 percent of neonatal patients who were residents of Central and West Harlem were either on Medicaid or uninsured. The overwhelming majority of this group of obstetric patients—94 percent—deliver in a hospital within the area, suggesting, again, that travel to an out-of-area hospital, such as the Roosevelt site, is unrealistic. Indeed, the report notes that women who are uninsured or on Medicaid are far less likely than insured patients to deliver at out-of-area hospitals. The report goes on to note that low-income women ''usually present at the obstetric facility closest to their residence and will not generally migrate from Upper Manhattan to Roosevelt Hospital.''[9] Moreover, although HSA did not note this, the proposed arrangement of services is likely to lead to discontinuity of care. Poor women are more likely to need emergency deliveries. Under these circumstances, even if they are receiving outpatient prenatal care at St. Luke's Hospital or another site sponsored by St. Luke's-Roosevelt, they are liable to end up at Harlem or Presbyterian Hospitals, where they and their history are unknown, thus complicating an already complex delivery.

Yet, in the face of the overwhelming evidence of the need for obstetric and especially neonatal inpatient services in Central and West Harlem that it had documented, and in spite of continued opposition from the community and local politicians, HSA in its final report recommended the relocation of services to the Roosevelt Hospital site. The rationalization? To do otherwise "may require the hospital to amend and resubmit its CON . . . leading to further delays in proceeding with the project . . . [and] would result in either significantly increasing project costs or decreasing project scope. . . ."[10]

In evaluating the options, HSA ignored the fact (although stated in the report) that consolidation of services at St. Luke's instead of Roosevelt would offer many advantages for the neediest residents of Upper Manhattan, including minimal disruption of utilization patterns and hospitalization closer to home for mothers and their infants.

The report also neglected the effect of the plan on other facilities. Instead, it off-handedly announced that "after consolidation, it is anticipated that many Medicaid/self-pay patients currently utilizing St. Luke's will migrate to other Upper Manhattan facilities [and] Presbyterian/Allen Pavilion, [and] Harlem [Hospital] . . . may be required to reallocate some of their bed capacity for Medical/Self Pay [sic] patients residing in these zip codes to insure access to inpatients [sic] services."[11] HSA thus sidestepped any consideration of increased costs to other facilities, provoking the New York City Health and Hospitals Corporation, the agency responsible for the city's public hospitals, to respond: "We simply do not have the resources to increase capacity further at the [Harlem Hospital] facility."[12]

HSA constructed a strained rationalization for its conclusions: "These data re-affirm that access to, and the availability of, inpatient obstetrical services is not a concern."[13] Resulting shortages of neonatal services could be addressed by expansions at Harlem and Presbyterian Hospitals, the report reiterated, assisted by creation of a perinatal regional transport system that would use ambulances to move sick babies from these communities to Roosevelt. Again, the ability and willingness of these hospitals to pick up the additional work load—not to mention the cost—were left unexplored.

HSA further rationalized that ambulatory care would be more effective than inpatient services in improving maternal and infant health in upper Manhattan. Furthermore, HSA decided, "the critical factor that will determine the actual impact of consolidation . . . is improved community education, outreach and prenatal care services."[14]

Trading in Services

This confidence in such "long-run" solutions is astonishing, given the inadequacy of the current prenatal and other primary care options in New York City. The community is being asked to trade in existing services for the promise of more and better services of another, more transient kind. They are apparently asking too much to have both inpatient and outpatient services. Yet, there is no reason to expect that the end result will be anything other than a loss of the inpatient services *without* development of the promised ambulatory services.

The planned abandonment by St. Luke's-Roosevelt has galvanized the community. It has continued to resist the proposal through the same coalition of community organizations that opposed the initial decision in 1986 to allow these services to be moved and whose pressure resulted in the study by the West Side/ West Harlem Community Planning Coalition and the HSA report that followed it. In November 1989, the coalition organized a public meeting attended by over 100 community residents to respond to the first draft of HSA's report. Essentially all the speakers at the meeting who were not connected to St. Luke's-Roosevelt considered both the plan to move services out of St. Luke's and the assessment conducted by HSA inadequate. Testimony was provided by a wide range of local political leaders, all of whom vowed to support the community in its struggle to keep the services at St. Luke's.

On March 4, 1990, 300 people marched and rallied to oppose, once again, the decision to remove these services from the community that so sorely needs them. The issue has received mounting press coverage and political support. The position of the community on this issue could hardly be more clear.

Despite the evidence and community sentiment, HSA refuses to consider the most reasonable option—consolidating services at the St. Luke's site—supposedly because it might require the development of a new CON. As this is written, the decision rests with Commissioner Axelrod, who could exert some leadership to resolve this issue. The formalities of CON review are part of the regulatory process that his department controls, and he has the ability to alter this portion of the plan. Instead, Axelrod has said that he will respond to the HSA report and recommendations, as well as the community opposition, in April, adding, "It doesn't necessarily mean that I will have a decision by then."[15]

In the meantime, the St. Luke's-Roosevelt modernization plan, which the community supports as necessary to ensure that St. Luke's Hospital will exist for them in the future, moves forward. Further delays simply mean that a decision to alter the original plans to fit current and projected needs becomes less likely as more of the project is completed. And the community is left out in the cold.

NOTES

1. "As a Hospital Grows, Debts Threaten It," *New York Times*, December 18, 1989, p. B4.

2. Gallagher, Peggy, "Back to the Drawing Board," *Health/PAC Bulletin*, 1986:16(5), pp. 7–8.

3. "Washington Heights/Inwood Neighborhoods: Assessment of Health Care Needs," New York: North Manhattan Health Action Group, February 1984.

4. Gallagher, Peggy, "The Presbyterian Story: The People Pull the Strings for a Change," *Health/PAC Bulletin*, 1986:16(5), p. 11.

5. Letter from Thomas Morris to Stephan Berger and Robert Gumbs, "Re: Ambulatory Care Network Corporation Development," October 24, 1989.

6. *New York Times*, March 9, 1989.

7. *New York City Community Health Atlas*, New York: United Hospital Fund, 1988.

8. Peggy Gallagher, op. cit.

9. Health Systems Agency, "Assessment of Maternal and Child Health Needs in Upper Manhattan," February 1990, p. 35.

10. Ibid., pp. 45, 108.

11. Ibid., p. 42.

12. Letter to Robert Gumbs, Executive Director of the New York City Health Systems Agency, from Raymond Baxter, December 19, 1989.

13. Health Systems Agency, op. cit., p. 100.

14. Ibid., pp. 87, 91.

15. *New York Newsday*, March 5, 1990.

THE LOSSES IN PROFITS: HOW PROPRIETARIES AFFECT PUBLIC AND VOLUNTARY HOSPITALS

Louanne Kennedy

At no time since their establishment have the nation's non-profit, voluntary, and public hospitals been swept by such radical change. Hospital care has entered a new stage, and these old actors must either adapt to it or disappear.

The impact of for-profit corporate chains on hospital care has been measured primarily in terms of the number of hospitals or beds they control. And, indeed, these chains have been growing rapidly. Arnold Relman, editor of the *New England Journal of Medicine*, has noted with alarm that if their expansion continues at the current rate, by 1990 they will own 30 percent of all hospitals.[1] The American College of Hospital Administrators has projected an even more remarkable figure of 60 percent market share by the year 1995.[2]

Whether or not either of these forecasts is accurate, the growth and consolidation of for-profit chains is of concern not solely because it is changing the ownership pattern of hospital beds, but because it is quickly causing what can be termed the proprietarization of voluntary hospitals, which means a fundamental change in their historic mission and function. The nation's public hospitals, meanwhile, are continuing to disappear, hurried into oblivion by the declining local government commitment to the provision of health care.

Although acute-care hospitals are most affected right now, the movement toward for-profit centralized ownership has progressed in nursing homes, psychiatric hospitals, home health care, health maintenance organizations (HMOs), and freestanding surgi-centers, and emergi-centers; this process has recently spread to alcoholism and drug dependency clinics, primary care centers, and medical equipment suppliers. (See Table 1.)

The Impact on the Voluntary Hospital Sector

The historic claim of voluntary hospitals has been that they provide necessary community health services. In reality the care they have offered has often been determined by research and teaching priorities, particularly in major metropolitan areas dominated by medical schools and large teaching hospitals. However even if community service was only a byproduct in such institutions, at least it existed. In many localities throughout the country where academic medicine was absent, community service was minimal. In others, non-profit institutions did provide care otherwise unavailable to those with limited insurance coverage or

Table 1
Multi-Unit Providers

	Chains	Units/Offices
Hospitals (US)	179	1,926
Shared services organizations	106	9,562
Alliances	6	500
Department control managers	74	6,411
Psychiatric hospitals	25	154
Alternative services*		
Run by hospital chains	90	758
Run by other chains	31	226
Nursing homes		
Run by hospital chains	30	239
Run by other chains	24	2,079
Lifecare centers		
Run by hospital chains	21	47
Run by nursing home chains	9	29
Home healthcare agencies		
Full service	11	1,261
I.V. therapy	4	175
Health maintenance organizations (US)		
Run by hospital chains	11	12
Run by other chains	13	134
Rental dialysis centers	6	267
Surgery centers	8	82
Dental clinics		
In retail stores	6	73
Franchisers	7	140
Subtotal	663	24,075
Groups sponsoring hospitals	58	244
Total	721	24,319

* Freestanding centers other than surgery centers.

Source:
Modern Health Care, May 1984 and August 1983

ability to pay. Today the new corporate chains are taking over voluntary hospitals in even the smallest cities, and where they do remain independent, nonprofit institutions—and some public hospitals—are increasingly adopting the practices of proprietary hospitals, eschewing community responsibility in their pursuit of solvency.

This phenomenon has an impact far greater than the proprietary hospitals themselves do because voluntary and public institutions still provide most hospital care; the voluntary institutions alone account for two thirds. In 1982, the for-profit institutions accounted for only 9 percent of all non-federal acute care beds, a share up only 1.2 percent from 1975.[3] This apparent stability is, however, deceptive. The proprietary sector is now dominated by chains rather than individually owned facilities, corporate giants with far greater ability to distribute costs, gain access to capital markets, and diversify into other health care ventures.

Currently 475 centrally managed corporate chains own, lease, or manage 7,602 hospitals, nursing homes, lifecare centers, home healthcare agency offices, and physicians' offices. Another 58 organizations, mostly Catholic orders, sponsor 244 hospitals.[4]

Of these, 179 manage acute-care hospitals. (Table 2 describes the 10 largest corporate, secular non-profit, and religiously-affiliated chains.) Between 1979 and 1983, the secular non-profit chains have added the most beds, followed by the investor-owned chains; the number of beds in religious and public hospitals has dropped.

When proprietaries alone placed primary emphasis on profit and fiscal management, there were safety valves in the voluntary and public sector to assure minimum care levels. Now that voluntaries are following their lead, whatever possibility many people had of finding accessible, high-quality, accountable care is fast disappearing.

Historically, their care was arranged through cross-subsidization, both between individual institutions and at the community level. Premiums paid by subscribers to Blue Cross and private insurors have subsidized care for the medically indigent to some extent. Indigent care also tended to be distributed: implicitly or explicitly, patients were sorted so that no single voluntary hospital was responsible for all the non-paying or low-paying patients. Certainly this balance was an uneasy one; some hospitals shouldered much greater burdens than others. Particularly in areas with sizable numbers of public hospital beds, some voluntaries were able to more nearly sidestep the responsibility. Nevertheless, even in the current period of intensifying cost containment pressures, voluntary hospitals could reasonably have been expected to maintain a significant role in providing care for the uninsured, and voluntary hospital lobbies have continued to support some form of national health insurance as a way of socializing the cost of this care. However, the tide among voluntary hospitals has shifted towards proprietarization, instituting the classic business strategy of seeking a more and more selective market of patients at the expense of community services.

Public Hospitals Disappear

In some cases, proprietarization involves an actual takeover of a public or voluntary institution; in others, it is indirect, effecting a fundamental realignment of values.

When the Coweta County, Georgia, public hospital was suffering from internal problems and inadequate funding, public officials chose to abandon this county hospital rather than raise taxes to cover the need. Despite opposition from a group of Georgia Legal Services clients and initial Health Systems Agency opposition, the state approved the county's application to sell the hospital to the Humana Corporation. The effects of this transfer were soon clear:

• Under an agreement with the county, a dollar amount was established to provide indigent care. This sum immediately proved to be far less than was needed, but when it is exhausted the uninsured are given only emergency care —as defined, narrowly, by the Humana staff.

• As a hospital which had received funding under the Hill-Burton Act, Coweta County was obligated to provide care to the medically indigent until 1997; this obligation ceased within the sale.

• Far from enhancing cost-effectiveness, the sale has increased the cost of care. One new expense is interest payments. Humana borrowed $9 million at 17 percent interest to purchase the hospital. Interest payments now account for 15.8 percent of operation expenses, or $52 per patient day, compared to 2.2 percent, or $5.92 per patient day, under public ownership. Some of the capital outlay has gone for new facilities and equipment, but access to these services is limited.[5]

Although Coweta County's experience is not unique, proprietarization more commonly takes less overt forms. Tampa General, the public hospital in Tampa, Florida, is one example. In 1983, hard hit by loss of paying patients to the new Humana Women's Hospital and voluntary institutions which had adopted aggressive marketing tactics, it developed a two-track strategy. First, it has adopted a policy of turning away medically indigent and Medicaid patients whose cases are not urgent. (Florida Medicaid rates are below those of other third-party payers such as Blue Cross.) Second, it has embarked on a major construction program to provide new beds for well-insured patients.[6]

A Voluntary Diversifies

In 1981 Dayton Hospital, a voluntary non-profit facility in Dayton, Ohio, was in serious straits. Its occupancy rate was low; its assets were declining; it had difficulty borrowing money; it didn't have the funds to purchase equipment its physicians deemed absolutely necessary; and its physicians who also had attending privileges at other institutions often sent their well-insured patients to them.

To reverse this downward spiral, the Board of Trustees established a Marketing Department to seek out better insured Daytonians and identify new services that would be attractive to patients and physicians. The new department developed an ambitious plan, which included a new hospital with new technology. Three years later, Dayton Hospital had:

• Developed a for-profit subsidiary which purchased a nearby proprietary nursing home and an alcoholism clinic.

• Formed a group to sell management services to other hospitals in trouble.

Dayton Hospital is considering the purchase of one of its management contract clients, a voluntary hospital in Gainesville, Florida.

• Achieved an AA rating from a major brokerage house, which has enhanced its ability to borrow for capital expenditures and lowered the interest rates it must pay.

• Boosted physician morale. Delighted with the new patient population, new equipment and new physical plant, most now believe they are attached to the "best" hospital in Dayton.[7]

The Seven Choices

These three cases indicate some of the responses to the growing concerns about fiscal accountability in a competitive, cost containment environment. In the decade ahead, public and independent voluntary hospitals will face the following choices: 1) seek acquisition by a for-profit or non-profit chain; 2) diversify and expand vertically; 3) merge; 4) hire contract management; 5) take forceful measures to maintain current market share; 6) convert into another type of institution; 7) close.

Not all of these strategies are available to every type of institution. For example, public hospitals are unlikely to be in a position to diversify and expand and are more likely to seek acquisition or contract management. Moreover, as the three cases described above demonstrate, none of these potential strategies are based upon providing low-cost care to the poor and uninsured.

Why Is Proprietarization Occurring?

The accelerating trend toward proprietarization is encouraged by a number of factors, including changing ideologies, the unequal mobility of hospitals, and changes in reimbursement policies.

The role of ideology. The commitment to the public delivery of services has historically been limited in the U.S. In the 1930s, the New Deal programs to solve the problems of the Great Depression included public sector financing of delivery of education and health as well as construction projects. Once again in the 1960s the public sector was expanded to deliver health, employment, and community services. In both the 1930s and the 1960s public financing of services was the result of powerful social movements among the poor demanding them. However, these periods of expansion are aberrations, running counter to the dominant ideological premise that public delivery of services is worse, i.e., inefficient, plagued by incompetent workers, and costly, while services provided by the private sector are efficient, cost-effective, and responsive to the demands of the market.

Since the election of President Reagan, assertions of the superiority of private ownership have become even more insistent. Pressures to contract with private firms for delivery of services ranging from garbage collection to social programs have intensified. Behind the rhetoric of "public vs. private" lies the real issue: whether poor and working people get care.

The provision of health services has always been marked by an uneasy balance between public, voluntary, and proprietary interests, with the voluntary non-profit hospitals dominant. However in the 1970s and the 1980s mounting pressure to control costs has shaken their dominance and further marginalized the public institutions. Both government and industry have seized upon marketplace competition as the answer to rising costs.

Unequal mobility. Voluntary hospitals are usually associated with a particular community. Private hospital chains—actually large, national corporations—are in the business of buying and building facilities in areas where market analysis indicates the presence of a substantial insured population. They have almost complete freedom to go into places with a favorable state regulatory climate and high population growth. As a result, they are heavily concentrated in the South and the West, regions where population and economic growth has been rapid in recent years: 73 percent of the beds owned by the nation's five largest private firms are located in the South and another 20 percent in California. This has given these companies a steadily increasing patient base and made them essentially recession proof.[8] David Jones, Chairman and Chief Executive Officer of Humana, is one of many corporate officials who expect investor-owned chains to continue to expand most vigorously in the Sunbelt, where population growth runs ahead of the national rate. Although many executives are predicting an increase in private management of urban public hospitals in the North and the Northeast, they do not foresee any dramatic growth in their ownership of northern urban hospitals.[9] Jones points out that the high cost eastern states such as Massachusetts, New York, and Maryland also have the most "oppressive" regulations and cites their tightened planning restrictions as further reasons for staying out.

David Williamson, Executive Vice President for domestic development at Hospital Corporation of America, agrees that "By and large, the future growth of the industry will be in dynamic states where the population is growing . . . and in those states that decide to modify punitive state regulations." He added that HCA's pursuit of growth opportunities will continue to be "principally in the hospital sector of the health care field and not in diversification." HCA, he elaborated, expects to replace and/or build 2,500 to 3,500 hospital beds per year, and it is currently targeting public hospitals "whose life cycles have ended, and that are without the resources to finance the replacement of their facilities."[10]

As the easier markets in the Sunbelt are saturated, the industry is likely to pursue management contracting and acquisition more aggressively, because Certificate of Need laws make construction of new hospitals difficult in heavily bedded areas. Another possibility is accelerated diversification. National Medical Enterprises, for example, is acquiring and building nursing homes, psychiatric hospitals, and homecare agencies.

Voluntary hospitals generally lack mobility, although some have moved to more well-to-do suburbs—creating serious problems for the patients left behind. Many institutions that remain in areas of declining population and income are adopting restrictive access policies in the name of financial solvency. Others that continue to serve everyone in their community regardless of ability to pay face bankruptcy. Most of the 25 hospital closures in New York City since 1975

Table 2

Top 10 Hospital Operators by Type, in 1983*

	Beds		Units	
	1983	1982	1983	1982
Investor-Owned				
1. Hospital Corp. of America	52,913	47,415	363	325
2. Humana Inc.	17,704	16,786	89	90
3. American Medical International Inc.	14,274	12,623	104	95
4. National Medical Enterprises Inc.	9,576	8,919	63	64
5. Nu-Med Inc.	5,696	5,403	21	11
6. Lifemark Corp.	5,074	4,334	30	28
7. Republic Health Corp.	3,335	895	29	10
8. Universal Health Service Inc.	2,732	1,573	23	12
9. American Healthcare Mgmt. Inc.	2,704	1,857	25	15
10. Hospital Mgmt. Professional Inc.	2,654	1,799	21	13
Total	116,662	101,604	768	663
Secular Non-profit				
1. Kaiser Foundation	6,576	6,583	28	28
2. Fairview Community Hospitals	3,842	3,536	46	42
3. Intermountain Health Care Inc.	2,953	2,887	23	23
4. Health Central System	2,769	2,689	20	20
5. SunHealth	2,685	2,143	27	23
6. Health Frontiers Inc.	2,611	2,662	34	35
7. Lutheran Hospitals & Home Society of America	2,451	2,232	45	45
8. Affiliated Hospital Systems	2,179	1,960	24	23
9. SamCor	1,604	1,564	9	7
10. HealthOne Corp.	1,455	880	5	3
Total	29,125	28,226	261	249

Table 2 *(cont.)*
Top 10 Hospital Operators by Type, in 1983*

	Beds		Units	
	1983	1982	1983	1982
Catholic				
1. Sisters of Mercy Health Corp.	5,889	5,760	28	25
2. Sisters of Mercy of the Union	4,356	4,166	14	14
3. Sisters of Charity Health Care System	4,306	4,336	13	14
4. Hospital Sisters Health System	3,719	3,731	13	13
5. Sisters of Providence Health Care System	3,428	3,218	14	13
6. Catholic Health Corp.	3,335	3,003	24	19
7. Holy Cross Health System Corp.	3,089	3,062	11	10
8. Franciscan Health System	3,012	2,877	11	11
9. Anellia Domini Health Services Inc.	2,903	2,933	10	10
10. Sisters of Charity of Leavenworth Health Services	2,454	2,397	9	8
Total	36,491	35,483	147	137
Other Religious				
1. Adventist Health System/US	10,633	10,536	74	76
2. Methodist Health Systems Inc.	3,692	3,275	16	12
3. Lutheran Hospital Society of Southern California	2,373	2,615	11	12
4. Evangelical Health Systems	1,634	1,634	5	5
5. Harris Methodist Health System	1,603	1,221	12	10
6. Baylor Health Care System	1,497	1,425	6	5
7. Baptist Medical Center	1,351	1,152	5	5
8. St. Luke's-Roosevelt Hospital Ctr.	1,315	1,316	3	3
9. Southwest Community Health Services	1,201	1,269	12	13
10. Methodist Hospital of Indiana	1,190	1,190	2	2

Public

	Beds operated	Beds managed	Facilities operated	Facilities managed
1. NYC Health & Hospital Corp.	7,778	7,919	11	12
2. Los Angeles County—Dept. of Health Services	4,506	4,902	6	7
3. North Broward Hospital District	1,262	1,253	3	3
4. Peoples Community Hospital Authority	1,236	1,236	5	5
5. Fulton-DeKalb Hospital Authority	1,204	1,204	2	2
6. Harris County Hospital District	804	774	3	3
7. Hospital Commission of Prince George County	791	791	2	2
8. Wake County Hospital System	656	656	2	2
9. Spartanburg General Hospital System	617	617	2	2
10. Alameda County Health Care Services Agency	600	600	2	2
Total	19,454	19,952	41	43

Contract Managers**

	Beds operated	Beds managed	Facilities operated	Facilities managed
1. Hospital Corp. of America	22,642	18,828	169	144
2. Nu-Med Inc.	4,815	5,291	12	10
3. Catholic Health Corp.	3,335	3,003	24	19
4. National Medical Enterprises Inc.	3,269	2,691	22	23
5. SunHealth	2,685	2,143	27	23
6. Hospital Management Professionals Inc.	2,654	1,799	21	13
7. Fairview Community Hospitals	2,606	2,300	39	35
8. American Medical International Inc.	2,137	2,119	13	13
9. Lutheran Hospital Society of Southern California	2,124	1,960	8	5
10. Geisinger Medical Mgmt. Corp.	1,123	1,039	6	4
Total	47,915	41,004	342	294

* Largest systems based on number of U.S. and foreign acute care hospital beds operated in 1983.
** Largest managers of U.S. and foreign acute care hospitals based on number of beds-managed facilities in 1983.

Table 3
Hospitals in Multi-Institutional Systems

Total

Year Type of System:	Beds 1979	1983	% Change	Hospitals 1979	1983	% Change
Investor-owned	90,580	123,810	36.7	695	869	25.0
Secular non-profit	56,398	86,266	52.9	301	583	93.7
Religious	106,062	87,826	×17.2%	455	415	×8.8%
Public	21,718	20,646	×4.9	59	49	16.9
Totals	274,758	318,548	15.9%	1,510	1,916	26.9%

Owned

Year Type of System:	Beds 1979	1983	% Change	Hospitals 1979	1983	% Change
Investor-owned	58,000	86,128	48.5	395	595	50.6
Secular non-profit	50,775	69,886	37.6	245	374	52.6
Religious	100,389	78,319	×21.9%	391	327	×16.4%
Public	21,619	20,646	×4.5	57	49	14.0
Totals	230,783	254,979	10.5%	1,088	1,345	23.6%

Managed

Year Type of System:	Beds 1979	1983	% Change	Hospitals 1979	1983	% Change
Investor-owned	32,580	37,682	15.6	300	274	-8.7
Secular non-profit	5,623	16,380	191.3	56	209	273.2
Religious	5,673	9,508	67.6%	64	88	37.5%
Public	99	0	×100.0	2	0	-100.0
Totals	43,975	63,570	44.5%	422	571	35.3%

Source:
Modern Health Care, April 1981 and May 1984

are due to bankruptcies, caused in large part by their willingness to serve increased numbers of uninsured patients.

Changes in reimbursement policies. For many years hospitals were cushioned by cost-based reimbursement, under which they were reimbursed for whatever they spent on patient care. Those days are clearly over. As controls on reimbursement have tightened, mostly through government efforts, voluntary hospitals have been acting more like proprietary hospitals than ever before. For the proprietary sector, prospective payment systems such as diagnosis-related groups (DRGs) have been a boon. According to John Hindelong, Director of Research at the brokerage firm Becker Paribas and a leading health care analyst,

DRGs are "now seen as a system that does what it's supposed to do—that is, increase profits to the efficient provider of health-care services."[11]

Nonprofit Chains and Subsidiaries

As competitive pressures mount, many non-profit hospitals are setting up for-profit subsidiaries and/or multihospital systems and chains of their own, which then often initiate diversification schemes "to work out of the corner they've been pushed into by government constraints and increased competition."[12] Typically, they form for-profit subsidiaries to supplement the revenues from their non-profit hospital operations. Some non-profit systems are even considering offering stock in these subsidiaries, a move that would further blur the once clear-cut line between for-profits and non-profits.

Intermountain Healthcare Inc., a voluntary chain in Salt Lake City, now has three for-profit subsidiaries. One offers insurance; another provides shared services; the third, a professional services corporation, will manage operations such as clinics, outpatient surgical centers, and occupational medicine programs.

The Health Central System in Minneapolis is also in the midst of corporate restructuring. Like Intermountain, this 23-hospital group is diversifying into the insurance business. It also plans to manage three housing centers for the elderly. Research Health Services in Kansas City completed a reorganization in 1982 and is moving into the commercial laboratory business. The Alexian Brothers of America, Inc., in Elk Grove Village, Illinois, is also restructuring. According to Sam Torres, Vice President of Alexian Brothers Health Management, the religious systems now "understand that being competitive and being growth oriented is compatible with being church oriented . . . We can't afford to sit quietly and allow the proprietaries to take over health care—including us."[13]

In the coming years consolidation of the voluntary hospital industry is likely to continue through the demise of the weaker institutions, or their absorption in the expanding non-profit and for-profit chains. Their growth, in turn, is certain to be accompanied by diversification into non-hospital based services, including surgi-centers, emergi-centers, and alcoholism, drug, obesity, and wellness clinics.

The Impact on Health Care Services

A judgment as to whether this trend toward proprietarization should be encouraged or discouraged ought not to depend on an uncritical ideologically-based belief, but on a pragmatic assessment of its consequences for health care services—in particular on access, costs, quality, and accountability.

Access. The proprietary sector has made it clear that it feels little or no obligation to serve the medically indigent and only limited obligation to serve Medicaid patients. Nationally, the for-profit chains have a much smaller proportion of Medicaid patients than the average hospital. In states such as Texas, Tennessee, and Florida, which have low Medicaid reimbursement, less than 3 percent of their patients are covered by it, while in California, which reimburses for the care of Medi-Cal patients at a rate close to that offered by other third party payors, 11.45 percent of their patients qualify.[14] Similar practices are now followed by voluntaries, who rationalize them as good management practices necessary for economic survival.

Quality of care. Little is known about the quality of care in proprietary hospitals. In general it appears to be adequate. The problem arises at the system-wide level and is related to the proprietary policy of "skimming the cream"— attracting patients with the easiest diagnoses, and leaving more complicated, poorly insured cases to the public hospitals and those voluntaries still willing to take them. There is also some evidence that for-profits retain certain complicated but financially rewarding patients who may be more appropriately treated elsewhere.

Another problem arises when a hospital company acts to improve the profitability of the mix of services at a particular hospital it owns or manages. This may entail emphasizing the profitable services (e.g. surgical as opposed to medical, ancillary as opposed to routine, simple operations as opposed to complicated, etc.), increasing the intensity of care with new services and technology, and adapting the services offered to the demographics of the market area. These practices reflect a conscious decision to focus on profitability of services rather than medical necessity. There is also pressure to curtail or eliminate services that may be required in the community but not at a level sufficient to yield a profit. For example, certain ophthalmology services and therapeutic radiology.

The new DRG method of Medicare reimbursement will probably exacerbate these trends. It is also evident that physicians will be pressured to make their practices fit the demands of the market or the reimbursement system rather than a professional standard as, however imperfectly, they have in the past.[15]

In all community hospitals, both profit and non-profit, overall length of stay is declining, along with ratios of full-time equivalent personnel and staffed beds. This is a direct result of efficiency demands that may well bode ill for quality of care. The decline in length of stay poses particular hardship for the elderly. However, to the for-profit sector, this decline is a measure of increased efficiency and profitability:

> Declining length of stay increases profitability because, when you think about a hospital visit most of the actual business occurs in the first couple of days—surgery, intensive care, diagnostic testing, etc. The last part of the stay, convalescence, does not generate a lot of revenues. So if you cut that out, you don't lose profits . . . efficient hospitals are going to make more money for doing the same amount of work. An inefficient hospital is going to be paid less money for doing the same amount of work . . . From a parochial investor's perspective on these companies [for-profit corporate chains], being paid more for doing the amount of work because they are efficient is what [DRGs] really amount to.[16]

These criteria, obviously, do not take into account whether the elderly have sufficient resources for a nursing home nor whether they have family or community support to provide care. (Investment firms usually go on to encourage stockholders to purchase nursing home stocks, particularly those of the larger chains such as Beverly Enterprises, because DRGs are likely to increase the nursing home population.)

Personnel cutbacks are also common. Full-time staff are being replaced with part-timers who work without benefits and are called in only when needed.[17] This shift in staffing may be a reasonable response to demands for cost efficiency, but it is not based upon a professional judgment of the best method of providing patient care.

Costs. Data from several studies show that, when adjusted for case mix, costs and charges measured on the basis of either patient days or admissions are higher in for-profit hospitals. Lewin and Associates found that "the investor-owned hospitals priced their services considerably higher with respect to their costs than did the not-for-profit hospitals, and therefore generated higher profits.[18] Pricing differences between the groups were small for routine services (room and board) and very large for several ancillary departments."[19]

In those ancillary services such as blood transfusion and diagnostic radiology where the private chains just about broke even, the researchers found little or no difference from voluntary chains in the number of units of service delivered per patient day or per admission. Therapeutic radiology, a service which invariably runs at a loss, was virtually unavailable in investor-owned hospitals. On the other hand, the units of service per patient and per admission are higher in the corporate chains than in the voluntaries.

Pattison and Katz conclude that "there is a tension between profit maximization and medical practice in these hospitals."[20] The introduction of DRGs may change the precise manner in which hospitals maximize profits, but the drive to emphasize lucrative services and diminish or abandon unprofitable ones will continue.

Physician accountability. Physicians working in for-profit chains may experience increased pressure to practice in a manner that enhances profits; some may be more influenced by these corporate demands than they are by peer standards. Of course, the criticism that some physicians require more visits and more tests than necessary to increase their income is not new.

"There are," as Luft points out, "many gray areas in practice where any number of diagnostic tests and curative actions at widely different cost may be given with no scientific evidence indicating which is preferable . . . despite this physicians may have strong preferences concerning these alternatives and . . . there may be a correlation between economic incentives and these preferences." For example, "A great debate continues over whether certain types of coronary diseases are best managed surgically or medically . . . Yet in each situation, individual physicians tend to prefer and use one mode of treatment and do not behave as though there is a gray area that research evidence does not resolve."[21]

Although it cannot be argued that proprietarization gives birth to profit consciousness by doctors,[22] what is new is the systemic incentives that encourage such behavior in these institutions and the direct conflict they pose between professional principles and business ideology.

Conclusions

Considerable evidence indicates that the growth of the for-profit sector has reduced access, raised costs somewhat, and lessened physician accountability to professional standards. Whether the quality of care, for those who get it, has been affected remains undetermined.

As we have seen, the expansion of the private chains is also negatively affecting the performance of voluntary and public hospitals. What can be done to reverse these trends and to encourage hospitals to respond to community health needs rather than immediate fiscal pressure?

To begin developing solutions, we must consider the roots of the problem. First, between 25 and 40 million Americans have no health insurance. Universal health care coverage is not only just and ethical, it may also be essential to the preservation of the nation's voluntary and public hospitals, which serve the broad health needs of the public.

Second, differences in rates of reimbursement encourage skimming of more lucrative patients and dumping of poorly insured patients on the dwindling number of hospitals willing to serve them. This inequitable pattern could be alleviated by all-payer, uniform systems of reimbursement—which have already been enacted in some states and proposed nationally.

Third, insurance coverage must be sufficiently comprehensive to ensure that patients are likely to receive appropriate care rather than a treatment, often more expensive, which happens to be the only one covered by insurance. All-payer systems, now in place in a few states, that reimburse hospitals for uncompensated care are a progressive move toward universal coverage, but affect inpatient care only. These programs should be expanded to include more states and outpatient care—for the medically indigent as well as others.

Fourth, we ought to have a National Hospital Policy similar to the National Blood Policy of 1974, one which defines minimum standards of access, quality, and cost and is monitored to guarantee that low cost is not the sole criteria of excellence.

Universal coverage, uniform reimbursement rates, and comprehensive services are the characteristics of a planned, national health care system. The United States is the only industrialized nation aside from South Africa without a program embodying these fundamental characteristics. Although currently far from the top of the American political agenda, such a national program for financing and planning health care services represents the best hope of preventing the complete transformation of our health care institutions into businesses that court and serve only the wealthy and well-insured.

This is not the costly approach it is often depicted to be. In the long term, by relieving the financial pressure on those hospitals that serve everyone, and distributing the costs of caring for the uninsured equitably, a national program offers the best prospect for reducing the costs of care—and for providing quality care for all.

N O T E S

1. Arnold Relman, "Investor Owned Hospitals and Health Care Costs," *The New England Journal of Medicine*, vol. 309, no. 6, August 11, 1983, p. 370.

2. *Hospital Week*, The American Hospital Association, vol. 20, no. 33, August 17, 1984, Chicago, Illinois.

3. *Hospital Statistics*, American Hospital Association, 1983 Edition, pp. 5–6.

4. Laviollette, R., *Modern Health Care*, May 1982.

5. Linda Lowe, "Sales of Strapped Public Hospitals Bode Ill For Poor," *Atlanta Constitution*, October 1, 1982. See also "Consumer Testimony Opposing the Sale of a Public Hospital in Georgia to a For-Profit Corporation," Georgia Legal Services, Atlanta, Georgia, 1982.

6. "Public Hospital Limits Care to Tampa's Poor," *American Medical News*, April 20, 1984, vol. 27, no. 16, pp. 1 and 21.

7. Ibid.

8. Robert Sonenclar, "Investing in Health Care," *Financial World*, vol. 153, no. 16, July 25–August 7, 1984, pp. 12–16.

9. Marilyn Mannisto, "For Profit Systems Pursue Growth in Specialization and Diversification," *Hospitals*, September 1, 1981, pp. 71–76.

10. Ibid.

11. Sonenclar, op. cit.

12. Laviollette, op. cit.

13. Ibid.

14. Robert V. Pattison and Hallie M. Katz, "Investor Owned and Not-for-Profit Hospitals: A Comparison Based on California Data," *New England Journal of Medicine*, vol. 309, no. 6, pp. 347–353, August 11, 1983.

15. Ibid.

16. Sonenclar, op. cit.

17. *Trends*, American Hospital Association, Office of Public Policy Analysis, no. 82, September, 1984, Chicago, Illinois.

18. Lewin and Associates, "Studies in the Comparative Performance of Investor-Owned and Not-for-Profit Hospitals, vol. 4. The Comparative Economic Performance of a Matched Sample of Investor-Owned and Not-for-Profit Hospitals," Washington, D.C., Lewin and Associates, Inc., 1981.

19. Ibid.

20. Ibid.

21. Pattison and Katz, op. cit.

22. Ibid.

EXCLUDING MORE, COVERING LESS: THE HEALTH INSURANCE INDUSTRY IN THE UNITED STATES

Donald W. Light

Private health insurance is one of the largest institutions in the United States and growing rapidly. At the end of 1988, more than 211 million Americans depended on its protection from serious financial loss in return for $149.4 billion paid in premiums. Slightly more than one-third of this amount went to non-profit Blue Cross/Blue Shield (BC/BS) plans, and slightly less than two-thirds to commercial companies. This total is double that of 1980 ($70 billion), which was in turn more than triple the 1970 figure ($20 billion).[1] Additional premiums paid to self-insured plans and health maintenance organizations (HMOs) come to $73.7 billion in 1988, up from $17.3 billion in 1980, and were too insignificant to measure in 1970.

Through various devices used to avoid insuring high-risk individuals or paying out on claims, the insurance industry has instituted a spiral of exclusion and discrimination, so that those who need coverage most are likely to get the least and pay the most for what they get. Because these practices are inherent in competitive private insurance, it seems that as long as private health insurance companies are permitted to exist, universal health insurance is unlikely to succeed.

Origins of Health Insurance

Health insurance in this country has arisen in three basic ways: 1) people come together to help each other when illness or accident befall them (mutual benefit); 2) the state provides protection in order, among other things, to promote social harmony and a healthy, productive work force (social benefit); and 3) health care providers seek a system to guarantee payment of their bills. The American medical profession quelled attempts at mutual benefit insurance near the turn of the century and blocked the government from providing universal insurance, so that little health insurance existed before the Depression outside of certain company plans in isolated or dangerous industries.

In the late 1920s and particularly in the 1930s, when medical expenses seemed so high, hospitals, medical societies, entrepreneurs, employers, and employee groups invented a wide variety of schemes for paying medical bills.[2] The American Hospital Association set out to find and sponsor a non-competitive, non-profit insurance plan that would cover only hospital expenses, a plan that spread to most states as a multi-hospital prepayment plan called Blue Cross.[3] Thus, American health insurance began as a provider-driven system to get bills paid. Several years later, when the medical profession saw that Blue Cross was working well, it started Blue Shield plans to help patients pay their doctors' bills.[4]

The Blue Cross/Blue Shield plans were predominantly community rated but covered only groups that could pay the premium. Community rating means that everyone in the plan pays the same premium for the same benefits, as opposed to risk rating, in which premiums are based on the health risks of the individual or group. Thus, most Blue Cross plans combined a spirit of mutual benefit insurance for subscribers with professional benefit insurance for health care providers, but they did not address the need for social benefit insurance for the entire population.

A fundamental change occurred as health insurance spread rapidly. BC/BS plans went from covering 6.0 million people in 1940 to 38.8 million in 1950 and 58.1 million in 1960. Commercial plans grew faster still, from 3.7 million in 1940 to 37.0 million in 1950 to 69.2 million in 1960.

Besides reimbursing hospitals and doctors for what they actually charged rather than offering a limited package of covered services, commercial companies underbid BC/BS plans by focusing on groups of healthy, working people, beginning the erosion of community rating. The market was so large and expanded so rapidly that this erosion proceeded slowly until the 1970s, when the market became relatively saturated. Since then, and with increasing intensity in the 1980s, the health insurance industry has become a contest to see who can avoid higher risk individuals or insure them without paying out much in claims, creating a spiral of exclusion and discrimination as companies hone their practices finer and finer to exclude ever more people or health conditions. The stakes are high, because only 1 percent of the market (population) generates about 30 percent of all costs, and 5 percent generates about 50 percent. Driving the market is what could be called the Inverse Coverage Law: The more coverage people need (because they are at high risk or sick), the less likely they are to get it and the more they are likely to pay for it.

The Theory of Risk Rating

The object of commercial insurance is to calibrate premiums, exclusions, and other policy features as finely as possible to the risks of its policy holders. Behind this rational economic theory is a theory or vision of the just society, a libertarian ethic that holds it is unjust to force one person to help pay for another person's needs or welfare.[5] Charity is fine, but taxes or mandatory community-rated insurance are unjust, because they force one person to give up some of his or her freedom to pay for ameliorating the miseries of another.

In contrast, a social ethic[6] would hold that health fundamentally affects the just distribution of opportunities and resources, and therefore equal access to services that minimize the adverse effects of ill health is a prerequisite of the just society. This concept is embodied in the common view of insurance as a system for spreading serious losses over as wide a population as possible. Ironically, however, the concept that "good" and "efficient" insurance calibrates premiums and coverage according to risk factors as accurately as possible leads to no insurance at all, because then there is no risk to be spread around—the fundamental purpose of insurance. And, by creating hierarchies of risk that declare a growing number of conditions as "uninsurable" and limit coverage by risk, private insurance companies are breaking down the social function of health insurance, even for the middle class.

The language of commercial insurance contains two important terms that go along with the notion of risk rating as "good insurance." The first, "medical underwriting," refers to practices by which insurers discover risks and illnesses in applicants so that they can avoid covering them, or charge more, or appear to cover them while minimizing the claims paid out. Thus, the industry uses the term underwriting to mean the opposite of its common definition of financial support—a kind of Orwellian doublespeak to obscure that what is really taking place is medical "undermining" through underinsuring. Medical undermining is the central vehicle for carrying out the Inverse Coverage Law.

The second concept is "moral hazard." This strange term refers to the danger that policy holders may exploit their policy and the insurance company by becoming more careless once covered, either by taking greater risks than they would have before coverage or by defrauding the insurer. Such actions would not only alter the risks being insured but also the losses being claimed. Insurers are quite moralistic about moral hazards; they claim they are perpetrated by manipulators and people of bad character. But while such behavior occurs with a certain frequency, the remedies for moral hazard fall most heavily on those with genuinely serious problems.

Missing from the vocabulary of the insurance industry is a term for a complementary set of actions by insurers who sell policies under false pretenses, deny valid claims, delay payments for months, insert complex provisos that few policy holders understand, charge risk groups much more than their risks warrant, and the like. If insurers face what they call "moral hazard," then policy holders face what could be called "moral abandonment" by insurers they assume to be honest.

Risk Rating in Practice

How does the insurance industry implement its policy of risk rating which leads to the spiral of exclusion and discrimination? Risk rating as an overt policy comes in several forms. In a recent national survey, commercial insurers said they charge *higher premiums* for a growing list of conditions, including such common ones as allergies, asthma, back strain, alcohol or drug use, hypertension (even when controlled), arthritis, obesity, and mild psychoneurosis.[7] They write special clauses within policies to *exclude coverage* for people with cataracts, migraine headaches, back disorders, varicose veins, chronic sinusitis, knee problems, and other disorders (see sidebar). They *deny coverage* to people with ulcerative colitis, diabetes, cancer, epilepsy, alcohol or drug abuse, severe obesity, and, of course, AIDS. Insurance companies also *redline entire industries,*

RISK CLASSIFICATION OF HEALTH CONDITIONS BY COMMERCIAL HEALTH INSURERS

Higher Premiums	Exclusion Waiver	Denial
Allergies	Cataract	AIDS
Asthma	Gallstones	Ulcerative colitis
Back strain	Fibroid tumor (uterus)	Cirrhosis of liver
Hypertension	Hernia (hiatal/inguinal)	Diabetes mellitus
(controlled)	Migraine headaches	Leukemia
Arthritis	Pelvic inflammatory disease	Schizophrenia
Gout	Chronic otitis media (recent)	Hypertension
Glaucoma	Spine/back disorders	(uncontrolled)
Obesity	Hemorrhoids	Emphysema
Psychoneurosis (mild)	Knee impairment	Stroke
Kidney stones	Asthma	Obesity (severe)
Emphysema	Allergies	Angina (severe)
(mild - moderate)	Varicose veins	Coronary artery disease
Alcoholism/drug use	Sinusitis, chronic or severe	Epilepsy
Heart murmur	Fractures	Lupus
Peptic ulcer		Alcoholism/drug use
Colitis		

Source:

AIDS and Health Insurance, Washington, DC: Office of Technology Assessment, 1988.

such as beauty shops, hotels, restaurants, trucking companies, and even law firms, hospitals, and nursing homes (see sidebar).

One cannot assume that these practices are based on solid empirical and statistical analysis. Groups find that they receive quite different rates from different insurers, a phenomenon that is rarely scrutinized by a regulatory body but which suggests that the actuarial science of risk rating and its application are far from scientific. Aside from the ways in which marketing and profit strategies may affect such premiums, when researchers ask insurance companies to rate the risk of the same cases, they give widely different answers.[8]

Even if one embraces the libertarian ethic of risk rating, evidence indicates that it is not done fairly. For example, the BC/BS plan of New Jersey decided in 1988 to risk rate its community-rate pool. It issued page after page of specific weight factors by age, sex, and county of residence; yet it turned out that these weights had no empirical basis.[9] The weights included inexplicable patterns, such as women age 35 being charged 30 percent more than men in one county but being charged no more in another county. Yet no official questioned them, including the professional staff in the Department of Insurance, which approved all of them without exception. Only a suit mounted by a coalition of citizens' groups determined that they were all illegal (see ''NJ Citizens Stop Blue Cross Discrimination,'' *Vital Signs*, Winter 1990).

Several new practices designed to reduce costs are intensifying risk rating without necessarily being identified as such. In *within-group underwriting*, insurers are going into small and even middle-sized groups (of up to 100) to risk rate individuals. Up to now, individuals with health problems who were in an existing group were covered once they passed the initial waiting period. However, a group premium can be lowered if exclusion clauses are written for preexisting conditions or if certain people within the group are denied coverage altogether. By 1987, a national survey of mid-size to large employers found that 57 percent used preexisting condition clauses. Insurers use them on nearly all small groups under 50, which make up over 80 percent of all businesses.[10] A 1988 survey of insurers by the U.S. Office of Technology Assessment found that three-quarters of commercial insurers and Blue Cross plans either screen for high-risk members of groups or plan to.[11]

Renewal underwriting is another example of doublespeak. Although the term suggests that a policy holder will be financially supported once again, in practice it means that each time the policy is renewed, the insurer goes through the group to identify anyone who has acquired a new risk or medical problem that warrants exclusion or denial.[12] In addition to those denied coverage by this practice, some 10.8 percent of the labor force changes jobs each year and therefore is subject to initial waiting periods that are part of almost all private insurance.

In what can be called *policy churning*, insurers, their agents, and employers are joining hands to cut costs at the subscribers' expense.[13] While "churning" a stock portfolio generates more commissions, policy churning aims to keep the premiums low by having employers change policies each time the initial waiting period runs out. Waiting periods are a principal reason why first-year premiums are low, because anyone in the group with medical problems gets no coverage for that problem during that time. While originally instituted to reduce "moral hazard," waiting periods combined with policy churning mean that nobody with a medical condition at turnover time ever gets covered. The practice also generates a handsome first-year commission for insurance agents, whose job it is to help employers find the least expensive policy, and the insurer has few claims to pay out. In short, everybody wins except the sick who do not time their medical problems or pregnancies precisely, and the health care providers left with unpaid bills.

Genetic and biological research will soon enable insurers to greatly refine and expand risk rating to cover large segments of the population. Genes or genetic markers have already been found for a long list of diseases, and evidence of hereditary patterns has been found in a still longer list.[14] Although the goal of this research is prevention and treatment, its results can be used by insurers and employers to screen out people with risks. Massive screening already takes place for employment and life insurance. Screening to deny health insurance is a natural, if ironic, next step. In addition, the insurance industry is constructing more sophisticated models that combine the weighted product of multiple risks, such as being female and the daughter of a mother who had multiple sclerosis. About 700 insurers share such data through a central data bank known as the Home Office Reference Laboratory.[15]

These activities already are creating a new class of people who are neither sick nor well but "at risk," which can be seen as "a new medical limbo between health and illness."[16] Although the scientific probability of an individual's contracting a given condition may be small and is often the result of interactions

EXAMPLES OF INDUSTRIES DEEMED
INELIGIBLE FOR HEALTH INSURANCE
UNDER SELECTED COMMERCIAL PLANS

Amusement parks
Aviation
Auto dealers
Barber and beauty shops
Bars and taverns
Car washes
Commercial fishing
Construction
Convenience stores
Domestic help
Entertainment/athletic groups
Exterminators
Foundries
Grocery stores
Hospitals and nursing homes
Hotels/motels
Insurance agencies
Janitorial services
Junkyards/refuse collection
Law firms
Liquor stores
Logging or mining operations
Moving companies
Parking lots
Physicians' practices
Restaurants
Roofing companies
Security guard firms
Trucking firms

Source:

Promoting Health Insurance in the Workplace: State and Local Initiatives to Increase Private Coverage, Chicago: American Hospital Association, 1988; and interviews with insurance companies.

with other factors, when in doubt the institutional dynamics of risk rating lead insurers to exclude people with these conditions. Yet recent research shows that even age and sex explain little of the variance in medical expenditures because there is as much variance in expenditures within such groups as between them.[17] Thus, risk rating creates a hierarchy of statuses, albeit biased and inaccurate, from admirable and desired to outcast.

Containing Costs

Besides risk rating, insurers use a number of devices that they claim are cost-containment measures independent of risk rating, since they apply to all holders of a given group policy. These include *waiting periods* (usually 12 months) during which new enrollees get no coverage for pre-existing conditions; *deductibles* (usually $500); *copayments* (usually 20 or 50 percent) that the policy holder pays of any stipulated bill; and *payment caps* per treatment, per year, or per lifetime. However, because the impact of these measures is proportional to the medical expenses of subscribers, they are a de facto form of risk rating. These measures can be designed with such a goal in mind, as when inadequate coverage is offered for mental health services or nursing home care.

The growth in these strategies for containing or shifting costs by thinning coverage has been phenomenal. In one of the few longitudinal data sets assembled, Hewitt Associates found that between 1982 and 1987, the percentage of salaried employees in large firms who had to pay a deductible rose from 29 to 65 percent, and the percentage of plans covering all surgery dropped to 15.[18] By 1990, only 5 to 10 percent of all firms did not require employees to pay part of all bills, usually 20 percent up to a ceiling of $1,000 to $2,000.[19]

As means for containing costs, however, these measures do not work very well because patients have little control over costs, particularly for serious problems. The main effect of such strategies is to shift significant amounts of medical expenses back to the individual, so these practices only "save money" in the sense of reducing the amount of claims paid by the insurer. Deductibles and copayments reduce minor discretionary visits of the "worried well," but they also reduce preventive visits and early detection of problems. Whether this saves money or not in the long run is a complex question that depends on many factors.[20] Patients with more serious problems, however, face complex and anxious decisions over which they have little control.

At the macro level, competitive risk-rated health insurance increases overall costs. First, it simply shifts more of the cost to higher risk groups and individuals. This means that about half the employers in a metropolitan area pay more than the overall average. Second, the additional costs of creating thousands of different policies, marketing them, evaluating bids to choose one, monitoring them, and handling hundreds of different claims forms adds at least 8 percent to everyone's bill.[21] Third, insurers create such a bewildering array of policy variations that it becomes very difficult to compare them, even for companies with full-time benefits officers. Finally, the competitive risk-rated market pits one employer against another and thus prevents united efforts to manage health care costs. This causes everyone to be worse off over time as health care expenses continue to rise at about twice the rate of general inflation. Most effective measures, like the total budget caps and fee schedules used by other countries, are not possible unless buyers are united.[22] Finally, the deregulated market, where true competition cannot often take place, lures fraudulent operators to offer shell policies that in fact pay no claims at all.[23]

The other reason given by insurance companies for using these measures is to reduce so-called reactive risk—that created by actions of policy holders. Aside from elective visits, however, there is little evidence that reactive risk by patients is a serious reality. While the owner of a building might think, "Now that I have fire insurance, I'll get this building torched," it is difficult to imagine a person saying, "Now that I have health insurance, I'll damage my body and see if I can run up large medical bills." Even acts of neglect, such as not keeping the roof of a building in good repair, do not make sense in health care because the property is the owner's own body and psyche.

The reality of cost containment is that the large number of people with ongoing, preexisting medical conditions over which they have no control who are excluded from coverage during waiting periods is far greater than the number of people who wait to get insurance until they become ill or pregnant. And once insured, people's ability to shop by price or to decide whether a given additional procedure is necessary or not is very limited. Indeed, no other industrialized nation uses waiting periods, deductibles, or co-payments to any significant degree, and yet all have been much more effective at controlling medical expenditures than the United States.[24]

Avoiding Payments

The spiral of exclusion begins with de jure risk rating, continues with de facto underinsuring by shifting portions of medical bills back to patients, and ends with strategies to avoid paying claims. The bottom line of many risk-rating and cost-shifting measures is to reduce the number of claims paid. Evidence from the field indicates that insurers, under the pressure of competition and cost containment by employers, are reducing claims in still more underhanded ways.

One method is creating *elaborated rules for claims eligibility* which, if not followed, disqualify a legitimate medical procedure from coverage. Physicians and patients constantly battle these fine-print provisions, which seem to be appearing with increasing frequency. For example, some policies stipulate that a patient must call a number within 24 hours before an operation to confirm it. Many patients are so anxious and so busy during those 24 hours that making such a call is the last thing on their mind. In one such case, a former student failed to call as she made complex arrangements for her family and job and now faces $11,000 of uncovered bills. Her new policy with this "gotcha" clause had recently been written by her employer with a new insurer to slow the rise of medical costs. Her employer is a hospital.

An increasing number of insurance companies also seem to practice *claims harassment*, with employers as consenting partners.[25] Some companies are known to deny all claims on the first round and then see how many policy holders have the time, organization, and persistence to fight the denial. Making patients responsible for their claims is itself a form of harassment, since it pits the least-skilled, least-experienced party in the health care transaction against the insurance company. Very few other nations involve patients in claims at all. Forms that are difficult to read or understand, requirements that the patient must coordinate a claim with providers, and claims departments with too few telephone lines are other common forms of harassment. All are probably quite effective in both delaying payments so the insurer can gain a few months of additional interest on the funds and reducing the claims finally paid.

A related phenomena might be called *exclusion by association*. Patients who have exclusion clauses that deny coverage for medical expenses of a chronic condition report that their insurers extend the denial to other medical problems the insurer claims are related. For example, a diabetic with an exclusion clause for her diabetes contracted heart problems. The insurer excluded the medical bills from payment because the heart problems were "associated" with her diabetes. This woman has managed her diabetes for 20 years and thus coped with the exclusion of her diabetes from coverage; but the invocation of "exclusion by association" threatens her ability to afford care for grave health problems beyond her control.

Discrimination

All of these practices systematically discriminate against disadvantaged minorities, older workers, those with chronic conditions, lower income workers, and employees working for small establishments.[26] They also discriminate against groups that include individuals defined as high risk, because employers are reluctant to hire them. The trends of unemployment, poverty, and the shift to industries that have poor health insurance all contribute to the spiral of exclusion.

The overall impact of these practices appears to be extensive. As of 1984, about 56 million people, or a quarter of the population under 65, were estimated to have inadequate coverage for major medical expenses.[27] A recent study found that 46.8 percent of all unpaid hospital bills in a large Midwest sample came from patients who had health insurance.[28] Coverage is probably even thinner for doctors' bills.

"High risk" and "uninsurability" are not categories in nature but artifacts of the risk-based view of private insurance. In effect, risk rating is the negative commodification of pain, suffering, and disability. It is the process of pricing both the present and future value of illnesses so as to calculate the importance of *not* selling coverage for them.

Crisis and System Failure

What are the institutional dynamics by which "good" commercial health insurance drives the industry to exclude more and more conditions and claims? The crisis of the capitalist economy[29] has prompted employers, as well as the state as the largest insurer of all, to overcome all forms of resistance[30] and transform themselves from passive payers to active buyers intent on stopping the fastest-rising cost in their budgets.

For this and other reasons, a growing number of corporations are becoming self-insured, and this has shocked the health insurance industry.[31] It has meant a mass exodus of large corporate customers and the reduction of insurers to mere administrators, if anything, of health benefit programs. It put insurers on notice that they would have to work hard for any market share they earned.

Service institutions, like insurers, now compete to avoid people with unprofitable disorders. Ironically, costs increase. According to Estes and Alford, "State costs are rising both as a result of the costs of competition, privatization and pluralistic financing, and from the additional costs incurred by the state's necessity to subsidize the most difficult (and least profitable) clients who are being dumped on the public sector as too costly for either the nonprofits or for-profits to treat or serve."[32]

The result is that health insurance companies, as a population or system of organizations, are undermining their own legitimacy by insuring less and less of the population's health risks by acting as "good" insurers are supposed to act.

With each passing year, the risk rating and cost shifting intensify. Thus, the appearance of AIDS throws the insurance/delivery system complex into crisis.[33] Rising costs and greater dependence of everyone on insurance intensify the impact of inadequate or no coverage. Medicaid serves as a large catchbasin at the bottom of the health insurance system.

It is increasingly clear that the only viable alternative is national health insurance. However, all the prevailing proposals retain competitive commercial insurance companies. Moreover, none of them address the drive of those companies to avoid high risks and minimize claims payments, even if direct risk rating were prohibited. Only a plan that eliminates the commercial factor has a chance of providing equal access to health care regardless of risk.

NOTES

1. *1986–1987 Source Book of Health Insurance Data*, Washington, DC: Health Insurance Association of America (1988), pp. 9, 28.

2. Williams, Pierce, *The Purchase of Medical Care Through Fixed Periodic Payments*, New York: National Bureau of Economic Research, 1932; Burrow, J. G., *Organized Medicine in the Progressive Era: The Move Toward Monopoly*, Baltimore: Johns Hopkins University Press, 1971; Goldberg, L. G., and Greenberg, W., "The Emergence of Physician-Sponsored Health Insurance: An Historical Perspective," in Greenberg, ed., *Competition in the Health Care Sector: Past, Present, and Future*, Germantown, MD: Aspen Systems, 1978; and Starr, Paul, *The Social Transformation of American Medicine*, New York: Basic Books, 1982.

3. Rorem, C. Rufus, *Non-Profit Hospital Service Plans*, Chicago: Commission on Hospital Service, 1940; and Reed, Louis, *Blue Cross and Medical Service Plans*, Washington, DC: Federal Security Agency, 1947.

4. Reed, op cit.; Anderson, O. W., *Blue Cross Since 1929: Accountability and the Public Trust*, Cambridge, MA: Ballinger, 1975; Law, S. A., *Blue Cross: What Went Wrong?* New Haven: Yale University Press, 1975; and Starr, op. cit.

5. Nozick, Robert, *Anarchy, State and Utopia*, Oxford, England: Blackwells, 1974.

6. Rawls, John, *A Theory of Justice*, Cambridge, MA: Harvard University Press, 1971; Daniels, Norman, *Just Health Care*, New York: Cambridge University Press, 1985; and Daniels, "Insurability and the HIV Epidemic: Ethical Issues in Underwriting," *Milbank Quarterly*, 1990:68, pp. 497–525.

7. *AIDS and Health Insurance*, Washington, DC: U.S. Office of Technology Assessment, 1988.

8. Neil, H. A. W., and Mant, D., "Cholesterol Screening and Life Assurance," *British Medical Journal*, 1991:302, pp. 891–893.

9. *Community Rate Schedules and Development*, Newark, NJ: Blue Cross and Blue Shield of New Jersey, 1988.

10. *Indemnity Plans: Costs, Design, and Funding*, Princeton NJ: Foster Higgins, 1990.

11. *AIDS and Health Insurance*.

12. Nadel, M. V. "Health Insurance: Availability and Adequacy for Small Businesses," Washington, DC: U.S. General Accounting Office, 1990; and *Health Insurance: Cost Increases Lead to Coverage Limitations and Cost Shifting*, Washington, DC: General Accounting Office, 1990.

13. Ibid.

14. Stone, Deborah, "At Risk in the Welfare State," *Social Research*, 1989:56, pp. 591–633; and Hunt, Morton, "The Total Gene Screen," *New York Times Magazine*, January 19, 1986.

15. Stone, Deborah, "AIDS and the Moral Economy of Insurance," *American Prospect*, Spring 1990, No. 1, p. 64.

16. Ibid., p. 62.

17. Cave, Douglas G., Schweitzer, Stuart O., and Lackenbruch, Peter A., "Adjusting Employer Group Capitation Premiums by Community Rating by Class Factors," *Medical Care*, 1989:27, pp. 887–899.

18. *Salaried Employee Benefits Provided by Major U.S. Employers in 1982–87*, Chicago: Hewitt Associates, 1988.

19. Sullivan, C. B., and Rice, T., "The Health Insurance Picture in 1990," *Health Affairs*, 1991:10(2), pp. 104–115.

20. Russell, L., *Is Prevent Better Than Cure*? Washington, DC: Brookings Institution, 1986.

21. Woolhandler and Himmelstein, "The Deteriorating Administrative Efficiency of the U.S. Health Care System," *New England Journal of Medicine*, 1991:324, pp. 1253–1258.

22. Glaser, William, *Health Insurance in Practice*, Jossey-Bass, 1991.

23. Meier, B., "A Growing U.S. Affliction: Worthless Health Policies," *New York Times*, January 4, 1992, pp. 1, 46.

24. Glaser, op. cit.; and Scheiber, G. J., and Poullier, J. P., "International Health Spending: Issues and Trends," *Health Affairs*, 1991:10(1), pp. 106–116.

25. Grumet, G. W., "Health Care Rationing through Inconvenience: The Third Party's Secret Weapon," *New England Journal of Medicine*, 1989:321, pp. 106–116.

26. Trevino, F. M., Moyer, M. E., Valdez, R. B., and Stroup-Benham, C. A., "Health Insurance Coverage and Utilization of Health Services by Mexican Americans, Mainland Puerto Ricans, and Cuban Americans," *Journal of the American Medical Association*, 1991:265, pp. 233–237; Saywell, R. M., Jr., Zollinger, T. W., Chu, D. K., MacBeth, C. A., and Sechrist, M. E., "Hospital and Patient Characteristics of Uncompensated Hospital Care: Policy Implications," *Journal of Health Politics, Policy and Law*, 1989:14, pp. 287–307; Wenniker, M. B., and Epstein, A. M., "Racial Inequalities in the Use of Procedures for Patients with Ischemic Health Disease in Massachusetts," *Journal of the American Medical Association*, 1989:261, pp. 253–257; and Farley, Pamela, "Who Are the Underinsured?" *Milbank Memorial Fund Quarterly*, 1985:63, pp. 476–503.

27. Farley, op. cit.

28. Saywell et al., op. cit.

29. O'Connor, James, *The Fiscal Crisis of the State*, New York: St. Martin's Press, 1973; Offe, C., *Contradictions of the Welfare State*, Cambridge, MA: M.I.T. Press, 1984; and Harrison, Bennett, and Bluestone, Barry, *The Great U-Turn*, New York: Basic Books, 1988.

30. Alford, Robert, *Health Care Politics: Ideological and Interest Group Barriers to Reform*, Chicago: University of Chicago Press, 1975.

31. Goldsmith, J., "Death of a Paradigm: The Challenge of Competition," *Health Affairs*, Fall 1984:3(3), pp. 5–19.

32. Estes, C. L., and Alford, Robert, "Systemic Crisis and the Nonprofit Sector," *Theory and Society*, 1990:19, p. 175.

33. Perrow, Charles, and Guillen, Mauro F., *The AIDS Disaster: The Failure of Organizations in New York and the Nation*, New Haven: Yale University Press, 1990.

THE THREAT AND PROMISE OF MEDICAID MANAGED CARE: A MIXED REVIEW

Ronda Kotelchuck

Capitalizing on a highly unusual political consensus, the New York State Legislature in the spring of 1991 quietly adopted one of the most sweeping changes in the state's Medicaid program since its inception. This change, if carried out as designed, has the potential to significantly reshape New York State's health system, either for good or for ill.

The Medicaid Managed Care Act of 1991 requires that within five years, half of the 2.9 million poor New Yorkers who receive Medicaid be enrolled in managed care programs. To achieve this ambitious goal, the counties that administer the program will clearly eventually have to make it mandatory. For these clients, Medicaid will no longer purchase individual medical services on a fee-for-service basis. Instead it will pay a single price for a complete package of services. No longer will it pay physicians, clinics, hospitals, and other providers directly for the services they produce. Instead, it will pay plans—health maintenance organizations or HMO-like organizations—that will be responsible for providing all services to which Medicaid recipients are entitled (with the exception of long-term care, which will remain unchanged).

The Medicaid Managed Care Program is a major departure from previous New York State health policy. It will severely limit freedom for Medicaid recipients to choose their own providers, and it will sanction a fundamentally separate system of care for the poor. It will introduce incentives to reduce not only the cost of care, but the use of services as well. It will inject competition into New York's largely nonprofit, highly regulated health care environment. It will create a major new player in New York's health system—the plan or HMO—and impose this player between the Medicaid program and medical providers. And, finally, it will create enormous demand for the most precious of commodities in New York—primary care providers willing to serve poor populations.

New York's Medicaid Managed Care Program offers an ambiguous mix of opportunities for improving care for the poor and threats to its access and quality. The threats and problems are serious enough that, given a choice, few advocates for the poor would have opted for managed care as good social policy. In New York State, and increasingly in other states as well, however, Medicaid managed care is no longer a policy choice. It has become a fact. Moreover, it is a fact that is unlikely to be reversed, at least in the near term.

What should people of conscience and of action do in the face of this new reality? Unless one thinks managed care can and should be turned back, the question now becomes: How can the threats that managed care poses be contained, minimized, and eliminated? What new opportunities does managed care offer for building a system that will guarantee accessible, appropriate, and high-quality care for the poor?

Why Managed Care Passed

The consensus to enact New York's program stemmed from its double promise of reducing costs, while simultaneously improving the quality of care offered to Medicaid recipients, as well as from the growing aura of managed care as a free-market panacea to the entrenched problems of the health system. Its authors also saw managed care as the last and best hope for saving the embattled Medicaid program.

Cost Savings

The promise of cost savings was clearly the strongest motivating force behind passage of the Medicaid Managed Care Program. New York's $14 billion Medicaid program is enormous, and spending, rising at 20 percent a year over the last two years, is widely perceived to be out of control.

Unlike most states, where the federal and state governments share Medicaid costs, in New York a third party, the county, pays 25 percent of the cost, adding strong local support for cost cutting as well. New York City, for example, which encompasses five counties, pays $2 billion, and many counties pay as much as 30 percent of their tax dollars to support their share of Medicaid.

The problem of Medicaid spending was set in bold relief in the spring of 1991, when steep recession engulfed the entire northeast region of the country. New York City found itself mired in the second year of a major fiscal crisis, and the state for the first time faced a major budget deficit of its own. Calls for "structural reform"—that is, cuts that would permanently reduce spending—joined with an increasingly ugly ideological climate to make the Medicaid program particularly vulnerable. Eleven years of the Reagan-Bush victim blaming and racial and class polarization set the stage for attacks on social spending. Moreover, the rapidly declining standard of living and the hardships of recession on the middle and working classes made additional taxation unthinkable. In no way could a social program for the poor, of the size and growing at the speed of Medicaid, be held harmless through a round of major budget cuts. The only issue was how, not whether, the program was to be cut.

Cuts in programs such as Medicaid can be targeted in four ways: tightening eligibility of recipients for the program, eliminating benefits covered by the program, cutting prices paid to the providers, and reducing utilization of services by recipients. Traditionally, New York City, the state assembly, and the governor, all dominated by the Democratic party, have tended to line up in defense of Medicaid recipients, staunchly opposing reductions in eligibility and benefits and favoring cuts to providers. The conservative, Republican-dominated senate, on the other hand, siding with the hospital and provider interests, historically has taken the opposite tack, preserving reimbursement to providers at the expense of recipients.

Reimbursement paid to providers in New York State has already been highly controlled, however, removing it as the most likely candidate. Physician fees are second lowest in the country, causing the virtual withdrawal of private physicians from the program; outpatient rates have been frozen since 1981 and are now the single largest source of hospital financial losses; and the rate of increase in reimbursement to hospitals for inpatient stays is already among the lowest in the country.

By contrast, utilization of Medicaid services in New York is very high. Those eligible for Medicaid in New York, for example, use 2,600 hospital days per thousand people compared to 760 days for non-Medicaid patients and 15 ambulatory care visits per year, compared to a national average of 5.3 visits. Utilization is particularly high among one group of Medicaid recipients, those on Home Relief (single adults), who use 4,440 hospital days per thousand and average 30 visits per year.

An earlier program adopted in 1989 for Home Relief recipients and extended in 1990 to all Medicaid recipients targeted reductions in utilization and paved the way for managed care. The Medicaid Utilization Threshold (MUTS) Program imposes fixed limits on the number of pharmacy and outpatient services Medicaid will cover for each recipient. As cost-cutting pressures intensified, it became clear that MUTS would be extended to include more and more services, and the limits would also be ratcheted down. Managed care offers an attractive alternative to the arbitrary limits of the MUTS program, by using individual case management by a physician or other "gatekeeper" to control and decide what services are needed.

Managed care was the near-perfect political compromise. The program targets reductions in utilization, while preserving eligibility, benefits, and, in the first instance, rates. Its impact on both recipients and providers is attenuated, lessening the political resistance of advocates for both groups and definitely posing it as the lesser of the four evils.

The program's advocates in the legislature viewed managed care, with its powerful political consensus, as a strategy for preserving Medicaid in the face of fiscal and political attack, rather than a major cost-cutting tool. Under the cost-control rubric, managed care could be used to preserve benefits and eligibility that would surely be lost to the rest of the program. Wisely, they assumed no immediate savings to the state, unlike their New York City colleagues, who eagerly rushed to project $30 million savings in the city share of Medicaid alone (and a total savings of $100 million) in the first year.

Improving Care

If its business approach, financial incentives, and cost-cutting potential made managed care attractive to conservatives, its potential to improve care for poor people appealed powerfully to liberals and others. Supporters of managed care articulated a devastating critique of the care Medicaid currently provides. Not only does it spend enormous amounts of money, but Medicaid purchases care that is fragmented, inappropriate, and incapable of meeting the exploding health care needs of New York's poor communities.

While managed care may limit the patient's freedom to choose a provider, under the current system this freedom is an illusory one. Medicaid recipients are free only to choose among Medicaid mills, weeks if not months spent waiting for an outpatient appointment, or an overcrowded emergency room. They cannot choose the kind of care that will address their needs.

The missing ingredient is primary care. Extraordinarily low Medicaid physician rates (currently $11 per visit) have driven private physicians from low-income communities, with the exception of a few who practice in Medicaid mills. Study after study has documented the lack of primary care physicians available to New York's low-income population. The most notable of these, released by the Community Service Society in 1989, surveyed primary care physicians practicing in nine low-income communities. After factoring out those who did not meet basic standards of primary care, the study found *a total of only 28 primary care physicians serving 1.7 million people.*

The consequences are evident. Hospitalization rates for conditions treatable by primary care, such as asthma, diabetes, and hypertension, are nearly four times higher for Medicaid patients (35.2 admissions per thousand) than they are for others (9.60 admissions per thousand). They constitute nearly 20 percent of all admissions, and the proportion is growing.

Lack of primary and preventive care played an important role in New York City's recent hospital overcrowding crisis, which at its height threatened access to care for everyone, regardless of class or status. During 1989 and 1990, in-patient occupancy soared to over 100 percent in many of New York's major hospitals, and emergency rooms backed up, with patients often waiting days for admission. The gridlock is largely attributable to the urgent and growing health care needs of the poor, many of which could have been addressed at an earlier stage, less expensively, and more appropriately by primary care.

In contrast to the current system, managed care promises to purchase the product most needed by the poor—a comprehensive and coordinated package of services whose centerpiece is primary care.

The Panacea

The final selling point for managed care was its growing aura as a panacea for the ills of the health system. If planning and regulation characterized health policy in the 1970s, and competition dominated the 1980s, the 1990s are fast becoming the decade of managed care.

New York is the first in a rush of financially beleaguered states joining the 6 that already rely heavily, if not solely, on managed care for the delivery of Medicaid services. Another 27 are experimenting with Medicaid managed care demonstrations. Managed care both for Medicaid and for privately insured beneficiaries appears to be the single strongest point of agreement between Republicans and "pay-or-play" Democrats—those who favor a payroll tax on employers who don't provide insurance to cover the uninsured. And the nation's newspaper of record, *The New York Times*, never misses a chance to lobby for "managed competition," even if its editors are hard put to explain exactly what this is. Managed care is well on its way to taking on an ideological life and becoming a bandwagon of its own.

Payment Mechanism

The boldest departure of the New York State Medicaid Managed Care Program is in its payment mechanism. Instead of paying for individual services as they occur on a fee-for-service basis, under managed care the state will pay a single price per enrollee—or capitation rate—representing the average cost of the entire package of services covered by Medicaid (with the exception of long-term care, which is excluded from managed care and will continue payment on its current basis). While the program allows for two other forms of payment (capitation for primary care services only and continued fee-for-service payment with a monthly case management fee), full capitation is the model heavily favored by the state.

Capitation is paid to a plan, which can be an HMO or a prepaid health service plan (a Medicaid-only HMO-like organization). The plan either directly provides the required services (primary, specialty, emergency, and inpatient care and a variety of other services) or contracts with a network of other providers to do so. The plan selects these providers based on their availability, convenience, and price.

Managed care reverses the financial incentives of the traditional fee-for-service system. Under the latter, a provider is paid every time a service is rendered, and thus benefits from providing more services. Under managed care, the plan is paid a fixed sum, and must provide all the care required regardless of cost, thus placing it "at risk." If the cost of providing the required services is less than the capitation rate, the plan profits. If it is more, the plan loses. This creates incentives for plans to reduce the use of expensive services, to compete for healthier enrollees, and to seek low-cost participating providers.

Managed care is both an extension and the culmination of the movement to fixed pricing in health care represented by DRGs (diagnostic related groups) for inpatient care, AVGs (ambulatory visit groups) for outpatient care, and RUGs (resource utilization groups) for long-term care.

Model of Care

The New York State program specifies a laudable model of care. Under managed care, each recipient must be assigned his or her own primary care provider. The patient will see the same provider, visit after visit, creating the opportunity to build a meaningful relationship in which the provider gets to know the patient and his or her family and social context. Appointments must be available within a maximum of four weeks for a new patient and within two weeks for followup care.

When needed, the provider refers the patient for specialty care, but afterward the patient and the relevant information are returned to the primary care provider for followup and ongoing care. The primary care physician also admits the patient to the hospital, follows him or her during the stay, and continues to provide care after discharge. Patients can call their primary care provider or a backup physician 24 hours a day to ask questions and seek advice. Care outside the plan must be authorized, or it will not be reimbursed. Thus, with the exception of genuine emergencies, other providers will generally refer the patient back to his or her plan.

To reinforce this model of care, the state has issued strict standards for who qualifies as a primary care provider. Providers may be physicians, nurse practitioners, or physician's assistants and must work at least half time in the managed care program. Physicians must be board certified or, if board eligible, be certified within five years in a primary care specialty. They must also have admitting privileges and attend their patients when hospitalized. Providers must offer 24-hour telephone access for patients and must also offer evening and/or weekend hours.

Responsibility for the Program

Counties are responsible for implementing and monitoring the program. (In the case of New York City's five counties, the city itself is responsible.) In each of the first five years the state will designate 20 counties to participate; each county must then submit its own plan specifying how it will reach the goals of enrolling 10 percent of the Medicaid population in the first year, 25 percent in the third, and 50 percent in the fifth year. Although these targets are extremely ambitious, no penalty or enforcement is built into the legislation if they are not achieved. The state can intervene if a county refuses to participate or does not submit a satisfactory plan.

Counties bear first-line responsibility for assuring the quality and accessibility of care under the managed care program. Together with the state, they approve which plans will be allowed to participate and the particular arrangements these plans propose for providing the care. Counties are also responsible for the enrollment process as well as for monitoring the plan's operations to ensure that quality, continuity, and access to care are acceptable.

Patients' Rights

While counties may make the program voluntary for recipients, the extremely aggressive enrollment targets ensure that the Medicaid Managed Care Program will eventually be mandatory. Under a mandatory program, recipients must be offered a choice of three plans within a geographically accessible area, and within each plan, a choice of three primary care providers. Recipients can change plans after the first six months and can change their primary care provider at any time for cause.

Managed care is to include all four categories of Medicaid recipients (Aid to Families with Dependent Children; Home Relief; Blind, Aged, and Disabled; and Medicaid only). Particular recipients may be exempted from the program, however, including those who can demonstrate a pre-existing relationship with a primary care provider, and those with conditions considered incompatible with managed care. The managed care program guarantees most recipients six months of coverage even if they lose Medicaid eligibility during that period.

The Plans

A managed care plan in its essence is an insurer. It can function solely as insurer or it can also deliver services. Plans can be health maintenance organizations (HMOs), which can serve anyone, or prepaid health service plans (Medicaid-only HMOs). They can be profit-making or nonprofit. Establishing an HMO or PHSP is a lengthy and expensive process, requiring millions of dollars and frequently years of work, guaranteeing that only a limited number of such programs will attempt to participate.

The largest managed care plan currently serving Medicaid recipients in New York City is the Health Insurance Plan of New York (HIP), a nonprofit HMO and one of the country's oldest and largest. Over the last several years, different groups within New York City's health system have developed plans to allow their constituents to participate in managed care demonstration projects. Thus, community health centers have formed nonprofit plans in the Bronx (Bronx Health Plan) and Manhattan (Centercare); the Greater New York Hospital Association is forming its own HMO, as is the network that makes up the Catholic Medical Center. The Health and Hospitals Corporation, the city's municipal hospital system, will utilize its own HMO (the Metropolitan Health Plan). The county medical societies in both Manhattan and Brooklyn are also developing plans. Empire Blue Cross/Blue Shield, as well as commercial HMOs, such as US HealthCare, Oxford, Total Health, and Cigna, will participate, at least minimally. And finally, for-profit Medicaid managed care firms from outside of New York, such as Managed Health Systems, which operates the Health/PASS program in Philadelphia, will enter the New York market.

Building Primary Care

New York State's poor lack primary care because this type of health care has been starved for resources and made the lowest priority of New York's health system. Only 4 percent of the statewide Medicaid budget is spent on primary care. Over the long run, Medicaid managed care holds the potential to build primary care capacity by increasing resources for primary care, opening up access to commercial HMOs for the poor, and creating demand for the increased training of primary care providers.

Increased Primary Care Resources

Capitation pays a fixed sum for a package of services and leaves the issue of how and how much the plan will pay for each service to the plan's discretion. Thus, capitation makes possible a reallocation of tertiary care resources into primary care, which the state, for political reasons, has been unable to achieve. Plans are free to enhance primary care services and pay primary care providers at higher rates as they wish, financing these additional costs from savings in expensive specialty, emergency, and inpatient care. Similarly, plans can finance health prevention, health promotion, and social services not previously reimbursable under Medicaid.

Managed care does this by quietly removing the locus of decision making about allocation of resources between primary and tertiary care from the level of state policy, where an unorganized and largely low-income constituency for primary care comes up against politically and economically powerful hospital interests supporting tertiary care. It moves these decisions to the invisible hand of the managed care plan and the physician case manager, both of which have incentives to reduce expensive tertiary services. In addition, capitation largely delegates rate-setting responsibility from the public policy apparatus of the state to the privacy of the individual plan. Thus, the Medicaid Managed Care Program could be viewed as an end-run around a historic impasse created by entrenched and powerful hospital forces.

Managed care also offers an end-run around a second deadlock in state primary care strategy—the question of the appropriate vehicle to deliver primary care. Should the state vest the chief responsibility with hospitals and academic medical centers, knowing that primary care will never be their priority and risking that funds will be dissipated in supporting medical education, research, overhead, and other objectives? Or should it rely on entities dedicated solely to primary care, such as neighborhood health centers or private physicians, which have no such conflicting priorities but which are small and unstable and where quality of care is much harder to regulate? Managed care simply bypasses this debate, adopting instead the plan as the chief vehicle and reducing hospitals, health centers, and private physicians to the role of contractors.

Mainstream Access

As a means of expanding primary care capacity, the state intends to "mainstream" Medicaid patients into commercial HMOs, opening up primary care resources that would ordinarily be available only to more affluent patients. The seeds for this policy were planted in 1986 when the state for the first time broke with its historical opposition to all for-profit HMOs by allowing proprietary HMOs to enter the New York market. The quid pro quo, however, was willingness to enroll Medicaid recipients. This provision has remained unenforced while the fledgling industry got its start. Now the state is calling home the industry's promises. In its 1992 session, the legislature passed a measure heavily penalizing plans that do not enroll a minimum percentage of Medicaid recipients. Overnight, commercial HMO interest in Medicaid recipients skyrocketed.

Enrollment of Medicaid recipients in commercial HMOs is a mixed blessing, however. First, the financial incentive aside, commercial HMOs—many of them independent practice associations (IPAs), which contract with physicians in private practice—have little experience and even less desire to serve poor patients. Second, Medicaid recipients are quite different than commercial enrollees in their health status and needs, their health-related social problems, and their care-seeking behavior. Medicaid patients require a very different approach in terms of both education and intervention and the resources that must be invested in both.

Primary Care Training

The Medicaid Managed Care Program creates a new opportunity to address the supply of primary care providers. It intensifies pressure on the state's medical schools and academic medical centers to train primary care physicians. Medicaid recipients are the major training resource for both. As the single largest hospital payer, Medicaid is an important revenue source, both for New York's major academic medical centers and for the municipal and community hospitals with which they are affiliated. The threat of losing half of this patient population is a powerful one, offering important leverage for change.

The six medical schools run by the New York State university system should be most subject to pressure. Despite their public funding, they are currently indistinguishable in their mission, their recruitment priorities, their program, or their product from the state's private medical schools.

Finally, unlike the medical profession, which must be browbeaten against its perceived self-interest into meeting primary care needs, mid-level professions face no such conflicts or obstacles. Nurse practitioners, physician's assistants, and nurse-midwives are dedicated to the delivery of primary care, and they are far quicker and less expensive to train than physicians.

Threats to Care

If managed care offers a number of new opportunities to improve care for the poor, so too does it pose a variety of threats to the future quality and accessibility of that care.

Financial Incentives and Competition

The most pervasive and troubling threat is generic to managed care and goes to the heart of the payment mechanism. Can the natural consequences of an incentive to underservice be corralled and channeled into providing a high-quality and accessible model of care? And will a competitive environment ever be compatible with serving the needs of the poor?

Managed care creates a financial incentive to decrease costs, largely through reduced use of expensive services. While this incentive can support a good model of care (for example, reduced utilization through good primary and preventive care), it can far more easily promote the opposite. Plans can reduce utilization in far cheaper, quicker, and more certain ways, both by design and by default. They can rely on screening and control of utilization to deny authorization for care; long waits for appointments or discourteous service to discourage patients from seeking care; and inadequate telephone lines or insufficient numbers of operators to make it impossible for Medicaid enrollees—many without telephones in their home—to gain access to the system.

Most seriously, however, good care for Medicaid recipients is certain to cost more in the short term, not less. While some Medicaid recipients may overutilize medical services, the vast majority underutilize them, discouraged by the overwhelming obstacles they face. Good managed care plans will reach out to these recipients and, in so doing, will tap into long pent-up health care needs. Bad plans, however, will reap pure profit from such underutilization. While it will be argued that competition among plans for enrollees will discourage these abuses, the freedom of the patient to change plans is highly constricted, and information about available alternatives and how to make the change is complex and forbidding.

All that stands between a dubious incentive and its natural consequences— between a good model of primary and preventive care and a mediocre or scandalous one, between willingness to treat all patients and skimming of healthy patients, between appropriate service and underservice—is the regulatory capacity and disposition of the state and the local county. Not only are these as yet undetermined and untested in the New York program, but the future does not bode well. Additional regulation flies in the face of a new, antiregulatory environment and will require the commitment of additional resources just when the state and counties are cutting administrative staff and budgets and moving rapidly toward deregulation.

Speed of Implementation

Just as Medicaid Managed Care has the potential in the long run to build primary care capacity, so the lack of such capacity in the short run poses a major roadblock to implementation and a major threat to quality of care under the system. Qualified primary care providers do not and will not exist in sufficient numbers to enroll half of the Medicaid population in five years. Nor does this timetable allow for the complex task of reorganizing the massive hospital outpatient clinics upon which the poor overwhelmingly now rely for care.

Rather than investing resources to create the needed capacity or reconsidering the timetable, however, the state is instead crafting a variety of measures that will support or even accelerate the speed with which managed care will be implemented. First, Governor Mario Cuomo is proposing to take over the 25 percent share of Medicaid costs now paid by counties. Savings to localities are tied directly to the number of recipients enrolled in managed care in the first four years of this eight-year proposition. New York City has unrealistically estimated that it could achieve $90 million in savings in the first year, causing some forces to call for an immediate mandatory program.

Second, in exempting Medicaid recipients who enroll in managed care from Medicaid cuts enacted in the 1992 session, the state legislature created a cameo of the compromises that an unreasonable timetable will entail. Because there is little capacity to enroll recipients in actual managed care programs at present, the state instead allowed them to sign up with "medical care coordinators." These can be either private physicians or outpatient clinics and are not subject to the strict standards of quality and access required of plans.

Under the pressure to enroll patients, will the state and city relax the program's standards for access and quality? If the state compromises to accept outpatient departments, could Medicaid mills be far behind? Has a tacit strategy decision been made to forcibly reorganize the system first and only then address the problems of quality and access? If this is true, will managed care have a long run? These questions remain as yet disturbingly unanswered.

Less Money for Care

Not only will access to good primary and preventive care for underserved populations cost more, managed care will actually mean fewer resources available for direct care. First, the state will deduct a guaranteed savings off the capitation it pays to the plans—a discount ranging from 5 to 15 percent of the expected average annual cost of treating the patient. Then the plan must pay for its own administrative expenses, which range anywhere from 15 to 27 percent, including the cost of administration, finance, marketing, patient and provider relations, information systems, reserve funds, re-insurance for high-risk patients, and quality assurance and utilization review programs. Finally, any surpluses or profits also come out of the premium received by the plan.

Beyond the plan, the Medicaid program must finance the cost of additional staff at both the state and local level to implement, administer, and monitor the managed care system, while continuing to operate the fee-for-service system. Thus, managed care typifies and accelerates a disturbing trend in the larger health system in which less and less money goes to the direct provision of care and more and more goes to administration and monitoring.

Two Systems of Care

The original vision was that New York State's Medicaid program would remove financial barriers to health care for the poor. By offering insurance coverage to the poor, Medicaid was supposed to assure them same access to services as the more affluent. The actuality fell woefully short of the ideal, particularly for ambulatory care, where physician fees and outpatient rates have been frozen at unrealistic levels. The inpatient rates Medicaid pays to hospitals, however, are equal to those of private insurers as a result of New York State's "all payer" approach to inpatient reimbursement. Consequently, two-thirds of all Medicaid inpatients are treated by the private sector.

Managed care closes the door on this vision of one system. It undermines the all-payer system and accepts that Medicaid patients will be treated in different settings and systems. The prospects for quality and access are not reassuring, since separate never turns out to be equal.

Reducing Costs

The Medicaid Managed Care Program was sold on its promise to control Medicaid costs. What are the prospects?

Limited Savings, Total Control

Managed care, by establishing a fixed price system, shifts financial risk to the plans and gives the state nearly total control over what it pays out. In addition, the state achieves an immediate and guaranteed savings of 5 to 15 percent, since the capitation rate it pays to plans is based on the average historical cost per Medicaid recipient, less this discount. The state at any time can ratchet down this capitation rate, although it is unlikely to do this in a period in which it wants to encourage program expansion and development.

The largest potential savings—those resulting from reduced utilization—remain within the plan as an incentive and are not available to the state. Plans can achieve substantial savings over the first several years by eliminating excessive and inappropriate utilization through case management and the provision of primary care. These are one-time savings, however, and once excess utilization has been squeezed out, costs will continue to escalate at their previous rate.

The Real Causes of Medicaid Increases

Managed care cannot possibly address the most important causes of increased Medicaid spending in New York State, however, because the real causes lie outside the populations served by managed care.

First, fully half of all Medicaid dollars pay for long-term–care patients, many of whom are middle class and either ''spend down'' or divest their resources to become eligible for Medicaid. Yet, at the legislative level, no one wants to pit the needs of the poor against the elderly. Concern about cost cutting has cut deeply enough for legislators to bite the bullet with their poor constituents, but not with their elderly or middle-class ones. Second, after 20 years of stability, the number of people on Medicaid has begun to increase notably over the last several years, reflecting increasing poverty and unemployment.

Finally, spending has also ballooned recently because the state has become very adept in exploiting the Medicaid program, with its 50 percent federal matching funds, to pay for programs that previously depended entirely on state or local funding. Thus, Medicaid has assumed the cost of many mental health and mental retardation services, as well as vast portions of bad debt and charity care at the state level and indigent care for New York City's Health and Hospitals Corporation. But legislators do not make fine distinctions in their zeal to cut spending, and the Medicaid poor take the fall.

Preserving the Medicaid Program

While managed care has not kept the wolf from Medicaid's door, so far it has largely preserved benefits for its enrollees. After cutting over $800 million from the state's share of Medicaid in 1991, the state legislature came back in 1992 for another $1 billion. Most but not all of these reductions avoided direct impact on patients. Nevertheless, the arbitrary limits on outpatient and pharmacy services imposed by the MUTS program were made more restrictive and were extended to all recipients. Medicaid recipients will for the first time begin paying co-payments out of pocket on inpatient, outpatient, and pharmacy services. And payments for inpatient care for Home Relief recipients will be limited to 32 days per year. With the exception of the last, managed care enrollees have been spared all these cuts.

Progressive Agenda

Medicaid managed care, with all the threats and problems it embodies, might not have been the preferred option for progressive forces. Nevertheless, it appears to be here to stay. The resulting agenda for progressive forces in New York State is clear. Most immediately, we can utilize the formative period in which the program is being shaped and implemented to make sure that protections for patients' interests are built in. Prevention before the system is in place will be far easier and more effective than cure after the fact.

At the local level, this means lobbying to ensure that marketing practices are honest, that patients truly understand their choices, and that plans do not "cherry-pick" good risks while avoiding the bad; it means making sure that patients know and understand their rights; that programs to monitor quality and accessibility are well funded, rigorous, and meaningful; that standards of care are not compromised; that plans willing to reinvest their surpluses in enhanced quality and expanded primary care are encouraged and predatory plans are excluded from the program; it means translating complex and confusing regulations and plans so that community and advocacy groups understand the issues and can deploy their influence and resources effectively. The program is being implemented by professionals who have the best of intentions. Progressive forces can at least assure that these intentions are supported and institutionalized in the program.

Progressives would be remiss if we did not go beyond a reactive stance, however. New York State's managed care program has broken through important barriers that blocked the development of primary care to create an enormous new demand for primary care. The urgency of New York State and New York City in implementing the program offers important new leverage in promoting primary care and reshaping the health care system.

Progressive forces must also use this opportunity to make sure that managed care is defined to be primary and preventive care, not control and screening systems. We must then lobby to assure that resources are invested in new primary care capacity and that the necessary numbers of primary care physicians, nurse practitioners, and physician assistants are trained. If we can pursue this agenda and exploit these opportunities, we will guarantee that, whether it succeeds or fails, New York State's Medicaid Managed Care Program will leave a legacy much closer to the health system we envision.

GREAT EXPECTATIONS

The Politics of Biotechnology

Eric Holtzman

Most critical public discussion of "genetic engineering" and of other biotechnological matters, has focused on obvious "hot" issues—public and environmental safety, possible ethical problems in applications to humans, and the peculiarities of patenting living organisms and life processes.

Fueled largely by the momentum of the environmental and antinuclear movements, and the resurgence of religion, a vague undertone of disquiet has developed.

Much of the debate, however, has centered on peripheral and short-term questions. This is unfortunate, since biotechnology has potentially explosive economic and political aspects—far from all of which are necessarily to be feared or opposed. Agricultural and medical practices are likely to be dramatically changed and important new productive capacities unleashed with major consequences, perhaps especially for the Third World. Concrete questions about who is to control biotechnology and how this control is to be exercised are already looming, promising struggles and shake-ups.

The discussion that follows is written from the vantage-point of a university-based cell biologist. Inevitably its perspective develops out of experience with biology in the U.S. I am aware of the ambiguities of technology and of the evils attendant upon overrelying on technical solutions to solve social problems. I do, nevertheless, believe that much of biotechnology should be greeted as potentially liberating, and as difficult to assimilate within current economic frameworks.

The idea that new technologies are to be resisted, reflexively, because the history of the last century teaches us that technologies tend to run out of control is both ahistorical and beside the point. Such positions do simplify matters and help energize opposition. They eliminate the need to weigh benefits and risks, or to evaluate the economic, political, and cultural forces that underlie particular developments. But this approach tends to be based too heavily on fear, which can disable as well as mobilize.

Moreover, many of the most important issues raised in terms of risks are really forms of fundamental questions about how economic and political power is exercised and who, legitimately, has the right to make decisions with potentially broad social effects. I believe such questions are more fruitfully posed as such, rather than in the more mystifying terms of technologies running out of control.

What's New

Our vision of biotechnology is dominated by news of progress in sophisticated genetic manipulation. In fact, recent advances are much broader-based and include many less spectacular, but still very useful, improvements in our understanding of cells and organisms and in our capacity to work with them.[1] With increasing ease, rational approaches can be constructed to deal directly with diverse problems that researchers hitherto grappled with clumsily or in hit-and-miss fashion. The combination of versatility, relative simplicity, and potential low costs is the basis for the promise of biotechnology. These attributes also generate the growing pressures on current practices in research, the control and transfer of information, and structures of production and distribution.

Modern biotechnology draws heavily on longstanding, sometimes quite ancient, methods of agriculture, medicine, and industry. Selective breeding and related procedures, based on an increasingly refined understanding of heredity, have been fundamental to the establishment of present-day food crops and herd animals. Medicine has applied biotechnological approaches to produce vaccines and antibiotics for decades; medical personnel also use biologically based diagnostic procedures and extract drugs and hormones from biological sources. The production of alcoholic beverages is only the most widespread of a varied group of microbiologically based industries; sewage treatment is another.

As would be expected, the recent upsurge in biotechnology has largely flowed within agendas and production methods originating in this long history. This "conservativism" is likely to diminish as the possibilities arising from recent research are explored and exploited.

What is new intellectually is the sophistication of techniques for manipulating biological material directly at the genetic level and the capacity to engineer particularly convenient cell populations—principally microbes and cell cultures—to produce materials that were previously available primarily from markedly less convenient, or inherently limited sources.

In the laboratory genetic engineering of bacteria has produced hormones and other medically or industrially valuable proteins of higher organisms. Hybrid cell lines, produced by fusing different cell types, have been used to generate monoclonal antibodies useful in diagnosis and therapy. Animal embryos, including those of humans, have been transferred and stored. The study of the cell and molecular biology of plants have come of age.

All this has excited enthusiasm which has carried over to a range of other activities in search of strains of organisms, enzymes, and other biological materials for industrial, medical, and agricultural use. This enthusiasm and the confidence that biological approaches have tremendous potential are probably the most important products generated thus far.

Many people, however, are convinced that this potential is primarily for disaster. Public doubts have centered on the possibility that laboratories might accidentally create microbial "gypsy moths" which would escape, propagate, and wreak havoc—cause cancer, an exotic plague, or devour oil fields.

This concern has been raised in the scientific community as well. When recombinant DNA techniques (the foundation of genetic engineering) were first developed as research tools, a broad and highly influential body of biological researchers imposed its own system of precautions and controls. Under the auspices of the National Institutes of Health (NIH), these restrictions by and large held sway for several years. Some communities, including Cambridge, Massachusetts—an early center of genetic engineering—attempted to develop their own regulations for research and applications of the emerging technologies.[2]

The Decline of Regulation

No disasters occurred. Recombinant DNA techniques proved to be immensely powerful research tools. A few studies evaluating potential dangers produced reassuring results. Soon the scientific community decided that the fears were exaggerated and that all but a few of the usual applications of the techniques were safe. In the space of a few years virtually all the controls that had been imposed were effectively lifted. (The NIH did retain a review panel, one of whose jobs is to regulate field tests of engineered organisms; more will be said about this below.) At this point those few individuals in the scientific community who still argue in favor of controls must endure heavy opprobrium from their colleagues.

In truth, most applications of the procedures are as safe as more familiar industrial techniques, few laboratory uses pose much danger, and the possibilities of accidentally producing a monster are very low. But it should also be recognized that the regulatory structure was razed so quickly in part because people were impatient to get on with research.

Competition heightened the urgency. There were fears that some states, localities, and nations would gain a significant edge in attracting researchers by promising much laxer regulation. As the commercial potential of the new methods became increasingly real, this was no longer an academic question. Another factor was the strong, not entirely groundless, fear of regulation in our society.

This history has had several important consequences. One is that although the issues of regulation were debated primarily in terms of laboratory research, the outcome, a system of minimal regulation, may well be carried over to regulation of commercial activities despite the very important differences in scale and spirit between research laboratories and commercial enterprises.

The NIH is encouraging private genetic engineering corporations to seek approval voluntarily from the NIH field-test panel before testing engineered organisms outside the laboratory. However, the NIH panel is already facing familiar company demands that significant portions of the proceedings be conducted in secret, as well as charges of conflict of interest.[3]

Congress is eager to step in, but its major concerns are stimulating investment, opening foreign markets, emulating aspects of Japanese government-industry cooperation, and taking up issues which carry political mileage such as possible "engineering" of humans.[4] The Environmental Protection Agency's view of its responsibilities is not yet known.

Another legacy of the history of regulation is that the issues were framed and resolved in terms of accidents and exotic laboratory creations. It is, however, not genetic accidents that should concern us most, but deliberate misuse of the

new techniques and more mundane matters such as disposal of wastes and occupational safety. During the recent period relying on self-discipline, there have
been a few publicized (and probably a few more unpublicized) violations of the
rules by scientists whose only likely rewards were the ability to publish research
findings a few months earlier. Temptation to cut corners and bend the rules will
multiply with the addition of potential commercial advantages in speed in getting
to market and minimization of costs. Recent history is not reassuring when such
stakes are involved, especially when production is shrouded under the argument
that irreplaceable "trade secrets" are at stake.

Dangers could, of course, be premeditated. Biological agents designed to
devastate crops, herds, or humans can be created more readily than ever. It
would be naive not to believe that this has played a role in both the Reagan
administration's drive to relegitimize the Pentagon's chemical warfare programs
and its claims that our "enemies" are using biological weapons—with the clear
implication that we must rid ourselves of awkward and restrictive treaties so we
can increase our own capabilities.

Another quite serious negative consequence of the history of regulation was
that the embryonic experiments in modifying relations between the public and
research scientists were terminated just when they were beginning to produce
valuable results. The regulations were formulated and imposed at the federal
level, essentially administratively, and they were relaxed in similar manner. In
the discussions of local legislation and regulation it was evident, in at least some
cases, that laypeople in local government were quite capable of weighing expert
advice and making well-reasoned judgments. This experience, which might well
have turned into an exceptionally creative two-way interplay between science
and society, was rendered irrelevant. The overblown notion that scientific matters are particularly difficult for legislators and the public to understand has been
perpetuated. In addition, the precedent was set for minimizing local regulation
of biotechnology.

Finally, this history gave scientists the sense—partly false, but with some
real substance—that the emerging technology is truly theirs to control and dis-
pose of. This, I believe, colored subsequent events—especially the auction of
scientists and research departments that followed court decisions establishing
that products and procedures of the new biology can be patented.

The Rise of Commercial Exploitation

During the past few decades, virtually all of the significant frontier research
now being applied as biotechnology has been funded by the federal government
through the NIH and the National Science Foundation. The fruits of this research
represent a remarkable collective effort, involving major contributions from tens,
perhaps hundreds, of laboratories and thousands of people in several countries.
Even though these laboratories and scientists were professing traditional competitive and individualistic attitudes and often engaged in frantic races to be first
with a new finding, the structure and practices of research were highly cooperative operationally: information, organisms, and biochemicals were shared to
an extraordinary degree. Furthermore, through peer review and related practices

the scientific community held considerable control over the directions research took; within understandable limits this control was exercised reasonably democratically.

Commercial exploitation of biotechnology, on the other hand, involves a rapidly growing number of competing private corporations. Some are well established pharmaceutical and agricultural giants. Others are new research and production companies, many of which sprung up in the giddy investment period of 1981–82, when it seemed that millions of dollars in venture capital were available to anyone who wished to incorporate for genetic research.

This explosion of private investment fulfilled the theory under which the government supported basic research: public funding would ultimately bring practical benefits, with the private sector developing their commercial potential and reaping the profits.

There has been a bit of concern that the increased interpenetration of the academic world and the commercial sphere will unduly distort university life, subject graduate students to new forms of exploitation, perhaps choke off some of the openness and cooperation through which biology has thrived, and diminish government funding. There has also been some discussion in Congress about the degree to which government funds for basic research should be available directly to private, profit-making, high-technology enterprises, as well as about existing legislation aimed at providing research funds to relatively small businesses. Still, it is remarkable how little scientists and the public at large have been disquieted by the appropriation of a body of knowledge produced by a large scientific community, with public funding, for private economic advantage benefiting only a very few scientists and institutions.

The lack of concern with such issues in the scientific community has multiple roots. In some measure it reflects the involvement, actual or hoped for, of significant numbers of the intellectual leaders of modern biology in commercial ventures. Another factor is the lack of obvious, available alternatives to commercialization through private corporations and the numerous precedents for this route.

But equally important are the traditions of science itself, especially the pattern of competition, publication, recognition, and reward. The history of progress in lines of research fades rapidly from view as the latest results and interpretations accumulate. In publications and grant applications the sense of building on past accomplishments of others is much less evident than the stress on what is new and what disagrees with past viewpoints. Access to publicity via the proper journals, meetings, and connections plays a very important role in deciding who gets credit for what.

Small wonder then that it appears natural when scientists who take the most recent step in a line of research scramble, successfully, to establish claims to commercial profits that are actually derived from the entire chain of research and hence the accumulated effort of many other people.

Furthermore, for all the effective cooperation among laboratories and the widespread networks of communication upon which progress has depended, biologists, like other scientists, lack organizations or other means for effectively promoting or even debating their common political and economic interests and concerns. Professional societies are grossly underdeveloped in this area and relatively powerful and influential groups such as the National Academy of Sciences are both too non-representative and too self-selecting to create a sense of actual operational community. The American Association for the Advancement of Science has more potential along these lines, but it is not regarded in the research community, at least its natural scientist component, as a "spokesperson." The fragmentation of the scientific community reflects, in part, strong traditions of individualism and scepticism toward anything that smacks of trade unionism, and the widespread conviction that the present system is reasonably just in rewarding merit. Such judgments have long been recognized as major determinants of the attitudes of intellectuals in societies like ours. It is also true that relative to sectors of society hard hit in recent years science, especially branches with military applications, has been well treated. This creates a feeling that those who speak for science are doing as well as can be hoped in influencing decisions.

The Distortion of Academic Life

The rush by private corporations to develop biotechnology has led them to establish various arrangements with academic institutions. These arrangements are initiated, most often, to obtain some form of privileged access to new findings, or sometimes to personnel. They provide significant amounts of money for basic research at the institutions in areas of general interest to the sponsoring corporations.

In addition, new private research enterprises have been intensively recruiting well established scientists and new graduates to work on lines of research with potential for profit.

Inevitably, these developments will alter the structure of scientific research. They do have some quite positive facets: formidable intellectual resources are being focused on important practical problems, redressing biases in favor of basic—"purer"—aspects of science. Nice as it is to think of universities as truly independent havens of seekers after intellectual beauty, this is belied by their history. While traditions of academic freedom and the degree of university independence that does exist are very worth preserving, they are not inevitably threatened by vigorous concern with the needs of the broader society.

Still, the relatively rosy view of commercialization ignores the overarching problems arising from the roles and power of large corporations. More narrowly, there is certainly need to brake the intrusion of the corporate drive for profit or control into the academic world, and to protect the endangered public investments, which have been essential to maintaining diversity of activities and viewpoints in academia. Most directly threatened are the long-run health of biological research and the traditions of open exchange of information and open sharing of materials.

For the time being, corporations have been satisfied with relatively unrestrictive arrangements in their support of basic research at universities; limitations on publication or discussion are modest. Because the fundamental information is so widely available and the general nature of the problems most immediately challenging is so widely known, commercial control of research and information poses complex difficulties for the private sector. Moreover industry and the new research enterprises need ready access to fundamental research underway around the world and would hesitate to disrupt the flow by raising their own barriers.

The new research enterprises have constituted themselves with large enough groups of scientists to ensure vigorous interchange in-house. Some arrange extensive programs of seminars and visits from outside as well to keep abreast of the latest findings.

However even with the most optimistic assumptions about corporate self-interest in not killing the goose that lays the golden eggs, it is inevitable that much information and research material of the kind hitherto freely circulated among scientists will be sequestered entirely or enter public circulation at a much slower pace. This may occur minimally with respect to fundamental information about the nature of genes, but clearly it will apply to precisely the sort of details about convenient short cuts, tricks in procedure, useful materials, and the like that can be crucial to the success or speed of research. Much of biotechnology will be very difficult to "protect" with patents or comparable legal devices—too much information is already broadly available, there are too many alternative routes to the same goal, and too much of the most difficult fundamental work has already been done. Thus commercial success will depend largely on corralling talent and on relative speed in getting to market and maneuvering once there. This is already true in sectors of agriculture and the pharmaceutical industry. It is hard to imagine that niceties such as openness about tricks of the trade or sharing helpful mutant cell lines will survive such pressures indefinitely.

The future role of the federal government is also in doubt. The Reagan administration has been very concerned with keeping technology and information under wraps to maintain the American superiority considered vital to profits. It has already made several classification and secrecy forays into the academic world, purportedly to protect militarily sensitive technology.[4] Given the importance of agricultural and medical exports to the national economy and American influence abroad, it is not surprising that government and corporate policymakers are obsessed with our supposedly slipping world supremacy in generating new ideas in such fields. Their temptation to "protect" discoveries by restricting the extensive international communication and cooperation that has characterized biological research will be very strong.

Prospects in Underdeveloped Countries

Given the centrality of agriculture in much of the Third World, biotechnology offers considerable promise for aiding in economic development and in the solution of health problems.

Many of the most important applications are relatively simple and inexpensive and do not require detailed mastery of all the most recent advances or elegant solution of remaining problems at the fundamental level; there are already plenty of scientists in many of these countries capable of doing much of the work if given the resources. Cuba, for example, is very actively pursuing a host of agricultural and medical projects; some of these, such as work to improve animal feeds and livestock breeding, are already paying off. For Third World countries to succeed with reasonable efficiency, however, they must have access to precisely the kind of information most likely to be increasingly restricted—practical details about the handling of economically important organisms.

BOOM AND BUST AMONG THE BIOTECH BLUE (AND RED) CHIPS

Those who wish to follow the growth and development of biotechnology are better served by a subscription to the *Wall Street Journal* than one to the *New England Journal of Medicine* (*Science* and *Nature*, it is true, are required reading). Speculation—scientific, journalistic, and financial—is fast overwhelming the healthy scepticism of traditional medicine.

Gene-green fever began seriously in October 1980 when Genentech, the San Francisco gene splicing firm, opened its first public stock offering at $35 per share and watched the price leap to $89 the first day. The company got $36 million in new capital.

Five months later the Cetus Corporation of Berkeley, CA raised $115 million in the largest initial public stock offering in U.S. corporate history. Other biotech companies, including Enzo Biochem, Genetic Systems, Biotechnics, Ribi Immuno Chem, Biotech Research, Bio Response, and Genetic Engineering have enjoyed similar meteoric rises in their stock prices; as a group they outpaced the bullish 1983 market by some 40 percent.

But all that splices and clones is not green and gold. Southern Biotech, a Tampa, FL, firm, filed for protection under Chapter 11 of the Federal Bankruptcy Act in June 1982 with $1.4 million in liabilities. This despite a successful blood component and interferon business. Toronto's Bio Logicals lost almost $1 million in 1980.

The brokerage firm E. F. Hutton also spoke too soon. DNA Science, its biotech holding company venture that was supposed to spawn subsidiary corporations wherever the hunted scientists were, spent two years getting organized and recruiting the prestigious Weizmann Institute of Science in Israel, the Battelle Memorial Institute of Columbus, OH, UC San Francisco's Dr. John Baxter, and Nobel laureate Christian B. Anfinson. The entire project then collapsed when Johnson & Johnson entered as a major investor and in exchange for its $5 million demanded exclusive marketing rights for any projects developed. Other investors and the researchers involved weren't interested on that basis.

Who's Who Among the Biotech Companies

Company	Leading Scientist(s)	Major Shareholders
Biogen (Geneva, Switzerland)	Walter Gilbert Phillip Sharp	Schering Plough, Inco (Int'l Nickel)
Cetus (Berkeley, CA)	Peter J. Farley Stanley Cohen	Standard Oil of Indiana, Standard Oil of California, Nat'l Distillers & Chemicals
Collaborative Research (Lexington, MA)	David Baltimore	Dow Chemical, Green Cross (Japan)
Genentech	Herbert Boyer	Lubrizol
Genex	J. Leslie Glick	Koppers Co.

—Hal Strelnick

Subtler problems also hinder their efforts. Too often the most experienced and best equipped scientists in the Third World received their training in industrialized nations and imbibed the perspectives and interests prevailing there. As a consequence they lack the motivation and the orientation necessary to tackle unglamorous but vital local problems. In addition, since so much of genetic engineering is publicized in terms of success in being first with the most elegant solutions to the most basic problems, it is often hard for Third World researchers to build up their self-confidence. A sense of facing very bright, very rich competitors who have all the advantages can be disheartening even if the problem at hand is actually of little or no immediate interest to these "rivals." There are also problems in developing self-reliance among people with habits of purchasing "better" solutions from the industrialized world and receiving "aid" of various sorts from foreign agencies.

Matters, however, will not stand still. Difficult choices will be forced upon the countries of the Third World. One very probable effect of advances in biotechnology will be exacerbation of several focal imbalances in their relations with the industrialized countries. The Third World constitutes a crucial market for precisely the sorts of products and production techniques biotechnology is likely to affect first—agricultural materials such as foods, seeds, and fertilizers; and pharmaceuticals and related medical materials. The poorer nations are also an essential source of land, labor, and raw materials. In the short term, we can expect intensification of phenomena already underway in many of these countries: changes in patterns of landholding and crops, with attendant massive social upheaval; struggles between locally-owned industries and multinationals; competition among the industrialized countries; sales of products prohibited or restricted in the industrialized countries; and the flight of multinational capital to friendly, low-wage havens.

Longer-term prospects depend on the political future most centrally on the degree to which countries of the Third World achieve governments committed to autonomous national development accompanied by broad social welfare.

The prospects also depend on whether some of the more dramatic possibilities of biotechnological agriculture are realized. It is not unimaginable, for example, that products now fundamental to the economies of various Third World countries such as sugar and some petroleum derived chemicals will some day come to be produced by quasi-industrial microbiological techniques. This would render current production methods and sites increasingly unnecessary, and perhaps even obsolete.

More certain is that in the medium term, many of the diseases of humans, livestock, and plants that still afflict the Third World will become much more susceptible to large-scale amelioration or eradication, at least insofar as scientific understanding of the responsible organisms and etiology is concerned. It will be increasingly obvious that the major problems are how to mobilize interest in the necessary research and how to overcome political and economic impediments to adequate public health measures, agricultural improvement, and veterinary programs.

Possibilities at Home

As already mentioned, the recent history of biology provides some interesting lessons concerning how curiosity is constituted and constrained. Our society evolved mechanisms, based on relatively generous support, appreciable autonomy, and relative democratization of opportunity, which unleashed remarkable scientific capabilities. There is much to learn from this experience of value in organizing intellectual work and maintaining high morale and productivity in many sorts of contexts and societies. On the other hand, scientists have effectively been insulated from control over and concern with practical applications of their work. Buttressed by the prevailing mechanisms for recruitment, training, and socialization of scientists, this has ensured that the issue of private appropriation of the collectively-produced, government funded body of knowledge would not arise with any insistence.

It is disconcerting, but instructive for understanding the contradictory psychology of the middle class, that at a time when the very idea of government involvement in society is under heavy attack as inevitably ineffective and wasteful, almost no one offers in rebuttal the exceptional success of the government-mediated planning and investment that started, in the case of biology, over a century ago. What remains to be seen is how scientists will react to a future which will bring sharp decreases in autonomy and in funding for many of them, as well as an atmosphere in which suspicion, secrecy, and occasional fraud are apt to increase markedly.

There is at least some hope for the development of countervailing movements within the scientific community, which does still retain a strong commitment to cooperation, openness, and international collaboration, and has potential political and economic leverage.

It would require implausible levels of conspiracy and control to keep biotechnology completely confined within present balances of economic and political forces. The experience of the last decade with electronics, especially computers, and with copying machines demonstrates how very difficult it is to entrap new technologies within the bounds of the legal devices constructed principally to protect previously dominant commercial interests—especially while at the same time supporting "free market" economics and international competition. An intensive effort is underway to devise patent and copyright formulas that will "properly" reward innovation in biotechnology.[5] This may help funnel some profits to "deserving" scientists, universities and corporations, but at very least there is likely to be a long period of sustained, international competition which will be only minimally constrained by domestic law. U.S. antitrust laws are already being reinterpreted and reframed to facilitate cooperation in research among otherwise competing companies.[6] Competition is heating up among the U.S., the Western European countries, and Japan—one interesting question that will probably be answered is whether countries like the U.S. which have a "lead" in the research end of biotechnology will be able to translate this into continued economic supremacy.

More concrete issues may soon emerge. Given the large social investment in the underlying research, public contention could arise over what products are brought to market and at what prices. This debate probably will concern medicine first. A likely harbinger of things to come, with resonant implications for the Third World, is the delay in aggressive development of a potential malaria vaccine caused by disputes over licensing rights.[7] The potentials exist for dramatically lowering production costs for a variety of medical materials, increasing supplies of presently very scarce resources, and evolving effective, inexpensive diagnostic procedures. How these enter and alter medical practice cannot be clearly foreseen yet, but they almost certainly will contribute to the already heated ferment over the costs, organization, accessibility, and effectiveness of modern medicine.

In agriculture, the issues concerning Third World countries outlined above will be paralleled in industrialized countries; these are already foreshadowed in discussions of policies about diet, land and water use, natural vs. chemical pest-control, chemical fertilizers, and the like. Differences will probably gradually intensify as it becomes clearer that fewer and fewer choices are dictated by biological necessities and more and more by political and economic decisions.

It would be foolhardy to predict how all this will turn out. I started with the conviction that the engineering of organisms could prove an appreciably more versatile, more productive, and less distorting approach to important facets of certain large-scale economic activities when compared with the elaborate interference with environments these activities entail today. Whether these possibilities are realized depends principally upon the political future, but biological scientists have fewer justifications than ever for pretending that their laboratory life is separable from what goes on outside in the "real world."

It seems to me that scientists have particularly strong stakes and responsibilities in several of the key issues that will determine the short-term future of biotechnology.

Paramount among these are matters of secrecy. Practices that inhibit or close off the flow of information either within national scientific spheres or internationally must be combated on grounds of both their practical effects and their violation of longstanding principles.

More positively, scientists and their institutions should vigorously support the few efforts now being made to organize international mechanisms which would facilitate the spread of biological information and personnel to Third World nations. These initiatives are being developed through the UN, scientific institutions of individual Third World countries, and internationally funded laboratories.[8] There is a longstanding tradition—albeit one mixed with paternalism—of small-scale efforts of these sorts. Not surprisingly, the official response of the U.S. and other industrialized countries towards proposed large-scale projects in spreading knowledge related to biotechnology has been unenthusiastic and dilatory. The projects have also suffered from the usual sorts of disputes among the Third World nations themselves over matters such as where new facilities should be sited.

BETTER LIVING THROUGH BIOTECHNOLOGY

What are the products promised by genetic engineering and biotechnology that have Wall Street and medical science pacing expectantly in the delivery suite waiting room?

The hope (and hype) embraces almost every commercially significant organic chemical from methane (a major component of natural gas) to perfume, as well as diverse biological "factories" such as dioxin-eating and hormone-producing bacteria. Last year the FDA approved distribution of human insulin produced by a genetically engineered bacterium. Biologically active agents such as interferon (naturally produced only in such minute quantities that its use in cancer and other treatment is prohibitively expensive) might be similarly "manufactured."

Design of such "magic bullets" is rapidly moving from the drawing boards to laboratories and hospital wards. Among these exciting most interest are hybridothas, fusion of antibody-producing white blood cells (lymphocytes) with permanently-growing white blood tumor cells (myelomas), that will indefinitely produce a single, highly specific (monoclonal) antibody that can recognize types of cells targeted for diagnosis or treatment.

University of Minnesota doctors have already tried this approach to protecting leukemia patients with bone marrow transplants against rejection of the body by the transplants (graft versus host disease). Monoclonal antibodies have also been used in conjunction with radioisotopes to identify cancer cells missed by other techniques.

Gene splicing may alter existing vaccines, provide new protection against existing infections, and facilitate production of existing pharmaceuticals. A New York State Department of Health scientist searching for a vaccine against herpes has just developed a technique that might one day lead to a universal vaccine, incorporating into the current smallpox vaccine (vaccinia) genetic information which will stimulate the body's immune reaction to a host of viruses, bacteria, toxins, and parasites.

Below is a list of potential biotechnology products and their markets, determined by the proprietary research of Genex, one of the new biotechnology companies. These data were published in 1981, which is a long time ago in this field.

Scientists should also lose their inhibitions about publicly defending the benefits of public investment. They may well be driven to do so if they want to save their research programs and the educational and other institutions in which many of them work. If optimistic, one can imagine that this will lead many of them to question the policy of giving away the fruits of decades of biological research to enterprises whose primary interest is their own economic success.

One of the few beneficial aspects of the Reagan administration's remodeling of the U.S. is likely to be widespread interest in experimenting with new forms of regulation and with new modes of interaction between the public and the private sectors. Despite their relative quiescence, there is a broadly based sense among scientists that what is happening in their professional life and surroundings is distasteful and threatening; this sense is a potential source of energy.

Allowing the market to be the principal determinant of what is produced with the new techniques, and what the products will cost, would have predict-

Biotechnology Products

Product Category	Product Lines	Current Value ($ million)	20 Year Projected Market
Amino acids (food enrichment and flavoring)	9	$ 1703	$5110
Vitamins	6	668	—
Enzymes (catalysts, drugs)	11	218	—
Steroid hormones (e.g. cortisone)	6	377	—
Peptide hormones (e.g. insulin)	9	264	1000
Short peptides (e.g. sweeteners)	2	4	2100
Nucleotides	2	72	—
Miscellaneous proteins (e.g. albumin, interferon)	2	300	1000
Antibiotics	4 (classes)	4240	—
Pesticides	2 (classes)	100	—
Methane	1	12,572	—
Organic chemicals: alephatics	24	2738	—
aromatics	10	1251	—
Inorganic chemicals (ammonia and hydrogen)	2	2681	—
Gene preparations	3	0	100
Viral vaccines	9	N.A.	—

Source:
Office of Technology Assessment, *Impact of Applied Genetics: Micro-Organisms, Plants, and Animals.* Washington, DC: Government Printing Office, OTA-HR-132, April, 1981.

ably unfortunate consequences, but this is not inevitable. There are, after all, major social movements demanding better nutrition, cheaper and more accessible medical care, improvement of the workplace or environment, and the like. As they come to understand that the new biological technologies can contribute to the goals they seek, they are very likely to press more constructively for socially responsible use of these technologies.

Specific issues where the concerns of such movements parallel those of scientists concerned with the long-term integrity of their fields and institutions have begun to surface. For instance, a recent suit to enjoin the NIH from permitting field tests of genetically engineered microorganisms has sharply questioned the capacity of scientists with commercial connections or the desire for such connections to disentangle their own self-interest from their judgments about proposed tests, especially when the discussions are carried out in secret.[9]

Such issues have many contradictory features, and it is unlikely that many scientists will be comfortable allied to movements with tenets and practices that seem unscientific and obstructionist, or to groups so reflexively hostile to ''scientific progress'' as many are at present.[10] But we are only at the beginning of what promises to be a long period of tumult. Just as we hope that scientists will come to understand their roles and possible obligations better, so we can hope that progressive movements will realize that fears of ambiguity and the new can lead to the surrender of what could and should be contested terrain.

NOTES

1. A helpful brief review is Abelson, P.H., ''Biotechnology: an overview,'' *Science* 219:611. 1983, The entire issue in which this appears (vol. 219, no. 4585) consists of articles outlining the range of current biotechnological approaches.

2. Holtzman, E., ''Recombinant DNA: Triumph on Trojan Horse,'' *Man and Medicine* 2:83, 1977.

3. Fox, J.L., and Norman, C., ''Agricultural Genetics Goes to Court,'' *Science* 221:1355, 1983; and David, P., ''Suit Filed Against NIH,'' *Nature* 305:262, 1983.

4. Garmon, L., ''How the New Congress Will Legislate Biotech,'' *Bio/technology* 1:27, 1983.

5. For a curious illustration see Kayton, I., ''Does Copyright Law Apply to Genetically Engineered Cells,'' *Trends in Biotechnology* 1:2, 1983.

6. David, P., ''Antitrust Restraint Is on the Way Out.'' *Nature* 304:4, 1983.

7. cf. ''NYU's Malaria Vaccine: Orphan at Birth?'' *Science* (News and Views column) 219: 466, 1983.

8. See, e.g., Dickson, D., ''UNIDO Hopes for Biotechnology Center,'' *Science* 221:1351, 1983; and ''Nairobi Laboratory Fights More than Disease,'' *Science* 216:500, 1982.

9. Boffey, P.M., ''Plan Gains for First Outdoor Test of Genetically Engineered Plant,'' *New York Times*, Sept 23, 1983: p.B7.

10. See, e.g., the editorial and discussion of the NIH suit in *Nature* 305:347, 349, 1983.

THE DRUG MANUFACTURING INDUSTRY: A PRESCRIPTION FOR PROFITS

STAFF REPORT
OF THE
Special Committee on Aging
United States Senate

United States Drug Prices Versus
Other Industrialized Nations

Prescription Drug Price Inflation

Background

Despite decades of pleas from millions of chronically ill Americans of all ages and their representatives inside and outside of the Congress, the pharmaceutical manufacturing industry has refused to moderate its pricing policies. For over 2½ years, the majority staff of the Senate Special Committee on Aging has been investigating prescription drug prices and methods to contain prescription drug price inflation. This section provides some current data on prescription drug price inflation in the United States.

Finding 1: During the 1980s, at a time when the overall health care inflation rate has more than doubled the general inflation rate, the pharmaceutical inflation rate has exceeded even this seemingly out-of-control health care inflation index (Chart 1). On average, pharmaceutical inflation rose almost *20 percent (185. percent)* more each year than medical inflation during this time period.

Finding 2: From 1980–90, while the general inflation was 58 percent, prescription drug price inflation was 152 percent, almost three times the rate of general inflation[1] (Chart 2).

Finding 3: In the face of last year's unprecedented Congressional scrutiny and criticism of drug price inflation, the drug industry not only has maintained but increased the rate of inflation on its products in 1991. During the first 6 months of this year, the overall annualized general inflation rate was 3.3 percent, while the annualized prescription drug inflation was *almost three and a half times* this, a staggering 11.2 percent[2] (Chart 3).

CHART 1
PRESCRIPTION DRUG PRICE INFLATION
SHARPLY OUTPACES MEDICAL INFLATION

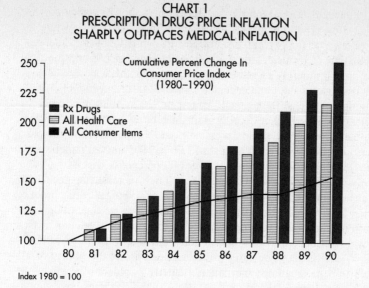

Index 1980 = 100

Source:

Senator David Pryor, Senate Special Committee on Aging, June 1991

CHART 2
PRESCRIPTION DRUG INCREASES
OUTPACE INFLATION

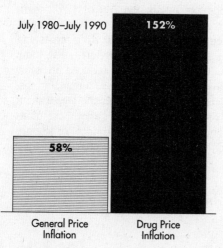

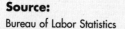

Source:

Bureau of Labor Statistics

Finding 4: Recent data released by the Bureau of Labor Statistics indicate that prescription drug price inflation is accelerating. In August 1991, while the general inflation rate was 0.2 percent, prescription drug inflation was 1.3 percent, six and one-half times as much. This 1.3 percent increase in prescription drug prices was the largest monthly increase for the last 8 months.

Finding 5: Because of the unprecedented increases in drug product costs, a prescription product that cost the average American $20 in 1980 now costs the average American $53.76. If pharmaceutical manufacturers continue to increase drug prices in the future at the same excessive pace that they have in the past, this $20 prescription drug product will cost $77.06 in 1995 and an unbelievable $120.88 in the year 2000—an increase of over 600 percent (Chart 4).

Alternatively, if drug manufacturers had kept price increases at pace with current general inflation (CPI-U) projections, the same 1980 $20 drug product would only cost $49.72 in 2000, only two and a half times as much. Unfortunately, there are no signs that the drug industry plans to limit its price increases to CPI-U or even the medical care inflation index anytime in the near future.

Finding 6: While prescription drug price increases affect the ability of all Americans to afford medications, the nation's elderly population continues to be the hardest hit by skyrocketing drug costs. For example, studies have shown that expenditures for prescription drugs represent the highest out-of-pocket medical care cost for three of four elderly Americans. In addition, a recent report by the Congressional Budget Office (CBO) found that 60 percent of Medicare enrollees face potentially catastrophic out-of-pocket expenses, either because they have no supplementary Medicare coverage or because their supplemental coverage does not include prescription drugs. The report suggests that financial risks could be limited for enrollees by including coverage for prescription drugs in the Medicare program.[3]

Finding 7: Since enactment of the Medicaid Prudent Pharmaceutical Purchasing provisions of the Omnibus Budget Reconciliation Act of 1990, there have been reports—most recently confirmed by a September 18, 1991 General Accounting Office report about Department of Veterans Affairs drug prices and by a September 1991 HHS Office of the Inspector General report—that some pharmaceuticals with which they have traditionally negotiated reduced prices or discounts. These buyers include hospitals, health maintenance organizations, community health centers, and other Federal purchasers such as the Department of Veterans Affairs and the Department of Defense. It appears that these manufacturers are using the Medicaid rebate law as an excuse to eliminate or sharply reduce the discounts that they have given to other purchasers and to pad their already enormous profit margins.

Pharmaceutical Industry's Profitability

Background

The pharmaceutical industry had distinguished itself as one of the very few recession-proof industries in the United States. Year after year, the pharmaceutical industry has been able to impress Wall Street by posting industry-leading

CHART 3
PRESCRIPTION DRUG INFLATION
1991–1ST HALF

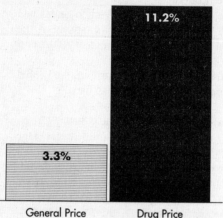

3.3%   **11.2%**

General Price   Drug Price
Inflation   Inflation
        (Annualized)

Source:

Bureau of Labor Statistics

CHART 4
A $20 DRUG INCREASES 604% TO $120 BY YEAR 2000*

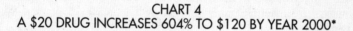
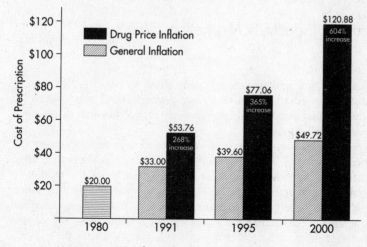

*Assumes current rate of general and pharmaceutical inflation through year 2000.

Data Source:

Congressional Research Service

double-digit profit margins that dwarf all other industries in the United States. Recent evidence suggests that this trend continues unabated. While Americans have never been critical of an industry making profits, they are growing extremely weary of having the most vulnerable populations of our society underwrite these excessive and unconscionable profits.

Finding 1: While the average Fortune 500 industry in the United States had an average profitability of 4.6 percent in 1990, the average profitability of the top 10 drug companies more than tripled that amount: 15.5 percent[4] (Charts 5 and 6).

Finding 2: In 1990, the pharmaceutical industry led all industries in the United States in the three most commonly used profitability measures [5] (Chart 7).

1. As a *percentage of return on sales*, the pharmaceutical industry's first-rank profitability measure (13.6 percent) is more than three times the average industry's profitability by this measure (4.1 percent).

2. As a *percentage of return on assets*, the pharmaceutical industry's first-rank profitability measure (13.1 percent) is three times the average industry's profitability by this measure (4.8 percent).

3. As a *percentage of return on stockholder's equity*, the pharmaceutical industry's first-rank profitability measure (26.4 percent) is more than twice the average industry's profitability by this measure (13 percent).

Finding 3: A drug industry analyst recently predicted that the pharmaceutical industry's profits will climb at a staggering rate of 18 percent each year over the next few years as a result of the upcoming introduction of some extremely high-priced new drug products to the market. As a result, he forecasts that the average pharmaceutical manufacturer's revenue will increase 15 percent this year and 14 percent next year.[6]

Pharmaceutical Industry's Marketing Excesses

Background

Excessive sales, marketing and advertising expenditures by pharmaceutical manufacturers substantially contribute to high drug prices in the United States. A reduction in these expenditures would significantly reduce the cost of pharmaceutical products for all Americans.

Because the drug industry has become very proficient in developing an excessive number of "me-too" drug products—that is, drug products that offer little or no therapeutic advance over those that are already on the market—manufacturers invest substantial financial resources on marketing to convince health professionals that their new drugs really do make a significant contribution to the drug therapy arsenal. Recent data clearly indicate that drug manufacturers continue to inflate drug prices higher and higher to pay for their lavish and expensive marketing and advertising campaigns.

Finding 1: In 1991, according to the pharmaceutical industry's own data, drug manufacturers will spend $1 billion more on marketing and advertising

CHART 5
DRUG COMPANY PROFITS: 1990
PROFITS AS % SALES

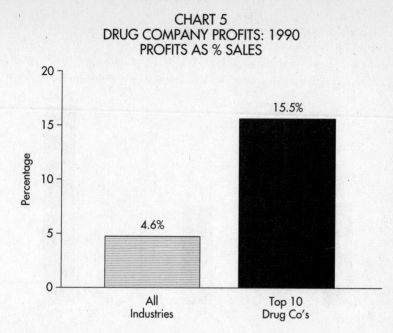

Source:

(The 1991 Business Week 1000)

CHART 6
DRUG COMPANY PROFITS: 1990
PROFITS AS % SALES

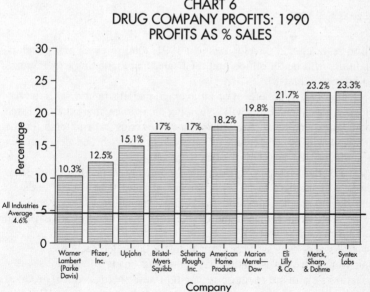

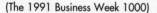

Source:

(The 1991 Business Week 1000)

CHART 7
PROFITABILITY OF THE PHARMACEUTICAL INDUSTRY 1990

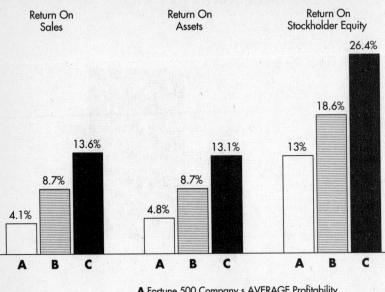

Return On
Sales

Return On
Assets

Return On
Stockholder Equity

26.4%

18.6%

13.6%

13.1%

13%

8.7%

8.7%

4.1%

4.8%

A   B   C   A   B   C   A   B   C

A Fortune 500 Company s AVERAGE Profitability
B Second Most Profitable Industry
C Pharmaceutical Industry (N.B. ranked #1 in each category)

Source:
Fortune Magazine, April 1991

than it will on research and development. In 1991, total research and development expenditures will be $9 billion and total sales and marketing expenditures
will be $10 billion[7] (Chart 8).

Finding 2: In 1991, as a percent of an average manufacturer's sales, advertising and marketing expenditures will constitute, on average, more than research
and development expenditures. Advertising and marketing expenditures for the
average company will be 25 percent of sales while research and development
expenditures will be 22.5 percent of sales (Chart 8).

Finding 3: For the average pharmaceutical company, expenditures on sales
and marketing will increase faster as a percent of sales than expenditures on
research and development. Sales and marketing expenditures are expected to
increase 15 percent, while research and development expenditures are expected
to increase 13.6 percent (Chart 9).

Finding 4: As shocking as these drug industry compiled facts are, the ongoing Aging Committee investigation has found that many of the dollars that
drug manufacturers claim are spent on research of new pharmaceutical products
are actually spent on marketing research. This research is unrelated to the purpose for the research credit; that is, encouraging the development and discovery
of new drugs. These so-called "research" activities help the companies collect
the data they need to design their lavish marketing and promotional campaigns.

CHART 8
DRUG MANUFACTURERS—1991

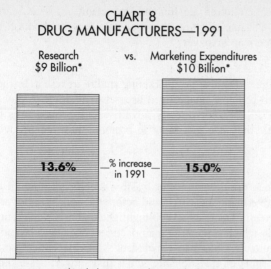

Research   vs.   Marketing Expenditures
$9 Billion* $10 Billion*

13.6%   _% increase_   15.0%
         in 1991

Represents percent by which R&D expenditures and sales and marketing
expenditures were expected to increase in 1991.

*Projected for 1991

Source:

Forbes Magazine, April 15, 1991, based on information provided by the Pharmaceutical Manufacturers Association

CHART 9
DRUG MANUFACTURERS—1991

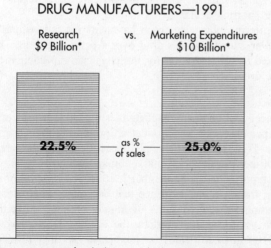

Research   vs.   Marketing Expenditures
$9 Billion* $10 Billion*

22.5%   as %   25.0%
         of sales

Represents percent of total sales expected to be spent on R&D and sales
and marketing in 1991.

*Projected for 1991

Source:

Forbes Magazine, April 15, 1991, based on information provided by the Pharmaceutical Manufacturers Association

Such marketing research expenditures are lumped into claimed research and development expenditures, and manufacturers are then able to write them off at a significant cost to the American taxpayer.

• Some drug manufacturers disguise postmarketing studies as research studies, and use these studies to promote unapproved uses of their drugs to physicians. Because manufacturers may not directly advertise unapproved uses of their products to physicians, they use this route to promote these unapproved uses to prescribers.

Finding 5: Not only does the drug industry waste a significant amount of dollars on marketing and advertising, hearings held before the Senate Labor and Human Resources Committee in December 1990 highlighted abusive marketing and promotional practices in which some drug manufacturers engage to promote their products. The Committee's Chairman concluded: "Pharmaceutical companies are spending larger sums on questionable tactics that subvert basic standards of medical practice, tempting doctors with lavish vacations, gifts, and cash payments."[8]

Examples:

• Drug manufacturers sponsoring all-expense paid "educational symposia" for physicians and their spouses to plush resort locations.
• Manufacturers giving physicians the chance to win expensive tickets to prestigious entertainment or sporting events.
• Drug manufacturers offering physicians cash payments for prescribing a certain amount of a particular manufacturer's drug over a period of time. The payments are often disguised as remuneration for the physician's participation in a "clinical trial" for the drug.

Finding 6: One pharmaceutical company executive estimated that his company spends at least $100 per physician per product on promoting their drugs. According to a 1989 *New York Times* article, pharmaceutical manufacturers spend approximately $5,000 per physician on marketing and advertising.[9]

Finding 7: Recently, as reported in the September 7, 1991, *Washington Post*, the Food and Drug Administration found evidence that one major pharmaceutical manufacturer is spending substantial sums of money on promoting the company's drugs that have yet to be approved by the agency. Doctors were offered free dinners and $100 gift certificates for medical books in return for attending a meeting and discussion session about these unlicensed products. In addition to this being an example of how some drug manufacturers engage in questionable and even potentially illegal marketing activities (Federal law prohibits drug companies from promoting drugs that have not yet been approved by the FDA), it is yet another example of the amount of money that drug manufacturers waste on marketing and promoting their products.[10]

Specific Comparisons of Drug Prices Between the United States, Canada, and Europe

Background

A 1989 report of the majority staff of the Special Committee on Aging reported that Americans pay over 50 percent more than Europeans for the same prescription drug products. Recent data indicate that there continue to be wide discrepancies between prices paid by Americans for drugs and prices paid by Europeans and Canadians for the same prescription drugs. This section examines some of the differences in drug prices between the United States and other industrialized nations, and examines the wide price differences on specific drugs between Canada and the United States.

Finding 1: Although analysis on this subject differs, there is no question that Americans continue to pay extraordinarily higher prices on almost all brand name prescription drugs than do citizens of other industrialized nations.

• Another analysis of prescription drug prices in seven European countries, published in 1990 by the *Farmindustria*, the Italian Pharmaceutical Manufacturers Association, shows that Americans pay over three times more than the average European pays for prescription drugs[11] (Chart 10).

• According to the Office of the Inspector General's March 1991 study comparing Canadian and European drug prices with US drug prices, the average American citizen pays 62 percent more for prescription drugs than the average Canadian citizen and 54 percent more than the average European citizen.[12]

Finding 2: If State Medicaid agencies had access to prices that the pharmaceutical industry makes widely available in Canada (and other countries), State Medicaid agencies and American taxpayers would annually pay an estimated $474 million less for brand name drugs used in the Medicaid programs. Of this amount, $261 million would be federal savings and $213 million would be state savings.[13]

Finding 3: If all U.S. citizens had access to the prices that American drug manufacturers make available to other Western, industrialized nations, billions of precious health dollars could be saved by acutely and chronically ill Americans of all ages, health care institutions, such as hospitals and HMOs, health care insurance plans, and taxpayers.

Finding 4: Not only do Americans pay substantially higher prices for drugs than Canadians and Europeans, the most significant drug price inflation increases in the United States occur on the same products for which Americans already pay substantially more than Canadians.

• While the average American had to already pay 277 percent more than the average Canadian for Flint's Synthroid in 1989, the company also forced the average American to swallow a 22.2 percent price increase for the product between 1989 and 1990.

• Wyeth-Ayerst not only charged Americans 233 percent more than Canadians for Premarin in 1989, but between 1989 and 1990, the company raised the price 19.7 percent.

• Parke-Davis charged the average American 322 percent more than the average Canadian for Dilantin in 1989, and has also raised the price 19 percent between 1989–90.

• Wyeth-Ayerst charged the average American 682 percent more than the average Canadian for Ativan in 1989, and has increased the price of the product almost 80 percent between 1985 and 1990.

Canada—A Case Example of How a Drug Price Review Board Contains Drug Costs

Background

Price negotiations between the drug manufacturers and the health care systems of the various Canadian provincial governments help to produce lower costs for some pharmaceuticals in Canada. However, these negotiations are not the primary reason for lower drug costs in Canada. The creation of a Canadian Patented Medicine Prices Review (CPMPR) Board in 1987 has made the most significant contribution to restraining prescription drug price inflation in that nation. It is important to note that a national health care system is not a prerequisite for the establishment of this Board because the Board not only helps to contain costs for government purchasers, but for private payors as well.

Finding 1: While drug product inflation has been running at three times the rate of general inflation (CPI-U) in the United States over the last 10 years, Canadian prescription drug price inflation (CPI-RX) has been much more moderate, and has even decreased over the last 4 years[14] (Chart 11).

Finding 2: From January 1983 until December 1987, before the CPMPR Board was created, the pharmaceutical component of the Canadian Industrial Products Price Index (IPPI) increased by an annual average rate of 7.1 percent, while the Canadian CPI-U increased at an annual average rate of 4.3 percent. (The IPPI measures the prices of both patented and off-patented drugs.) After establishment of the Board, from December 1987 until August 1990, the pharmaceutical component of the Canadian IPPI increased much less than the January 1983–December 1987 period (5.5 percent per year), in spite of the fact that the Canadian CPI-U increased to 4.7 percent during that same time period.[15]

Finding 3: The CPMPR Board ties prescription drug price increases to increases in the Canadian consumer price index. If the Board finds little justification for the price increase or the excessive launch price of a new drug product, it can remove or shorten the period of market exclusivity of the drug being sold at an excessive price.[16] The Board works in the following manner:

1. The CPMPR Board is not a drug price control body; it is a drug price review body. The pharmaceutical industry in Canada is free to charge whatever

CHART 10
INTERNATIONAL DRUG PRICE COMPARISON

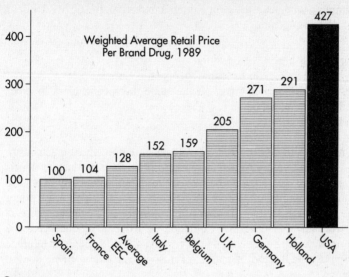

Weighted Average Retail Price
Per Brand Drug, 1989

Source:

'*Indicatori Formaceutici*', annual survey of *Farmindustria*, the Italian pharmaceutical manufacturers association, published 1990

CHART 11
PERCENT YEAR TO YEAR CHANGE IN THE INDEX
VALUES FOR CPI AND PHARMACEUTICAL
COMPONENT OF IPPI (BASE 1986=100)

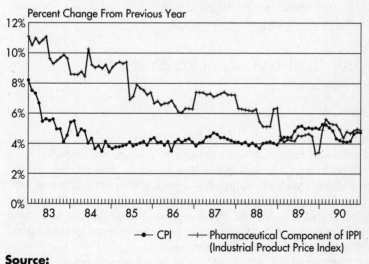

Percent Change From Previous Year

CPI   Pharmaceutical Component of IPPI
(Industrial Product Price Index)

Source:

Statistics Canada

price it wishes for its products. However, that price is subject to review by the Board to determine whether it is "excessive."

2. In determining whether a price on a drug is excessive, the CPMPR Board considers the following factors:

- the 5-year pricing history of the drug;
- the prices of other drugs in the same therapeutic class;
- the prices of the drug and others in the same therapeutic class in other developed, industrialized countries; and
- the Canadian CPI-U.

3. The CPMPR Board has adopted a "voluntary" enforcement mechanism. It is designed to encourage drug manufacturers to price their products at levels which are not excessive, using the guidelines above. When potentially excessive prices are identified, drug manufacturers are given the opportunity to bring prices in line with the Board's guidelines. To date, this voluntary enforcement approach has helped to restrain both drug price inflation on existing products and the launch prices on new drug products. However, the CPMPR Board's ultimate remedy is to remove the period of market exclusivity for a drug being sold at an excessive price.

Finding 4: While drug manufacturers have been increasing prices in the United States at three times the CPI-U over the last 10 years, in Canada, pharmaceutical manufacturers have indicated that they are prepared to restrict price increases in that country to changes in the CPI-U.[17]

Finding 5: Even with the moderating of drug price inflation in Canada, the pharmaceutical industry has made a commitment to increase its research and development spending in Canada by 10 percent by 1996, indicating that drug companies can still invest in meaningful research and development without charging excessive prices for prescription drugs.[18]

Drug Industry's Billion-Dollar Non-Research Oriented Tax Break

Background

It is fairly well known that the pharmaceutical industry receives hundreds of millions of dollars in tax credits and subsidies for researching and developing new pharmaceutical products. Few Americans are aware, however, of the fact that the pharmaceutical industry is, by far, the leading benefactor of a generous, non-research and development oriented tax windfall credit called the Possessions Tax Credit (as provided in Internal Revenue Code Section 936). The Section 936 Tax Credit provides an income tax exemption for business income earned in Puerto Rico and other US territorial possessions.

The stated purpose of the credit is to "assist the US possessions in obtaining employment-producing investments by US corporations," and hence stimulate economic development and jobs.[19] Although the stated purpose of Section 936 is meritorious, its terms provide no direct incentives to generate jobs. Instead, the credit rewards the generation of income in the territorial possessions. Particularly at a time when prescription drug price increases are tripling the general inflation rate, the non-research based tax subsidization of extraordinarily profitable drug companies which are extremely capital intensive rather than labor intensive seems highly questionable.

Finding 1: Nineteen pharmaceutical firms accounted for almost half of all the Section 936 Tax Credits claimed by all US manufacturing companies between 1983–87.

• During that time, these credits have resulted in tax savings of over $5 billion to the drug industry, or 45 percent of all the Section 936 Tax Credits claimed by all US industries. The credit was worth at least $1.4 billion to the drug industry in 1987. The Congressional Research Service estimates that the credit was worth $2 billion to the drug industry in 1990.

Finding 2: The Section 936 Tax Credit contributes to the drug industry's already overflowing coffers and substantially reduces the pharmaceutical industry's tax payments to the Federal Treasury.

• According to a recent Congressional Research Service report, drug companies pay taxes at a level that is lower than the average for US firms. The study said that the 1987 effective tax rate for pharmaceutical firms was 22.14 percent, compared to 24.72 percent for all firms. The same study indicated that the Section 936 Tax Credit had a dramatic effect on reducing the taxes paid to the federal government by the drug manufacturing industry. The credit reduced the effective tax rate of drug firms by an average of almost 9 percentage points.[20]

Finding 3: The Section 936 Tax Credit is an inefficient and very costly method of promoting jobs in the pharmaceutical industry in Puerto Rico.

• Recent data indicate that, on average, the pharmaceutical industry receives a Section 936 tax benefit worth $57,761 per employee that they hire in Puerto Rico. The average salary of a pharmaceutical industry employee in Puerto Rico is only $21,180, meaning that the average pharmaceutical company receives a tax credit that is 264 percent more than the average salary that they pay[21] (Chart 12).
• Other industries manufacturing in Puerto Rico receive much more reasonable Section 936 tax credits as compared to the pharmaceutical industry. For example, the next highest 936 tax benefit received by an industry manufacturing in Puerto Rico is the $20,611 per employee received by the machinery industry, which is $37,150 less than the average 936 tax benefit of the pharmaceutical industry. The textile industry and the apparel industry both receive a benefit worth $3,295 per employee, while the leather products industry receives a benefit of $3,567 per employee[22] (Chart 13).

CHART 12
AVERAGE DRUG INDUSTRY POSSESSIONS TAX CREDIT
PER EMPLOYEE ALMOST TRIPLES ACTUAL SALARY PAID

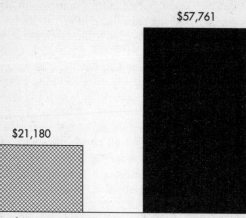

$57,761

$21,180

Average Salary Paid Per Employee
in Puerto Rico by Drug Industry

Average Tax Benefit Received
by Drug Industry Per Employee

Source:

Dept. of the Treasury

CHART 13
DRUG INDUSTRY POSSESSIONS TAX CREDIT PER
EMPLOYEE FAR EXCEEDS OTHER INDUSTRIES' CREDITS

Industry Receiving:
A—4th Highest Possessions Tax Credit Amount
B—3rd Highest Possessions Tax Credit Amount
C—2nd Highest Possessions Tax Credit Amount
D—Highest Possessions Tax Credit Amount

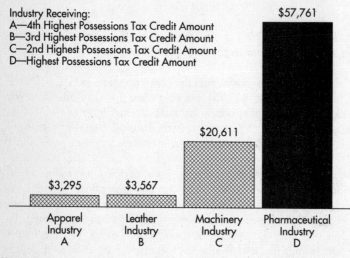

$57,761

$20,611

$3,295 $3,567

| Apparel Industry A | Leather Industry B | Machinery Industry C | Pharmaceutical Industry D |

Source:

Dept. of the Treasury

Finding 4: There is no evidence to suggest that the multi-billion-dollar taxpayer-funded Section 936 Tax Credit that Americans bestow on the pharmaceutical industry each year results in lower drug prices to the American consumer.

Finding 5: Most of the companies who have manufacturing operations in Puerto Rico have added little to the therapeutic arsenal over the past 5 years, while reaping significant tax breaks from the Section 936 Tax Credit.

• Only four New Molecular Entities (NMEs) of significant therapeutic gain have been developed since 1985 by the 19 pharmaceutical companies that have manufacturing operations in Puerto Rico.

• Five of the 19 companies with manufacturing operations in Puerto Rico have not brought a single new pharmaceutical product to market since 1985.

• Of 47 new products brought to market by pharmaceutical companies with manufacturing operations in Puerto Rico, almost 60 percent have been rated as having little or no therapeutic gain.

Finding 6: The pharmaceutical industry uses the Section 936 Tax Credit more intensely than any other industry in the United States.

• One measure of the value of this credit to an industry is to compare the value of the credit as a percent of the assets of an industry. Data for the period 1983–87 show that the tax credit contributed 1.654 percent to the pharmaceutical industry's assets, which was 20 times that of other manufacturing industries that claimed the credit, and 92 times that of all corporations that claimed the credit. A recent Congressional Research Service report concluded that, "compared to other industries, the pharmaceutical industry's use of the possessions tax credit is particularly heavy."[23]

Finding 7: The attractiveness of the Section 936 Tax Credit has lured US mainland jobs to Puerto Rico.

• A tax incentive as generous as the Section 936 Tax Credit is an attractive incentive for US companies to transfer jobs to Puerto Rico. A study entitled "The Impact of Section 936 on Manufacturing Jobs in the Mainland United States: Case Studies," prepared by the Midwest Center of Labor Research, documents thousands of mainland jobs which have been transferred to Puerto Rico. Twenty-five cases of plant closings and major layoffs were reviewed involving 21 different companies. Thirteen cases involved a direct and complete transfer of jobs from the mainland to Puerto Rico. The remainder of the cases in the study shows a transfer of jobs to multiple locations, including Puerto Rico. It is important to note that representatives of beneficiaries of the Section 936 Tax Credit strongly dispute this study. They claim that the mainland plant closings were business decisions made exclusive of the attractiveness of the Section 936 Tax Credit, and further, that the Section 936 Tax Credit actually creates jobs on the mainland. Regardless, it is clear that this issue certainly merits further study.

High Drug Prices Produce Few Breakthrough Drugs

Background

America's drug manufacturers argue that high drug prices are needed in this country to fund the research and development of new pharmaceutical products, which, they contend, is a very expensive, risky, and uncertain business. However, as previous sections illustrate, high prices, profits, and tax subsidies are producing many more slick and expensive marketing campaigns than they are truly significant breakthrough drug products.

Finding 1: Drug manufacturers that have either brought few if any new drug products to the market over the last 5 years *or* that have few if any new drug products in the research pipeline, resort to frequent and excessive price increases as a mechanism to maintain their high profitability.

Finding 2: The highest prescription drug price inflation occurs on drugs that have been on the market for many years, for which research and development costs have long since been recovered.

Examples:

- Tylenol with Codeine (a widely used moderate pain killer), manufactured by McNeil Pharmaceuticals, has been on the market since 1977, but has had cumulative price inflation of 128.5 percent since 1985, an average of 16 percent each year. McNeil has not brought a new molecular entity to market in the last 5 years.

- Synthroid (a thyroid replacement therapy), manufactured by Flint, has been on the market since 1938. The product had a cumulative price increase of 104 percent since 1985, an average of 15.5 percent each year. Flint has not brought one new molecular entity to market in the last 5 years.

- Premarin (an estrogen replacement therapy) and Inderal (a heart medication), both manufactured by Wyeth-Ayerst, have been on the market since 1956 and 1967, respectively. Since 1985, Premarin went up in price 131 percent, an average of 21.5 percent each year, and Inderal went up in price 112.4 percent, an average of 17.1 percent each year. Before the companies merged, Wyeth brought one new molecular entity to market. However, Ayerst has not brought a new molecular entity to market in the past 5 years.

- Dilantin (an antiepileptic drug), manufactured by Parke-Davis, has been on the market since 1953. Since 1985 it has gone up in price 69 percent, an annual average increase of over 11 percent. The company has not brought a new molecular entity to market in the last 5 years.

Finding 3: It is possible for a pharmaceutical manufacturer to maintain profitability, bring new drugs to the market, and refrain from charging excessive inflation. For example, Merck Sharp and Dohme, the world's largest and most research-intensive pharmaceutical manufacturer, brought 8 new molecular entities to market between 1985 and 1990, voluntarily limits its annual price increases to changes in the CPI-U, and was still able to maintain significant profitability (see Chart 6).

Conclusion: Policy Options

Background

For years, Congress has raised concerns about skyrocketing prescription drug price inflation. It was not until last year, however, that Congress passed legislation that took a substantive step toward addressing the problem. As a result, the $5 billion Federal-State Medicaid program, serving our Nation's poor and disabled, will no longer be forced to pay the highest prices in the market for prescription drugs.

During the debate surrounding the Medicaid drug rebate law, drug manufacturers frequently stated that the 1980s represented an anomaly. They said that drug price inflation that doubled and tripled the general inflation rate would not continue, and gave many in Congress the impression that they had received the message that drug cost increases of the past would no longer be tolerated. Sadly, however, if current trends continue, and as this report illustrates, it appears that the 1990s not only will be a price inflation encore, but may well surpass the unacceptable performance of the 1980s.

Attempting to shame the drug manufacturing industry into being responsive to the needs of the American public is obviously not working. Reasonable but concrete proposals, therefore, must be advanced that more effectively and fairly deal with the drug pricing problem. The following recommendations are offered in that spirit.

Relating to Pharmaceutical Access and Cost Containment Mechanisms in the United States

Recommendation 1: Because drug manufacturers are able to reap substantial tax breaks from the use of the Section 936 Tax Credit (Possessions Tax Credit), with little if any benefit to the American public, the Congress should enact legislation that would reduce the Section 936 Tax Credits of a drug manufacturer that inflates its US drug prices higher than a certain percentage of the Consumer Price Index (CPI-U). Taxpayer-underwritten financial rewards—such as tax subsidies—should be linked to acceptable and achievable performance standards.

Recommendation 2: Any revenue achieved through the Section 936 Tax Credit reform as outlined in Recommendation 1 (and directly attributable to excessive and inflationary pricing practices of drug manufacturers) should be directed to a new Federal Prescription Drug Trust Fund. This new Trust Fund would be used to establish a Medicare Outpatient Prescription Drug Demonstration Project. Revenue from the Trust Fund could also be used to target special populations of Medicare beneficiaries, such as those served by community health care centers.

Recommendation 3: The Secretary of the Treasury, acting in consultation with the Secretary of the Department of Health and Human Services, should be required to submit an annual report to Congress on all the Federal subsidies, grants, and tax incentives given to the pharmaceutical industry, and make an assessment of whether these Federal subsidies are being used in the most efficient manner by the pharmaceutical industry.

Recommendation 4: The Secretary of the Treasury, acting in consultation with the Secretary and the Department of Health and Human Services, should assess the advisability of developing a program that would restructure pharmaceutical product research and development tax credits so that they are based on the therapeutic innovativeness of the products that are brought to market. Drug companies that consistently bring few or no breakthrough drugs to the market and produce medications that largely duplicate what is already available should not be rewarded to the same degree as those manufacturers that do.

Recommendation 5: The Secretary of the Department of Health and Human Services, acting in consultation with the Commissioner of the Food and Drug Administration, should develop a program that identifies and makes public the role of the Federal Government in bringing each new drug and biological to the market. In instances in which there is a significant Federal role in bringing a new product to the market, the Secretary (or another federal agency) should seek to be a co-licensee of the product with the pharmaceutical manufacturer.

Recommendation 6: The Secretary of Health and Human Services should conduct a study to determine the feasibility and advisability of establishing in the United States a Pharmaceutical Products Price Review Board, similar to the one that has been established in Canada. The Board would provide a mechanism to insure that the American public is paying a fair, reasonable price for its pharmaceutical products. In so doing, the Secretary should determine how best to have manufacturers justify domestic pricing practices on existing and new drug products, especially where there are wide discrepancies between international and domestic drug prices. To encourage voluntary compliance, the Secretary should determine the feasibility of giving the board the authority to limit market exclusivity on certain drugs whose manufacturers refuse to price their products responsibly.

Recommendation 7: Broader-based, Congressionally mandated studies are underway to determine if the pharmaceutical manufacturers are responding to the Medicaid rebate law's "best price" provision by excessively raising prices to pharmaceutical purchasers such as hospitals and HMOs. If this is the case, Congress should amend the Medicaid rebate law so that the rebate is based on a "best price" anchored to a certain date in time, increased each year by changes in inflation. This approach was advocated in the Medicaid Anti-Discriminatory Drug Price and Patient Benefit Restoration Act of 1990, since it would maximize Medicaid savings on prescription drugs and would make it extremely difficult for drug manufacturers to use the Medicaid law as the cover for increasing prices to other drug purchasers.

Recommendation 8: To protect smaller, non-Medicaid federal purchasers, such as the Department of Veterans Affairs, the Department of Defense, and community health centers from excessive prescription drug price inflation, Congress should enact legislation that meets or exceeds the inflation protection now being given to Medicaid, the largest federal purchaser.

Relating to International Pharmaceutical Prices

Recommendation 1: As a condition of selling pharmaceuticals to federal government agencies and health care programs, each pharmaceutical manufacturer should be required to report annually to the federal government on the prices that it charges for its pharmaceuticals in other industrialized nations.

Recommendation 2: As an alternative to anchoring the Medicaid rebate price to a certain date and indexing it to inflation, Congress should consider enacting legislation that would base the Medicaid Prudent Pharmaceutical Purchasing program's rebate level on the ''best price'' that a manufacturer sells its drugs to other Western industrialized nations, such as Canada or European countries. Such a provision would substantially increase State and Federal Medicaid drug program savings, and would negate any rationale for manufacturers to blame the Medicaid law as the reason for increasing prices to other domestic pharmaceutical purchasers, since Medicaid's ''best price'' would not be based on a domestically determined price.

Recommendation 3: The Secretary of the Department of Health and Human Services should report to Congress on why prescription drug prices and prescription drug inflation are so much lower in other industrialized nations. In so doing, the Secretary should examine how other industrialized nations, such as Germany, are addressing the problem of prescription drug price inflation to determine what applicability, if any, their approaches could have in the U.S. health care system.

NOTES

1. Congressional Research Service (CRS) memorandum and personal communications on prescription drug price inflation prepared for the staff of the Senate Special Committee on Aging, July 29, 1991.

2. Ibid No. 1.

3. "Restructuring Health Insurance for Medicare Enrollees," Congress of the United States, Congressional Budget Office, August 1991.

4. The 1991 Business Week 1000.

5. Ibid No. 4.

6. *Fortune* Magazine, July 15, 1991.

7. *Forbes Magazine*, April 15, 1991.

8. Senate Labor and Human Resources Committee hearing on Advertising, Marketing, and Promotional Practices of the Pharmaceutical Industry, December 11, 1990.

9. *New York Times Magazine* "Pitching Doctors," November 5, 1989.

10. *Washington Post*, "FDA Will Probe Smith Kline on Pitch for Unlicensed Drugs," September 7, 1991.

11. Indicatori Farmaceutici, June 1990. Annual report produced by the Italian Pharmaceutical Manufacturers Association.

12. Department of Health and Human Services, Office of the Inspector General. "Strategies to Reduce Medicaid Drug Expenditures." March 27, 1991.

13. Ibid No. 12.

14. Third Annual Report of the Canadian Patented Medicine Prices Review Board, December 31, 1990.

15. Ibid No. 14.

16. "Price Review in Canada: The Role of the Patented Medicine Prices Review Board." An address given by Wayne Critchley, Executive Director, Patented Medicine Prices Review Board. Toronto, Ontario, Canada, November 8, 1990.

17. Ibid No. 16.

18. Ibid No. 16.

19. CRS Memorandum on Possessions Tax Credit prepared for the staff of the Senate Special Committee on Aging, May 20, 1991.

20. Ibid No. 19.

21. Department of the Treasury, Operation and Effect of the Possessions Corporation System of Taxation—6th Report, March 1989.

22. Ibid No. 21.

23. Ibid No. 19.

THE COMMODIFICATION OF WOMEN'S HEALTH: THE NEW WOMEN'S HEALTH CENTERS

Bonnie J. Kay

The health care facility is often located in a homelike setting that has been renovated to include meeting rooms for workshops. The office is comfortably furnished, softly lit, and redecorated with green plants and women's art. The accoutrements of service include unusually long appointments, access to one's medical records and history forms, explanations of prescribed tests and drugs, reports of laboratory test results, even when normal, and prices quoted in advance.

Such amenities characterize the new women's health centers that have appeared in growing numbers during the last five years. Could it be that mainstream medical care has finally responded to the demands of the women's health movement for the demystification of medical care, respect for the patient, and control by women over the medical decisions affecting their health care?

A closer look reveals that the services many of these women's health centers offer are directed only at a select segment of women: those who pay—or have health insurance that does. The target group is usually in their 20s and 30s, college educated, and employed. They are interested in maintaining a healthy lifestyle and peruse the popular press for articles on premenstrual syndrome (PMS), endometriosis, breast cancer, osteoporosis, and the like. Few have had contact with women's groups that address the political issues related to women and health care. The services these women receive at women's health centers frequently cost more than they would at a private doctor's office—the extra time spent with a clinician is expensive.

The gentle atmospherics, "paddle fans, herb teas, and green plants," that invite women "to relax and make themselves at home"[1] are the marketing tools of the 1980s. In contrast to 20 years ago when the women's health movement articulated its critique of the medical care system, women are now consciously recognized by medical centers, nonprofit hospitals, and proprietary health care companies alike as a large and lucrative market.

Cultivating a Clientele

In many respects, these women's health centers should be viewed as part of the larger development of ambulatory care centers by hospitals, promoted as a means to cultivate a clientele who will use the hospitals' inpatient services in the future. Estimates of the number of ambulatory centers in the United States range as high as 4,000, including both hospital-owned and independent, for-profit centers.[2] Primary and urgent care centers account for the bulk of these, but the greatest growth over the previous year has been among single-purpose centers, including diagnostic imaging centers, health clubs, and cancer care centers. Many of the services in these specialized settings are targeted at women: screening for breast cancer and osteoporosis, women-only alcohol treatment programs, mental health and stress-management workshops, PMS and gynecological care, and nutritional counseling and exercise. In fact, a 1984 survey by the American Hospital Association of over 3,000 hospitals with health-promotion programs found that 49.9 percent provided programs especially designed for women, frequently in the form of women's health centers.[3]

One recent issue of the local newspaper in Ann Arbor, Michigan, featured advertisements from three area hospitals with women's health programs.[4] Two announced public lectures on topics such as "Menopause: A Time of Changes, Challenges and Growth" and "Women and Estrogen: A Part of Your Life." The third program offered "Women's Night Out for the Health of It," complete with dinner at $19.50, featuring a former columnist for the *Detroit Free Press* lecturing on "In Search of Intimacy."

On the surface it appears that the health needs of women have finally become a legitimate item on the medical care system's agenda. "The Health Industry Finally Asks: What Do Women Want?" trumpets *Business Week*, adding as its response, "New services are springing up for female patients fed up with conventional care."[5]

Yet, while the services provided as part of these women's health programs are no doubt useful to some of the women who can afford them, these women's health centers are also offering up a more subtle form of the exploitation that the women's health movement initially opposed, in which health care is defined as a commodity to be marketed and sold for maximum profit to the provider, rather than a need to be filled for the benefit of the individual. Women are seen as easily manipulated by superficial accommodations (the "paddle fans, herb teas, and green plants") with the ultimate aim of filling maternity and surgical beds to maintain the financial viability of the medical institution. A center's existence is assured as long as it can document referrals to hospital services and it doesn't alienate local physicians or invade their turf.

As the medical system recognizes "women's health" as a legitimate area for research and treatment, it "medicalizes" women's normal life processes, such as birth, menstruation, aging, and even eating. They are redefined as pathological events, subject to the expertise of physicians for diagnosis and treatment. The understanding of these life events, which have strong political, economic, and social aspects and influences, is limited to the medical arena.

Whereas demystification of medical care was the central tenet of the women's health movement, the new women's health centers promote *re*mystification. The very language of social change has been coopted to fit new attempts to maintain the status quo or to further develop a class-based health care delivery system. The most obvious example is the use of the phrase "women's health center'' itself, borrowed from the alternative groups that formed the basis of the women's health movement.

The Women's Health Movement

The women's health movement expanded the analysis of the U.S. health system offered by the social change movements of the 1960s. The larger movement focused on the neglect of preventive care; physician-induced, culturally induced, and socially induced illness; and the economic inequalities of society as reflected in the health care system. The women's health movement added to this an emphasis on the imbalance of power in the medical system along gender and class lines—among health workers and between providers and clients. This critique viewed relationships in health care as reflections of relationships in the broader society. Its analysis of the medical practice model, for example, revealed a compliant, passive patient facing a dominant, usually male, authority figure in those areas of health care that are exclusively female: routine obstetrical and gynecological care.

Women's health groups were the visible part of this critique and formed a major force for promoting social change and raising the consciousness of women. Some groups chose to provide health services to women directly, while others organized to collect, evaluate, and disseminate information on providers of women's health care.[6] These groups emphasized a non-hierarchical structure, shared decision making, and a holistic approach to health. Groups that provided services sought to demonstrate, by example, an alternative to the existing hierarchical and class- and gender-based medical system. Good examples are the Feminist Women's Health Centers in Los Angeles and Chico, California; Portland, Oregon; Concord, New Hampshire; and Atlanta, as well as the Emma Goldman Clinic in Iowa City. Groups that provided information focused on using economic pressure as a means to institute change from within by directing women to providers who shared the movement's values and reflected those values in the provision of services. The Chicago-based Health Evaluation and Referral Service (HERS) has existed since 1973 using this approach.

In contrast to the challenge the women's health movement presented, today's women's health centers are mere fronts for the medical care system, more palatable entry points into the realm of medical care. A central tenet of the women's health movement was the personal empowerment that resulted from taking control over choices affecting one's health, in the broadest sense of the word, and most important, being able to define what those choices were. For instance, if abortion services are not available for women, being able to choose between an illegal abortion and carrying an unwanted pregnancy to term is not a meaningful choice. Similarly, if a woman's options for childbirth are limited to choosing between a hospital with a high rate of cesarean sections and one with a slightly lower rate, when what she really wants is a home birth, she is not truly exercising control over her health care.

It is this aspect of choice that is glaringly absent from the recent-day women's health centers and health programs. These centers may treat clients in a polite, respectful manner, and individual women may feel personally in control of the circumstances of their health care, but broadly speaking, control remains with those who define the underlying purposes of the new centers and their programs. And hospital administrators are quite forthright about these purposes: to enhance the hospital's public image, to fill hospital beds, and to promote the financial status of their institutions in what they perceive as a competitive market.

The Health Sector as a Marketplace

During the late 1970s, as health economists and policy analysts searched for ways to explain and contain continually spiraling health care costs, the notion of the health sector as medical marketplace became increasingly popular. The Reagan administration's dramatic cuts in support for health and social services in 1981 and its clear preference for strengthening ties with the profit-oriented business sector provided the right climate for transforming health care services into commodities not unlike chewing gum and automobiles. The non-profit medical sector responded by adopting management models from the business sector that emphasize efficiency and profitability rather than equity as criteria for deciding what mix of services to provide and to whom they should be provided.

Under these circumstances, the traditional distinction has been blurred between the *need* for health services, a concept based on health status compared against an accepted standard, and the *demand* for health care, that is, which services health consumers will pay for. The push to ensure economic viability in an environment of decreasing economic support from the public sector has meant that health providers have redefined necessary health care as services that consumers are willing to purchase at a price at least high enough to cover the costs of production. If that price is too high for some (i.e., the poor), it doesn't matter as long as the numbers willing to pay are sufficient to cover costs.

Thus, health needs are determined not by the health status of various groups in a community but by the preferences of the community's paying customers. Whereas (at least, in theory) community health planners attempt to assess health needs in order to recommend appropriate health services, determining the preferences (redefined as "needs") of paying health consumers is the major focus of health care marketing. The replacement of "health planning" with "health marketing" over the past several years succinctly illustrates the shift from equity to efficiency as the criterion for deciding which services are made available and accessible and to whom. Health care is whatever people will pay for—a commodity for sale. And who are viewed as the traditional buyers in our society? Women, of course.

Women as Health Care Markets

Women use a lot of health and medical care. They consume about 60 percent of all health services in the United States. Over 60 percent of all surgery is performed on women. Women schedule one-third more office visits to physicians than men and return for a repeat visit 6 percent more often.[7] As mothers, women also direct the medical care of their families. As one "health promoter" puts it, "If the hospital treats mom, the rest of the family will follow closely behind."[8]

Capturing the "women's market" is seen by many providers as critical to the continued economic viability of their organizations in these days of declining inpatient censuses. Articles in the health trade magazines talk about "market segmentation" (dividing patients into young, middle, and mature; or employed and not), and development of "product lines" (for example, breast diagnostic programs, PMS screenings, and osteoporosis examinations).[9] A text on *Marketing Women's Health Care* asks, among other questions, "Why is attractive decor as essential as technical competence in attracting women patients?" and "How can you turn a maternity stay into a long-term relationship?"[10] Another book, titled *Reaching Women: The Way to Go in Marketing Healthcare Services*, discusses "strategies used to win over women consumers and keep them coming."[11]

Hospitals are chastised for "missing out on the women's market" by continuing to view women's health as restricted to the maternal role and reproductive system. Instead, women's health centers are touted as presenting a "bold new strategy" that will allow a hospital to "differentiate itself from the competition."[12] Sally Rynne, a popular consultant to many hospitals interested in developing programs aimed at attracting women, identifies a host of advantages for hospitals undertaking to develop women's centers, including profitability, increased demand for inpatient services from referrals from the centers, a wider scope of clients beyond those seeking obstetrical services, and the ability to capture new sources of potential patients.[13]

Redefining the Agenda

The medical sector has taken the concept of empowerment and redefined it to mean providing information about which choices to make; these "choices," it turns out, have been reduced to services that can return a profit. Not only do women's health centers narrowly circumscribe the agenda for those who can afford to pay, but they completely exclude those women who lack income or insurance to pay for those services.

Information has become a marketing tool for attracting clients to a particular provider. Women's health centers are primary outreach tools for hospitals. Public lectures on topics such as PMS, osteoporosis, and stress—issues that have been used in the past by the women's health movement to raise the consciousness of women about the social and political aspects of their experiences—are now marketing magnets. And, of course, the context in which such information is presented is much narrower, generally focusing on medical aspects and biological explanations and ignoring social, economic, and political issues.

Women's health centers don't make money on educational services. They are "loss leaders," used to enhance the parent hospital's public image and develop a pool of paying customers who will be more inclined to use the more lucrative, technologically intensive inpatient services should the need arise. And the need will arise, based on the medical system's discovery and redefinition of a growing number of women's common life experiences as medical problems amenable to medical intervention.[14] Along with birth and menstruation, eating, aging, and economic stress have become popular as medical issues.

In the short term, more work needs to be done to sensitize women to the more subtle forms of exploitation by the medical system. Locally, alternative women's health groups (they still exist and are more prevalent than many realize) can be effective in pressuring the new women's health centers to broaden their focus beyond paying clientele and open their medically focused educational activities to include discussion of alternatives to traditional medical approaches.

In the long term, however, the transformation of women's health services into salable commodities is simply a symptom of a larger ill that cuts across gender lines. Broadly speaking, health needs are defined by the preferences for health services of those who can pay for them. Those who cannot are pushed to the periphery of a health system that increasingly relies on economic class as the basis for allocating its resources. The continuing struggle for social change must develop support for the idea that health is a public good (to use the economists' phrase), and medical marketing plays an unhealthy role in its delivery. Making commodities of health services denies health care to all those who cannot pay for it and perpetuates a health policy that serves the few at the expense of everyone else.

NOTES

1. Rynne, S., "Attracting Women—Have You Got What It Takes?" *Hospital Forum*, March/April 1985, p. 64.

2. Lutz, S., "For-profit Chains Retreat from Ambulatory Business; Not-for-profits Slowly Fill Void," *Modern Healthcare*, June 3, 1988, pp. 74–80.

3. Kernaghan, S., "Women's Health Centers: Early Predictors," *Factbook*, Chicago: Center for Health Promotion, American Hospital Association, 1986, p. FB 101.

4. *Ann Arbor News*, March 5, 1989, pp. F4–5.

5. Deveny, K., "The Health Industry Finally Asks: What Do Women Want?" *Business Week*, August 25, 1986, p. 81.

6. Simmons, R., B. Kay, and C. Regan, "Women's Health Groups: Alternatives to the Health Care System," *International Journal of Health Services*, 1984:14(4), pp. 619–632.

7. Steiber, S. "How to Plan to Tap into the Women's Health Market," *Health Care Marketer/Target Market*, April 14, 1986, p. 7.

8. Kernaghan, S., op. cit., p. 101.

9. Steiber, S., op.. cit., p. 7.

10. Dearing, R., H. Gordon, D. Sohner, and L. Weidel, *Marketing Women's Health Care*, Germantown, MD: Aspen Publishing Co., 1987.

11. Alpern, B., *Reaching Women: The Way to Go in Marketing Healthcare Services*, Chicago: Pluribus Press, 1987.

12. Rynne, S. "The Women's Center: A Bold Strategy," *Health Management Quarterly*, Fall/Winter 1985, pp. 12–17.

13. *Ibid.*, pp. 15, 17.

14. Reissman, C. "Women and Medicalization: A New Perspective," *Social Policy*, Summer 1983, pp. 3–18.

THE FALL AND RISE OF THE HOSPITAL WORKERS UNION

Upheaval in the Quiet Zone: A History of Hospital Workers' Union, Local 1199, by Leon Fink and Brian Greenberg. University of Illinois Press, 1989.

Sumner M. Rosen

When the authors of this important and interesting study completed their manuscript in 1988, Local 1199 faced an uncertain future. The charismatic and effective leadership group headed by Leon Davis had been succeeded by new leaders, whose decisions and style had placed in jeopardy the very survival of the hospital workers' union. Officially known as the Drug, Hospital and Health Care Employees Union, it is an institution that in its prime had earned the loyalty of its members and the praise of a liberal and socially conscious community hungry for inspiration from a labor movement that had largely lost its luster.

Local 1199 could cite Dr. Martin Luther King, Jr., as one of its most supportive advocates. Its Bread and Roses project had developed a range of activities in theater and the arts reminiscent of the pathbreaking work of the International Ladies Garment Workers a generation earlier. In an increasingly dismal labor scene, this union had been the shining exception, but its effectiveness and reputation had been severely damaged, and its ranks were ridden by division and badly demoralized.

Beginning with the election of Dennis Rivera as president after this book was written, and the union's brilliant and successful campaign in the summer of 1989 to negotiate a new contract with the city's private voluntary hospitals, the situation has changed. In many respects the new leaders—including a few figures from the earlier period—have established themselves as effective and energetic. They have brought the union out of its state of peril into a new period of strength and restored its earlier image among the liberal and progressive community.

Writing in 1988, Fink and Greenberg necessarily ended on a note of uncertainty, caution, and concern. Otherwise, *Upheaval in the Quiet Zone* is indispensable for anyone who wants to understand this chapter in labor history. As a narrative it is gripping and dramatic, told both in the authors' clear and cogent style and through the words of many rank-and-file members, whose memories, emotions, and life stories add a rare and moving dimension. As analysis and assessment it is mostly, though not always, on target. It joins a small, select library of works that bring us directly into the lives of working people and their unions, such as the study by Jewell and Bernard Bellush of the American Federation of State, County and Municipal Employees Union (AFSCME) in New York (*Union Power and New York: Victor Gotbaum and District Council 37*) and Eric Mann's story of United Auto Workers Local 645 in Van Nuys, California (*Taking on General Motors: A Case Study of the UAW Campaign to Keep GM Van Nuys Open*).

The Context of the Crisis

In addition to the drama of the story it tells, a major strength is the book's clarity in putting 1199 into historical, political, and ideological context. It makes clear that the crisis in the period following Davis's retirement had multiple roots. One of the most important was the "charismatic patriarch" style that Davis, like Cesar Chavez of the United Farm Workers, maintained. This leadership style created and sustained a vacuum where new, younger leaders should have been learning their lessons and building their own power base among the members.

Another source of the crisis was the erosion, both in the nation and in New York, of the sustaining power of the civil rights movement and the image of the hospital employees as the exploited and victimized members of the work force. This image had energized organizing, mobilized broad support, and isolated and embarrassed the affluent members of hospital boards of trustees. A third was the linked phenomena of escalating health care costs and the fiscal crisis of New York City in the mid-1970s. Their combined effect was to end the process by which the costs of contract settlements between 1199 and the voluntary hospitals were passed through to the public and private insurance payers through hospital reimbursement rates set by New York State. A fourth factor was the erosion of the union power base in New York City. This power had been channeled in support of 1199 by Harry Van Arsdale in his capacity as president of the Central Labor Council and confidant of governors and mayors. It had been central to 1199's organizing successes of the late 1950s and thereafter.

Fink and Greenberg don't state it explicitly, but the original leadership of 1199 never fully understood the meaning of these changes and was not able to adopt the union's essential and by now deeply rooted style of mobilizing and wielding its strength to support new advances at the bargaining table. This failure left the union vulnerable both to external resistance and manipulation, and to internal division. The authors describe the consequences of this failure in a dramatic and telling fashion. They explain why and how Davis's cherished dreams of national unity among health care unions were blocked and frustrated by the maneuvers of 1199's parent union, the Retail, Wholesale and Department Store Union (RWDSU). Its leadership fostered internal dissident groups led successively by Doris Turner and Georgianna Johnson, each of whom became president of 1199, but failed to last.

The union that had presented such a hopeful image to those who had despaired of the labor mainstream in the United States seemed destined to end up not unlike the prescient model etched in 1947 by C. Wright Mills in *The New*

Men of Power: a routinized, bureaucratized, centralized, unadventurous shadow and caricature of its early life. Fink and Greenberg stress that in its heyday, 1199 was in many ways the living contradiction of these images of American labor, eliciting expectations from disenchanted liberals and ever-hopeful radicals that no institution, particularly one so small and unique, could possibly satisfy.

Having built a militant, energetic, effective instrument on a highly centralized basis, with real power exercised by a small group of skilled, dedicated, ideologically charged white males, Davis came to see that their departure might leave the union exposed to serious erosion. The authors quote him:

> I am beginning to appreciate some of the old conservative unions who expected the worker to stand up for his rights on his own. I am beginning to think that we . . . overservice the members. Members get a bellyache and two organizers are there to see what it's about. [That] doesn't build leadership, responsibility, and strength [p. 208].

The struggle to organize the workers in Charleston, South Carolina, in 1969 showed both the strength and the limitations of the organizing strategy that had worked so well in New York and in some other major cities where the union went, though not in all. Ultimately, the national union that Davis created achieved strength in some places, but it failed to build a national base prior to its absorption in 1989, mostly by the larger Service Employees International Union (SEIU) as well as by AFSCME.

Critiques and Changes

The record is fairly laid out and assessed equitably, judiciously, and honestly. The criticisms of 1199 that have been articulated by Health/PAC, by Elinor Langer, John Ehrenreich and Barbara Ehrenreich, and others, and fairly summarized here, deal less with the limits of the organizing and negotiating approach than with the union's refusal to lend its strength and standing to efforts to reform a health care system that is increasingly costing more and providing less, particularly to blacks, Hispanics, and the poor. The union's rationale was its self-definition as a defender of its members' rights. It either held aloof from policy struggles or, in some cases, actively resisted involvement by its members in these issues, even though they were in many ways part of the community of the deprived and the badly served.

During much of 1199's early period I was a close observer from the vantage point of my post in District Council 37 of AFSCME in New York City, which organized workers in the municipal hospitals in the 1960s, and I have some corrections and personal observations to offer. The book gives insufficient attention to the relationship, partly supportive and partly competitive, between the two unions and their contrasting leadership styles. The training and upgrading fund that 1199 negotiated followed and was adapted from the fund that DC 37 negotiated in 1967; I recall vividly the internal debate in 1199 about the benefits to be achieved and the psychological cost of failing to match the pattern. Unlike the DC 37 program, the one in 1199 never seriously addressed the barriers to job access and upward mobility that are built into the hospital industry; nor were the leaders ready to work cooperatively with employers in efforts to change these structures. Under the new leadership there are encouraging signs that this may be changing. Given the pace of change in health care organization, 1199, like other unions, will have no choice but to participate actively in such efforts if they are to prevent wholesale erosion of jobs, downskilling, and speedup.

The new leadership's success in raising the wages, standards, and career prospects of workers in home care is a sign of a greater appreciation of the importance of health policies and priorities than was ever evinced by the earlier leadership. This campaign involved coalitions, not with the traditional social movements, but with providers of care, educators, advocates, and others active in the health care debate. In this respect, the future may well depart from past patterns.

Leadership and democratic participation remain problematic. Davis always saw the internal structures as channels for organization, mobilization, and discipline, not for shaping decisions about strategy and direction. The latter were the role of the top leaders; to alter this was to risk division, weakness, confusion. Here again I would argue that DC 37, equally embattled (particularly during New York City's fiscal crisis), with a membership embracing a wide range of jobs, skill levels, races, and ethnic groups, demonstrated repeatedly that it is possible to achieve and sustain unity while practicing an authentic internal democracy. Local 1199's strongly centralized leadership was the product of the ideology of its founders as much as—perhaps more than—the specifics of workers, the work setting, or the economic and political situation.

My reservations about this book are minor in comparison to its many merits. (One quibble: Benjamin Buttenweiser's name is consistently misspelled; he was a key participant from the beginning as trustee of Lenox Hill Hospital and chairman of the New York Urban League.) The 44 pages of footnotes are worth perusing for many insights and observations. *Upheaval in the Quiet Zone* deserves high praise and wide circulation.

PERCENT OF BLACK AND HISPANIC WORKERS IN SELECTED HEALTH CARE OCCUPATIONS (USA, 1987)

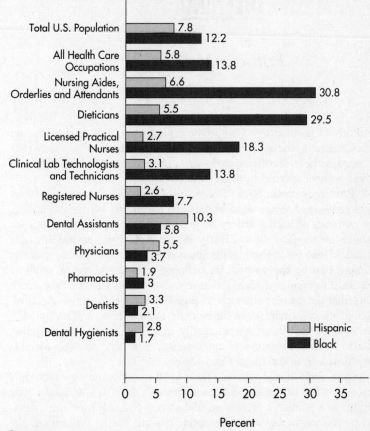

Sources:

US Department of Commerce, Bureau of the Census. Statistical abstract of the United States 1989, 109th edition. Washington DC, 1989: Table 2, p. 7; Tables 18, 20, p. 16.

US Department of Health and Human Services. Seventh report to the President and Congress on the status of health personnel in the United States. Washington, DC, March 1990; DHHS Publ. No. HRS-P-OD-90-1: Table IV-H-A-1, p. IV-H-8.

ORDERED TO CARE
DEMYSTIFYING NURSING'S DILEMMA

Patricia Moccia

Nurses are in a bind familiar to all who would nurture in our society, whether they be nurses, teachers, social workers, parents, or friends: How can they care for those in need without sacrificing their sense of self; and how can they care for their selves without sacrificing those in need?

Susan M. Reverby's recent book, *Ordered to Care: The Dilemma of American Nursing, 1850–1945*, helps us to understand the history of that bind. And, although the purposes of such a history do not usually include prescriptions for contemporary problems, Reverby so clearly identifies nursing's central dilemma in her work that it also contributes to discussions on how one of today's health care crises might best be approached. By defining nursing's historical problem as "being ordered to care in a society that refuses to value caring," she raises the possibility that the current shortage of registered nurses requires social reform in addition to, or perhaps even rather than, nursing reform. This by itself throws more light on the issue than practically any of the other, more popular, analyses. It also holds the promise of empowering those who struggle for progressive transformation in health care and society.

Reverby writes about nursing history from 1850 to 1945, during which time the act of caring for the sick changed from a woman's duty, to a woman's trade and occupation, to a woman's profession and career. Starting from the experience of nurses working in and around Boston hospitals during that period, she develops an analysis of its national implications. With nursing as a case study, Reverby also provides a much-needed connection between political histories of health care and the hospital system, such as *The Care of Strangers*, by Charles Rosenberg, and *Health Care in America: Essays in Social History*, edited by Reverby and David Rosner; the historiographies of nursing in a patriarchy, such as *Hospitals, Paternalism and the Role of the Nurse*, by Joann Ashley; and analyses of the work culture of nursing, such as *The Physician's Hand*, by Barbara Melosh.

The Nursing Shortage: Whose Side Are You On?

By now, the popular media has convinced all who look or listen that the nursing profession is in the midst of a crisis of numbers. Nursing positions in almost all the nation's hospitals go unfilled, and nursing schools face declining admissions, enrollments, and graduations. Thousands of dollars are being spent by private foundations such as Commonwealth and Pew to analyze the reasons for nurses' dissatisfaction; by professional and consumer-oriented organizations such as the American Nurses' Association and the National League for Nursing to market nursing as an attractive career option; and by trade associations such as the American Hospital Association to develop strategies to recruit and retain nurses as hospital employees. Even the federal government has finally decided to study the crisis, with a commission appointed by the Secretary of Health and Human Services to offer recommendations by the end of 1988.

Yet these intensive studies, all by interested parties, are peculiarly limited. They attempt to explain the shortage as the result of particular decisions by individual nurses, would-be nurses, and the nursing leadership. In the context of *Ordered to Care*, this approach seems curiously ignorant of the structural determinants of the problem. Despite the realities of daily life for nurses in hospitals, which Reverby so vividly depicts, serious proposals are still being prepared to find the few nurses who have left intolerable working conditions behind and entice them back to lives of subordination and personal and professional humiliation. Reverby carefully documents the fact that nursing students historically have been recruited from poor and working class families. Nevertheless, some still argue that, as a result of the women's movement, potential nurses are now choosing to study for MBAs or degrees in law and medicine. Yet we know that such programs are still protected by barriers of class and race from the majority of those in nursing's traditional labor pool. Again, Reverby exposes the hospital-based and controlled apprenticeship training that predated the current collegiate programs as a source of cheap and exploited labor, allowing institutions to profit without regard for the quality of nurses' lives either on or off the floors. Yet some still argue for a return to those days and ways in order to assure an adequate labor force for today's hospitals.

These arguments and proposed solutions share several themes. First, they lay the blame for the nursing shortage on nurses themselves: on those who choose not to be humiliated and overworked on a daily basis; on those who might have taken advantage of an opportunity to achieve more autonomy in their daily lives or more money, respect, and security for their families; and on those who have succeeded in moving nursing students away from oppressive training systems toward the relative, albeit limited, autonomy of educational models. In so doing, secondly, these arguments divert attention and responsibility from those who, like the American Medical Association and the American Hospital Association, benefit from an undereducated, divided, and subservient labor force.

Third, these analyses are critical of what they present as self-interest on the

part of nurses and the nursing profession. Nurses, they say, are willing to sacrifice the good of their patients for individual and professional advancement.
This assumes, falsely, that the nurse and the nursing profession ever had either
the sole responsibility for ensuring care in hospitals or the power to determine
how care was to be delivered. Finally, if heeded, these arguments would put
nurses ''back in their place'' and serve to reinforce and reproduce the authority
of those who currently control health.

Reverby pulls the veil from these illusions. She identifies nursing's ''crucial
dilemma.'' She presents the reader with ample evidence of nurses' struggle with
''the dichotomy between the duty and the desire to care for others and the right
to control and define their activity.'' Most significantly, Reverby exposes the
root of nursing's problems, those of the health care system, and perhaps even
those facing us as a civilization as ''the failure of our society to create the
conditions under which the desire to care can be valued.''

The Nursing Shortage: Qui Bono?

Conventional wisdom has it that correctly defining the problem will bring
you halfway to the solution. Mileage might be gained, then, by presenting the
nursing shortage not as a problem for nurses or for nursing, but rather as a
problem for the employer; that is, for hospitals and physicians. Reverby's history
tells us that, at least for the years between 1850 and 1945, nurses were clear
about what they wanted—a humane system for both patients and employees,
one that allowed dignity and integrity and respected the nurse's individuality
and autonomy, one that allowed people to care for each other. Today, as economic imperatives become ever more insistent, nurses are clearer and more
forceful about what it would take to keep them. Hospitals refuse to hear or to
heed. And so we have a nursing shortage.

Or do we? Since more nurses are working now than ever before, the problem
seems more one of increased demand than inadequate supply. In other words,
it's not that nurses are refusing to work, it's that the hospitals want more of
them—both literally and figuratively. The question then becomes: ''To do
what?''

As a challenge to the currently popular analysis that we are in the midst of
a nursing shortage, Dr. Nancy Greenleaf, Dean of the School of Nursing at the
University of Southern Maine, has argued that 1.8 million nurses ought to be
sufficient to meet the health needs of a nation with a population of about 250
million. She suggests that the roughly 1:150 ratio is only inadequate relative to
the needs of a health care system designed for profit, and that the ''shortage''
reflects the needs of the employer for more workers, not necessarily the needs
of people for more health services. Greenleaf poses two questions that lead to
entirely different discussions about the ''nursing crisis'' and entirely different
solutions: ''How have the benefits of the nurse supply been distributed?'' and,
''For whose benefit are those nurses working?''

To read Reverby is to find the answers to these two questions: The nursing
supply has been controlled by physicians and hospitals for the benefit of phy-

sicians and hospitals. She tells us that in 1878, "the demands of the hospital for a work force often overcame the nursing schools' abilities to educate their students." In 1910, "admissions to nursing schools were determined by hospital needs rather than educational standards."

Between 1920 and the mid-1930s, the growth of hospitals in the United States was dependent on student nurses to adequately staff the institutions. Reverby reveals that although graduate nurses achieved some degree of independence through private duty, the Depression forced them to bow, bitterly, to the pressures of physicians and hospitals and to accept the otherwise unacceptable working conditions offered to staff nurses in return for the security of steady, however meager, income.

Although Reverby's work stops at 1945, the attempts by organized medicine to control the education and supply of nurses have not. By crying "nursing shortage," medicine justifies its latest efforts to dominate and exploit. As a recent internal memo of the AMA's board of trustees reveals, organized medicine is so panicked or blinded by self-interest that it can on one hand acknowledge that "nursing has developed professional independence and authority over its own affairs," and on the other presume to interfere in this independent profession by recommending that the AMA set up nursing education programs and methods to accredit them. For these physicians, nurses are neither workers nor independent practitioners, but rather a "critical medical resource" in such short supply that critical care and medical surgical beds are being closed—and profits are being lost—in many parts of the country.

Nurses' Dilemma, Whose Failure?

Through this history of American nursing, Reverby makes several points about work, caring activities, and the position of women in society. Because of a society structured in such a way that human relations are distorted in the interests of efficiency and domination, the activities of nurturing and caring for each other are similarly distorted. As nursing work has traditionally been seen as women's work, its value reflects that of women in a patriarchy. How then can nurses and other women in such a position care for others without caring for themselves?

When nurses engage either of these struggles without engaging the other, and when they engage them alone, their efforts are confused and confusing. Their difficulties in advancing either their own or the patient's interests become the failures of individuals and evidence of the conservative nature of nurses. There is more opportunity for progressive social change when nurses look beyond their boundaries for either analysis or praxis. As Reverby says, "the dilemma of nursing is too tied into the broader problems of gender and class in our society to be solved solely by the political efforts of one occupational group." This re-framing of the nursing crisis is perhaps the greatest contribution of the book.

Though the voices of nurses are missing from this history, Reverby is aware of their value. She acknowledges her debt to nurses Sondra Clark, Nancy Green-

PERCENT DISTRIBUTION OF SELECTED HEALTH CARE PRACTITIONERS, BY GENDER (USA, 1986, 1988)

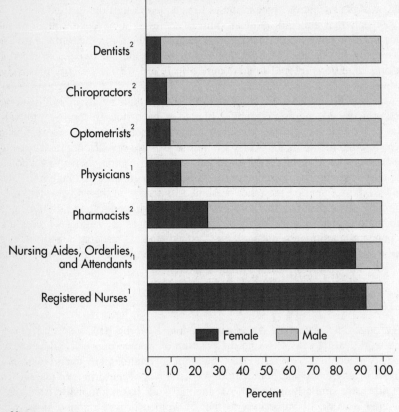

Notes:
1.*Data for 1986.
2.*Data for 1988.

Sources:

US Department of Commerce, Bureau of the Census. Male-female differences in work experience, occupation, and earnings 1984. Washington DC, 1987: Table G, p. 5. (Current Population Reports; Series P-70, No. 10).

US Department of Commerce, Bureau of the Census. Statistical abstract of the United States 1989. Washington DC, 1987: Table 152, p. 99.

US Department of Health and Human Services, Bureau of Health Manpower. Seventh report to the President and Congress on the status of health personnel in the United States. Washington DC, March 1990; DHHS Publ. No. HRS-P-OD-90-1: Table VII-A-6, p. VII-31; Table XI-A-2, p. XI-11; Table XII-A-2, p. XII-22; Table XV-A-3, p. XV-13.

leaf, and Karen Wolf for their willingness to share their experience of nursing with an outsider. Her gratitude is also evident in the degree of sensitivity and respect with which she treats her subjects. As nurses increasingly find and use their own progressive voices, they in turn will acknowledge their debt to Susan Reverby for this and other works.

NURSING AND CARING: LESSONS FROM HISTORY

Interview with Susan Reverby

The author of Ordered to Care, *Susan M. Reverby, now associate professor and director of the Women's Studies Program at Wellesley College, was a staff member at Health/PAC from 1970 to 1973. Until then, her only involvement with health care, aside from family dinner conversation (her father is a physician and her mother teaches human biology and medical technology), was a few weeks as a counselor in an abortion clinic. Health/PAC, she says, gave her an instant education. "I learned an enormous amount very, very fast about how the health care system works, about how to be a speaker, about how to think through issues, how to be an organizer, and I'm very grateful." The* Bulletin *recently asked her to comment on the nursing shortage, nursing history, and her experience with Health/PAC.—Ellen Bilofsky*

Health/PAC: *You're a historian. How did you get involved with nursing? Did Health/PAC have something to do with it?*
Reverby: Yes. I was hired in 1970 because of my interest in the abortion movement. When the person on staff who covered nursing left, it was a natural desk for me to take over, since I was the one with a degree in labor history and an interest in women. And I got fascinated, because I was a historian, by the history. I just fell in love. You couldn't not like them, and you couldn't not be interested in what they tried to do.

Eventually, I left Health/PAC because I was becoming the kind of academic intellectual who needed to have more of a grounding in the complexities of a topic. I was frustrated by what the kind of journalistic writing we were doing required me to do, which was to become an instant expert on some topic I knew nothing about in about three weeks. Frankly, we were often so rhetorical because we were trying to create a movement, and we didn't have the time to be careful sometimes about the complexities of historical change. That's a tension between intellectuals and activists. If you're faced with a problem here and now, you don't have the luxury of trying to figure out the niceties of the past. I felt then, and I certainly feel now, that it also led to a kind of screwed up politics, because if you don't really understand the complexities of the past then you really make political mistakes in the present.

I spent a year after I left Health/PAC trying to decide whether to go on for graduate training in health or whether I wanted to do history, and I decided I didn't want to go to my grave wishing I'd become a historian. So I completed my Ph.D. in American Studies.

Health/PAC: Ordered to Care *stops in 1945. Why didn't you bring it up to the present?*
Reverby: I knew the end of the story, because at Health/PAC I'd written about what had happened from 1945 on. And also because, like most historians, I made the argument that the seeds of the difficulty had been planted in the early years.

I end by talking about nursing's need to develop a language of rights around caring. I say two sets of things. One is that nurses have to develop a language about rights that doesn't mean just what you individually need but what we collectively need—what a communal set of rights would look like for nurses as a group to be able to care properly.

The second is that because the problems of nursing are so tied into the issues of women and of caring more broadly in the culture, nursing cannot solve the problem by itself. The only hope lies in a kind of alliance with other people concerned about what's happening to women and to caring issues in the culture more broadly. There have to be linkages in nursing school programs with women's studies, there have to be links in hospitals and with health consumers and with people concerned about what's going to happen in the hospitals to their loved ones. People have to understand what's wrong with the way the health system is set up now and what's wrong with the way in which nursing has been oppressed.

Health/PAC: *Do you consider nurses to be "professionals" rather than "workers"?*
Reverby: I think that the dichotimization of professionals and workers is arcane at this point, at least around nursing. It's an ahistorical question, because whether or not in the objective world you want to label nurses "semiprofessionals" or "workers," in terms of the way they're being educated and in terms of their consciousness, they consider themselves professionals. But what that means may have a worker consciousness to it. I don't mean to suggest that there's not a difference between being an aide and being a nurse. I just think you have to avoid a definition that has some academic sociological and political science meaning. You have to look at what meaning people give to the word themselves. There are different ways to act professionally. There are ways to be professional that also take into account what we would consider traditional worker consciousness. Being a professional does not negate organizing, or caring about anybody else in the hospital. It doesn't have to.

One of the things I tried to say in the book is where the limits of professionalization have been. But that doesn't mean I don't think some of that's important. I've shifted some ground on the B.S.N. issue over the years. I think that's probably where we went wrong in criticizing nursing when I was at Health/PAC. In 1972 I wrote against the B.S.N. degree as a requirement for entry into nursing practice because the line was that it was anti-working class.

Then a friend of mine said to me, "Do you think women shouldn't go to college?" And I thought, what a position for a feminist to take, that women who want to learn something should not go to college!

Health/PAC: *But there's a difference between helping women to go to college and requiring a college degree to become a nurse.*
Reverby: Right. But there are ways in which you could build ladders in nursing that would give them that. There have to be ways in which college programs are brought to the hospital to give people the kind of broad base that a college education gives.

One of the things I argue in the book is that class so divided nurses historically that gender couldn't unite them. I think that the whole issue of class and race as dividers, as in any women's community, has to be dealt with politically by nurses. We have to acknowledge what it means to help other women move from diploma degrees to B.S.N.s. The health system is only very slowly learning to really value increased clinical skills. We mainly reward people who move *out*, from the bedside into teaching or into administration. But that's true of any kind of service work in this society. At the university we don't reward people for being good teachers, we only reward them if they write a lot of books.

Health/PAC: *Then you're suggesting that we reward people adequately just for being good nurses?*
Reverby: Oh, absolutely. That's the first step. If nurses' starting salaries were $40,000 and went up to $80,000, you'd have no nursing shortage tomorrow. But it's not just money, and that's certainly clear when you talk to nurses. One of the things that's important has to do with what kind of control people have over the job, how they're perceived, whether they're taken seriously as professional colleagues in the hospital. Those issues sometimes speak louder than the money.

Health/PAC: *What's creating the nursing shortage? Is there really a shortage?*
Reverby: I think it's complicated. I don't follow the current numbers enough to argue whether the bodies are actually missing or not. I think there's what I call a cultural crisis in caring in general, for which women, rather than the structures that created the crisis, are being blamed. We are being blamed for not caring enough, or for not being willing to sacrifice ourselves. The culture has created a crisis in caring by not rewarding caring work in emotional, financial, and status ways. That's causing the crisis, not because women have abandoned their caring role.

Health/PAC: *You wrote in one of your Health/PAC articles in 1972 that the "disproportionate number of women [in nursing and other health care positions] reflects the fact that women have few other choices." Well, women now have a lot of other choices. Is that helping to cause the nursing shortage?*
Reverby: Oh, sure. I think you'd be naive to not admit that. I'm a health professions advisor at Wellesley, and I've only seen one student who said she wanted to go to nursing school. The problem often is that many students think

the only way to make it is to become a corporate vice president, that somehow being a nurse is not something valuable.

Health/PAC: *Since nursing has traditionally been a working class profession, are the women who traditionally went into nursing really going into law and medicine?*
Reverby: Some. And some are going into banking jobs, real estate, social work. We know that there's a decline in nursing school enrollments. They're going elsewhere. Some. Not all. But that's always been true. Historically, in the twenties lots of women went elsewhere, other than nursing, into secretarial jobs because they paid better.

Health/PAC: *Do you think that bringing in men will help the profession?*
Reverby: No, I don't, because I think it's a gendered profession. It's not a question of the bodies and their genitalia in the profession, it's a question of how the culture perceives the work. So more men in it are not going to matter, and in fact more men in it means they just become the administrators. Men tend to rise faster and push faster for the administrative jobs, and they get them. It's the type of work that's an issue, and how the culture links caring work to women's work and assumes it to be natural that women do it.

When the media talks about the shortage, all it does is bemoan the problem, but it doesn't really talk about solutions, or it ends up blaming women for the problem. The subtext is, "Gee, women shouldn't do this. Women shouldn't be abandoning us. Mommy didn't do it right." Rather than, "*Why* isn't Mommy doing it?"

Health/PAC: *Let's talk about solutions.*
Reverby: There ought to be joint education between doctors and nurses. Doctors ought to be required to take an introductory nursing theory course, so that they have some sense of the profession and what its history and demands and needs are. It would help a lot if they knew something about it other than what they see on the hospital floor. There have to be real linkages between women's studies programs and nursing schools. There have to be real linkages between women's groups and organizations of concerned consumers and groups of older people with nursing. If you think about who gets sick, in the end it's older women who are in the hospital. There have to be those kind of linkages. I don't think nursing can do it alone. We all have something to gain. We all get sick and die, every single bloody one of us, and at some point, we're going to come in contact with nursing.

Health/PAC: *What about unionization?*
Reverby: I think it helps. I don't think it's the only answer. Bread and butter issues are important, but if the unions don't bargain over control of the work process, there are still a lot of problems. Because it isn't just money that's the issue in nursing.

I think a way to go is to increasingly value the nurse clinician and to reward people for increasing clinical skills on the hospital floor. But it will also take giving nurses at all levels more control over their workplace. They need to have a say over pace, scheduling, and what they're allowed to do.

Health/PAC: *Can nurses continue to become more specialized and increase their knowledge and their technical skills and still give good bedside care?*
Reverby: That's always been the tension. Yes, I think so. I think that it has to be thought through and it has to be rewarded.

Health/PAC: *What's your prognosis? Is the nursing shortage going to change the status of the profession?*
Reverby: It's actually quite a crucial time for nursing. In the past, medicine has often pushed for an increased division of labor, so that you get more practical nurses, more aides, more technicians. And whether nursing is going to be able to hold on to the need to have more highly educated people, I don't know. The latest AMA language about what they think will be the solution sounds just like what Charles Mayo proposed in 1921. What the AMA proposed is that we should train more ''subnurses,'' in the term Mayo used. Back to the hospital, technicians, people who come in and all they do is give shots. People to give out meds, as if there was nothing else involved except handing somebody a bunch of pills to swallow. There has to be some long, hard thinking between groups of consumers and nursing leadership and medicine in the hospitals. It's starting to go on, but it's not going on enough yet. And that's why starting by changing some of the thinking in the medical and health administration schools is really crucial.

Otherwise, you'll see the hospital looking more and more like a nursing home; that is, one or two highly trained R.N.s at the top and then lots and lots and lots of L.P.N.s and aides running it. And I think we will all suffer. It doesn't mean aides and L.P.N.s don't often give very good bedside care. But there's a special knowledge that comes from a broader education that nurses bring as well.

One of the other things we'll probably end up seeing is a real two-class system—a lot of very highly paid technical people on one end and lots and lots of temps, lots and lots of foreign nurses, and lots of confusion in the hospital. And we all have a lot to lose by it.

Health/PAC: *How would health care have to change before nurses could be rewarded for caring?*
Reverby: I think our society will have to really think through what counts as caring. We need more studies on how caring and good nursing care really change things that could show how patient recovery is better. But it's going to be a long, difficult, political struggle. It isn't now, nor has it ever been, merely a question of not knowing how to do it. It's about having the political clout to make change.

Health/PAC: *Can the highly skilled R.N.s, the ''professionals,'' can they make alliances with the aides, the temps, the foreign nurses?*
Reverby: I think they've got to learn that if they don't they won't survive. That seems to be what the history teaches.

PEOPLE POWER VS. THE ALMIGHTY DOLLAR: HOW DEMOCRATIC MANAGEMENT CAN HELP TRANSFORM THE HMOs

Harry Krulewitch

I have spent over ten years working as a physician in democratically managed health care clinics in the Midwest and on the West Coast, and two years working for a large HMO in Minneapolis; in short, I have been exposed to the extremes of health care delivery available in this country.

My experiences in Minnesota have shown me that HMOs have little to do with health, are not interested in illness prevention and health maintenance, and are poorly organized. Their goal is to maximize enrollment and invest profits. I have seen HMOs systematically cut back on health education because it is not immediately profitable, sabotage independent community programs, and avoid any position on critical health care conflicts within the community. I have seen them refuse to either reduce premiums or pay bonuses to physicians at the end of fiscal years in which they reported handsome surpluses.[1]

Many people consider Minneapolis to be the center of the HMO movement. Indeed, our ten HMOs control 41 percent of the health care market in the Twin Cities. Physicians in private practice can also participate in so-called preferred provider organizations (PPOs), in which physicians provide services for reduced fees in return for a steady source of patients. Private physicians in the area depend on referrals from HMOs and PPOs for 60 percent of their practice. Ninety-five percent of all Twin City physicians belong to at least one of these organizations.[2]

It's hard to convey the full impact of this system on our community. Every day our newspapers and television and radio stations deliver a barrage of advertising for HMOs. For-profit hospital systems compete throughout the metropolitan region, and all but one hospital has merged or been sold to one of these national chains. Rural hospitals are closing.

The impact on physicians would have been unimaginable 10 years ago. The physician who contracts with an HMO, PPO, or independent practice association (IPA) agrees to let the organization temporarily withhold a portion of his or her fees. Holdbacks for primary care are typically from 10 to 20 percent; specialists must tolerate holdbacks of between 40 and 50 percent. Theoretically, most or all of this money is returned to providers at the end of the year, but if the company did poorly, much of it can vanish with the year-end accounting reports from the central HMO office. In 1986, 40 percent of physicians in the Twin Cities saw their income decline at least 10 percent in this way. Some saw their income cut in half.[3]

In the Belly of the Beast

How has the HMO system affected me personally? I worked for two years for an HMO organized around a staff model, where physicians are employees. During that time I was often told to do my work and go home and not ask questions about management. I saw physicians presented with 10 to 25 percent salary cuts and was then told that such contract violations constituted an incentive program. During a fiscal quarter when the HMO was running at a deficit, I saw an entire department of nurse practitioners laid off without warning on the day before they were to begin a citywide prevention program, essentially because they were the least organized group of providers. I was told my own pay raise would be withheld because I had organized a meeting of nurses, physicians, and clerical workers to discuss morale. The meeting, I was told, was critical of management and circumvented the standard channels of communication.

There was little flexibility or innovation where I worked, and little understanding of how to run a good clinic or build a health team. Despite a huge number of managers, morale was low and staff turnover high. Physicians felt captive. They had traded control over office and practice for benefits, repayment of their medical school loans, time off, and a secure income. When management began to consider laying off workers and cutting salaries, physicians were unable to organize themselves or confront management directly.

Physicians are recognizing that a transformation is underway. As cost containment fails, premiums rise, and income drops, it becomes apparent that the corporate system is generating huge profits at the expense of both the patient and provider. Some physicians are organizing challenges to the IPA's to question the legality of their management structure and obtain access to their books. Some are investigating the possibility of unionizing. Others are trying to lobby the legislature to pass laws that would enable physicians to engage in collective bargaining without violating antitrust laws. Many are merging their practices so that solo and small groups are disappearing. Some doctors are dropping out, bitter and frustrated.

No one can say for certain whether for-profit corporations will succeed in taking control of our health care. What's already clear, though, is that the struggle between providers and corporations is transforming a cottage industry into a corporate system. We can debate the quality of care that's resulting, but HMOs are clearly much more effective at managing money and generating profits than the old provider system, and any health planner who does not appreciate this transformation is making a big mistake.

In this struggle over who should control our health care system, only two alternatives are ever presented: providers or corporations.[4,5,6,7] But there is a third choice, although no significant policy currently being put into practice gives any legitimacy to it. The public is capable of and has the right to own and manage its own health care resources, and it is this alternative that we must fight for.

Health and Empowerment

It was my experience, in 11 years of work in participatory systems, that democratic ownership and participation can encourage community members to make fundamentally different choices about the use of their health care resources. I have seen democratic groups use resources for education, prevention services, home care, and community economic development, to establish neighborhood councils, and even to support a local nursing strike. The combination of personal self-care, community self-reliance, and worker self-determination can turn a health clinic into an agent for social change.

Democratic ownership is a complex issue, and dear to me personally. Despite its failures and problems, democratic management was the structure that most helped me to change my idea about what good care is and how a management system determines the quality of care. Collective work helped me to develop skills in communicating, sharing, listening, and cooperating. I learned to respect the contributions of others, and I could then apply those skills when working with patients. I continue to provide traditional clinical skills and diagnoses, but by using even a few learning skills and promoting a few prevention concepts, I can begin to change my role as a physician. I find the transition from authority to facilitator personally rewarding.

In the late 1970s I worked in a community-owned, worker-managed clinic in Oregon, which delivered integrated, holistic care. There, rather than making decisions for patients and controlling the course of their visits, the staff spent time educating them. By validating their concerns, exploring what physical, nutritional, socioeconomic, and emotional factors were involved in their illnesses, and which of these they could be responsible for, we attempted to empower them. We helped patients use cooperative skills—respect, communication—in interacting with their families, teaching them the power of those skills to affect their health and, ultimately, their community. In this way family medicine can be a model for larger social change.

Prevention services and self-care advocacy were important allies in this process: we supplemented our care with an outreach program to local communities and business. We formed a Health Action Council to bring health issues to the attention of local government. We trained block workers in leadership and self-care, devising procedures through which these workers could represent their communities in raising issues with the clinic's board.

Surviving the Lean Years

Of course, the maintainance of our democratically controlled clinic took an incredible amount of energy from its members. As the clinic grew more successful, democratic management became more and more difficult. When professionals were brought in to provide some business skills, conflicts arose between them and the original members, from whom they had very different values and perceptions of the role of management. Had we been able to orient the newcomers to our style of democratic management, we might have been able to work things out. Instead, the conflicts, coupled with cuts in funding, led to the clinic's eventual decline.

I see now that any democratic group that wishes to survive needs to commit itself to ongoing analysis of economic and political conditions. I have seen other democratically managed systems dissolve under the complexity of today's sophisticated health care delivery system, unable to make fiscal projections or coordinate complex billing reimbursements. The inability to accept clear lines of authority and establish effective business plans has destroyed them. But more than the lack of skilled fiscal and technical managers, the inability of people to cooperate and work for each other became insurmountable during difficult financial times.

The bottom line for the health planner, and particularly one who supports democratic control, is: Will the care be better in a democratic system? When the patient goes out the door of a clinic in our democratic health system, will she or he have had better medical care?

Redefining the Doctor's Role

The physician has a crucial role in answering these questions. At the heart of the medical system is the interaction between two people: patient and provider. The quality of that interaction is how we will measure that system; beyond any bureaucratic reorganization or national policy, it is in that setting that our efforts will be judged. That interaction, in workplace and in examining room, can be the place where we begin to create a new model of health care. Will it be oppressive or liberating? Insensitive or compassionate?

Today, the doctor-patient relationship is forged in our medical schools and residency centers, where the training is highly structured and extremely rigid. Doctors train in multimillion-dollar institutions amidst great poverty and suffering. The work is hard, often violent, chaotic, depressing, and frustrating. The glaring contradictions involved force many physicians to set their own survival above anything else. Distrust, isolation, cynicism, and arrogance are rampant. The authority physicians are taught to assume helps them remain insulated from their surroundings during these difficult years, but leaves them incapable of working in a cooperative setting. Physicians trained in such traditional systems are not likely to be interested in sharing control with patients. Where trust, intuition, communication, and caring are not valued, physicians are unlikely to empower others through their efforts to heal.

Democratic systems create new problems. The physician's is not a rotating position that is easily shared. Patients expect and need continuity of service. Yet physicians in democratic management systems face hostility from their professional peers and animosity from their own co-workers still dealing with repressed anger from previous encounters. The challenge is to build a system that can allow physicians to retain their proper sphere of responsibility without leaving them or others in the system unaccountable.

Change from Within

There are great obstacles to building any system of democratic ownership or management. These include the powerful, who will fight for the perpetuation of their privilege and profits; the complexity of the system itself, with its numerous reimbursement, therapeutic, and management modalities; and the communities that feel threatened when cultural standards are questioned by democratic initiatives and consequently will not give their support to them. Most of all, though, the obstacles lie within us, because we have little skill in nurturing or cooperating with and trusting each other.

But as public dissatisfaction with corporate medicine grows, as physician-patient interaction is reduced to a product-and-sales approach, patients will realize that their physicians have also lost control. There will be more opportunity for change. That change could be democratically driven, or it might come through massive federal reform, or worse, through support for greater subsidy of the privatization of the industry.

I do not know how we will get to a democratic system. But there is a lesson to be learned from dance therapy: support precedes movement. Democratic strategies need to be nurtured at many different levels, and in many regions, through citizens' groups, unions, coalitions, networks, and legislation. We need health providers, health planners, managers, and administrators who have studied and worked in well-organized research centers dedicated to studying the issue of democratic control. University and graduate schools need to develop programs around such a curriculum, and we need working models to challenge our imagination.

Physicians need to justify their leadership by promoting alliances with their patients and the communities they serve, not by fighting for a return to the days of provider control, and not by accepting corporate control as the only other option. The kinds of physicians who will do that are most likely to come from those communities that have encouraged democratic programs to grow. If democratic health systems are to evolve, they will emerge from personal, local, and regional efforts that give credibility to the idea of public ownership of resources.

NOTES

1. Miller, M. "Minnesota Health Care Markets: Cost Containment and Other Public Policy Goals," *1984 Report to Legislature, Minnesota Department of Health*. Reported in the *Minneapolis Star and Tribune*, 11/28/84, Section 1B.

2. *Reece Report*, Vol. 1, No. 3, June/July 1986, p. 11.

3. *Ibid.*, Vol. 1, No. 2, May 1986, p. 6.

4. Murray, J. "A Comparison of Patient Satisfaction Among Prepaid and Fee for Service Patients," *The Journal of Family Practice*, February 1987, p. 203.

5. Kennedy, L. "The Losses in Profits—How Proprietaries Affect Public and Voluntary Hospitals," *Health/PAC Bulletin*, Vol. 15, No. 6, Nov./Dec. 1984, p. 5.

6. "Medical Discord: Some Doctors Assail Quality of Treatment Provided by HMO's," *The Wall Street Journal*, Vol. 67, No. 235, 9/10/86, p.1.

7. "Doctors Will Review HMO's Effect on Care." *Minnesota Medical Association Annual Report*, 1986. Reported in the *Minneapolis Star and Tribune*, 5/3/86, Section 1B.

SECTION IV

COMMUNITY RESPONSE AND INNOVATIVE POLICY

INTRODUCTION

Nancy F. McKenzie

The progressive response to terrible times is often not easy to discern. This is particularly true in the arena of health care delivery because health care not only fulfills medical needs—it defines them. Without an independent understanding of what needs individuals have or the precise techniques or organization of care that could provide for them, it is difficult for citizens to assess health care. The situation becomes more complex when a society is so divided by class that it has separate institutions for the delivery of services.

Because health care delivery in the United States is now separate in financing, as well as in access to basic services, it is easy for the middle class to assume that sound fiscal policy will bring health care to all. Alternatively, it is clear to those working with communities not welcome in the majority of care facilities that, without a radical change in the institutions of health care, a change in fiscal policy will only serve to enhance revenues for providers and will not substantially extend health care to those most in need. President Clinton's offer of "Managed Competition" in the face of a national tuberculosis epidemic is but the latest example. Progressive health policy must bridge the divide that exists between those who are traditionally served by our health care institutions and those who are not.

This section refers specifically to communities and to innovative policy that principally comes from their attempts to provide for their own health care needs. It places its emphasis upon communities and their providers rather than on officials or health care policymakers in an attempt to go beyond the history of misinformation and dis-empowerment that has been the legacy of health care institutions in the United States—especially during the years of the "new federalism."

In the early 1980s, the American public accepted the fiction that health care was costing too much and that this was the fault of the public sector programs. Limits to health expenditure in federal programs were created and the country began to get used to the notion of "cost containment" as a fiscal fact of medical reality, especially for poor people. Public health was considered a luxury; disease prevention, a too-liberal rejoinder to the permissive sixties. Public health programs died; prevention was no longer a medical goal; new epidemics of tuberculosis, syphilis, measles, all came second to the continued creation of acute care technology and ideology.

It has taken a few years for the "new federalism" of the Reagan/Bush years to put the nation into a state of medical emergency. Due to the dismantling of safety net programs, the undoing of federal oversight and federal funding for worker safety, environmental and health programs, and the *vast* increase in the numbers and types of poor populations in the United States, the country has subdivided and now contains a developing country seeking relief within its own shores.

Not only has there been no agency with enough political will to respond to millions of homeless, undernourished, un-immunized, infectious individuals, there are no longer even the structures of care for chronic disease, for the disabled, for long-term care. All have been neglected during the gold rush of the last two decades for hospital expansion and physician entrepreneurship (brought into existence, in part, by the Medicaid and Medicare programs) in everything from diagnostic equipment to nursing homes. Consequently, not only do we not have a public health policy or a set of institutions whose primary job it is to oversee the nation's health, our teaching institutions no longer even produce enough basic care doctors to deal with poor communities.

In the United States today, we face a future of epidemic diseases that we have neither the research capability nor the basic care or housing infrastructure to respond to. According to *Science*, the United States has lost almost twenty years of public health and research expertise in tuberculosis alone. Our prevention and treatment programs in New York City, where tuberculosis is 45 times the national average, are not as good as those in *most developing countries*.

Those most negatively affected by the irrationality of the current health care system in the United States are the poor who have multiple health problems caused by the conditions of their lives—conditions which complicate an otherwise clear story of medical neglect.

The health emergency for poor individuals in the United States has not been announced, for there has been no one in the "Beltway" (otherwise known as Washington, D.C.) that cared enough to sound the alarm. The heads of all Congressional committees, recipients of hundreds of thousands of dollars from the major health PACS, have not sounded the alarm for reasons of self-interest. Between 1980 and 1990, over $27 million dollars went to Congressional representatives from *one* of the four health industries: pharmaceuticals, physician associations, insurance corporations, and hospitals.

For the 10-year period between 1980 and 1990, the United States Congress and all state legislative bodies, in full knowledge of the international scandal of our infant and maternal mortality rates, lack of housing for individuals with HIV, a growing tuberculosis epidemic, and millions of individuals without health care access, dealt with the health care crisis by devising further strategies of "cost containment." State budgets, strapped by the withdrawal of over 50 percent of federal funds for health care, created everything from *caps on hospital stays* for the poor and elderly to *rationing preventive health care for women and children*. Hundreds of programs designed to prevent catastrophic illness and disease in the most vulnerable *were cut*. Tuberculosis monies were ended. Immunization began to be publicly de-funded. Clinics closed, hospitals in poor neighborhoods in urban and rural areas closed, departments of health cut services and were transformed from community epidemiological oversight and intervention centers into single-function testing sites for sexually transmitted diseases. Medicaid eligibility showed a frightening disparity between states, who pay 25 percent of its funding. In 1990, a family of four in Alabama was eligible for Medicaid only if they made under $1,700 a year, while a family in Vermont was eligible if they made under $7,500. All manner of stratagems were used to keep individuals from utilizing their public programs. Medicare has become a virtual sea of paperwork. Medicaid has developed into a labyrinth of documentation and intrusion, and has been used by Medicare recipient nursing homes to supplement their income. Only 40 percent of Medicaid funds in 1991 went to poor people. And only 40 percent of the eligible poor were covered under Medicaid.

Those who were "policy analysts" in the 1980s tended to be careerists, more businessmen and -women than health experts, and they spent most of their time developing hidden "cost containment" strategies for all of the public programs, leaving in their wake bureaucratic structures so tied to "disinformation" that it is now virtually impossible to make heads or tails of whole agencies specifically designed to serve the poor. The social service institutions are places of intentional under-service, designed to disguise the lack of meaningful structures of rescue and care. The *official* health care movement in America has been largely a financial movement—a consumer movement which seeks to make health care more "affordable" through payer schemes. It has not been a movement that seeks to make anyone accountable for a system of health care delivery that neglects the ordinary while profiting from the extraordinary. This movement has not been a citizens' movement in the sense that "citizen" carries any weight in the political policies that are developing. Rather, it has been led by an agenda for change in insurance tailored by corporations and lobbying groups who are currently designing a health payer system largely for the well-employed. They studiously avoid the notion of a national health care system or the universal right to health care. Finally this year, in response to the Clinton task force proposals, a citizens' health movement, calling for substantial changes, has emerged. (See "Change the Health Care System? How UHCAN," p. 645.)

If anything can change the substance of the delivery of health care in the United States, it will not be policymakers. It will be the AIDS epidemic, the outrage among women, particularly women of color, over the reproductive cancers and issues of prenatal care, and the increased numbers of people negotiating a life around disability and around issues of homelessness, drug use, homicide, and suicide.

No one, except communities themselves, their providers, advocates, and representatives seem to want to face the sheer redundancy, irrelevance, and malfeasance of the American health care system. Those who do and have spoken to the outrage of our current health care system (like Health/PAC) rely upon struggling communities for guidance to make the conceptual stretch to meaningful change.

AIDS and the follow-up by epidemiologists charting its spread have highlighted the extent to which hundreds of thousands of individuals in our cities are without social networks, housing, education, or jobs, and are almost beyond hope or health. They are not portrayed this way in the American media but are instead stigmatized as drug-using criminals. Because of their marginality, help for these individuals comes largely from within their own ranks and from community advocates who attempt to procure and provide services for the individuals' physical and mental needs.

These make up a vast network of people entirely politicized by death and suffering who do not have the professional smugness of the unscathed but who understand the issues of health care as being closer to civil rights than to finances. This is a kind of health activism that occurs in small community groups struggling to stay ahead of two epidemics (HIV and, now, tuberculosis) that are killing thousands of individuals, and social policy producing unemployment, housing displacement, and drug-related poverty that is making streets and shelters, prisons and hospitals substitute for communities, jobs, and housing.

It is among communities and in their most radical measures that health care delivery finds its reformation. The accomplishments are not seamless, nor do they lend themselves to generalization. But it has, in the national economic crisis of the 1990s, become evident what people can do for people; what advocates can do for patients; what services lawyers can procure; what suffering humane providers can help their patients avoid; what bureaucratic red tape social workers can cut through for clients; what vision patients can have of their rights, their deaths, and the quality of their time left given the institutional space and community support to do so.

In their corner of political action and outright service, whether this corner is geographical or conceptual, communities carve out issues which the national debate has left unaddressed. They fill in gaps unseen by "policymakers" and they offer resistance to what many consider to be the "medicalization" of ever-worsening social conditions. Demonstrable change has come from the "new urban activism," from AIDS activism and its treatment and research alternatives, from the "empowering" strategies of self-help in the National Black Women's Health Project, in the "harm reduction" movement, from activists in the disability movement, from traditional providers who see beyond "business as usual" service, and from the political activism of health care unions.

Tony Bale opens this section with an editorial on "Activism in the New Urban Health Crisis" (p. 406), which accompanied a special edition of the *Health/PAC Bulletin*, from which many articles in this section are taken. Bale speaks directly to the health crisis in American cities outlined in the preceding sections of this book. He points to a "social transformation" that has already occurred within groups committed to providing care "where the need was greatest, when it counted, doing what had to be done." And indeed, many articles in this section graphically describe individuals motivated by the moral imperatives of direct service in "makeshift" structures for those imperiled by a new level of poverty and affliction in America. But Bale also calls for a "shared understanding" and a "unifying political vision" of the altered conditions of peoples' lives and of the reforms that can address them—a political vision that has yet to occur.

Few movements have had to be as innovative or as resourceful as those that work with homeless individuals. According to the Legal Services Homelessness Task Force, National Housing Law Project,[1] there are about twice as many very low-income families seeking housing as there are available affordable units, with the number of very low-income renter households exceeding the number of units by a national average of 93.7 percent.[2] According to one report, 84 percent of the cities surveyed reported an average 26 percent increase in the demand for assisted housing in 1987.[3] From 1970 to 1982, many cities lost from 50 to 85 percent of their single room occupancy (SRO) facilities,[1] and the General Accounting Office (GAO) estimated that these losses totaled 1.1 million units.[4] These hotels are a traditional source of low-cost housing for single low-income people.

Over a third of homeless individuals are women and children. Another third of them are seriously ill and in need of primary health care, mental health counseling, or drug treatment. In "Rethinking Empowerment" (p. 409), Cheryl Merzel (in introducing presentations at an empowerment and housing conference held in New York City in 1991), speaks to the paradox of self-help programs. The paradox exists in the fact that these alternative programs presume that energies will be more devoted to small, local acts of delivery than to a larger political change that might make them unnecessary. Of the panelists, Sally Guttmacher and Jeremy Leeds ("Empowerment," p. 412) reflect on the apolitical history of the term. Gwen Braxton ("Well-being Is Our Birthright," p. 416) outlines the philosophy and strategies for self-help in the Black Women's Health Project. In "Knowledge Is Power," (p. 420) Gabrielle Immerman writes about self-help in a women's shelter in New York City. And finally, in "Housing and Empowerment" (p. 427), Ellen Baxter speaks about the power of a lease to the individuals in a project she heads who find housing for themselves and work cooperatively to run and pay for it.

"In the Role of the Disability Movement in Health Care Reform" (p. 433) Bob Griss articulates the extent to which disabled individuals must be the bellwether for an improved health care system and offers a more concrete understanding of what are the true issues of health care reform. The issues are as much about access as about liberation; about civil rights as about patient rights; about self definition as about medical condition. These issues are further explored by the two Health/PAC articles on Sharon Kowalski and her lover Karen Thompson, who struggled against the twin disenfranchisements of lesbian families and disability.

The political activism of HIV tells some of the story of how access to health care can evolve into questions of the content and effectiveness of health care itself. In looking back on the first decade of AIDS, it is instructive to see the movement as it developed from an assertion of civil rights to medical discourse.

Once people with AIDS began to be recognized as sick people and to receive health care that was dominated by the controversial use of anti-viral treatment, the issues of treatments themselves emerged. This involved going beyond pure cellar interdiction of the virus to enabling clinical treatment of the myriad infections that dominate the medical lives of people with HIV. Out of this has come an understanding of HIV as a chronic condition—a more generic way of regarding the disease, and also a "code" for the numerous medical access and civil rights issues that emerge out of the myopia of our provider defined, acute care health care system.

General health issues are regarded monolithically by public health experts and the health establishment only so long as the definitions of health needs remain the province of experts. As soon as communities are empowered enough to have a say in their own health needs, the understanding of health needs changes and reflects the needs that exist in the lives of the affected.[5]

In her article "AIDS at the Beginning of the Second Decade" (p. 457), McKenzie discusses the development of the HIV epidemic and its influence on American medicine on the occasion of the Sixth International Conference on AIDS. Nick Freudenberg, in "Teaching to Live: Learning from Ten Years of AIDS" (p. 466), and "Know News: Reassessing Communities" (p. 471), reflects on the meaning of AIDS activism for the notion of community development.

The disability and chronic care movement is one that seeks to address the ways in which health care in the United States not only neglects the majority of conditions that keep people from getting on with their lives, but, when it engages them, does so in such a way as to make the problem worse rather than better. This is highlighted by "Home Is Where the Patients Are: New York's Home Care Workers" (p. 448), in which Barbara Caress speaks to the important struggle of the Health and Hospitals Union (1199) to get a union for under-paid home care workers, and also by Jean Stewart, at the end of this chapter, whose "voice" piece, "The Troublesome Cripples of Orlando: Disability and Activism" (p. 499) gives us a glimpse of another kind of activism. In this powerful article we witness the attempt of disabled veterans of nursing homes to focus upon the ways in which health care delivery is skewed for the enormous profits of the nursing home industry, not only to the detriment of effective health care treatment, but to the civil rights of individuals who are imprisoned, often for life, simply because they require help with dressing.

Since "empowerment" may be an equivocal term for the "self-help" necessitated by failed institutions, and may point to the need for individuals to fight their victimization in regimes that deprive them of the right to housing, to jobs, to food, to treatment, and to self-determination, a more political term might be needed. Given the background of so much harm caused by the last 10 years of federal neglect and resulting attack upon the poor, as well as the development of epidemics and lack of infrastructures that keep people from receiving help, "Harm Reduction" (discussed by Rod Sorge in "Harm Reduction: A New Approach to Drug Services" p. 484) might, in fact, be the rallying cry of the new health reform movement. "Harm reduction" engages not only the conditions of people's lives but those conditions as they are systematically developed, and then medicalized in a political war against the poor, the sick, the "uncooperative" unemployed, homeless and malnourished individuals, or those who are disabled and who quarrel with their incarceration.

Chronic conditions are individuating conditions—the condition of people's lives, rather than their bodies. Chronic conditions are the "way we live now" of any group of people joined together in devising strategies of maintenance and enablement whether they emerge out of the activism of AIDS, women and cancer, the disability movement, or homeless individuals who create living spaces for themselves. "Community health," the term of the civil rights health movement of the 1960s, has given itself over to people without "communities" of any kind (in the geographical sense) other than those based upon affinities of struggle. Thus the AIDS and the disability movements have taught the nation again, in the 1980s and 1990s, what African Americans have known for decades. And the new warriors, in forging health care responses to the conditions of their lives, have made the nation think seriously about the extent to which medical care is necessary when home care or community support is truly the issue. But, more than this, their struggles exemplify the extent to which health care must be "community-driven" rather than "provider-driven." It must be developed out of the multiplicity of needs that people bring to the doors of health care, as well as the conditions of their lives that prompt those needs. No institution, particularly one that is designed primarily for profit, can devise the essential means for individuals to negotiate their lives and their health with the effectiveness of communities who have developed their own "safety nets" in the storms of economic crisis.

Innovation can occur within traditional structures of health care delivery when providers take into account the individuals and the situations of their lives as they devise strategies for caretaking. In "Successful Strategies: Meeting the Needs of Children in Adversity" (p. 473), Lisbeth Schorr speaks to the ways in which conventional providers can be innovative in reaching the children they wish to help by more broadly defining the tasks that lie before them. Highlighting the fragmentation that is now inherent in our health care system, Dr. Schorr calls upon individuals to figure out ways around dysfunction institutions to bring cohesion to the care for sick and poor children. And in "Media Scan: The View from Olympus" (p. 482) by Hal Strelnick we get the view of a physician who works in broken neighborhoods, contrasted with his academic counterpart who sees nothing but the abstract policy of "business as usual." In this article we can view both sides of the chasm that exists between the innovation of communities and the fiscal policy of academic policy makers. (In Section V, "Another Kind of Bronx Cheer," (p. 574), we will have an extended discussion of Dr. Strelnick's clinic as a structure that allows for the development of adequate health care delivery.)

Now that the nation has finally rejected the Republican dismantling of the federal government, it is entirely possible that not only communities, but whole cities will begin to regard the health care needs of its constituents as the highest priority and fund some of the programs and humane strategies outlined in this section. No country in the world is more in need of a health care system focused upon individual need than the United States. And no country in the world is more blind to the fact that such a system has its nascent concept already operative in its shelters, its soup kitchens, its unions, its drug addiction activists, and its disabled individuals.

N O T E S

1. Unpublished communication from Mary Ellen Hombs, Director, Homelessness Task Force.
2. Hombs, Low Income Housing Information Service (LIHIS) estimate, 1992.
3. Hombs, Conference of Mayors, *Growth of Hunger*, p. 43.
4. Ibid., p. 23.
5. Nancy F. McKenzie, "HIV and the Role of Community," in *AIDS: Social, Political, Ethical Issues*, New York: Meridian, 1991, p. 494.

ACTIVISM IN THE NEW URBAN HEALTH CRISIS

Tony Bale

It is time to appreciate and learn from the powerful work of a new generation of urban health activists. The articles in this issue of the *Health/PAC Bulletin* lead me both to honor the activists' commitment and talent and to look for a more encompassing political project that builds upon their diverse experience.

In contrast to the health activists of the 1960s, who were embedded in a movement pressing for broad-based, grass-roots democratic social transformation, the new generation came to political awareness over the course of the 1980s more through engaging the immediate survival needs of people around them, as well as their own. Often out of public view, working in the margins of the health care and related systems that responded to conditions of newly intensified suffering, the new generation was motivated less by theory than by the moral imperatives to help and heal. They responded to their personal needs to act, to do what one can, to try and make a difference, while people around them were dying, being denied vital care, losing their homes, being destroyed by drugs and violence, and becoming infected with deadly diseases at a horrifying rate.

The new generation, seeking out communities others actively avoided, has developed respectful ways of working with people in marginalized and threatened communities that the mainstream health care system, with its elitist and technocratic orientation, disparages, when it provides service at all. Some have made the transition from movement volunteer to professional in an organization they helped build; many have developed programs that have been influential far beyond their small size. All can say that in the midst of the urban health catastrophe we are living through, they have been where the need was greatest, when it counted, doing what had to be done.

The articles in this issue illustrate some of the character and accomplishments of the new urban health activists. Building upon the experience of the sixties generation, empowerment became their distinctive, unifying goal. The activists understand empowerment as expanding the sphere of personal choice, building support systems, such as self-help groups, and feeling rooted in communities of oppressed people in struggle for their dignity and health. Only individuals who are truly empowered—through adequate information and the space to make meaningful choices, a strong social support network, and connection to broader struggles of the communities to which they belong—are regarded as fully free to seek health.

Working with people where they are at, which often means in desperate and difficult circumstances, the new activists seek to build on peoples' strengths, while addressing their immediate needs for food and shelter, access to health services, and preventing infection with the HIV virus. They seek to provide immediate help in a way that gives people a sense of their own power and enlists them in the fight for more. A common thread connects the self-help groups of the Black Women's Health Project, the counseling of battered and homeless women in shelters by the Women's Health Education Project, the politically conscious AIDS education described by Nick Freudenberg, the work of activists like Rod Sorge who took it upon themselves to challenge the law by distributing clean needles to intravenous drug users, and Ellen Baxter and her colleagues' work converting abandoned buildings into affordable housing for people without homes. All combine elements of personal transformation, provision of help in a nonhierarchical and noncontrolling way by virtual peers, and identification with communities in struggle.

Not surprisingly, given the pervasive individualism of the dominant culture and the difficult political times, the work of the new generation of urban health activists falls most heavily on the side of personal rather than political empowerment. Building lasting support structures that empower people to engage in prolonged struggle for collective transformation remains a distant goal. The most apparent strengths of the new activists are their energy, commitment, and ability to develop small-scale practical models to address pressing needs. Yet the social space, the political conjuncture, in which they work does not have a name, let alone a coherent set of shared understandings that could help them forge a common political project. Nor are the activists able to draw upon the kind of organized political vehicle that would allow them to move from trying to keep things from getting worse to starting to attack the root causes of the health problems they confront.

It is time to give a name to the altered conditions of suffering and death that the new generation of urban health activists has responded to. It is time to break through some of the silences imposed by various professional, academic, media, and, yes, community and left political discourses, to begin to name and describe the core of the social transformation the new activists work within. I believe many urban health activists already feel a need to understand the connections between the elements in the kind of familiar litany invoked by Emilio Carillo, former head of the New York City Health and Hospitals Corporation, when he told a congressional committee in 1990 of the impact of the drug epidemic: "New York endures a much larger share of the costly public health consequences of this epidemic: increased violence, AIDS, homelessness, seriously ill newborns, overcrowded hospitals and compromised care."

All these elements are linked; all are part of an ensemble of suffering and death that has struck New York and other cities in recent years. It is the new urban health crisis, the complex catastrophe that forms the unacknowledged context for much of this work. The crisis builds upon growing economic, racial and spatial polarization, intensified poverty, and badly organized and overloaded service systems. The core of the new urban health crisis is the ensemble consisting of the interrelated conditions of HIV and other infections, homelessness, violence, drug use, and mental illness. The new urban health crisis spirals through individual lives, social networks, and communities to produce a more extensive, more visible and palpable, more deadly and senseless pattern of suffering and death in the cities. A newly expanded system of services and social control becomes prominent in the crisis management of people variously regarded as at risk, sick, and dangerous.

Within the crisis, urban health activists develop and advocate models of care and service that draw upon and expand the abilities of people in difficult circumstances to control their lives. They struggle against the alternative: models of collective policing and crisis management of objectified persons addressed principally as threats to public health and the social order.

The new urban health crisis, located largely in low-income minority communities, is, I believe, the major health event of our time. Those working within it are well positioned to reflect upon its distinctive structure of suffering, service, and struggle. Working from a shared understanding of the new urban health crisis could help infuse the organizing and programs of the dispersed activists with a unifying political vision. We lack critiques that point toward a full understanding of the altered conditions we are living through; a richer understanding of the current conjuncture could help inform the analysis and practice addressing the many segmented problem areas of the crisis. By naming it, analyzing it, debating it, and developing a political response that ties disparate issues and struggles to a common vision of individual, networks of solidarity, and community transformation, activists can inject their agenda more fully into the political life of the nation. Urban health activists need to be heard loudly in the national health care reform debate, where the urban agenda is largely absent.

The convulsive urban health transformations of the 1980s have thus far produced little in the way of shared analysis among health activists. The time is right to reflect on this experience, to develop a political response from within the new urban health crisis that addresses the broad social changes needed to end it. The *Health/PAC Bulletin*, with its origins in sixties activism, has recently reported and reflected on this new terrain, giving voice to the concerns of the new generation of urban health activists. As this exploration continues, we invite your ideas and your help.

RETHINKING EMPOWERMENT

Cheryl Merzel

Editor's Note: The following five articles are presentations at a Health/PAC forum in 1991 on "Women and the Meanings of Empowerment in Public Health."

Empowerment has become the latest buzzword in health education and social welfare policy in the United States. Although the concept was created by the left several decades ago, there is currently a new emphasis on empowerment among some progressives in the United States who are living and working in poor and minority communities. In areas ranging from teen pregnancy to housing development, the concept of empowerment is invoked to explain the failure of past policies and to point the way to solutions for dealing with the effects of poverty.

A fascinating offshoot of this phenomenon is the use of empowerment across the political spectrum. The right uses the term to define and promote its platform for counteracting the "dependency" of the poor supposedly created by reliance on public welfare programs. Jack Kemp, Secretary of the Department of Housing and Urban Development, has made empowerment the policy of choice for addressing urban problems. The federal Centers for Disease Control refer to empowerment as a method for educating about HIV and AIDS.

Obviously, empowerment cannot mean the same thing to such politically diverse groups. The significance attached to empowerment by its progressive adherents, particularly women of color, calls for a closer look at how they define the approach to understand why it is so important and to explore the possibilities of empowerment as an instrument for social change. The right's appropriation of the concept compels us to articulate the similarities and differences in its definition.

Empowerment as a Process

It was in this spirit that Health/PAC sponsored a forum last spring that brought together six women to discuss the meanings of empowerment in public health. The following articles by panelists Sally Guttmacher, Ellen Baxter, and Gwen Braxton are based on presentations given at that forum and present some of the issues surrounding the resurgence of the concept of empowerment. LaRay Brown of New York City Health and Hospitals Corporation and Marilyn John of J & B Health Consultants also participated in the panel, as did Stephanie Stevens of the Women's Health Education Project, which is featured here in

Gabrielle Immerman's article. Several themes emerged from the forum. First, self-esteem is an essential element of empowerment. Although this may be reminiscent of the victim-blaming "culture of poverty" hypothesis, it also resonates with Jesse Jackson's "I am somebody" notion, as well as the consciousness-raising of the health groups that developed *Our Bodies, Ourselves*. Empowerment is a process, not a product, which has several levels. The first level is the realization that one deserves to have one's needs met and that one is capable of making decisions in order to fulfill one's needs. The second level is knowing when and how to use this newly discovered voice, and the third is using the voice and wielding power. Thus, there must be an evolution of personal empowerment first before political empowerment can be developed. But, we should not overlook that the converse is also true. Powerlessness does not occur without structures of oppression.

Another theme raised at the forum was a critique of traditional health education models that emphasize compliance with predetermined standards of behavior and ignore the full context of the lives of the poor and people of color. As one speaker noted in reference to the patients' rights movement among the mentally ill, "at times, *non-compliance* is empowering." Others agreed that empowerment is not intended to be a tool to achieve increasing compliance with professionally accepted standards; it is a process by which people make decisions that are right for them. Among these groups, empowerment is viewed as a means of resisting the passive and dehumanizing patient and client roles engendered by the social service and health care systems. The welfare bureaucracy in particular was repeatedly referred to as a source of oppression that disempowers poor women and women of color.

Sally Guttmacher and Jeremy Leeds provide a thought-provoking critique of the concept of empowerment. They ask the important question of how people can be empowered when in fact they lack real political power in a society. The authors trace the historical impact of empowerment movements in health, education, and welfare. They conclude that although these movements have raised important issues that have not been addressed by the traditional left, they have been ineffective in creating social change because they focus on the paternalism of welfare state institutions and leave underlying political structures unchallenged. In this sense, there is a similarity with the right's targeting of the liberal welfare state in its critique of anti-poverty policy. While the tension between individuals and institutions of social control may be unresolvable, the right appears to take the argument a few steps further and actually blame these individuals for the perpetuation of poverty. Whereas empowerment movements of the past may have ignored oppressive social structures, the right refuses outright to recognize the class-, race-, and gender-based roots of inequality.

In her article, Gwen Braxton of the New York Black Women's Health Project identifies the mentality of helplessness as a product of poverty, racism, and sexism. Through the process of empowerment, individuals are liberated from that helplessness to make their own decisions and implement them to the fullest extent possible. For Braxton, health is a holistic state that encompasses the physical, emotional, interpersonal, and political. The health problems of African-American women derive both from their social conditions and their internalization of these conditions. In order to improve their health, therefore, women must first empower themselves to take control over their lives.

In a discussion of empowerment for the homeless, Ellen Baxter states what is obvious but is all too often overlooked: having a home is empowerment. Without stable housing and a home, a person is disenfranchised. Baxter provides an enlightening "how-to manual" for developing supportive, community-based and tenant-managed housing that doesn't segregate people by socio-medical diagnosis. She speaks of the bureaucratic barriers to creating such housing, including a social service system that is committed to keeping people in a transitional state until their personal problems are solved, rather than seeking to develop supportive housing alternatives that provide additional social services as well.

Gabrielle Immerman discusses the Women's Health Education Project (WHEP), which works with women in shelters for the homeless in New York City. This organization was developed by holistic health practitioners working in traditional community clinics who became frustrated with their inability to prevent poor health among their patients. They created a program of women— practitioners and clients—working together to form health education focus groups dealing with self-help and preventive health care. Like the Black Women's Health Project, WHEP sees empowerment as a means of facilitating a woman's decision making and providing her with knowledge of options so she can make her own choices. In this context, WHEP informs women about alternatives to the alienating, fragmented, acute-illness oriented health care system.

From Personal to Political

The current empowerment movement recognizes the need for political activity on a broader level, but it is tethered by the many factors that make it difficult for the poor to organize. Whether these new organizations can develop into a movement is a question that remains to be answered. Their self-help groups bring to mind the consciousness-raising groups of the feminist movement, which also started on the personal level before developing to the political. Another, more recent model of evolutionary empowerment is the gay community's challenge to the health care system spurred by the HIV epidemic. Following this example, a new patients' rights movement is growing among people with cancer.

Although it may be argued that all these movements can only be effective in forcing reform rather than true transformation of the system, the discussions of empowerment in this issue make clear that such changes can appreciably improve the daily lives of the many people who struggle just to get by. And in so doing, empowerment may not need to develop into its own movement in order to be part of a larger political process. By helping people achieve a sense of human dignity and worth for themselves and for others, empowerment may be the first step toward political awareness. And that would be an ironic legacy for Jack Kemp and his ilk.

EMPOWERMENT: A TERM IN NEED OF A POLITICS

Sally Guttmacher and Jeremy Leeds

After approximately 25 years, "empowerment" as a movement or concept doesn't have much to show for itself. This is in stark contrast to a promising beginning, when various disciplines and social forces—feminism, community psychology, education, progressive health movements—seemed to find in empowerment an embodiment of the new attitudes to authority. But in fact, it could be argued that the biggest boost for "empowerment" in at least the past decade came when Jack Kemp, Secretary of Housing and Urban Development in the Bush administration, appropriated the term as the watchword of his housing policy. We hardly need to point out that this isn't what the original "empowerment" advocates had in mind! It does no good to say that this is not "really" empowerment. What empowerment "really" is has not been sufficiently established, and Kemp unfortunately has as much of a claim on it as anyone.

The impasse facing empowerment as an organizing concept in health and mental health provision calls for an evaluation. We are not arguing that empowerment is dead or irrelevant. Many of the contributions in this issue show that valuable activities are being performed by dedicated organizers and community members under the empowerment label. However, after 25 years, the term has not been adequately defined; and the concept has not become a dominant force in social change movements, let alone a decisive force in any area of social struggle. Why is this so?

There are several weaknesses in empowerment as a concept. These are the unresolvable lack of clarity in its definition; the parasitic relationship of empowerment to the liberal welfare state that characterized American government in the middle of this century; problems with the "power" component of empowerment as an overriding concept; lack of clarity about the relationship—desired and actual—of the empowered individual to the community; and a failure to acknowledge and attempt to have an impact on real power. At the same time, the questions and problems that gave rise to the notion of empowerment are still there, no matter how inadequate the current answers are; and we thus still have a long way to go.

The provision of health, educational, and psychological services has traditionally been seen as fundamentally a one-way transaction, in which a relatively passive subject is helped by the ministrations of the authority and expert. The relationship between the "helping professional" and the client, however concretely helpful, always runs the risk of fostering a dependence that in the long run hinders the client's independent evaluation and action. Illich has made this point in examining the traditional doctor-patient relationship.[1] In the field of social criticism, Lasch makes the case that "the school, the helping professions, and the peer group have taken over most of the family's functions," and that, while possibly humane in intent, such usurpation has debilitated those it means to protect.[2] In political action, "community control" movements, typified by the Black Panther Party's medical and breakfast programs and the calls for community control of police and education, saw the goal of building an alternative and more progressive source of resources for poor and oppressed communities as in some fashion a foundation for a new society. In the women's health movement of the early 1970s, demands for women's control over aspects of medicine pertaining to female reproduction sought to challenge the dominance of males and professionals in a key sphere of control of women's lives. As one of this paper's authors said in 1979,

> Although the concepts of self-help and self-care can be easily perverted and coopted, especially as a rationalization for cutting back on services, they also offer individuals a constructive way to decrease their dependency both on health care professionals and on traditional health care institutions.[3]

The concept of empowerment was originally an attempt to codify the spirit of these and other such responses to the problems of overprofessionalization, mystification, inadequate service delivery, and lack of control over key aspects of oppressed peoples' lives. "Power" as an overriding concept was woven into the fabric of the new "helping relationship." Conflict over power and control, sometimes including conflict with the helper, was often seen as therapeutic for the individual. In community psychology, empowerment was sounded as a call to replace the "paternalism" of other models of service delivery.[4] In education, specifically concerning literacy, Freire has argued that the learning process must be a transformative one that includes the subject's becoming an engaged opponent of oppressive social structures.[5] In short, "empowerment" was initially a concept relating the "personal" to the "political," in the sense that it was a statement about a new concept of the everyday life goals embedded in social struggle, and vice versa.

Weaknesses in the Concept

From the beginning, however, the concept has been fraught with contradiction and unclarity. While Kiefer expressed a need for greater clarity of definition,[6] others were less bothered by the impreciseness. "We do not know what empowerment is, but like obscenity, we know it when we see it," wrote one commentator.[7] (Given recent developments in the Supreme Court, this is a rather unfortunate analogy.)

A second problem has been the possible contradiction between empowerment as a psychological feeling of potency and empowerment as actual power acquired from access to resources. The question continues to arise, even in the context of the contributions in this journal: just what do the "empowered" have power over?

From the perspective of the 1990s, we think it is clear that the key weakness in empowerment is that the background has shifted and exposed the context-dependent nature of the concept. Empowerment was a response to perceived inadequacies and paternalism, in various forms, of the liberal welfare state, as implemented by Democratic administrations from Roosevelt to Johnson (and administered more or less uninterruptedly by Nixon, Ford, and Carter). With the dismantling of this welfare state, or at least of liberalism as the country's dominant ideology, empowerment is often uncomfortably unable to differentiate itself as an ideology from the budget-cutting, "bootstrap," "self-help," "thousand points of light," anti-government-spending philosophy of the Reagan Republicans. Thus, Kemp's ability to claim it for his own. In these times, therefore, instead of being seen as an alternative to dominant government practices, empowerment often shades into making a virtue of necessity, of at the very least not coming to terms with government's outright abandonment of the poor.

Ironically, then, it appears that empowerment had its greatest impact when it was fighting its original opponent, the liberal welfare state. Now that liberalism has suffered a major defeat, at someone else's hands, a large part of its *raison d'etre* has vanished.

Empowerment in Context

It is time to examine the message, the morality, the vision we want to put across, and to determine the place that power has in this context. Power itself is a problematic concept. Power over what? to what? for what? "Power over one's own life" is a good slogan, but not good enough. What is the context? Is the power to be exercised in the context of a community? If so, what kind of community? Whatever the answers to these questions, is power, however defined, the value to which we want to accord pride of place? What about freedom, happiness, equality?

Furthermore, in a world to be hoped for, will we not be entitled to, and even encouraged to, cede some of our power to others who can help and care for us in ways we cannot for ourselves? To put it bluntly, in some situations we have a right and need to be passive and dependent and to expect that those who care for us, including government, will be humane. Alternative institutions and caretakers in the community, however empowerment-oriented, who must care for the needy without the requisite material support are at best a stopgap—often an essential one—but not the basis of a health care policy.

This leads to the larger political problem with empowerment. For many people at this time, the authorities to whom one would cede such power are not benevolent. But most community activists who promote the concept of empowerment in its current forms accept this larger power as a given and attempt to work around it. For example, the goal of a number of projects is to tie clients into social welfare programs that frequently leave them feeling frustrated and powerless rather than empowered. The small community focus and veritable siege mentality that accompanies much of today's empowerment rhetoric is a product of the hostile environment over which, sadly, community activists have little control at this time. But "working around" this problem can only get us so far. The real questions of power and control remain to be addressed.

Like many of the social movements and theories that arose in the struggles of the 1960s, the notion of empowerment has thrown a light on problems that had been ignored or inadequately addressed by the traditional left. In brief, it brings us to question the relationship to be desired between the leaders and the led and between the individual and the community. What are the limits of benevolent assistance?

Empowerment is likely to remain a contested concept and therefore an ambiguous one. Its positive legacy is a dedicated group of organizers and practitioners, a way to look at and evaluate programs and movements, and a persistent set of difficult but vital questions.

NOTES

1. Illich, Ivan, *Medical Nemesis*, London: Calder and Boyars, 1975.

2. Lasch, C., *Haven in a Heartless World*, New York: Basic Books, 1979, p. xiv.

3. Guttmacher, Sally, "Whole in Body, Mind and Spirit: Holistic Health and the Limits of Medicine," *The Hastings Center Report*, August 1979, pp. 15–21.

4. Swift, C., "Empowerment: An Antidote to Folly," in Rappaport, Swift, and Hess, eds., *Studies in Empowerment: Steps Toward Understanding and Action*, New York: Haworth Press, 1984, p. xi.

5. Freire, Pablo, *The Pedagogy of the Oppressed*, translated by Myra Ramos, New York: Continuum, 1970.

6. Kiefer, C., "Citizen Empowerment: A Developmental Perspective," in Rappaport, Swift, and Hess, eds., op. cit., pp. 9–36.

7. Rappaport, J., "Studies in Empowerment: Introduction to the Issue," in Rappaport, Swift, and Hess, eds., op. cit., p. 2.

WELL-BEING IS OUR BIRTHRIGHT: THE MEANING OF EMPOWERMENT FOR WOMEN OF COLOR

Gwen Braxton

The Brooklyn-based New York Black Women's Health Project is a chapter of the National Black Women's Health Project (NBWHP), which was founded in 1980 by Byllye Avery of Atlanta, Georgia, as a way of filling the void in both the mainstream health care system and the feminist health movement regarding the specific needs of African-American women. According to Avery, health education is "not just about giving information; people need something else. . . . We are dying inside. . . . Unless we are able to go inside ourselves and touch and breathe fire, breathe life into ourselves, [of] course, we couldn't be healthy. [We] started working on a workshop that we named 'Black and Female: What Is the Reality?' This is a workshop that terrifies us all. And we are also terrified not to have it, because the conspiracy of silence is killing us."

The NBWHP attempts to break this conspiracy of silence by giving African-American women an environment of supportive self-help groups in which women are able to express the whole of the condition of their lives and share their feeling with others who understand what it is like to be Black and female in this society. A basic philosophy of the organization is that health behavior is not simply a matter of knowing what to do or not to do and then making "rational choices"; rather, individual health reflects personal and social circumstances. Poor women often know the "facts" but feel powerless to make changes because their lives are conditioned by many levels of oppression and despair.

People are born with many powers, including the power of self-healing. I was over 30 before I understood what power is or that I was powerful. I was very interested in but confused about being a human being. I didn't even know what feelings were. I was disconnected from myself. I thought feelings were somewhere out there in my "soul" and not related to my body.

Human beings are born powerful and, given the appropriate care and environment, will increase this power. We focus on what infants can't do and fail to notice that they have the necessary resource to get others to help satisfy their basic needs for food, care, exploration, attention, physical affection, human interaction, and so forth. That is power—the ability to satisfy our basic needs. When we are children, the adults around us unintentionally interfere with the development of this power. How? Listen to what they tell us: "Hush, now don't cry, there's nothing to cry about. Come on eat all of this it's good for you; I've been slaving over this food for you. Don't talk so loud. Walk, don't run; you're going to hurt yourself. You can't wear your hair like that. I'm tired, it's time for you to go to bed. Do what I say or I'll spank (punish, or stop loving) you. Shut that child up; give her a pacifier. There's nothing wrong with him, he just wants some attention. Don't pick that child up, don't play with that child, you'll spoil her. The family is your only protection against the dangerous people in the world. Keep the things that happen in the family secret. Don't be so emotional. Keep your feelings to yourself. Don't brag; be modest, be humble. You can only be affectionate with the family you were born into, the person you marry, and children.''

All of this is contrary to what healthy human beings need. We need to feel good about ourselves, whoever we are, to be able to identify and to satisfy our own needs.

Empowerment is the process in which we take back our power by exercising it. We have to know what our feelings are and express them regularly, passionately, appropriately. Expressing our feelings enables us to think clearly so that we can live well, solve any problems that arise, have healthy, cooperative relationships with other humans, dream, and continue creating a world suitable for humans and other living entities. Poverty and systemic and internalized oppression are the root causes of Black women's poor health and distress as well as the hopeless, powerless feeling that we are unable to take effective action in our own lives.

Self-Help for Self-Empowerment

The Black Women's Health Project helps Black women reclaim and exercise our power. The primary work that we do is to teach women to organize self-help groups. These groups are intended to promote health and well-being; they are not organized around a particular problem. Each group meets once a month. Women begin to talk about their lives. We talk about health, about relationships, about whatever we need to talk about. We express our feelings freely, all of them. We cry; we laugh; we encourage people to express their anger. We encourage people to sing, dance, and express physical affection; to appreciate themselves and each other; and to appreciate people who are close to them. We learn how to listen to ourselves and each other. We talk about how we were raised, how we raise children, and how we interact with people as well as what's needed to create environments that will help us develop into healthy human beings. We encourage women to use these skills with their families, on the job, at school, in all their relationships.

We define health broadly not just in terms of physical health or freedom from disease. We provide health education around diverse topics, including racism, sexism, violence, poverty, sexual health, reproductive rights, nutrition, stress management, fitness, disease prevention, parenting, relationships, homophobia, empowerment, addiction, AIDS, money—all forms of oppression. We help people learn about their bodies to know themselves and to understand what we need in order to maintain healthy individuals and communities.

Our approach sometimes makes fund raising difficult. If we were willing to have an alcoholism program, a drug program, a teen pregnancy prevention program, we would be able to get money for each for a limited time. But our program of promoting health and well-being, if fully implemented, would enable Black women to prevent the diseases and problems that are causing illness, disabling conditions, early death, and unhealthy relationships and allow us to be more effective in solving local and global social problems that we continue to struggle with. Our Love, Intimacy, and Sexual Health Program is not an AIDS 101 program; we promote a holistic comprehensive vision that includes self-help, empowerment, nutrition, stress management, sharing experiences about incest, rape, violence, dreams, sexuality, love, intimacy, basic information about sexuality, sexually transmitted diseases, addiction, AIDS, negotiating safer sex, grief, pleasure, information, shared experiences and feelings, increased self-esteem, and ongoing emotional support through group participation.

The Black Women's Health Project also works with Black men and with women of all races to show them how to organize groups. We've done a lot of work with young people. As an organization, we need to develop the capacity to have enough trainers (both within and outside the organization) to do this work throughout all the communities in New York City. We advocate for policies and programs that will enable people to get healthy and stay healthy.

One of the things we have *not* succeeded in doing, which is part of the goal of the organization, is community and political work in addition to the personal work. At some point, we hope that members of self-help groups will notice that women in the group, their families, and their communities have similar problems and will begin to develop strategies for solving community problems. We are still a young organization. We know that the personal and the political work are both necessary to solve our problems. We focus first on the personal level because that's where empowerment begins. Changing ourselves is essential to social change.

Reclaiming Our Power

The way that I use the word empowerment is different from the way I hear most people using the word. One way that is different is that I know we were all born powerful and that we can reclaim that power by exercising it; it's self-empowerment. All human beings have the power to satisfy their individual and collective needs. Whether we are professionals or not, each of us needs to be working on ourselves to take back our own power and use it in our lives. If we don't do this, we are not going to be able to help anybody else reclaim their power. We have to model what we want others to do and accept that it will be different when exercised by others. Each of us has to distinguish between our own needs and the needs of others individually and collectively.

For example, suppose an organization has a program with measurable objectives that 150 people will use condoms and practice safer sex, and so on. The director says she wants to empower her clients to fulfill these objectives. That's not empowerment. The organization needs to determine what its needs are and how best to satisfy those needs, and the workers and clients need to determine *their* needs and how to satisfy those.

For you and I to assist others in reclaiming their power means we do whatever is necessary for them to make the best decisions that they can make for themselves with the resources that they have or have the ability to develop. This means that you and I have to accept that they might not make the decision that we want. They will make mistakes despite our advice and learn from their mistakes. I haven't met anyone who wanted to get AIDS, but because their priorities are different, their decisions will be different than our decisions for them. The program may not achieve its measurable objectives, and may lose its funding. That's a separate issue, it's not about the clients' empowerment; it's about the organization's empowerment! Organizations need to ask what we need to do differently to accomplish our measurable objectives, to satisfy our basic needs, to empower ourselves.

Empowerment means creating a space in which a woman can say, "It's all right for me to think about myself, not just my family; it's all right for me to say I need help." You have to create an environment in which people can say, "I'm infected, but right now I need food," or "I have to talk about being raped before I can begin to heal and talk about safer sex, condoms, or my needs."

Sometimes I have blamed myself, others, or the society for the problems I see in the world. This was not helpful. Someone told me that I was 100 percent responsible for the whole universe. That's very different from blaming myself. It's hopeful; it means that I can use my intelligence and creativity to think about solutions and make a commitment to solve the problem with the help of others who also accept 100 percent responsibility for the universe.

Empowerment means that we have the ability and the responsibility to be fully human, exercising all our powers: intelligence, love, creativity, problem solving, healing, energy, passion, and humor to create healthy individuals, healthy communities, and a healthy world able to solve human problems as they develop.

KNOWLEDGE IS POWER: THE WOMEN'S HEALTH EDUCATION PROJECT

Gabrielle Immerman

Health care in the United States has become an unabashedly capitalistic enterprise. This country boasts some of the most advanced medical technology and techniques in the world, provides some of the finest medical care, and stands in the forefront of medical research. And these resources are all within the grasp of any individual, with only one condition—the ability to pay.

Anyone with sufficient means has virtually unlimited access to private doctors and hospitals and a plethora of extraordinary options for meeting his or her health needs, including an array of alternative practices from around the world. However, the poor—and the vast majority of families living in poverty in this country are headed by women—are economic prisoners of a huge, impersonal, bureaucratic medical system that is proving less and less effective in meeting the needs of the clients for whom it ostensibly exists. As one resident of a New York City shelter for the homeless described the process of obtaining health care, "The ones that are really in need are the ones who go through so much hassle with it. The ones that really don't need it or take advantage of it, they slide through like *that*. Yes, they do. No problems whatsoever."

To be able to get their health needs met under such a system, individuals must be knowledgeable both about their own health and about negotiating that system. Yet, to poor women whose daily lives consist of a struggle just to obtain the basic means of survival, such knowledge would seem to be a luxury.

"These women just want to get through their daily lives," explains childbirth educator Allison Jucha. "They want to get their checks, get their food, get their kids off to school, and they would like a little peace. The last thing on their minds is 'Gee, I ought to read up on this new measles vaccine.' Which is not to say they're not smart, they're not willing to have the answers, they don't ask the right questions—it's just that I don't think they've been treated as if there's a benefit to having knowledge."

In fact, for women with little or no income, such knowledge "is not a luxury—it is a necessity," asserts Stephanie Stevens, Executive Director of the Women's Health Education Project (WHEP). Founded on this principle, WHEP's goal is the empowerment of women with little or no income. WHEP achieves this empowerment by helping women obtain the knowledge they need, enabling them both to more effectively utilize the existing health care system and to transcend that system wherever possible by taking responsibility for their own and their children's health needs.

WHEP was first conceived in April 1988 when the Learning Alliance, a nonprofit education organization in New York City, sponsored a day of workshops by and for women on self-help health care. Women in battered and homeless shelters were specifically invited, and their costs were covered by a grant from the Leonard Stern Foundation. Many were prevented from attending by a variety of factors, however, including the fear of running into someone who had abused or battered them and the difficulty of traveling with small children. Those who did attend spoke of the urgent need for access to self-help information for women in the shelter system.

The organizers of the day of workshops were struck not so much by the lack of information among women in the shelters, but rather by their lack of access to it. These organizers came together to form the Women's Health Education Project as a liaison between women health practitioners, lay specialists, and educators in New York City on the one hand, and the women in the shelters who could benefit from their knowledge on the other. WHEP has become a coordinating center for a network of women in the New York area with fields of knowledge ranging from gynecology and obstetrics to Shiatsu massage, nutrition, and aerobics. Thus far, WHEP workshops have reached as many as 500 women in a dozen different shelters on topics including self-help gynecological care, prenatal care, child care, stress management, self-defense, AIDS prevention, lesbian health care and support groups, and herbalism.

One of the most effective aspects of WHEP's programs is that they are dictated solely by the needs of the shelter residents, as expressed by the women themselves. WHEP operates with a collective philosophy, prompting the sharing, rather than the preaching, of knowledge. "That's really what makes it different from the other groups," points out Tina Zarillo, Director of Women's Survival Space, a shelter in Sunset Park, Brooklyn. "The residents have the choice to pick and choose what they'd like, and whether or not to attend it. WHEP hooks them up with what *they* want, not what *we* want—with what *they* have identified their needs to be." The agenda is created solely by the women involved; workshops are mutable and change constantly with the input of the participants. They also continue only as long as there remains an interest; this may mean a single workshop or a continuing series, depending on the needs of shelter residents.

Health Problems in the Shelters

Women housed in the New York City shelter system live under enormously stressful conditions that only begin with the homelessness or abusive situations that bring them into the shelters. The "Tier 1" or congregate shelters into which most homeless women are first placed are crowded, unsafe, barracks-like facilities. They are ridden with crime, most notably widespread sexual abuse and drug use. Tier 2 shelters—more apartmentlike housing—are generally smaller, more private, and better equipped, but living in them still entails the stress of a transient lifestyle—stays are limited to 90 days—and the paperwork and logistical maze of city-run services. Many women are single parents, often of several children, which means they serve as care givers 24 hours a day, and this complicates their needs for housing and other resources.

The circumstances of life in the shelters can bring on a host of illnesses and problems that go well beyond the routine health needs of most women and children, including depression, drug addiction, malnutrition, stress-related health problems, and increased vulnerability to HIV and AIDS and other disease. And yet the public health care system, the only option available to low-income people, particularly the homeless, in New York City, is painfully stretched beyond its capacity and resources, hopelessly underfunded, and is being gutted by further slashing of city and state budgets.

Public health services present myriad other difficulties for shelter residents attempting to cope with their health problems. Overwhelmed clinical facilities is only one of many obstacles encountered by shelter residents. Often when low-income patients are admitted to care, they are not given the treatment or rights afforded to paying customers. Medical histories are frequently lost or not kept at all during a client's involvement in the shelter system.

The public health care system, moreover, is based on a fundamentally wrong-headed policy of responding to specific symptoms and illnesses that have already developed rather than providing preventive and holistic care to maintain a healthy body. Allison Jucha is critical of the prevailing medical approach. "Doctors study dead bodies. That's what they know. By which you're telling people, 'I'm going to treat your symptoms, not your whole person, not your body, not your social climate, not your financial problems, not your emotional state.'" By spot-treating only specific illnesses, this approach leaves preventable problems such as stress untreated until they manifest themselves in more severe chronic medical or social conditions.

In the face of such obstacles to effective medical care, staying healthy becomes that much more of a necessity. Yet the residents of shelters are restricted in their ability to care for their own and their children's health by the twin poverties of money and knowledge. The lack of money blocks access to private doctors, alternative treatments such as herbalism, Eastern techniques, and homeopathic medicine, and the education and resources that would bring the women knowledge of the importance of such factors in the on-going process of staying healthy as nutrition, exercise, and emotional well-being.

WHEP in the Shelters

Allison Jucha has been offering workshops on a wide range of child-related issues in the Springfield Gardens, Queens, family shelter since February 1991. Although it is home to 65 homeless families, medical care at the Springfield Gardens Shelter consists of a weekly visit by a single doctor, a general practitioner whose infrequent contact with the shelter residents and overwhelming workload make him ill-prepared for the specialized pediatric needs he encounters at the shelter. Based on his diagnosis, Allison Walker, a resident of Springfield Gardens, treated her infant son's respiratory infection as a common cold for several weeks before finally taking him to a nearby clinic. "I walked in the door and they took one look at him and told me he had pneumonia," she told Dr. Diane Gocs, Jucha's own pediatrician whom she brought in to lead a workshop last April. All nine women attending Dr. Gocs's workshop voiced a need for on-site pediatric care. Currently, the only practical alternative to the shelter's visiting doctor is a trip to one of two nearby clinics, which, like all public health facilities, are so overextended as to have little or no time for individualized, personal care or questions.

At Women's Survival Space, a shelter for battered women and their children, which provides residents with counseling for domestic violence, advocacy for obtaining housing, help in getting legal and public assistance, and numerous other concrete services, WHEP provides a means of broadening the range of services the shelter can offer. "I think all of us feel that although these women and families are coming in as victims of domestic violence, we cannot isolate that issue," says shelter director Zarillo. "A lot of them are coming in pregnant who have never seen a doctor, have never had prenatal care, don't know what it's like to go to the gynecologist, don't know how to raise or take care of children, so there's a lot of gaps we needed to fill."

Yet, when WHEP made its initial contact with Women's Survival Space early this year, the women expressed a need to address a more abstract, yet perhaps more fundamental issue—that is, the enormous stress that pervades and affects all parts of their lives. "You come in here so stressed out and so confused you don't know where you're *going*," says Joyce Jenkins, a resident of the shelter and active participant in WHEP workshops. "My life is turned completely upside down. I've left my home, I've left everything I have, all my belongings . . . and you come in here and you *need help*. And if they don't help you here, you go back."

At the residents' request, WHEP educators Karen Flood and Robin Bennett led a 10-week workshop on stress management, including sessions touching on herbal medicine and children's self-management. Next on the agenda, as requested by the shelter's clientele, was parenting skills. Jenkins explained the need for this workshop: "There are ladies in here who are taking full responsibility for their children for the first time in their lives. Everyone who has a baby is not automatically a mother. The instinct isn't always just naturally there—sometimes you need somebody to teach you." Aishah, a 24-year-old woman at Women's Survival Space has five children, ranging in age from newborn to 9 years old. She has never cared for her children on her own before. For her, discipline consisted of sending her children to her partner, who spanked them. "Nowadays spanking is 'corporal punishment' according to the laws of the Bureau of Child Welfare," Jenkins noted. "They say it's the worst thing you can do. Aishah needs to learn different types of ways to keep that positive side in there. Even though children do negative things, you still talk to them in a positive way."

Although WHEP is not the only source of this type of information, it appears to be the most personal and the most accessible for the residents. Jenkins, for instance, had taken a parenting skills class in Manhattan before she moved into the Brooklyn shelter. "There are places, but they're hard to get into. A lot of them don't go towards parents with older children—most of them are for teenage mothers with babies, things like that." It's hard to find a class for mothers of adolescents, Jenkins says. "You have to really dig deep, you have to really look, look, look, look, or have someone really looking into it for you."

Defining Empowerment

"Empowerment" is the ultimate aim of WHEP's efforts to transmit knowledge through its workshops, but what is the meaning of this elusive goal? Says Jenkins, "Whether you put different labels on the groups or not, all of it is empowerment, in different ways. It's all helping you to get back out there. It's all there in you. You just have to be shown that it is there. We *all* are somebody. But some people have been put down so much that they don't realize it anymore." For Jenkins, empowerment is self-esteem. "Mostly everything is talk," she chuckled. "But, you discuss how you feel about yourself, what you want to do with your life, how you were beaten down, and now how do we build it back up, and keep it there? How do we build up the children's self-esteem, so that *they* don't grow up feeling that their self-worth is less than what it should be?"

Like Jenkins, Tina Zarillo defines empowerment as a strong, positive sense of self. You can't be empowered, she feels, until you know who you are, and accept yourself, and love yourself, and connect with the ability to nurture yourself. "Empowerment education allows the opportunity for women to grasp that knowledge. A lot of women aren't given that opportunity and don't know that there's so many things out there that they need to learn about." Zarillo shies away from the dictatorial model of education; instead, she says, "being exposed is primary. That's what empowerment education is to me. It's not standing in front of a classroom, saying, 'I empower thee.' It's giving that information, it's sharing that knowledge. It's continually reinforcing, and giving choices, and presenting options so a woman can make a choice. And letting her know that she has a right to make the choice, and the ability to make the choice."

In WHEP's definition, knowledge is power. Learning to care for themselves and their children gives women control over their lives and allows them to better utilize or even transcend the current medical establishment. This may mean knowing to give chamomile tea to a child with an upset stomach, it may mean learning a breathing exercise to help soothe and relax in times of stress and tension. Empowerment may also simply mean knowing what questions to ask.

For Angela Golden, pregnant with her third child, and a resident of the Springfield Gardens Shelter for homeless families, empowerment has come in the form of learning that doctors are not gods, and that as a patient she has rights and power to choose what will happen to her. This was brought home to her specifically in regard to her forthcoming birth experience. "Some of the doctors have their rules, and when you get in the hospital, usually you have to listen to what they say." But, Golden says, she learned from Allison Jucha, her workshop leader, that "you don't—you can question." For example, in a childbirth preparation relaxation workshop, Jucha explained that there are a number of ways to avoid needing an episiotomy during childbirth, which is performed routinely by doctors. Golden, who had experienced much discomfort as a result of episiotomies during her first two births, was shocked and delighted to find that she could challenge her doctor's decisions. Armed with the knowledge of alternative birth positions and other helpful techniques, Golden felt capable of refusing to submit to an unnecessary procedure. "If they tell you one way, you can say, '*No*, I want it *this* way.' If we can stand up and talk about the things we don't want, then we're going to get what *we* need.''

Sisterhood and Support

Underlying all these ways of gaining strength is the crucial component of supporting one another. A sense of community, of *sisterhood*, is vital to the process of achieving self-awareness and power. "I like her," Angela Golden said of Jucha, her workshop leader. "She was very helpful. And she was very dependable. She didn't let me down. Even when I was the only one there, she *came*. It's really good to know that she cares.'' Zarillo mentions that the influx of people from "outside" is also helpful in combatting the sense of isolation often experienced by women living in the largely self-contained world of the shelter. And Joyce Jenkins made unmistakably clear the importance of the solidarity of the women's community. "Just by sitting in a group, knowing that other women are going through the same thing you're going through, it helps," she said. "It helps to talk. Even though I'm here with all these strange women, we have something in common. We understand each other. And we need each other.''

One powerful manifestation of this sisterhood among battered and homeless women is the desire to establish a support network that will outlast them in the shelters. At Women's Survival Space, the length of a woman's residence is limited to 90 days (with occasional extensions). Despite every effort, sometimes it is impossible to arrange a workshop before a particular woman's stay is over. For example, Aishah, the 24-year-old mother of five at Women's Survival Space, left before the parenting skills workshops she so badly needed began. However, knowing they may not benefit personally from a workshop doesn't stop the women from expressing their needs. Residents know or have learned that the problems they face are common to most of the women who pass through their shelter. Says Jenkins: "We're trying to keep it going for those that come behind us so that they can benefit as well, or even more.''

Self-Help and Self-Defense

By bringing women together to pool their resources, by working together rather than against one another, WHEP seeks not to topple the existing system, but rather to find ways of working effectively in and around it. WHEP recognizes the necessity of a massive restructuring of the health care system, yet works to ameliorate women's current situations. In the face of the health care catastrophe now gripping New York City, empowerment education, in this case focusing on self-help and preventive health care, may be the most effective defense we can offer the women of this city who are living in poverty. WHEP teaches women to navigate the existing system and finds creative ways for women to remain healthy, to remain *cared* for, to break free of their status as victims of a system that may be irretrievably overextended and unresponsive.

"It's very hard to 'empower oneself' when one is female in this society," concludes WHEP's Allison Jucha. "And you can't empower someone else.

However, you can keep offering and offering and offering the information, support, resources, alternatives, groups, organizations, phone numbers, ideas—whatever it is—that they can choose from, and thereby support them in their self-empowerment. Because it's always your own choice of what you're to do in life. But if you don't have choices because you don't *know* about choices, you can't do anything. You're stuck in a box.''

As members of the progressive health care and feminist movements we must be careful with the use of the word ''empowerment.'' Too often empowerment is twisted into indoctrination, credited to external forces—magnanimous benefactors of the poor and ignorant masses. Based on a belief that we all start out as strong, powerful beings but are beaten down by society and ideology, Gwen Braxton of New York's Black Women's Health Project offers a strong and simple definition of empowerment as the process of ''reclaiming the power you were born with.'' Empowerment must be *self*-empowerment—we can help each other toward it, but we cannot give it to anyone but ourselves.

HOUSING AND EMPOWERMENT

Ellen Baxter

I am one of a group of people in Upper Manhattan who take over abandoned buildings and convert them into affordable housing for homeless and low-income men and women. To someone who has experienced homelessness, a lease is one of the most empowering things one can extend.

In New York City there is a tendency to look past the issue of homelessness itself and to be more concerned about an individual's personal problems. This plays into the assumption that the homeless are largely mentally ill and/or drug addicted. And it means that rehabilitation and professional care receive primary attention. "Fixing" individuals becomes first priority, and the importance of housing is ignored.

There is heavy societal and institutional pressure to move people who are now homeless into what is called "transition," a state of personal rehabilitation that ultimately leaves them nowhere, since no decent, affordable housing exists. Once people have been "transitioned" through drug rehabilitation programs and are sober and clean for six or nine months, their only place to live, if they can't find work that pays well above minimum wage, is a shelter. Housing at public assistance levels cannot be found. But, in the shelters drug activity is common, and residents often feel that using drugs is the only way to survive under those conditions. So people end up back where they started.

About 12 years ago, a group of us in Washington Heights decided that the obvious solution to homelessness is housing. It's a simple concept. We had seen abandoned buildings and had the idea to fix them and move people in. Most of us weren't even familiar with what a mortgage was, but we began to meet with public agencies to discuss the notion. We'd go to meetings where everybody was talking mortgages and loan requirements, and we would nod and agree. Some people at those meetings with cynical views argued that poor people would never pay rent, that they would wreck their own housing, and that the effort was futile. Social service agencies pushed to have individuals segregated by category. The initial questions were: "Well, are you going to house homeless elderly people, or are you going to house homeless youth, or homeless single parents, or homeless mentally ill, or who?" Our idea was simpler than that. We wanted to house everybody.

Many of us were working other jobs and doing this on the side, continually trying to persuade our employers that it was in their interests to support this kind of work. After a lot of red tape and countless discussions to circumvent numerous obstacles, we found an abandoned building and went to the Department of Housing Preservation and Development. This began another series of seemingly endless meetings. Finally, I think mostly out of no longer wanting to meet with us, the housing officials told us the next place to go. We kept meeting with bureaucrats until they agreed in 1983, about three years after we began the process, to give us a mortgage attached to federal Section 8 rent subsidies. We were then able to get a bank loan for renovation, and we incorporated ourselves as a not-for-profit group. A *pro bono* lawyer filed the papers in Albany, and we were on our way.

With the mortgage, the bank loan, and a state grant, we renovated the building and moved in 55 homeless people, most of whom had been living in shelters and the streets. The construction alone took a very long time, a year and a half more than we expected, which left a tenant's association of homeless people ready to move in long before the building was done. So we rented a city-owned apartment around the corner from the building and used it as a place where people who were living in the streets and shelters could come to use the shower, use the address for mail, use the stove, keep their belongings, and have a weekly meeting and dinner.

At these meetings, people would talk about the difficulties of being homeless. They talked about racism, drug addiction, and sexism. Many of the individuals who had lived in institutions such as jails and shelters, or in foster care for extended periods, were not practiced at sitting down and talking with the opposite sex and people of all racial groups to discuss cooperative living goals. The meetings were interesting, and the waiting time gave us a chance to agree among ourselves that coexistence regardless of individual differences was desirable.

Finally, in 1986, as the construction neared completion we urged the contractors every week to move along. We began picking out rooms where tenants would eventually live. Our efforts have worked out well. There are 55 tenants in this building, which is called The Heights.

Housing is an opportunity. It is a place where basic needs can begin to be fulfilled, where one has friends and can restore abilities and develop new ones. It's a place where the government will allow kids who are in foster care to visit. If someone gets sick at the Heights and needs to go to the hospital, there is cab fare at the front desk so people don't have to take an ambulance. It is a supportive place for people to live, where they make their own decisions.

Participation in any part of running the Heights is not required. You can live there, pay your rent, come and go, and not be part of the tenant's association or the tenant patrol. Some people are very active in the management of the building, some are not. But the tenants alone are responsible for the building during evenings and weekends. There is no staff present at these times and, despite others' views of them as chronically mentally ill or having risky backgrounds of substance abuse, tenants manage the building quite well.

This arrangement is not without conflict. There are people who won't go into a room with other people because they don't get along. There are individuals with peculiar habits that may stay up all night. But when such situations arise, they are dealt with and resolved, and when individual behaviors don't interfere with the rights of others, the best approach seems to be to do nothing at all.

The building has common spaces all over it—lounges were built on each floor because fire department regulations require a double means of exit in buildings. The lounges are places where there is usually someone willing to play cards if you can't sleep, and someone to talk to. There is a tenant patrol 24 hours a day, seven days a week. The tenant patrol attends to everything from overflowing toilets and other problems with the physical plant to people problems.

Based upon our experience with the Heights, we got a second building, the Stella, in 1988 for 28 homeless men and women. We were again able to persuade the city to let us do integrated housing and not separate people solely by special needs categories. And again, individuals were given leases. People stayed, and the tenant patrol matured and stabilized. After that we got two more and, later, a fifth building. There are now five buildings in Washington Heights and Upper Harlem, accommodating 220 men and women, all of whom have leases.

The buildings are legally protected as low-income housing for a minimum of 30 years. The non-profit ownership and management entities are obligated to preserve their futures beyond this time.

Government agencies provide essential capital financing, but often discourage non-profit initiatives in housing. There is a group of women in the Bronx who have been working hard to get housing, for example, and I believe this may be their third year of effort to secure an abandoned property on their block. The bureaucracy can work against these kinds of community initiatives, despite the fact that owning and managing housing can be quite simple. You pay Con Ed, you pay the telephone bill, you pay your insurance bill, people pay rent. If someone stops paying rent, the tenant's association has tremendous power, far more than any landlord would, to get it paid. It takes a while for some individuals to get into the habit of paying rent. Some people pay irregularly, but this can be managed as long as the majority of tenants are behind the effort.

Sometimes not-for-profit groups who develop homeless housing fall into the trap of becoming more like a private landlord than like a community housing sponsor. When non-profit organizations are in antagonistic or adversarial relationships with tenants, they lose the support necessary to maintain quality building services and a solid rent roll. I think a constant collaboration with tenants develops one's appreciation for the benefits of tenant-managed housing. Too often organizations will hire security firms who clearly don't have any long-term interest or investment in the project. It doesn't seem to work as well. Tenants are much better placed to assume responsibility for their own housing.

The Committee for the Heights Inwood Homeless (CHIH) has eight staff people now. Four of them are superintendents and maintenance people, and two help with the books, managing the bills and the paper work that the city and state require for this kind of effort. A project director oversees all management responsibilities, resolves problems and interacts daily with the staff of Columbia University Community Services (CUCS), the agency that provides on-site social services to tenants in all the buildings. I receive a salary from the Community Service Society, a large social welfare organization. CHIH has a remarkably small staff to be managing 220 units. We could not sustain the housing without the services provided by CUCS. And, so long as the skills and capacities of the tenants are promoted, it's quite adequate.

Developing housing is not really a difficult thing to do. Not that much technology or expertise is involved. The process teaches you what you need to know. It takes so long to do anything in the city that, even if you don't know how to undertake a certain stage in the process, you figure it out along the way. You meet with architects and lawyers and contractors and argue over details. Being a part of the debate is educational and exciting.

Providing housing is very satisfying and a terrific base for other kinds of service provision. It's concrete, and it's encouraging for people to have their own housing and to watch it being built. People's involvement in the operations of housing can also be invigorating.

Bureaucratic obstacles surface regularly, and sidestepping these can be tricky. Angry people in crisis can occasionally be destructive in housing, and the forces of substance addictions can prey on many. Still, the great majority of tenants can be relied on to steer a course of cooperative and decent housing.

HEALTH INSURANCE COVERAGE FOR PEOPLE AGES 16–64 BY DISABILITY STATUS, OCTOBER TO DECEMBER 1988

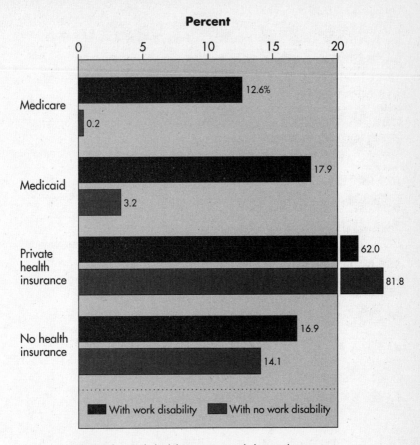

Percent

Medicare	12.6% / 0.2
Medicaid	17.9 / 3.2
Private health insurance	62.0 / 81.8
No health insurance	16.9 / 14.1

■ With work disability ■ With no work disability

Note: The "work disability" category includes people reporting a disability that prevents them from performing at least some types of work. Many people with a work disability are employed.

Robert Wood Johnson Foundation, 1991

Source:

US Bureau of the Census. *Health Insurance Coverage: 1986–88.* Current Population Reports. Series P-70, No. 17. Washington DC, 1990. Table 1, p. 17.

DAYS OF RESTRICTED ACTIVITY
BY RACE AND INCOME, 1988

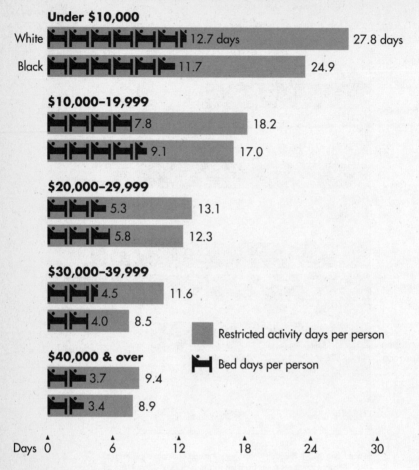

Under $10,000
White · 12.7 days · 27.8 days
Black · 11.7 · 24.9

$10,000–19,999
7.8 · 18.2
9.1 · 17.0

$20,000–29,999
5.3 · 13.1
5.8 · 12.3

$30,000–39,999
4.5 · 11.6
4.0 · 8.5

Restricted activity days per person

Bed days per person

$40,000 & over
3.7 · 9.4
3.4 · 8.9

Days 0 · 6 · 12 · 18 · 24 · 30

Robert Wood Johnson Foundation, 1991

Source:
Unpublished data from the US National Center for Health Statistics, Division of Health Interview Statistics, Illness and Disability Statistics Branch.

THE ROLE OF THE DISABILITY MOVEMENT IN HEALTH CARE REFORM

Bob Griss

Uniqueness of a Disability Perspective

Despite the recent spate of hearings that Congress has held on national health care policy, most of those invited to testify represent the interests of the private insurance industry, employers, medical providers, or government agencies. Occasionally, a consumer with a disability has been invited to describe how they have been victimized by pre-existing condition exclusions or financially impoverished by catastrophic health care expenses.

A consumer perspective is largely ignored because in the present system the employer is regarded as the actual consumer even though private health insurance accounts for less than one-third of health care expenditures (see *WfW*, Jan./Feb. 1991, p. 24). Moreover, policymakers are seeking to facilitate a political solution to the multi-sided health care crisis among the major stakeholders in the health care system. Given the constellation of political interests poised to influence national health care policy on Capitol Hill, policymakers have tended to favor a restriction on the scope of health care coverage as a way to maximize cost containment, while extending basic coverage to the 37 million uninsured persons, rather than restructuring the health care system.

Unless the disability community can help refocus the goals of the health care debate from extending the present system of inadequate acute care to 37 million currently uninsured persons to one that expands the definition of "health," the national health care policy which Congress adopts will continue to ignore many of the health-related needs of persons with disabilities or chronic illness. The disability community can warn the American public and our policymakers about the major barriers to access, adequacy, and affordability in the existing private and public health insurance systems.

Strategic Role of Disability Movement

The disability movement could be a powerful force in reexamining health care financing policy for several reasons. First, people with disabilities are highly vulnerable to the limitations of both public and private systems as they are squeezed between a private system which is designed to charge according to an assessment of risk and a public system which subsidizes health care according to age, poverty status, family structure, and an inability to work.

Secondly, people with disabilities know better than anyone else the limitations of trying to address their chronic health care needs in a health care financing system that was historically developed and remains principally organized to deliver acute health care.

Thirdly, disability cuts across class lines encouraging all people to consider what kinds of health care they would want for themselves and their family members when they become disabled or develop a chronic health condition and no longer view themselves as "temporarily able-bodied" (TABs).

Fourthly, the disability movement is the most logical consumer group to make health care the civil rights issue for the 1990's. Access to health care and personal assistance services are the two critical issues needed to assure full implementation of the promise of ADA. Unions have a tendency to see rising health care costs as a threat to their wages, and employers view it as a threat to their profits and to their ability to compete with other employers who face lower health care costs either in this country or abroad. But people with disabilities and chronic illness understand how obstacles to health care can prevent participation in employment, limit community activities, and disrupt family life.

Obstacles to Overcome

Before the disability movement can be taken seriously in the health care debate, it will have to overcome several obstacles. One is that different disability organizations must not focus just on their specific health care needs, but must be as united as we were in the passage of the ADA and must support the changes which are critical to the health care needs of other groups as well. For some groups the most critical health care takes the form of mental health services, while for others it is rehabilitation therapies, prescription drugs, or assistive technology. We cannot allow ourselves to be "divided and conquered."

Secondly, the disability organizations must join forces with chronic illness organizations who happen to represent a far larger constituency of persons who are equally vulnerable in our acute-care oriented health care system. Thirdly, the disability movement must recognize that, however effective it has been in advocating for categorical solutions to other problems facing persons with disabilities, the national health care crisis requires a generic solution.

One of the reasons that the disability movement has not played this role is the long-standing aversion in the Independent Living movement to the "over-medicalization" of services. There is also a mistaken impression that most persons with disabilities are primarily dependent on public insurance. Approximately two-thirds of all persons with disabilities have some form of private health insurance. [This includes 64.2 percent of children with cerebral palsy and 49.3 percent of adults with cerebral palsy.] And those who are dependent on public programs, like Medicaid, face major cutbacks in their benefits as illustrated by the Oregon Medicaid rationing plan.

Another reason is that the disability community, like the larger society, is greatly divided into the "haves" and the "have-nots" with each individual concerned about his or her own health insurance plan. In addition, many national voluntary associations are afraid to alienate the medical community, which has traditionally opposed national health insurance.

Confronting Dilemmas

Because the current health care financing system is so unfair, almost any reforms look good by comparison, at least for some people. This creates a real dilemma for people with disabilities: Should we support a change that is less than ideal because it is better than the existing system, or withhold our support in favor of more far-reaching changes that would better address the needs of persons with chronic health conditions, even if there is a smaller chance that those changes will be adopted.

While the status quo is unlikely to continue because of the massive contradictions in the current health insurance system, the greatest danger from a disability perspective is in legitimating the rationing of health care before the structural changes have been made. This may take the form of permitting "barebones" health insurance policies which are masquerading at the state level under the banner of small business insurance reform or of rationing under-funded public programs on the basis of quality of life like the Oregon Medicaid rationing plan.

Shaping the Health Care Debate

Recognizing that the disability movement cannot influence health care policy without the support of other groups, it is important to consider how the disability movement can have its greatest impact. Certainly, every effort should be made to expose the inequities in the current system and the hidden costs which they impose on:

1. persons with and without disabilities as families struggle to pay out-of-pocket for necessary health care;
2. employers who cannot afford the health care that their employees and their dependents deserve;
3. under-funded government programs which serve as a safety net for persons who have been dumped out of the private health insurance system; and
4. the society in general when secondary disabilities are not prevented, or when people with disabilities are afraid to risk working because it might jeopardize their only access to health care.

But at the same time our greatest contribution may be in clarifying the principles which should guide our health care system. These include: 1) expanding the definition of "health" to include prevention services, rehabilitation therapies, assistive technology, and on-going health-related maintenance services; 2) distributing all health-related expenses equitably throughout the population; and 3) restructuring our health care delivery system to more effectively support consumer-directed chronic care management.

The United States is at a crossroads. Our health care policy will either legitimate retrenchment by rationing services to those least able to pay, or it will restructure our priorities so that more resources will be devoted to managing chronic health conditions and less will be consumed by administrative waste, excess capacity, and "medical recidivism" which consume vast quantities of acute care services for health needs which could have been prevented.

UCPA has prepared a detailed critique of the "play or pay" approach from a disability perspective which will appear in subsequent issues of *WfW*. For those who would benefit in seeing it now, it is available on request. Contact Bob Griss, United Cerebral Palsy Associations, Inc., 1522 K Street, N.W., Suite 1112, Washington, DC 20005. Tel: (800) USA-5UCP or (202) 842-1266.

THE FRAGILE RIGHTS OF SHARON KOWALSKI

Ellen Bilofsky

The ease with which any one of us could suddenly lose control of our lives and fall prey to the vagaries of our medical and judicial systems is underscored by the plight of Karen Thompson and Sharon Kowalski. The women, long-time lovers, were tragically separated following Kowalski's disabling automobile accident over five years ago. Although there are many lessons to be learned from this couple's fight to be reunited and to ensure Kowalski a voice in her own care, their story painfully illustrates the fragility of the claims gay and disabled people can make to health and legal rights in this society.

Kowalski, a 32-year-old physical education teacher, was paralyzed in a head-on car crash in November 1983. Two years later, her parents, acting as her legal guardians, forbade Thompson and others from visiting her and isolated her in a nursing home not equipped for intensive rehabilitation.

Donald and Della Kowalski reacted to the situation with denial. They denied that their daughter had ever been a lesbian and they appeared unable to cope with her profound disability. Faced with Sharon's paralysis, they contended that she now functioned as a child, even though others were able to communicate with her on an adult level without difficulty. They used this rationale to avoid letting their daughter make her own decisions about her treatment, her visitors, and ultimately her institutionalization.

Thompson's five-year legal battle—first for guardianship of her partner, then to ensure her adequate care and rehabilitation—has become a cause célèbre in the gay and disabled communities. Her recent success, after a string of legal defeats, in convincing a Minnesota court to move Kowalski from a nursing home to a rehabilitation center for intensive treatment and evaluation has focused broader national attention on the struggle for Sharon Kowalski's rights and for the rights of gay and disabled people throughout the nation.

Stymied by the legal system in her attempt to obtain some measure of self-determination for Sharon Kowalski, Thompson, although a private person, was compelled to make alliances and turn to political organization. Galvanized by Thompson's story, an unlikely coalition of gay and disabled rights activists spearheaded an energetic organizing campaign to mobilize public support and sympathy. Support groups to ''free Sharon Kowalski'' began springing up around the country. To activists for the rights of the disabled, the fact that a woman was virtually imprisoned in a nursing home simply because of her disability spotlighted the fragility of their civil rights. But the story of two lovers, torn apart, first by disability and then by prejudice, had its most powerful effect on lesbians and gay men, for whom it was an object lesson in the precarious nature of their ties under our legal system.

Thompson, with the backing of these support groups, confronted the forces of prejudice, custom, and a host of legal and medical barriers—including the courts' refusal to admit crucial evidence about Kowalski's competence. So, on February second of this year, when Thompson walked into her lover's room after a three-and-a-half-year separation, it was much more than a personal victory. It was a triumph over what Thompson calls the "white, heterosexual, able-bodied, Christian, male system" that had separated them. And it represented symbolic victories for the recognition of the relationships of lesbians and gay men and for the self-determination of disabled people. Karen Thompson's goal is to win a say for Sharon Kowalski in the direction of her own life and, ultimately, to bring her home. But whether or not she succeeds, her efforts have clearly gained a significance far beyond their effect on these two women and their families.

Coming Out

The complex ramifications of the case are revealed in the tangled history leading up to the recent court order that reunited the women. Kowalski and Thompson were lovers who had pledged themselves to be life partners, had bought a house together, and had exchanged rings as a symbol of their commitment. Although they had lived as a couple for almost four years in St. Cloud, Minnesota, where Thompson is an assistant professor of physical education at St. Cloud State University, only their closest friends knew about their relationship.

On a cold, drizzly Minnesota afternoon in November 1983, Kowalski was driving her visiting niece and nephew home, when a car driven by a drunk driver smashed into them. The accident killed her niece, severely injured her nephew, and left Kowalski comatose, brain injured, and ultimately a quadriplegic.

At St. Cloud Hospital, Thompson was initially denied access to Kowalski because she was not "family." Once admitted, Thompson remained at her lover's side, searching for ways to break through Kowalski's silence. It was Thompson who noticed the minute movements of Kowalski's right index finger, the first sign that, despite the doctors' skepticism, she might come out of her coma.

Thompson's constant presence began to disturb the Kowalskis, who asked her to stop spending so much time with their daughter. Fearing that she might be forbidden from visiting altogether, Thompson met with a psychologist at the hospital. On his advice, she wrote a frank letter to the Kowalskis explaining her lesbian relationship with Sharon, in the hope that it would help them understand and appreciate her unusual devotion to their daughter's recovery. Their response was anything but accepting. Debbie Kowalski, Sharon's sister, called at the request of her parents, and, as Thompson recalls, told her: "You are a sick, crazy person who has made up this whole story. . . . My parents never want to set eyes on you again!"

Fearful of losing access to her lover, Thompson filed in court for guardianship of Sharon Kowalski in March 1984. When the matter dragged on, Thompson settled out of court, hoping to avoid a protracted battle. The settlement named Sharon's father, Donald, a retired miner, as guardian. Although this would prove to be a bitter setback, it did not seem a defeat for Thompson at the time. The court recognized that she had a "significant relationship" with Sharon Kowalski and was a "suitable and qualified person to be guardian," and the settlement gave Thompson equal access to Kowalski's medical and financial information and assured her equal visitation rights.

In the first two years following the accident, Thompson continued to spend all her spare time with Kowalski to encourage her recovery, often staying with her from 6:00 A.M. until midnight and leaving only to teach her classes. In time, Kowalski was once again able to accomplish simple tasks, such as combing her hair, eating instead of being tube fed, and drinking from a cup. Perhaps most important, she began to communicate, first by moving her finger to indicate yes or no in response to questions and eventually progressing to typing out words and phrases and even speaking on occasion.

When, about a year after the accident, Kowalski was moved to a nursing home in Duluth, a three-hour drive each way from Thompson's home in St. Cloud, and Thompson could no longer spend the better part of each day with her, Kowalski regressed. Thompson maintained that her work with Kowalski reinforced the professional rehabilitation she received and enabled her to make the progress that she did. Notations in Kowalski's medical records, as well as the courtroom testimony of a few health care workers, confirm that she was indeed more alert and responsive around Thompson.

Separation

Soon matters got even worse for Thompson. In July 1985, Donald Kowalski, after trying unsuccessfully several times to bar Thompson from seeing his daughter, finally won unrestricted guardianship. The court reached its decision partly on the basis of testimony from medical experts (supplied by the Kowalskis' attorney) that Sharon Kowalski couldn't adequately understand her situation or reliably communicate her wishes. These physicians also supported the family's contention that Thompson's visits were causing Sharon Kowalski to become depressed. The court accepted their assessments despite the fact that none of these doctors had treated Sharon Kowalski on a regular basis or had ever seen her interact with Thompson.

In winning full legal power to direct his daughter's care without the previous limitations, Donald Kowalski also secured the right to decide who could or couldn't visit her. The Kowalskis immediately moved her to the Leisure Hills Health Care Center in Hibbing, which was closer to their home and even further from Thompson's. The move was permitted despite the fact that the court had previously ruled that this nursing home, which lacked appropriate rehabilitation facilities, was unacceptable for Sharon. The parents also ordered the nursing home to screen all of her visitors and expressly prohibited any communications from Thompson.

While Thompson appealed the court order, she was able to see Sharon Kowalski for one final six-day visit. She found her regressed and withdrawn. Her feeding tube was back in place, and her typewriter, her most important tool of communication, was missing. According to Thompson, on the last day of her visit, before she was permanently barred from the nursing home, Kowalski typed out these words on a typewriter provided by Thompson: "Help me. Get me out of here. Please take me home with you."

Competency Evaluation

The Kowalski family appeared to be forsaking any plans of continuing the rehabilitation of their daughter, who barely resembled the independent, active, able-bodied woman they remembered. One condition of the order granting Donald Kowalski unrestricted guardianship of Sharon Kowalski was that she be tested for competency within a year and every 6 to 12 months thereafter. Minnesota law specifically requires that a guardian, in addition to ensuring that there is adequate care and treatment, arrange for the regular evaluations of the competency of his or her ward. But it wasn't until Thompson filed a legal motion to have Kowalski restored to capacity (and thus regain decision-making power) that an evaluation was finally conducted, over the guardian's strenuous objections, in September 1988.

Clearly, as is so often the case, the court viewed the parents' guardianship as sacrosanct, despite their failure to meet the requirements of state law. Without Thompson's intervention, Sharon Kowalski might have remained perpetually confined in an inadequate nursing home. Thompson's persistence succeeded in preventing the courts and the family from locking the door and throwing away the key.

Five years after the accident and three years after Sharon Kowalski was confined to the Leisure Hills Nursing Home, a team of three physicians declared her officially capable of communicating and expressing her needs. On January 17, Sharon was sent to the Miller-Dwan Medical Center in Duluth for intensive rehabilitation and reevaluation. The Kowalskis protested the move, claiming it would disrupt Sharon's treatment, and the family physician, Dr. William Wilson, wrote to the judge, calling the move medically inadvisable.

Until the court approves other arrangements, the Kowalskis' guardianship remains in place, but Sharon has been able to see visitors with her doctors' approval. She quickly made it clear that she wanted to see Thompson. When Thompson was reunited with Kowalski on February 2, she found her excited, alert, and responsive, but confused and with some deterioration in her physical condition. After further treatment, the judge will evaluate Kowalski's ability to make decisions about her life and will decide on her future placement. Most likely this will be in a long-term rehabilitation center. Although guardianship is not an issue in the current proceedings, it is clearly in the court's power to further limit Donald Kowalski's control over his daughter and to grant her a greater degree of self-determination. Thompson says she hopes that as her rehabilitation progresses, Sharon Kowalski can be sent to a transitional center for independent living, with the goal of ultimately returning home.

Intertwining Prejudices

While Sharon Kowalski's fate is being decided by physicians, lawyers, and judges, a growing number of people who feel their lives could be affected by the outcome of this case—largely gay men and lesbians and disabled people—are fighting for the right to make such decisions themselves. Gay and disability rights activists say the issues of sexism, homophobia, and disability prejudice are inseparably intertwined in this case. Paula Ettlebrick, Legal Director of Lambda Legal Defense and Education Fund, a New York gay rights organization that has provided legal consultation to Thompson, says, "This case illustrates the worst of both homophobia and handicapism: the total disregard for Sharon as a disabled person and the total lack of respect or recognition of her relationship with Karen."

The blatant prejudice against homosexuality infected nearly everyone connected with the case: the parents, the judges, the doctors. It clearly prompted the judges to ignore the evidence on record that Thompson had a consistently positive effect on Kowalski's rehabilitation. And ultimately it was homophobia that isolated Thompson and prevented her from helping to rehabilitate Sharon Kowalski. It may be fair to speculate that the family's fear and loathing of their daughter's lesbian relationship compelled them to deny her needed medical care. As Thompson's lawyer, Sue Wilson, puts it, "The father would rather have her be in a nursing home and a vegetable than be a lesbian."

The denial of Sharon's rights to adequate rehabilitation constitutes disability prejudice, says Marilyn Saviola, Executive Director of the Center for Independence of the Disabled in New York and member of the New York Committee to Free Sharon Kowalski. "The fact, very simply, is that no matter if Sharon were a lesbian or straight, if she could speak, none of this would have happened to her," argues Saviola. "Her competency was being threatened because of her disability."

The point is well taken. After the accident, Thompson began to realize that Kowalski's disability radically altered how people viewed and treated her. Kowalski's parents—even her doctors and other health care professionals—assumed that because she could not speak or move, she was totally helpless. From her inability to speak, they extrapolated an inability to think. For instance, she has never been asked to testify in court or attend any of the hearings that have decided the course her life would take. Jerry Nuzzi, a member of the New York Committee to Free Sharon Kowalski and himself disabled with cerebral palsy, says, "I'm hoping that when the judge finally decides on her competency, she can be rolled into court, or, better yet, she can roll herself into court in an electric wheelchair, and she can tell the judge, either with a letter board or some other electronic device, 'Look, I am a human being. I am competent. I have to make choices on the way I live my life.' "

But as a disabled person, Kowalski was judged incapable of having legitimate desires of any kind, including sexual. Although Kowalski told Thompson that she still loved and wanted her, she was prevented from having any contact with her lover by her family, her doctors, and the court, all of whom rejected any notion that she might still think and feel like an adult woman. "What the hell difference does it make if she's gay or lesbian? . . . She's sitting there in diapers," Donald Kowalski once told reporters. Arguing in favor of the enforced separation, Dr. William Wilson, the Kowalski family physician, even testified in court that the previous relationship between Thompson and Kowalski created the potential for sexual abuse of the disabled woman.

A number of other medical personnel involved in Kowalski's care were also influenced by this combination of prejudices. Some were so blinded by Sharon's apparent helplessness that they assumed she had no potential for rehabilitation —something disabled rights activists say is not uncommon. Many hospital workers also assumed from the beginning that because Thompson was not "family," she had no right to be involved in Sharon's care and treatment. Even when they observed that Kowalski responded best in Thompson's presence, the majority of care-givers were hesitant to say so in court.

The issue of Sharon Kowalski's competence to make decisions for herself is, of course, central to the case. But the fact is, because of the weight given to the family's perception of her helplessness, Kowalski was never given a fair chance to demonstrate her capabilities. Again and again, her abilities were glossed over or ignored. Less than a year after the accident, Thompson made a videotape showing Kowalski answering questions, combing her hair, drinking from a cup, and playing checkers. At various times during her hospitalization and treatment, representatives of a local handicapped services program and the Minnesota Civil Liberties Union visited Kowalski. Each reported holding extensive conversations with her, which included, among other topics, discussions of her sexuality and requests for services.

The courts ignored or refused to admit this evidence of her competence (and denied her various requests) in favor of the testimony of medical experts who had never treated her. According to patients' rights advocates, judges often prefer to rely on the opinions of so-called neutral medical experts who spend a few hours with the patients, assuming that care-givers who come to know their patients will become biased and render an overly optimistic assessment of their abilities. The courts presumed Sharon Kowalski incompetent until proven competent, instead of the reverse.

Guardianship: Who Decides?

The Kowalski case clearly raises complicated questions about guardianship. For example, who should have the right to make vital decisions for someone who is deemed incompetent? The potential for abuse of the guardianship arrangement has sparked much debate in the gay community amidst its struggle to cope with the AIDS epidemic. While some may resist comparing Kowalski's situation to that of people with AIDS—since guardianship could be necessitated by any incapacitating illness or accident—the parallels are only too clear. Some people who have been disabled by AIDS have been forced out of the closet by their illness, only to be separated from their lovers by parents who have assumed guardianship. As in the Kowalski case, the courts will generally presume that a guardian should be a close family member, regardless of a disabled person's other significant relationships. Organizations like the Lambda Legal Defense and Education Fund are working to reform the marriage statutes to legally recognize lesbian and gay relationships.

But gay and lesbian activists point out that they are not alone in falling victim to the legal system's bias in favor of the traditionally constituted family. It is not difficult to imagine how unmarried heterosexual couples without legal ties to their partners could be affected. Nor is it improbable that a member of a long-separated couple might become injured and the former partner assigned as guardian. Elderly people are particularly at risk of being declared mentally incompetent when only their physical powers have waned. Even securely married couples are threatened, as was the case when anti-abortion advocates recently filed for guardianship of a comatose pregnant woman at a Long Island hospital. They tried to prevent her husband from approving an abortion for her that, he argued, had the potential to prolong her life. Although the plaintiffs had no relationship to the patient, and their motion was eventually denied, they nonetheless succeeded in delaying the abortion while they appealed the case to the Supreme Court.

A major objective of the support groups that have sprung up around the Kowalski case is to educate people, regardless of sexual orientation or marital status, to protect themselves from the possibility of similar abuses of guardianship arrangements by using a legal vehicle known as a durable power of attorney. A durable power of attorney allows a person to designate a proxy decision maker to act in his or her behalf should he or she become incapacitated. Similar in intent to a living will, it is called durable because, unlike most powers of attorney, it remains in effect even after the signer is mentally incapacitated. (Details of this procedure, whose legality varies from state to state, can be found in the appendix to the recently published book about the case, *Why Can't Sharon Kowalski Come Home?* by Karen Thompson and Julie Andrzejewski, Spinsters/Aunt Lute Book Co., San Francisco, 1988, or from the National Committee to Free Sharon Kowalski.)

One of the most disturbing aspects of the role of the guardian in this case is the extent of the control Donald Kowalski exercised in making decisions, such as limiting his ward's visitors, that went far beyond her medical needs. Kowalski was appointed his daughter's guardian because the courts presumed that, as a father, he had only her best interests at heart. Although his actions did not bear that out, the courts did not set limits on his power. In one of the many bizarre legal twists of the case, a Minnesota appeals court ruled that the Minnesota Patient Bill of Rights, which guarantees patients the right to choose their own visitors, applies only to health care facilities, not to guardians, and thus did not protect Sharon Kowalski. As the Minnesota Civil Liberties Union wrote in a friend of the court brief: ''The convicted criminal loses only his or her liberty; Sharon Kowalski has lost the right to choose who she may see, who she may like, and who she may love. . . . [T]he court . . . made no finding that it was medically necessary to terminate Ms. Kowalski's relationship with her friend although that was the obvious result of the order [granting Donald Kowalski control over visitation].''

Who Failed Sharon Kowalski?

When a person is incapacitated, as Sharon Kowalski was, the legal and health care systems are charged with protecting her and ensuring that she receives the best and most appropriate care possible. In Sharon Kowalski's case, the medico-legal system failed on both counts.

While the courts focused on the conflict between Kowalski's parents and Karen Thompson in this adversarial encounter, Sharon Kowalski's own health and legal rights were blatantly neglected. Societal prejudices were built into the court's assumptions that Sharon Kowalski was incompetent in all matters and that, in the words of attorney Sue Wilson, "father knows best."

The judges failed Sharon Kowalski by attending only to the evidence that supported their prejudiced assumptions. Health care workers failed Sharon Kowalski by allowing prejudice to blind them to Kowalski's progress and denying her the support she needed to continue. They failed to act as her advocate, permitting her parents to make decisions inimical to her recovery without protest.

Existing protections for incapacitated individuals—such as patients' bills of rights and legal obligations imposed on guardians to have their wards tested periodically for competency and to provide them with adequate care—are insufficient as long as the courts enforce them selectively. We need to design and enforce policies that can preserve the rights of the family without abandoning the patient. A first step is to ensure that the courts consult the wishes of the patient whenever possible, not solely relying on the interpretation of the family or medical experts. Had they done so in Sharon Kowalski's case, her institutionalization might have been more rehabilitative and less like an incarceration.

Because the outcome of Karen Thompson's legal battle hinges on a judgment of Sharon Kowalski's individual competence and of her wishes, whether Thompson ultimately wins or loses in court will not change the central questions this case raises nor alter the relevance of the movement it has fomented. Even the most devastating decision, one that found Sharon Kowalski incompetent and allowed her father to retain unlimited guardianship, would not influence the competency evaluation of another disabled person in a similar situation. For Thompson to have won reentry into her lover's life and for Sharon Kowalski to have regained some control over whom she may see marks a recognition of both the legitimacy of gay relationships and the autonomy of disabled individuals that is precedent setting in this age of AIDS. But simply by sustaining their fight and being willing to make it public property, Karen Thompson and Sharon Kowalski have already won an important battle.

SHARON KOWALSKI AND THE RIGHTS OF NONTRADITIONAL FAMILIES

Ellen Bilofsky

Although Karen Thompson has finally been reunited with her lover, Sharon Kowalski, after nearly five years of enforced separation, she is still angry, still fighting to ensure her partner's proper care.

Thompson and Kowalski are lesbian lovers in Minnesota who were separated as a result of Kowalski's disabling automobile accident. The two primary issues in their struggle are the disabled woman's human rights—including adequate health care and a say in decisions affecting her—and Thompson's right, as an unrelated loved one, to be involved in her care.

As reported in the Spring 1989 *Health/PAC Bulletin*, Thompson fought a lengthy and bitter legal battle (with grass-roots support from gay and disability rights groups around the country) and eventually won the right to visit her lover. To prevent Kowalski's lesbian friends from seeing her, the injured woman's parents—her court-appointed guardians—had placed her in a nursing facility far from the home she had shared with Thompson. The nursing home was not equipped to provide rehabilitation for someone suffering Kowalski's degree of brain damage. Thompson's lawsuit also succeeded in enforcing Kowalski's legal right to be evaluated to determine her potential for rehabilitation and her ability to participate in decisions about her own treatment and life arrangements.

That Thompson prevailed over Kowalski's parents was a tremendous victory both for the rights of loved ones who do not fall under the traditional category of "family" and for the rights of disabled people to be taken seriously as competent human beings. Since the *Bulletin's* last report, the court has moved Kowalski to an extended care facility, where Thompson and other friends can visit her freely, and Kowalski has resumed her rehabilitation in preparation for less-structured care. The doctors who conducted Kowalski's court-ordered evaluation explicitly recognized her desire to return home to live with Karen Thompson again and set that as the goal of her rehabilitation. The National Committee to Free Sharon Kowalski, considering its purpose achieved, has disbanded.

Unfortunately, the fight for Sharon Kowalski's rights did not end there. Although Kowalski's father, Donald, asked to be removed as guardian because he was not happy with the changes in her situation, St. Louis County District Court Judge Robert Campbell has indicated off the record that he will neither restore Kowalski to partial competence nor appoint Karen Thompson as guardian in the elder Kowalski's stead. One woman proposed by the judge as a neutral third party and candidate for guardian approached Thompson to ask whether, if she got everything she wanted in terms of Kowalski's care, she would agree not to speak out about the case any longer. When Thompson refused to accept the condition, the judge, acting on his own volition, imposed a gag order on all parties.

The order was overturned on appeal as unconstitutional, but Thompson feels that it represents an attempt to contain the damage done to the court's and state's credibility by the negative publicity about Sharon Kowalski's neglect. And that neglect—a violation of her medical rights—has caused deterioration in Kowalski's physical and mental condition that can never be undone. For example, although she was able to bear weight on her legs soon after the accident, as a result of lack of exercise her legs no longer straighten and her feet are permanently bent back. Her motivation to learn new skills, such as using the speech synthesizer Thompson rents for her, is poor. After four years of isolation, says Thompson, "she doesn't believe in the future." Although Thompson can take Kowalski out of the institution on day passes, a staff member must accompany them because of the parents' fear of sexual abuse.

Despairing of getting an appropriate guardian for her lover, at the end of August 1989 Thompson filed for guardianship of Sharon Kowalski. "I will never again believe that my silence will protect me," she said. "That's what helped get us here" in the first place.

Legitimizing Nontraditional Families

Thompson hopes her case will make people aware of the need for legislation, like the proposed New York State "health proxy" bill, to prevent such tragedies from occurring again. This measure would allow an individual to designate someone—not necessarily a family member—to make decisions about medical treatment if he or she were to become incompetent. This is explicitly legal in only a few states, although in most other states it is possible to use so-called durable powers of attorney for the same purpose. The New York State bill, which is under consideration in the 1990 legislative session, also allows an individual to specify in advance treatment that the designated agent could authorize. Because such treatment could include terminating life-support measures, the bill has engendered considerable opposition from religious and right-to-life groups who oppose such practices, and its fate is uncertain.

At the same time, there is a growing recognition in society of the legitimacy of nontraditional families. In July 1989, the New York State Court of Appeals ruled that gay couples (and unmarried heterosexual couples) whose relationships met certain considerations, such as "exclusivity and longevity," could be considered family under New York City's rent-control regulations. Although the decision dealt with housing law, the case in fact stemmed from a health care crisis: the death of a man as a result of AIDS, after which his partner was threatened with eviction. The decision legitimizes gay relationships in certain specific situations, but it is not a recognition of gay marriage or its equivalent.

Although the court did not extend its ruling to cover any health-related benefits, New York City's then Mayor Ed Koch shortly thereafter issued an executive order granting bereavement leave to city employees who register their "domestic partners." The decision was again related to the AIDS issue, which has made more visible the suffering of gay individuals whose partners have died. The ruling also affects unmarried heterosexual couples, however, as well as other people who might be caring for an unrelated friend.

Koch sidestepped the issue of considering these "domestic partners" as family for purposes of health care coverage because of the substantial costs involved, leaving that issue for collective bargaining. The city's current policy is also being challenged in another law suit filed by the Gay Teachers Association on behalf of three New York City teachers. Their attorneys, the Lambda Legal Defense Fund, charge that the city discriminates in denying health benefits to their partners because of their marital status and sexual orientation. The case is currently before the New York State Supreme Court in Manhattan.

Six cities currently recognize some form of domestic partnership, including Berkeley, Los Angeles, West Hollywood, and Santa Cruz, California; Madison, Wisconsin; and Takoma Park, Maryland; and others are considering establishing such a category. However, in a recent referendum in San Francisco, the one city considered most likely to legitimize gay and nontraditional families, voters recently rejected the domestic partnership ordinance unanimously approved by the city's Board of Supervisors. The law would have recognized unmarried partners who registered with the city clerk as legally equal to married couples. In addition, it would have granted bereavement leave and hospital visitation rights to city employees in such domestic partnerships.

Activists attribute the San Francisco defeat to complacency in the face of a well-organized opposition, and don't expect the setback to be permanent. And, as the *Bulletin* went to press, two New York legislators have introduced a bill in that state to create legal domestic partnerships and prohibit discrimination based on marital status.

In the age of AIDS and openly gay relationships, it is no longer sufficient for the traditional family to set the parameters within which basic health care decisions are made. Cases such as that of Karen Thompson and Sharon Kowalski and the increasingly apparent burdens of partners of people who suffer from or die of AIDS-related illness have made clear the need to protect the rights of people who are not in traditional relationships.

HOME IS WHERE THE PATIENTS ARE: NEW YORK'S HOME CARE WORKERS' CONTRACT VICTORY

Barbara Caress

"Every morning I say to myself, 'There but for the grace of God . . .' " says Willie Sutton, a 45-year-old mother of two, whose job it is to care for an 88-year-old woman with severe heart disease and arthritis. Eight hours a day, five days a week, Mrs. Sutton gets her disabled, sick, and irritable patient toileted, bathed, dressed, medicated, and fed. In addition to her patient-care responsibilities, she cleans the apartment, does the laundry, shops, and cooks.

For her labors, Mrs. Sutton had been getting paid $4.15 an hour, with no overtime pay, no health insurance, no pension, and no job security. If her patient required 24-hour care, Mrs. Sutton was paid for only 12 of those hours.

Willie Sutton is one of an estimated 70,000 people who provide home care for New York City's sick, disabled, and elderly. I first met her two years ago, when I was asked to assist the staff of Local 1199, the 80,000-member health care workers' union that represents Mrs. Sutton and 20,000 other employees of the New York City home care system. The union, one of three representing home care workers in New York, sought a strategic understanding of the industry to arm it for an upcoming contract battle with the city and state. Despite the fact that I had no particular knowledge of home care, I thought my experience as a health policy analyst and planner in the city's health care system would provide a decent enough grounding to quickly figure it out. I was wrong.

I took the job already believing that whatever it was these workers did, they deserved a living wage. But before long, I discovered that this was more than a typical union struggle of health care workers. The more I learned about the home care system and the workers, the more appalled I became at the exploitive working conditions and the insecurity of their livelihood. They labor in a system built on the powerlessness of its mostly minority, often immigrant, and overwhelmingly female labor force. It is held together by the decency of the workers and their commitment to their patients.

The size and growth of the system was for a long time a closely held secret among a small number of state and city regulators. Few people knew much about home care, and even fewer cared about the plight of the workers. There was much to learn, much to be done, and there is still more that needs to be accomplished if these workers are to continue to make progress. What began for me as another job, another client, emerged as something far different. I was to become not merely an expert or technical advisor writing background papers or costing out settlements, but an advocate for a cause.

The Long March

On March 31, 1988, a jubilant Dennis Rivera, the executive vice-president of Local 1199, announced a stunning victory for that cause. Governor Mario Cuomo's administration, after long resistance, had just agreed to fund a 53 percent wage increase and to create a decent health insurance plan for the workers. (While the city controls the purse strings, the state is the major funder of home care services.) These long overdue gains were the fruits of the Campaign for Justice for Home Care Workers, launched and maintained through the joint efforts of Local 1199 and District Council 1707 (AFSCME), another of the unions representing the home care workers. In just over a year's time, it was joined by a coalition of the non-profit employers and virtually every local politician of even a vaguely liberal stripe. The workers, no longer invisible, were recognized and even celebrated by the city's major newspapers and television stations. Justice for home care workers had been transformed into a widely endorsed public cause.

While the victory was sweet, the workers had waited a long time for some meaningful benefit from their labor union membership. Fifty thousand of the home care workers employed through vendor contracts with the City of New York are represented by three prominent labor unions. Every three years, Local 1199 of the Retail, Wholesale Department Store Union (RWDSU), DC 1707 of the American Federation of State, County, Municipal Employees (AFSCME), and Local 32-B and 32-J of the Service Employees International Union (SEIU) independently went through the motions of negotiating new contracts. After nine years, the workers had gained an hourly wage rate of only 80 cents above the minimum wage. They had also won a small seniority differential and inadequate vacation and sick leave benefits.

This time around, the new leadership of Local 1199, recently elected after a bitterly fought campaign for control of the union, was determined to break through and get a contract that came closer to paying a living wage. The question was *how?*—how to force home care agencies, the city, and the state to spend far more than they wanted to for employees who worked alone in 50,000 different work sites? How to garner public support for people whose labors were all but invisible as they cared for poor patients in poor communities? How to win a radical change in wages and benefits for workers who could not use labor's most powerful weapon—the strike?

The Campaign for Justice for Home Care Workers was equal parts muscle and image. The muscle was flexed by two of the three unions, Local 1199 and DC 1707, who, with the support of Jesse Jackson, put their collective organizational and political clout on the line. And the image was the reflection of a well-coordinated media campaign to portray the plight of these workers as a matter worthy of widespread public support.

The Economics of the System

Following the scandals of fraud and abuse in New York City's nursing homes during the 1970s, publicly funded home care programs mushroomed as an alternative form of care for the chronically ill and the elderly. The president of the United Hospital Fund, Bruce Vladeck, summarizes the changes this way: "In a relatively short period of time we have transformed our entire system of care from one dominated by nursing homes to one in which a growing majority of services are provided to people in their own homes." The number of patients receiving home care doubled between 1980 and 1987. And, because increasing numbers of them required round-the-clock or seven-day-a-week care, expenditures grew fourfold—from $200 million to $800 million a year.

This transformation was spurred not only by fear of scandal but by the fiscal implications of New York City's changing demography. People age 85 and over are the city's fastest-growing population group, with their numbers expected to increase by 130 percent between 1980 and 2000. Without home care, half of them, or 90,000 people, would need to be in nursing homes. At the same time, after a slow-down in the 1970s, approvals for new nursing home construction were virtually halted in the early 1980s. In Brooklyn, the city's most populous borough, for example, no new beds have been added for 11 years. The current and foreseeable supply of nursing home beds has plateaued at about 40,000. The cost of supporting patients in these beds topped $1.5 billion in 1986, of which $1.2 billion was public money.

Home care is the long-term care analogue to hospital deinstitutionalization, costing about half as much as nursing home care. In 1987, approximately 43,000 New York City residents were being cared for daily in Medicaid-financed long-term home care programs at an annual cost of $700 million, compared to over $1.2 billion in Medicaid money spent for 38,000 nursing home residents.

Like many other of the best laid plans of New York's policymakers, the home care system is unraveling. Home care is a less costly alternative to nursing home or hospital care only if it is provided by low-wage earners for just a few hours a day. Without low pay, it's more costly. The reason is simple: one-on-one coverage is extremely labor intensive. Paying as little as $6 an hour for 24 hours of care would cost $144 a day or 50 percent more than the typical nursing home.

To keep home care cheap, wages had to be kept very low. But this strategy too has a price. Because there are numerous less-demanding jobs that pay equivalent wages, the home care industry faces a severe labor shortage. A 1988 report by a special New York State Task Force on Health Personnel documented a state-wide vacancy rate of 11.4 percent in home care positions, a shortfall even more severe than that of the much-publicized nursing shortage.

Defining the Problem

When the current leadership of Local 1199 assumed office in June 1986, the plight of home care workers was not first on their list. After an extremely combative campaign in which Georgianna Johnson unseated incumbent president

Doris Turner, the new union leaders faced a myriad of difficult problems. Chief among them was the challenge of negotiating a final contract for the hospital workers, an agreement that had yet to be completed despite a bitter, unproductive strike that stretched on for 47 days. The insurgent leadership inherited a union riven by deep political and ethnic divisions and almost equally divided between pro- and anti-Turner camps. The new leadership retained few of the old pro-Turner organizing staff, and only a handful of new staff members had extensive organizing experience.

In the home care area, the union's internal weaknesses were particularly acute. Neither of the officers assigned to home care had any special knowledge of the system or ties to home care workers. Aside from hiring new staff, their first order of business was to get to know the workers and develop an understanding of the industry's history and structure. Hard work and long hours accomplished the first. The latter I was able to help with. The story wasn't, as I had so confidently assumed, just another variant of health industry unionization. Home care workers, although 20,000 strong in the 80,000-member union, had been organized in a manner parallel to the growth of the system itself—that is, haphazardly, as a result of a weird confluence of factors.

New York City's massive long-term home care system was created in part by the welfare rights movement of the late 1960s, and its unionization was in part a creature of the city's fiscal crisis. Beginning in 1967, welfare rights groups, most notably the National Welfare Rights Organization (NWRO), mounted large-scale campaigns to maximize welfare entitlements. One of the little-known benefits included in New York State's Medicaid program was home care. As both a strategy and a service, NWRO organizers encouraged elderly and disabled Medicaid recipients to hire neighbors, often fellow recipients, as home care workers. These workers were, in effect, employees of the patients. They were paid by two-party checks issued jointly to the worker and client.

For a decade, the system grew in an unregulated, uncontrolled, and largely unnoticed fashion. Unnoticed, that is, until the inevitable scandal. In 1976–77, then City Council President Paul O'Dwyer exposed a system rife with bureaucratic incompetence, inefficiency, and outright fraud. Some workers waited months for their pay checks, and many checks were issued to non-existent workers.

City welfare officials considered three possible remedies. They could maintain the existing system with increased scrutiny and controls. They could hire home care workers directly as city employees. Or, they could find someone else to take responsibility for the workers. The first alternative was thought to be administratively unmanageable, and the second deemed too expensive at a time when city government was laying people off. The third alternative, contracting out the system, was considered the only practical choice.

With one throw, the contracting-out solution killed two tough political birds. In addition to bringing the home care system into line, it found a use for the remnants of the city's anti-poverty program, whose funds had just about dried up. On the advice of the Vera Institute of Justice, a local anti-poverty think tank, many of these programs were reincarnated as home care employment agencies. Ultimately, 62 nonprofit, community-based organizations became home care vendors. Each now has an annual contract with the city for a specified case load, ranging from 200 to 1,200. The contracts are tightly written and closely supervised by the city's Human Resources Administration. In effect, the agency directors function as contracted middle managers supervising a largely unskilled labor force of 50,000 people.

Caught in the throes of the city's catastrophic fiscal crisis and faced with threats of massive layoffs of its members, even New York's largest and most powerful nonuniform public employees union, District Council 37 of AFSCME, could do little to prevent the privatization of this growing city service. The union did not go beyond uttering the obligatory public outcries. But DC 37 did exact two promises from the city administration for its relative quiescence, one of great potential benefit to the home care workers, and one that threatened to undermine that advantage. First, the administration promised to facilitate whole-sale unionization of the new industry. And second, it made an unwritten pledge never to give larger pay increases to contractors' employees than were won by city workers.

While DC 37, fighting to stave off municipal bankruptcy, wasn't interested in organizing home care workers who were not public employees, three other unions were. Local 1199, the voluntary hospital and nursing home workers union, Local 32-B and 32-J, primarily a union of apartment house workers, and DC 1707, a smaller social service affiliate of the same AFSCME international as DC 37, had soon organized almost all of the home care workers.

If the development of the home care system was convoluted and complex, the needs of the workers, I discovered, were simple. When the last contract expired on June 30, 1987, most earned less than $7,000 a year. They had an inadequate hospital insurance plan with no medical, dental, or prescription benefits. They had no job security, no pensions, and were totally isolated from each other. Partly because of the agreement between the city government and DC 37, workers' wages had progressed, at an average rate of 5 percent annually, from minimum wage to $4.15 an hour. If one of the three unions became a little more assertive on behalf of its members, the city simply picked it off by imposing the least expensive settlement. All three unions had identical wage and benefit packages.

Finding the Right Allies

No one said home care workers were adequately paid, but just about everyone argued the impossibility of paying them much more. The critical problem was to develop a strategy that would make substantial change inevitable. To accomplish this, the Local 1199 leadership needed allies. The most logical allies were the two other unions that represented home care workers.

Although they initially had some doubts about the chances for success, DC 1707's executive director, Bob McEnroe, and its home care director, Josephine Lebeau, readily joined with 1199 to form the New York Labor Union Coalition for Home Care Workers. Together, the unions formulated a set of demands: $6 an hour, comprehensive family health insurance, pensions, job security, overtime pay, and industrywide seniority. Even more important than the joint demands, each union promised not to settle without the other.

While the unions were natural allies, coalitions, even between similar organizations, are very difficult to sustain. DC 1707, like 1199, styled itself as a progressive union—a champion of left causes and minority politics. This is not the case with Local 32-B and 32-J of the SEIU. The officers of 1199 and 1707 tried through every possible vehicle and intermediary to get the reclusive president of Local 32-B and 32-J, Gus Bovona, to join them, but Bovona rejected all overtures. Lawyers representing him at two meetings with 1199 and 1707 balked at any joint bargaining. At most, they would agree to a position paper spelling out "the problems of the workers."

Lacking a united front, the union coalition decided to seek the support of sympathetic local politicians. They first approached Manhattan Borough President David Dinkins. At the time, Dinkins was the only minority member of New York City's Board of Estimate, the upper house of municipal government. Astonished at the size of the industry and the widespread exploitation of its workers, Dinkins organized a public hearing to draw attention to their plight.

The hearing, held in April 1987, was dramatic enough to warrant the notice of New York's major media. The presence of several hundred minority women packed into the board's ornate City Hall chamber, the articulate voices of the workers, coupled with the support of the nonprofit, community-based agencies that employed them and the unions that represented them, made the telling of their plight extremely effective. "The only thing that I am asking for my work is to be respected, to be paid for my job, and to have some kind of services," Gwendolyn Rosemond told Dinkins and other Board of Estimate and City Council members in the crowded hearing room. It was a simple story. Home care workers perform significant, occasionally heroic work, for which they are abysmally paid.

Dinkins summed up his findings in an extensive hearing report: "I found the employment conditions of home health workers unconscionable," he wrote. "As a result of the hearing I am convinced that the present wages, benefits, working conditions and opportunities for advancement of the home care worker must be improved."

Just a month after the hearing, John Cardinal O'Connor and the Rev. Jesse Jackson met to jointly express their support for the workers' cause. While the media led with headlines about the newsmaking get-together of the politically conservative cardinal and the progressive reverend, the fact that the meeting was arranged by the unions and announced their endorsement of the Justice for Home Care Workers Campaign did not go unnoticed in City Hall or the governor's office. Later the same day, Jackson addressed a rally of about 6,000 home care workers and their supporters in front of City Hall. Just about every liberal and minority politician in the city jostled for space on the platform to reiterate his or her support for the workers.

These politicians, however, could not deliver a contract, nor could the nonprofit home care employers. That power lay in the hands of the Koch administration, even though the state's Department of Social Services actually sets the Medicaid reimbursement rates for the home care program and picks up 40 percent of the cost. The city's power lies not in its 10 percent contribution (the federal government pays the other 50 percent), but in its control of all the home care agencies' operations, from contracts to procedural details. Before the nominally independent employer agencies could sign a union contract, the Human Resources Administration, the city's massive welfare and Medicaid agency, had to approve its terms.

Despite the support of Jackson, Dinkins, and the Cardinal, the Koch administration was unwilling to meet the union coalition's demands. According to Koch's chief labor negotiator, Robert W. Linn, the city couldn't commit money for the home care contracts until it settled with the city workers' unions. When that would happen, Linn refused to hazard a guess.

Developing a Strategy

More than moral high ground and the support of selected politicians was needed to move city and state governments to take the union coalition's demands seriously. Union strategists, led by Dennis Rivera, Local 1199's executive vice president, felt it would be best to negotiate with the home care vendors and then present the contract as a fait accompli. With a concrete offer, to which the city and the state would have to respond, the union coalition would be in a better position to gauge the opposition and target its activities.

The coalition laid out its strategy to the most sympathetic of the home care vendors. At their suggestion, the coalition invited the Home Care Council, a trade association, to negotiate on behalf of its members. The council leadership balked, however. Never before had home care vendors entered into negotiations without the blessing and permission of their real bosses—the city's Human Resources Administration—nor did they feel comfortable negotiating as a group. To allay some of their anxiety and to get the process moving, the coalition agreed to develop a "joint position," not a contract.

The unions continued to treat the joint position talks as actual negotiations, however. They established a negotiating committee composed of workers from each of the agencies represented by the two unions. The committee laid out its positions and the members debated them. After the usual give and take of contract talks, the two sides arrived at a common position—$5.90 an hour, significant pay differentials for people who worked 24 hours a day (but were paid for 12) or people working on weekends and holidays, and the establishment of a comprehensive health insurance plan. They deferred agreements on pensions, job security, and overtime pay to the next contract.

The Home Care Council and the union coalition joined together under the unwieldy title of "Justice for Home Care Workers and Recipients." On January 11, 1988, they announced agreement on their "joint position." Simultaneously, they sent letters to the governor and mayor requesting approval and funding for the agreement.

Since the joint position was not a contract, neither executive had to reply. And neither did. Instead, each pointed a finger elsewhere. Conveniently forgetting that any agency signing without city scrutiny risked losing its vendor contract, city officials asserted that the issue was between the unions and the employers. The state's position, equally absurd, was that until the city's Human Resources Administration sought approval for new reimbursement rates, the state had no role to play. With both city and state maintaining the posture that someone else had to go first, the campaign was getting nowhere.

A more intensive, sophisticated strategy needed to be developed. The union-management group approached every significant elected official in the city. They sought and received endorsements from Andrew Stein, the City Council president; Harrison Goldin, the city's comptroller; four of the borough presidents; and numerous members of the City Council and the state legislature. But neither Koch nor Cuomo, whose endorsement would carry a commitment to fund the agreement, made public comment.

The coalition convinced a number of city and state politicians, religious leaders, and "power brokers" to phone the governor and the mayor. Word filtered back that they were now prepared to do something, "details to be worked out." Given the situation of most of the workers, "something" was not enough. The coalition was unwilling to accept anything short of the full agreement.

At one point Bob Linn, the city's chief labor negotiator, told coalition representatives that he would agree to whatever the state was willing to give. Two weeks later he withdrew that promise and offered instead a complicated plan whereby workers would receive an additional 20 cents an hour for each year of service. Linn got so carried away with the coalition's adamant rejection that he forgot who he was talking to. "You are going to drive this industry out of the city," he absurdly charged. Despite a few other off-the-record meetings, the city continued to stonewall.

To move the issue and force a response, the coalition developed a full-scale press campaign. Moe Foner, one of the labor movement's most experienced publicists, went to work, tirelessly convincing major newspapers to take up the crusade.

Foner, a former 1199 officer with great credibility among reporters and editors, was remarkably successful. After a series of sympathetic feature and news stories, the editorial writers waded in. "Nothing's dumber than saving pennies and wasting dollars," the *Daily News* editorialized on March 3, 1988. "Why get tight-fisted with home health care workers; who clearly have a strong case for a wage increase? Koch's stinginess could gut the system." The local CBS TV affiliate broadcast a highly sympathetic editorial, "Caring for the Caretakers," which was followed by a *Newsday* editorial declaring: "Stop the games: Penny pinching won't save a dime."

The turning point came on March 14, 1988, when the first of the coalition's ads appeared in the *New York Times* opposite the editorial page where, perhaps serendipitously, the *Times'* editors made their position known. "Can the city and state afford the $96 million it will cost over the next three years to improve the lot of the home care provider?" they wrote. "If they are truly committed to moving people out of poverty, the answer has to be yes. . . . If they want to enable people to stay home who otherwise have to enter expensive nursing facilities the answer has to be yes."

Pressured by an avalanche of political and media support, the governor's office began to move. "What do you want?" asked a senior member of Cuomo's staff. "Our agreement with the bosses," Dennis Rivera replied.

Victory

On March 31, a week after the overture, 4 days after Jackson's victory in the Michigan primary, and 19 days before the New York primary, Cuomo's labor commissioner, Tom Hartnett, worked out an agreement with Rivera and the coalition's chief negotiator, former Lieutenant Governor Basil Paterson.

Despite a price tag of $350 million spread over two years, Koch told the press he was "pleased." But 12 weeks of often acrimonious negotiations with the city and the vendors followed the March 31 announcement. Having been outflanked by the governor, the Koch administration continued to make trouble. Each time we thought the deal was made, it collapsed over disagreements between the city and state about how much it would cost. Until the city okayed the contract, the agencies wouldn't sign. Once during a discussion in Linn's office, I spent almost an hour arguing with a senior budget official about a penny difference in the cost figures, while Rivera, Paterson, Linn, and an aide watched in silence.

Once the money issues were resolved, each of the unions entered separate formal negotiations with the agencies' management. Allies became adversaries over such issues as paid release time for union delegates, guarantees of a weekend off a month, drug testing, and seniority rights. A full agreement was finally hammered out between Local 1199 and 22 home care agencies. DC 1707 has also completed negotiations, and workers in agencies represented by Local 32-B and 32-J will get the same wage settlement. At a meeting last June, Local 1199 home care workers ratified the contract by a vote of 849 to 9.

So Near, Yet So Far

Two months before the ratification, Local 1199 convened an emergency meeting of the home care workers after a disastrous session with the city. On a hot and humid night, 600 workers packed the union's auditorium on West 43rd Street in Manhattan.

I was standing downstairs when a small, 60ish woman approached me and inquired if I were a lawyer. I told her no, but asked if I could help. She told me she had worked seven days a week for five years because her boss had threatened to fire her if she took a day off. "Is that legal?" she asked.

I went back to the auditorium just as the meeting was ending. That day, April 4, was the twentieth anniversary of the assassination of Martin Luther King. As I elbowed my way through the crowd, someone began to lead the meeting in singing "We Shall Overcome." People linked arms and sang together.

Recalling that harassed worker's question, I thought, we have come so far, but we still have a long, long way to go.

AIDS AT THE BEGINNING OF THE SECOND DECADE

Nancy F. McKenzie

The Sixth International Conference on AIDS was not the lesson in polarization and frustration that its main participants—researchers, health care providers, and activists—expected it to be and that the national media widely reported. Traditionally, researchers functioning within institutions confront providers and advocates across a political divide. Not only did this confrontation not occur, but the advocates and providers seem to have enlisted the others in viewing and acknowledging the wilderness of care that forms the reality of HIV infection. Nor was the conference the medical "boat show" that characterizes most medical conferences in the United States.

The conference's theme—"Science to Policy"—immediately became ironic as the Immigration and Naturalization Service (INS) refused to alter its policy of prohibiting HIV-antibody-positive individuals and homosexuals from entering the country, despite nearly unanimous criticism from the international public health community and the boycott of the conference by over 80 organizations world-wide. No one at the conference remained unmoved by the wholly political nature of these restrictions or the fact that the waiver offered to those wishing to attend the conference included the requirement that all HIV-antibody-positive participants document that they could pay for the cost of medical treatment should they fall ill in the United States. Thousands of participants did boycott, and seats on conference panels were purposefully left unfilled and programs were printed with no presenter for a topic to indicate the extent of the boycott. The sheer crassness of the policy and the heartlessness of the health care waiver did more to politicize the conference than activist demands. And it provided an opening for a partnership between researchers and providers—a partnership that ultimately allowed Secretary of Health and Human Services Louis Sullivan's speech to be drowned out not only by ACT UP but by his own irrelevance.

From the beginning of the San Francisco conference, there was unity against the INS restrictions. Everyone seemed buoyed by sharing red arm bands against the policy and by ACT UP's invitation to 20,000 people to chant against screen displays of George Bush, who at that moment was attending a fundraiser for Jesse Helms, the author of the INS amendment. Granted, not every participant was happy with this heated involvement in American politics. But it was clear that most felt the need for the conference to achieve a sense of rationality or coherence at the heart of an extraordinary biologic, clinical, social, and political phenomenon. And, while coherence was not achieved, consensus was—consensus that the division between science and action can no longer be maintained, and that we are losing the battle against AIDS in prevention, treatment, and delivery terms.

Information Exchange

Scientific exchange, the rationale for this type of conference, occurred in the usual small but grand ways. As far as the formal sessions were concerned, ACT UP was right: Abstracts or paper exchange would have been more efficient. Most of the major papers had already been accepted months or even years previously and would be published after the conference in journals. The poster sessions—literal posters on which people put up abstracts of their latest research for one day only—were the most informative. They offered more descriptions of studies and treatment efforts than methodologically correct research. The topics were highly varied, and it was clear that health care providers and scientists were able in this way to conduct a dialogue and play out their hunches.

Within the presentation halls, researchers listened respectfully to their peers and to the latest advances in the esoteric development of possible vaccines and the biological modeling of the infection. Dr. Jay Berzofsky of the National Cancer Institute announced that we now know enough about immunology to develop an artificial vaccine. And there were some other new insights.

Jay Levy, professor of medicine at the University of California at San Francisco and one of the main researchers into human immunodeficiency virus (HIV), offered a very clear description of the history of HIV infection and indicated what many have been suspicious of: HIV can infect almost any cell. He had his doubts about a vaccine because of the emerging complexity of HIV. Most controversial of the research giants was Dr. Luc Montagnier of the Pasteur Institute and one of the identifiers of HIV. He now hypothesizes that HIV plus a bacterium-like microbe are *both* implicated in AIDS. His evidence is the extent of mycoplasma infection he has found in his patients and what the presence of mycoplasma does to replication of HIV. The implications of Montagnier's assertions were startling and angered many people at the conference. If HIV is an infection that may, in itself, be innocuous until it is booted into betrayal of the human organism by some other infection or co-factor, then the small minority of researchers known as the co-factorialists have been right all along: We should be researching more than HIV as a cause of AIDS. Poster presentations supported such a view. Many researchers have found that hepatitis and tuberculosis seem to exacerbate the presence of HIV itself.

ACT UP's Research Agenda

One of the main complaints at every AIDS conference from providers, people with AIDS, and activists alike is how little research on effective clinical (as opposed to purely biological) interventions is presented. In the same way that the panel on "Access to Health Care" was narrowly focused upon access to AZT, there were few panels on treatments for the myriad infections associated with HIV. Yet it is clear to every person with AIDS and every AIDS medical provider that the need to enhance the clinical research agenda is being eclipsed by the single-minded basic science agenda for "cracking the code" of HIV itself. Most of this year's new treatment findings promise help to asymptomatic infected people, and may be too late to save thousands of lives in limbo. The call to reorganize the health care empire and its basis in pharmaceutical research may seem a distant imperative from the front line of an epidemic, but this is precisely what will ultimately have to be done if we are to "treat" AIDS.

The most popular handout at the conference was ACT UP's Research Agenda—an extensive outline of the drugs that should be tested and the treatments that should be tried in parallel track designs and other configurations of research protocols. At the end of the conference, one newspaper editorial headlined its applause of ACT UP by naming its members the "Scientists from ACT UP." This was prompted, no doubt, by the Research Agenda, as well as by the address of Dr. Anthony Fauci, director of the National Institute of Allergies and Infectious Diseases, to the convention on the closing day. Fauci admonished scientists for not taking ACT UP and other activists seriously as contributors to research design. He also chastised ACT UP, however, for charging the scientific community with not caring about the HIV-infected.

The Toll Worldwide

There were many sad moments when the news of the health of various populations reached the auditoriums and spilled out into the halls of the Moscone Center, not the least of which was the mounting death rate from the Iran earthquake that week. A global epidemic of tuberculosis is being caused by the AIDS pandemic, according to Dr. Peter Eriki of the World Health Organization. In Africa alone there are over 2 million people infected with microbes that cause AIDS and tuberculosis. AIDS is creating an entire generation of orphans in the developing world.

One of the keynote speakers at the conference, Eunice Muringo Kiereini, Chair of the World Health Organization's Regional Nursing/Midwifery Task Force, pointed out that 3.5 million people are infected with HIV in Africa alone. Six hundred thousand of these are children under age 5, and child mortality may increase by 50 percent in the 1990s. In Brazil, teenagers are at great risk for HIV due to the practice of adolescent prostitution in the major cities. Both African and Latin American cultures still create obstacles to care. In Brazil, for instance, the Catholic Church condemns condoms, and condoms cost 41 cents —a prohibitive expense for a Rio street kid.

In the Soviet Union, physicians have identified seven women who contracted AIDS from nursing HIV-infected infants. The babies had contracted HIV from infected needles used in immunizations, and the mothers had abrasions on their breasts at the time of nursing. More positively, because the USSR expects the incidence of AIDS there to increase as *perestroika* increases exchange between East and West, the government plans to lift a ban against homosexuality so that the epidemic can be dealt with directly and with public participation.

US figures on HIV infection from the National Academy of Sciences have finally made official what the affected communities have been saying for years:

Women and children are at increasing risk due to the intravenous drug use of sexual partners and to the addictions of adolescents and women to alcohol, cocaine, heroin, and crack.

The cost of AIDS care in the United States (costs calculated within one of the most inefficient health care delivery systems in the world) was cited at $85,000 per patient. The figure totals $4.6 billion in 1990 for all patients. But, as some investigators pointed out, AIDS is really no more expensive a disease than cancer, and the care for a single premature infant in a neonatal unit can cost as much as $1 million.

In the face of the figures there was outrage that the private insurance industry seems determined to get out of AIDS coverage altogether. Data from San Francisco alone show that only about one-third of white individuals were insured in 1990, compared to one-half in 1983. Health industry consultants maintain that private insurance companies avoid paying for AIDS in any way they can.

On the question of access to health care for people with HIV disease, some other countries are doing better than the United States, but access worldwide nonetheless still generally depends on an individual's class. The developing world, including the Caribbean Basin and Africa, have practically no resources for responding to their exponentially increasing incidence of HIV infection. In Canada, hospital stays are handled by the government, but home care is not provided and depends upon private providers or volunteers. The US system was characterized as entirely "perverse" by Jean McGuire, the Executive Director of the AIDS Action Council in Washington. According to McGuire, it "provides the greatest availability of services . . . to the smallest number of people."

From Complacency to Outrage

HIV is a bio-medical event. AIDS is a medical event, and the AIDS epidemic is a socioepidemic—one so intertwined with political and social questions that it is a mockery to "scientize" it. The first session on AIDS prevention presented ten obstacles to a "national program." In typical sociobehavioral jargon, the first and major obstacle was listed as "complacency," as if sheer laziness of individuals, agencies, or government was the major enemy of the vulnerable, the sick, the dying—as if lassitude was the reason that the uninformed and uninvited remain outside the house of health care delivery.

At this kind of convention, the obvious becomes the obscure and, with enough awareness, becomes the obvious again, but perniciously so. And so it was that presenter after presenter talked positively about the latest strategy for detecting, measuring, and defining the behavior of intravenous drug users and how/why/when parenteral transmission takes place, as audiences sat in numbed and compartmentalized silence, with their helplessness to offer treatment for the addicted or to make their needle a clean one. Prevention issues, like issues of primary care and access, strain behind the gloss of technical abstracts so as not to slip into outrage and calls to activism.

As each day passed, however, there was less "complacency" and more outrage, and not only from activists. The conference organization, frustration with an epidemic beginning its second decade, and the location of the conference in San Francisco all had a hand in humanizing the sessions and making palpable not only the extent of grief with the hardest hit cities of New York, San Francisco, and Kampala, Uganda, but the extent of exhaustion and even humility that now characterizes scientists, providers, and activists. It's not so much that science and policy researchers and providers are "burned out." The unique blend of discriminations that accompanies the HIV-affected, which at previous AIDS conferences was the topic of a poster session, or, at most, one formal paper, was here a resounding item in every major official's speech. This was not merely because of the INS restrictions. Rather, everyone finally shared the realization (some, of course, much later than others) that not only is AIDS *not* a respectable illness worldwide, but that knowledge alone—the knowledge the world has surely gained in the past ten years—has not made a dent in the social lives of the affected. In fact, quite the contrary. As one American study showed, two-thirds of 1,000 medical residents interviewed in the United States prefer to avoid having an HIV-infected patient, and 25 percent went into medical specialties expressly to avoid such patients. The residents indicated that this was not out of fear but out of explicit disapproval and discomfort with homosexuality and drug use.

The Organization Worked

The organizers of this conference expected something to get done. The structure of the conference itself had vision, and it opened up the discursive space for things to happen. It is not surprising, then, that the conference developed a consensus on AIDS as a political problem. HIV-infected individuals were involved in every stage of the planning. Scientific sessions were interspersed with documents and presentations about the lives of the affected. Sessions were housed at the Moscone Center and the Marriott Hotel, but there were public sessions in communities at which major researchers and officials in the epidemic spoke and answered questions. Included among those who spoke at these local gatherings were Dr. Fauci of NIH and June Osborn, the president of the National Commission on AIDS. There was a daily conference newspaper about the day's happenings, including not just the presentations but also any demonstrations or political events happening around the conference. Local public radio stations provided a few hours of live coverage of the conference each day. Seven hundred and fifty people with AIDS were allowed to waive the $550 registration fee and attend the conference.

At each of the poster rooms there were cafes with coffees and teas so that one could do the daunting work of reading the data and then sit down with others and talk. In order to get to the cafeteria, one had to walk slowly through the booths of the non-profit and provider groups. One could not help but be challenged by the hundreds of small groups trying to reach the unreachable in a very large tragedy. The organization worked.

On the next to the last day of the conference, delegates joined activists in a demonstration through the streets of San Francisco. The march, estimated to have 10,000 to 20,000 participants, brought together those who had been demonstrating all week about lack of AIDS funding and resources in San Francisco

Incidence of AIDS as of June 1990

Location	AIDS Total Cases	Total Deaths
San Francisco	8,649	5,692
California	26,925	17,440
New York City[a]	27,137	16,141
New York State[b]	31,220	19,038
United States	136,204	83,145
World, reported	263,051	—
World, estimated	600,000	3,000,000

Source:

World Health Organization, June 1, 1990, unless otherwise indicated
[a] New York City Department of Health, June 1990
[b] New York State Department of Health, June 1990

with the scientists and providers attending the conference. The conference delegation was led by the co-directors of the conference, Drs. John Ziegler and Paul Volberding. Ziegler called it a "new era of cooperation," and continued, "I'm a totally different person as a result of this conference. I am much more concerned about social responsibility. . . . We're all in this together. Action equals life."

AIDS at the End of the First Decade

In its second decade, the AIDS epidemic has killed more than 83,000 Americans, and worldwide HIV has infected more than 8 million people. AIDS has created activists, and it has gained a reputation as the disease that brought about a small reformation in the delivery of health care in the United States through an alternative health model that is more community based and community led. This involves not only a new concept of support services and out-of-hospital care, but the way in which treatments get formulated and reach the communities that require them. Cancer activists apparently are now trying the techniques of AIDS advocates in Washington that have worked to shake up the bureaucracy in research on and approval of new drugs. Cancer patients are also getting drugs for opportunistic infections associated with immune-suppression years earlier than they would have had the epidemic not occurred. Of 18 drugs approved for early release by the FDA under a new ruling in 1987 after pressure from AIDS activists, 12 are for treating non-HIV-related infections, mostly cancer.

But, practically no attention was given at the AIDS conference to health care provision. Biomedical interventions had priority, and service provision was relegated to the non-profit organizations whose booths snaked through the hallways of the Marriott. Only San Francisco's provision of AIDS services was highlighted, for the obvious reasons that San Francisco hosted the conference, that it has been a city under siege for more than ten years, and has served as a model for coordinated AIDS health care responsiveness. There are many successful alternative HIV health care systems developed mostly by gay communities across America. HIV infection, like mental illness, drug addiction, disability, and cancer requires a fine coordination of services if those affected are to get on with their lives. The American health care system is a highly fragmented one, and its public sector, as well as the public entitlement programs that fund it, are in great disarray and near collapse. The need for coordination is even more urgent today than it has been in the past, due to the disappearance of basic care centered in the family physician or internist in solo or group practice. But these facts of the health care system in America were barely mentioned.

Organized care—care that is coordinated—is health care that is able to identify patients' needs as they move through the trajectory of sickness. It focuses upon different stages of illness that urgently require various medical, mental health, and social services. Ideally, it is community based and accessible geographically and culturally, since "needs" depend not only upon levels of morbidity and disability but also upon the strengths of social, familial, and community networks, as well as upon the commitment of caretakers and health institutions. These things AIDS providers have recently taught us, as have small advocacy groups for other populations in the past. But, in the present, the world owes a large debt for the leadership, advocacy, organizational skill, and incredible innovation of the Gay Men's Health Crisis and other organizations like it —the Shanti Project in San Francisco, BEBASHI in Philadelphia, the Minority Task Force on AIDS of New York—for providing a complex of services to thousands upon thousands of people with AIDS in the first ten years of the epidemic, as well as for providing educational and caretaking models for the world of the HIV-affected.

But one left the conference with the realization that there is still no coordination of research efforts nationwide for the study of treatments. To say the least, there is no federal effort to underwrite research and make sure that those who develop effective therapies or treatments do so in the interest of the infected and not in the interest of profits.

THE SAN FRANCISCO MODEL BURNS OUT

Even as San Francisco hosted the most informed conference on AIDS to be held anywhere, San Francisco's own ten years of effort to respond to its residents is coming unraveled. ACT UP's poster, "The San Francisco Model: A View of the Ruins," pointed to what providers and officials from San Francisco suggested in their conference presentation: The next ten years will be harder because those who were able to respond in the face of crisis can do so no longer. This is true for individuals, for families, for communities, and for cities like San Francisco. The San Francisco model, a model developed through the coordination of private and public funds, volunteer and municipal services, which places great emphasis upon following a patient's illness trajectory through myriad medical and social needs and which has set AIDS care delivery policy for the last decade is competing for a smaller and smaller slice of city funds.

San Francisco, the city with the highest rate of HIV infection in the United States, committed itself very early on to helping those affected by HIV disease. But even a community as large and as solidified around HIV as the city of San Francisco can go only so far in providing responsive, humane care to the sick. Services now are worn out, donations are dwindling, and there is pervasive burnout among the entire array of service providers.

Next year's goal is to bring in $154 million to San Francisco from public and private sectors. Last fiscal year, the city spent $25 million of its revenues on AIDS. State and federal allotments totaled $15.6 million. But projections show that the next four years will require $100 million for treatment costs in the city. "San Francisco has mounted an incredible crisis response, but it's lunacy to think we can continue with it," says Robert Munk, Executive Director of the AIDS Service Providers Association of the Bay Area. Even with the political will and an informed health care leadership, even with the affected communities placed at the center of health care delivery, an effective response to the epidemic cannot be carried out in an economic vacuum. (Some help may be forthcoming. Congress has just passed and George Bush just signed a bill to send AIDS Disaster Relief to the major cities affected by the HIV epidemic.)

The San Francisco experience reflects the state of health care in the United States. There is no public health agenda. And the era of relying on voluntarism for responding to the epidemic is over, if, indeed, it ever began in many cities and communities.

—N.M.

There was frustration that there is little acknowledgment of the underside of the epidemic—the conditions in which people with AIDS live—and the minimal and increasing lack of access to physicians and other health professionals (dentists, therapists, etc.), to home care workers, to clinical trials. There was no mention at the conference of the extent of the collapse of this nation's health care system—a system in which more and more of the sick are becoming the medically indigent, and one organized for acute care that is unjustifiably expensive for chronic care, a system in which most cities and rural areas have severe gaps in basic care, primarily to their minority populations. Even in San Francisco, where voluntarism has organized a model system of care, there were large demonstrations during the conference against the city about the neglect of people with AIDS—like a six-month waiting list for an appointment with a physician in the public hospital system.

The drug addicted got short shrift indeed. There is no realistic appraisal by any public agency of the extent of illness among intravenous drug users, their partners, and their children, or of the growing numbers of women and adolescents at high risk because of their addictions to alcohol and cocaine, heroin, and crack. There is no mention of the intertwining epidemics of drug use, homelessness, and HIV infection or the extent to which they are reflections of poverty.

There are no plans for drug treatment—none at all. And short-term preventive interventions such as education about cleaning needles or exchanging used ones for clean ones meets the same resistance that condoms do from the Catholic Church, despite the existence of effective risk-minimization programs around the globe through state-sponsored needle exchange programs.

Finally, it was apparent that a new triage is emerging. Where services exist they invariably shortchange the HIV-affected or involve trading-off human rights of the HIV-affected for services. New York State, for example, recently decided to allow the Catholic Archdiocese to build a 200-bed skilled nursing facility without offering safer sex education, condoms, reproductive information, or safer drug use education. (The facility still requires New York City approval.)

Conclusion

The Sixth International Conference on AIDS was the coalescence of separate actors in the epidemic largely because of what the first decade of AIDS activism, AIDS research, and AIDS treatment did not get accomplished. It is only in the context of the first 10 years of struggle that the historical event of the San Francisco conference became historic. It remains outrageous that after 10 years there is still a lack of acknowledgment of the extent of the epidemic and the sick who are infected.

Nevertheless, it seems now that the Sixth International AIDS Conference has more than a documenting role to play in the epidemic. This conference, in a piecemeal fashion, gained an identity as AIDS policymaker and political champion of the affected. Future AIDS conferences—whether in Florence in 1991, Harvard in 1992 (if not relocated because of the INS policy), or Berlin in 1993—will be less scientific conferences and more "conventions" of individuals joined together in a common battle.

TEACHING TO LIVE: LEARNING FROM TEN YEARS OF AIDS

Nick Freudenberg

June 1991 marked the tenth anniversary of the first report from the US Centers for Disease Control on a cluster of cases of an unusual immune deficiency among gay men. Ten years after this report, 200,000 men, women, and children in the United States have been diagnosed with AIDS; more than 100,000 have already died from the disease, and it is estimated that at least 1.5 million Americans are infected with the human immunodeficiency virus (HIV) that causes AIDS.

Much of the press coverage of the tenth anniversary of the CDC report, as well as the general media coverage of AIDS, have focused on the failures in controlling this epidemic. And those failures are certainly glaringly evident. Scientists have yet to develop an effective vaccine against AIDS or a medical treatment that will cure the condition. The virus continues to spread unchecked in many parts of the world. Here in the United States it has reached new populations in the last few years, including teenagers, women, homeless people, gay men outside big cities, and others. While gay men have shown dramatic reductions in risk behavior, many still relapse to unsafe sex. Likewise in ten years our country has barely made a dent in increasing the availability or effectiveness of treatment for drug abuse to slow the spread of the disease among intravenous drug users. Despite the development of a number of drugs that control opportunistic infections and improve the quality of life for people with AIDS, our health care system has failed to provide access to these new treatments to tens of thousands of people with HIV illness.

It would be a mistake, however, to conclude that the decade has been without success. In fact, failing to analyze what has been learned in the past ten years would deprive us of the opportunity to generalize those successes to other settings and to other diseases. By reviewing some of the accomplishments of AIDS prevention efforts, this article seeks to open a discussion that will help to define an agenda for AIDS prevention in this next decade and to apply its lessons more broadly to public health practice.

Community Organization

Perhaps the most dramatic accomplishment of AIDS prevention efforts is the extent to which the AIDS epidemic has involved new organizations with public health. Consider the following examples:

- A hair dresser in a beauty parlor in an African-American neighborhood in Charleston, South Carolina, educates her clients about AIDS and distributes literature and condoms.
- A community group in Brooklyn offers sessions on AIDS to livery taxi cab drivers so that they can discuss the issue with their passengers.
- The Service Employees International Union trains shop stewards on AIDS, offers workshops, and distributes materials on AIDS to its 800,000 members and has lobbied for stronger protection for hospital workers against occupational exposure to HIV.
- Gay bars, not only in New York, San Francisco, and Los Angeles, but also in Nashville, Salt Lake City, and New Orleans, offer workshops on safer sex and distribute condoms to their patrons.

Although community organizations have previously been involved in public health programs, never before have so many groups defined such a broad array of activities to combat a threat to health. What accounts for the unprecedented mobilization? Certainly the public perception that AIDS is a serious problem helps, and here the mass media have played an important role in putting the issue on the nation's agenda, even if the coverage was often sensational or simplistic.

Early in the epidemic, the gay community, the population hardest hit in the first decade of AIDS, set an example of community education and organization that provided models for other communities to emulate. The gay community's success in persuading Congress and state and local legislatures to appropriate money for AIDS prevention programs also provided a source of funding for community-based initiatives, even if such funding was inadequate and contained restrictions that compromised its effectiveness. At the same time, the reluctance of public health authorities to launch explicit and comprehensive prevention programs forced private groups to take the initiative, leading to more creative approaches.

When thousands of local, regional, and national organizations each launch their own AIDS prevention initiatives, there are both negative and positive consequences. For example, at the beginning of the second decade of the epidemic, the United States still lacks a coordinated and comprehensive national strategy for AIDS prevention. While the CDC has made some important efforts in this direction, it lacks the political support and the financial resources to carry out this role effectively. As a result of this lack of coordination, many groups duplicate each other's work, compete for limited resources, and fail to address the needs of those highest at risk.

On the other hand, the strategy—by default—of ''letting a thousand flowers bloom'' has provided a rich diversity of experience. While existing evaluations have yet to provide a body of literature from which conclusions can be rigorously drawn, some generalizations on education that makes a difference seem warranted.

First, small grassroots organizations have close relationships with their constituents that can provide context for ongoing discussions about drugs and sex. At least some church groups, homeless shelters, ethnic social clubs, and youth organizations in low-income and minority neighborhoods and around the country have integrated AIDS prevention into their existing work. These groups may be better able than larger service providers to engage people in the intimate dialogue needed to change risk behavior. Not surprisingly, these smaller groups are often less able to apply for and manage AIDS prevention grants offered by government and foundations and thus have trouble sustaining effective programs.

Secondly, people need intensive and continuing intervention in order to be able to initiate and maintain changes in behavior that reduce the risk of HIV infection. Whereas early AIDS education programs consisted of lectures and pamphlets, most AIDS educators now report that much more is needed. More experienced AIDS organizations such as Gay Men's Health Crisis and San Francisco AIDS Foundation are now establishing relapse prevention programs, designed to provide ongoing support to gay men for maintaining safer sex practices. Similarly, for drug users, the major lesson learned is *not* that drug users are uneducable about AIDS (a politically appealing lesson in some circles), but rather that they need a high level of support in order to make real changes in their lives. Thus, to be effective, AIDS prevention programs will need more, not less, support in the coming decade.

Finally, people are more willing to engage the issue of AIDS when it is connected to their other central concerns. In the early years of the epidemic, AIDS educators often approached their jobs with missionary zeal, seeking to convince everyone that this epidemic was a calamity that required immediate action. Those who were unwilling to take action were accused of being in denial, homophobic, and uncaring. While these charges may sometimes have had merit, the accusatory strategy was seldom effective in mobilizing people. Now, AIDS educators are more likely to discuss the relationships between AIDS and poverty, drug abuse, teen pregnancy, inadequate housing and health care, lack of sex education, and a host of other social issues. Whether someone decides to get involved in the issue of AIDS because they are worried about their children, because it is a racial justice issue, or because their religion calls for compassionate involvement with others matters little. By being able to engage people on a variety of fronts and at different levels of activity, AIDS educators have been able to reach a wider constituency.

Politicizing the Epidemic

Another important accomplishment of the AIDS prevention effort of the last decade has been its ability to link education for change in personal behavior such as the use of condoms and clean needles with organizing for social change, for example, more resources for prevention and laws against discrimination. Although most health educators agree that effective interventions must address both individual behavior and social factors, in practice, programs aimed at other diseases have tended to emphasize one or the other. Thus, most heart disease prevention programs help people to stop smoking, exercise more, and eat less fat but do not take on issues of work organization, environmental pollution, or access to primary care.

AIDS prevention programs, on the other hand, almost always combine risk-reduction education, advocacy, and community organization. Many AIDS educators will distribute condoms in the morning, write letters to legislators or collect signatures on a petition protesting exclusion of HIV-infected people from the United States in the afternoon, and run a support group for people with AIDS in the evening. By avoiding the pitfall of abandoning advocacy as services become more important, AIDS organizations have maintained a voice in the political arena. This integration of different levels of practice can serve as an important model for other public health campaigns.

The assaults of the Reagan/Bush administrations on social programs and social movements and declining support for public programs made the 1980s a decade of coalition building. The AIDS epidemic, too, spawned thousands of local, regional, national, and international networks and coalitions. Not only have these coalitions played an important role in securing funding for AIDS prevention and services, but they also provided a forum for addressing issues of class, race, gender, and sexual orientation that arose in the battle against AIDS.

The New York AIDS Coalition, for example, which represents more than 400 organizations involved in AIDS work in New York State, each year prepares a budget outlining the needs of its member organizations. The preparation of this document provides groups an opportunity to coordinate their efforts and to set broad priorities. It also helps to unify the lobbying efforts of its constituents. When the state government attempted to increase AIDS funding for minority organizations while cutting dollars for gay organizations, the coalition successfully resisted this divide-and-conquer strategy by insisting on increased funding for both populations.

Individual organizations, as well as coalitions, have provided platforms from which to discuss how issues of race, gender, and sexual orientation influence the fight against AIDS. Here, too, the overtly political nature of this discussion distinguishes AIDS work from other public health practice. Nearly every AIDS organization has discussed the role of gay men and lesbians, people of color, and women in educating people about AIDS, and these questions usually lead to debates about who controls the organization and the work. Some of these discussions, of course, have disrupted the work, but rarely have central issues of power and control been successfully swept under the rug.

The politicization of the epidemic has also affected community education. Any AIDS educator who has given presentations on the disease has had to answer questions about why this disease affects who it does, the role of the government in the epidemic's origins and control, the effects of discrimination, and the sexual double standard. There is simply no way to talk about AIDS without locating the epidemic in its larger social and political context. As a result, community AIDS organizations have provided tens of thousands of people an opportunity to consider the political dimensions of the epidemic and its impact on their lives. For health activists who have been trying to achieve this goal with regard to other issues for more than two decades, the success of AIDS education warrants serious study.

Integrating Prevention and Care

Still another success of the campaign against AIDS has been the integration of prevention of AIDS and care for those suffering from the disease within many organizations. Even though funding streams for prevention and medical care are almost entirely separate, many AIDS groups provide both sets of services. This approach has several advantages. Politically, it makes it more difficult to pit prevention against care, since advocacy groups understand the importance of both. It also gives organizations a more comprehensive understanding of the deficits in our present system of care, allowing them to develop a more holistic approach and sophisticated critique and alternative. For people affected by the epidemic, combining prevention and services in one organization also makes good sense because individuals and families often need a continuum of care, which is easier to obtain in one place than many.

In a recent essay, Jonathan Mann, former director of the World Health Organization's Global Programme on AIDS and currently the director of the International AIDS Center of the Harvard AIDS Institute, observed that ''no other disease in the world's history has challenged the status quo as AIDS has done.'' He speculates that when the story of AIDS is written, ''the discovery of the inextricable linkage between human rights and AIDS, and more broadly, between human rights and health care, will rank among the major discoveries and advances in the history of health and society.''[1]

For activists who have long been seeking to unite the struggle for social justice with the fight for the right to health care and a healthy physical and social environment, this terrible epidemic has provided an opportunity to raise these questions with a much wider constituency. In the first decade of AIDS, activists and educators have made important strides in realizing this potential. The challenge of the second decade is to translate this potential into a substantive public health practice.

N O T E S

1. Mann, Jonathan, ''The New Health Care Paradigm,'' *Focus: A Guide to AIDS Research and Counseling*, 1991:6(30), pp. 1–2.

KNOW NEWS: REASSESSING COMMUNITIES

Nicholas Freudenberg

Just as social scientists have pronounced the traditional community dead, a victim of urbanization and industrialization, health educators are proclaiming it the hottest thing since computerized instruction.

Disappointed with the limited effectiveness of programs aimed at changing individual behavior, these educators have given the community a new life as the fashionable arena for their interventions. Established community programs have attracted renewed interest and funding, and newer models have sprung up as well.

Is the community alive and well, or has it followed the mom-and-pop grocery into extinction?

Much confusion over the community's place and unique function as an agent of change stems from differing definitions of the word itself. The traditional community, in which residents share values, customs, and local institutions, has found no place in our cities, where socioeconomic and cultural differences among people living in a given geographic area are often as great as are their similarities. The separation of residential areas from places of employment, together with the rise of the mass media and the isolation they engender, have further loosened the ties that once bound people together.

Another, broader meaning of community has come into use. Under this definition, the word refers to a group of people with a common ethnicity, religion, or sexual orientation. We speak freely of the black, Hispanic, and gay communities, yet by doing so refer to groups spread throughout the socioeconomic spectrum. Meanwhile, the neighborhood has taken over many of the functions of the traditional community. Here, face-to-face contact exists and people use common stores, schools, churches, and health centers; it is this type of community on which I will focus.

Despite these problems of definition, the idea of community is all the rage. Cognizant of new research showing the importance of peer and social support in maintaining health, and desirous of the financial advantages of using existing channels of communication and networks of influence, health educators have become intrigued with the community as a level of intervention.

Until now, however, they have failed to realize the full potential of organizing in such a way. While community newspapers, local leaders, merchants associations, and health providers have been effectively enlisted in these campaigns, most of the projects aimed at reducing chronic disease, although ostensibly dealing with the community, actually emphasize the reduction of individual risk factors—cigarette smoking, high-fat diets, high blood pressure. Only a few have addressed institutional issues such as access to health care, stressful work conditions and the availability of recreational facilities.

In addition, health educators have generally been unwilling to engage in the adversarial tactics practiced by community organizers schooled in the radical movements of the past decades. This has had two negative effects. First, the efforts of educators have usually failed to attract the passion or commitment that more confrontational tactics arouse. More important, the failure to challenge the people who permit illness makes it difficult for educators to mobilize the political power needed to win significant improvements in public health.

That mobilization, getting communities to change communities, is surely difficult, but the AIDS epidemic provides an ideal opportunity to develop such an approach. Only by organizing people to demand the reallocation of public money, both within each community and at the state and federal levels, can health activists relieve the underlying conditions that have caused the rapid spread of HIV infection.

The community offers progressive health educators an important arena for linking their commitments to public health and social justice. The challenge in the years to come will be to translate these concerns, and this new interest in community, into sensible models that can be implemented around the country.

SUCCESSFUL STRATEGIES: MEETING THE NEEDS OF CHILDREN IN ADVERSITY

Lisbeth B. Schorr

Meeting the neglected and often urgent needs of poor children in today's climate of scarce and dwindling resources is a significant challenge, and it is intensified by the fact that simply expanding existing programs would have only limited impact. After eight years of studying successful interventions in the fields of health, mental health, education, child care, and social services that have actually improved long-term outcomes for children who are growing up in adversity,[1] it has become clear to me that we must do more than improve access to existing services. We must also bring about profound changes in the content and provision of those services. If we are concerned with how the health and well-being of disadvantaged children can be significantly improved, we must begin by thinking anew about just what it is that these children need access *to*.

Comparing successful and unsuccessful health programs for disadvantaged populations, it becomes apparent that the health needs of children that are not being well met tend to have certain characteristics. They are not exclusively biological; they don't inhere entirely within the child; they require collaboration between pediatricians, other professionals, and parents; and they require continuity in care-taking and the investment of time. Of course, these issues don't even arise for children who lack access to the system, who are excluded from entry by financial and other barriers.

Two examples may help to clarify these points. The first illustrates the prevailing approach to health care for the poor, and how it fails disadvantaged children even when services exist for them.

Gail: How Health Care Fails

Gail was 13, shy, and soft-spoken. While being teased by schoolmates on the playground, she fatally stabbed an 11-year-old boy. She wandered away from school, and, several hours later, confused as to her whereabouts, telephoned her grandmother to pick her up. Later, she had no memory of the stabbing, and only vaguely recalled the boy pointing a knife at her. Witnesses said the boy had been pointing a pencil at Gail when she stabbed him.

Some weeks later, an official of the juvenile court reviewed Gail's medical records at the local hospital. They showed that Gail had been seen there more than 30 times for problems ranging from sore throats to recurrent headaches. The juvenile court reviewer discovered, in the midst of the fat file, an inconspicuous note by a resident physician saying that Gail had twice lost consciousness for no apparent reason while being examined. The resident recommended an electroencephalogram to determine whether Gail was suffering from seizures. None was performed until after Gail had killed her schoolmate.

Gail's family, with little education and overwhelmed by other problems, had no idea what Gail's examination had shown or that follow-up neurological tests had been recommended. There had been no single professional with continuing responsibility for making sense of the many complicated factors in Gail's background. Until after the killing, no one took the careful history that revealed that Gail had been the product of a long labor and traumatic delivery, that her mother had had syphilis during her pregnancy, that Gail's behavior since kindergarten had oscillated between withdrawal and fighting, that Gail often flew into a rage for no apparent reason. Following such outbursts, Gail would feel tired and have to sleep—a history that might have suggested a psychomotor symptomatology. Subsequent to the stabbing, neurologists concluded that Gail probably suffered from a psychomotor disturbance, and that the killing may have been associated with a seizure. No one, of course, can say today how Gail's behavior might have been different had she had proper medical attention.

Mrs. Cross and Jeffrey: Services That Work

The second story, a happier one, illustrates many of the elements of programs that intervene successfully with disadvantaged children. It comes from a pediatric group affiliated with Sinai Hospital in Baltimore, where the staff prides itself on meeting needs beyond the biological, that extend beyond the individual child, that involve collaboration across professional lines, and that require time-intensive, flexible, and non-episodic responses.

I met Mrs. Cross, a fiftyish grandmother, and her grandson, 2½-year-old Jeffrey, when the pediatric group suggested I learn about their work by meeting with some of the families they serve. The pediatric group enrolls every baby born at Sinai Hospital whose family has no other source of care, and takes responsibility for providing comprehensive services for that baby. Jeffrey's mother had been diagnosed as schizophrenic some time before he was born.

"From the minute that baby was born, from the first second, they showed concern for him," was how Mrs. Cross began her conversation with me. "Everyone, starting with Dr. Straus [the group's medical director, who became Jeffrey's pediatrician at birth], knew what the situation was from the beginning. My daughter couldn't have had a doctor who paid her any more attention or cared more about that baby." With Mrs. Bruce, the outreach worker, and Mrs. Polen, the social worker, "it's really been like a chain of concerned people," said Mrs. Cross. "Whenever I saw a problem, I got on the telephone and called Mrs. Bruce and she came right out. I felt confident, knowing she would do that. And I'm sure she relayed what was going on to the doctor, because everybody at all times knew what was going on. We didn't have to always start over again, and repeat everything, like at other hospitals."

Mrs. Cross described her daughter Lena's recurrent hospitalizations and her deteriorating ability to care for Jeffrey. She consulted with Dr. Straus about

Lena's refusal to let Jeffrey take the antibiotics ordered for him, to let water touch him, or to feed him anything other than pizza and grits, and about whether it was safe to leave Jeffrey alone with his father when he came to visit. "It strengthened me," said Mrs. Cross, "to know that I could get professional advice from someone I could trust and who was aware of the situation. After a while, I came to see that much as I'd like to think Lena could care for her own baby, it was wishful thinking."

Mrs. Bruce came and talked to Lena about feeding Jeffrey properly and about his health and cleanliness, to no avail. The Department of Social Services sent somebody who told Mrs. Cross that "if Lena remained at home they would have to take the baby and put him in a foster home."

Step by step, Mrs. Cross reviewed how the clinic's outreach worker and social worker helped her get her daughter back into hospital care and get temporary guardianship of her grandson—a painful process that she could never have managed, she said, without the help of the pediatric group. "All these people know that this is a child that really needed special attention. Dr. Straus, you know, he really *knows* Jeffrey! And Mrs. Bruce, she really became like a member of the family. She was like Jeffrey's . . . I would say she was like Jeffrey's appointed mother from the hospital. She always came. One day we opened the door and the snow was knee high and icy, but there she was. She never, never failed to keep an appointment."

Who is to say which of the services the pediatric group provided to Mrs. Cross are medical services, which should be considered mental health services, which are social services, and which are really family support services? We do know that less than six months after this conversation, the heroic Mrs. Bruce had to be let go because there was no money to support outreach activities. We do know that what Mrs. Cross describes as "a chain of concerned people" goes far beyond some mechanistic coordination of services. And it would probably be safe to guess that the residents being trained in that pediatric group have a radically different definition of the content of high-quality health care from that of most physicians, in or out of training.

The Elements of Successful Programs

The Sinai Hospital pediatric group has many elements in common with other successful programs. In my study, I identified these elements through a detailed examination of 18 such programs in the domains of family planning, prenatal care, child health, family support, preschool, and elementary education. These programs had succeeded in lowering the incidence of what I labeled "rotten outcomes"—teenage childbearing, dropping out of school, and delinquency— or in preventing antecedent risk factors.[2] I called these "rotten outcomes" because of their lifelong consequences and the enormous toll they take on the youngsters, their families, and society as a whole. Although none of the three outcomes is strictly a *health* outcome, poor health and poor health care are implicated, both as precursors and as consequences.

I then analyzed the information I had collected from the successful programs to see what common patterns could be discerned. Four basic elements emerged as essential attributes of success.

Most successful programs, like the Sinai Hospital pediatric group, are *comprehensive and intensive*. They provide or offer a way into a wide array of services, delivered flexibly and coherently. Families that are already overwhelmed are not asked to negotiate a maze of fragmented services, each with its own eligibility determinations, waiting times, and application forms. Successful programs respond to the needs of families at times and places that make sense to the family, often at their homes or at neighborhood clinics and centers, rather than offering help only in places that are far removed—geographically and psychologically—from those who use them.

A second attribute that marks successful programs is *active collaboration across professional and bureaucratic boundaries*. These programs are able—usually through heroic efforts—to overcome the fragmentation that results from separate funding streams, separate and often conflicting regulations, and separate disciplinary approaches. Successful programs, whether they are built around health clinics, social agencies, settlement houses, or schools are somehow consistently able to remove some of the most burdensome barriers to the receipt of coherent services. In these programs, no one says, "This may be what you need, but helping you get it is not part of my job," or "This is outside this agency's jurisdiction."

A third attribute of successful programs is that they *deal with the child as part of a family and with the family as part of a neighborhood and community*. These programs take into account the real world of those they serve and recognize the centrality of strong family support in the life of a young child. The successful school enlists parents in collaborative efforts to give children reasons to learn. The clinician treating an infant for recurrent diarrhea sees beyond the patient on the examining table to whether the family needs help from a public health nurse or social worker to obtain non-medical services. A rural health clinic in Mississippi actually delivers clean water to families that can't get it any other way.

Finally, in successful programs, *staff have the time, training, and skills necessary to build relationships of trust and respect with children and families*. Professionals in these programs say they work in a setting that allows them to provide services respectfully and ungrudgingly, in an atmosphere of mutual trust. They stress their informal and collaborative posture, and emphasize the importance of one-to-one relationships, listening to parents and adolescents, and exchanging information rather than merely instructing.

Obstacles to Implementation

A number of troublesome paradoxes inhere in these critical attributes of success and represent obstacles to the widespread implementation of similar programs. Understanding these paradoxes helps to explain why successful models so often remain isolated and unreplicated, and why many efforts to build on past successes fail.

The most obvious obstacle is that the key attributes of programs that are successful in improving outcomes for disadvantaged children (comprehensiveness, intensity, flexibility, front-line discretion, informality, emphasis on personal relationships, and dealing with individual children in the context of family and community) are at odds with the dominant ways that most large institutions and systems function. Indeed, many institutions and systems, both public and private, have recently demonstrated an upsurge of interest in providing more effective and coherent services to children at risk and their families. Many are even prepared to modify long-standing traditions and rules governing the division of labor and turf among various professions and various agencies and systems. However, the needed changes strike them as so complicated, profound, and far-reaching that practitioners and administrators as well as policymakers seem to have a hard time moving beyond rhetoric.

Although these groups may in fact recognize that fragmentation of services interferes with the provision of effective services, they find it exceedingly difficult to overcome because it is typically the product of legitimate pressures such as the need for accountability or the demands of political forces—including single-issue advocacy—that are themselves becoming ever more fragmented as well as the exigencies of a reward system that puts a premium on ever-greater specialization.

In the crisis atmosphere created by scarce resources, years of budget cutbacks, the increase in the social disruption of families, the increased incidence of AIDS, drug addiction, child abuse, and childhood poverty, moreover, it is almost impossible to persuade beleaguered administrators and politicians to address issues of long-term change—change that promises few, if any, immediate pay-offs. Operating agencies fear that efforts at cooperation could diminish their already inadequate resources.

Politicians—and advocates—may also recognize the need for broad, systemic changes, but know that their success depends on being identified with crisply defined, easy to understand, incremental steps designed to reach clearly circumscribed, manageable goals.

The distinctive forms of programming that improvements in services to the truly disadvantaged often require constitute another obstacle to their implementation. There is a tremendous discontinuity not only between the needs of the most disadvantaged and those of the rest of society, but also between the services and programs that would meet those needs and what actually exists. For example, the staples of middle-class prenatal care—routine laboratory tests and regular monitoring of blood pressure and fetal growth—are not enough when the patient is a teenager who is poor, frightened, depressed, suffering from a venereal disease, and perhaps addicted or without a permanent home. We try to gloss over these differences in order to provide equity in benefits and services and to maintain broad political support for our efforts to serve these populations, but our failure to face up to the distinctive needs of those at greatest risk may have become counterproductive.

Possibilities for Change

Obviously, when we focus specifically on health needs and health services, the obstacles to devising large-scale programmatic responses to the broad spectrum of needs of poor children and their families are no less formidable. Many of the problems are similar; others are even harder to solve in the health policy context.

The predominant view of medicine, in which a problem is seen as medical and therefore within the physician's proper purview only if it can be approached by the theory and techniques of biomedical science, may help to explain why children and families at risk often derive little benefit from their encounters with the health system, even when they have them.

In the hierarchy of values or priorities in health, social services, and education, disadvantaged populations rank low; preventive services rank low; and, in medicine, the non-technological services essential to many successful preventive interventions rank low. When it comes to professional status and economic compensation, direct provision of basic services to the least powerful carries little prestige. There are no prizes for being willing and able to respond "transmedically" to what David Rogers describes as the "great untidy basketful of intertwined and interconnected circumstances and happenings" that often all need attention if a health problem is to be overcome.

Moreover, the reforms in health policy and health financing that are currently under consideration are unlikely to solve the health problems of truly disadvantaged children. Proposals to eliminate financial barriers to health care by creating a universal entitlement to insurance would alleviate some portion of the problems that disadvantaged families encounter in obtaining health care. But, as Eli Ginzberg has pointed out, "Quantity and quality would continue to depend on the availability of physicians, support personnel, bed capacity, equipment, and other critical inputs."[3]

To the extent that rationing or spending ceilings are imposed (through a national health financing system or through state programs), the health services that will flourish will probably continue to be biomedical responses to biologically defined problems, because they are at the core of what the medical profession values most.

Medicaid reforms that expand eligibility and improve reimbursement are even less likely to benefit the truly disadvantaged in the future. Fossett and colleagues concluded on the basis of their Chicago study that, even with such reforms, because of the increasing concentration of the poor and specifically low-income minority women in areas of concentrated poverty, the choice of providers for this population (in the absence of other kinds of intervention) will be increasingly limited to a small number of high-volume Medicaid practices, "where there is cause for concern about the quality of care."[4]

If health system reforms now on the horizon are unlikely to bring solutions, are there other avenues that could lead to substantial improvements in the health care of disadvantaged children? Leaders in the health field might do better to make common cause with forces *outside* the health system that are working to improve a wide range of services and institutions on which poor children and their families depend. A profusion of scattered efforts are now getting under way in school systems, human service agencies, child care, and family support programs and within state and local governments that are aimed at reducing the mismatch between successful services of all kinds and the traditional workings of large institutions. These may offer a more forceful wave of change to ride than the wave of health system reform.

It is clear from the findings already discussed that if the health care, schooling, and social services and supports that could change the prospects of these youngsters are to reach those who need them most, they must be coordinated and coherent, and provided with enough flexibility and skill to be responsive to the needs of individual families and the circumstances of individual communities. This cannot be done in large numbers of communities to serve large numbers of families without changes in the way money flows to local programs.

A Modest Proposal

An idea that may merit further exploration is the creation of a sort of flexible superfund, to support flexible intensive services for children growing up in areas of highest need. An initiating agency (which could be a state, the federal government, or even a large city) would attempt to persuade other agencies and jurisdictions to join it in ear-marking a certain proportion of expenditures (including funds that currently support health services, social services, schools, preschools, and the like), to support comprehensive, neighborhood-based services.

Together with similarly targeted funds from foundations, businesses, and non-profit agencies and institutions (which may not be large in comparative dollar magnitude, but would provide additional flexibility and public support), these funds would flow, unencumbered by the usual restrictions, into neighborhoods characterized by high rates of poverty and social need. To guard against the misuse of these funds, it would be essential to provide intensive and highly competent technical assistance and training to all eligible participant agencies and to maintain accountability through the rigorous use of outcome measures. Assessing effectiveness by measuring real-world outcomes rather than processes would help in making continuing mid-course corrections and in assuring funders that the program's purposes are, in fact, being accomplished.

The target population would be defined geographically to minimize the barriers to access created when eligibility is determined by such criteria as income, assets, or family status, and to take into account the powerful neighborhood-level influences—positive and negative—that affect children's well-being. The definition of eligible target areas could be made at a federal, state, or local level, possibly by census tract. Criteria would include high rates of poverty, unemployment, school dropout, teenage childbearing, welfare dependence, and single-parent families. A neighborhood focus would also make it possible to combine efforts to improve a broad range of effective human services with simultaneous efforts to improve housing, job training, public safety, and community and economic development.

A massive infusion of new funds to support a parallel service delivery system for the poor (which is how many of the early Office of Economic Opportunity programs surmounted systems barriers) is unlikely, as is massive and rapid systemic change to accommodate comprehensive, transdisciplinary, flexible, responsive services. This proposal, however, would keep the scale of the effort relatively modest by limiting it to support for services to children and their families living in areas in which the truly disadvantaged are concentrated. Because the initiative would be targeted to only a fraction of the poor, it would not be as threatening to scarce resources and to prevailing administrative and professional arrangements as a proposal involving larger numbers.

Although the proposed initiative would be relatively small in scale, it would hardly be trivial, because it would target the populations at greatest risk, in greatest need of high-quality services, and yet least likely to receive them under present circumstances. Furthermore, it would tackle the broad sweep of barriers to the improvement of services for disadvantaged children. It would also represent a sufficiently bold departure from "business as usual" that it might attract the kind of talented and committed individuals who could make an initiative like this work.

The rewards to local communities of participating in the program would be only partially in the form of new funds. The additional attraction would be in the more favorable conditions under which funds would be made available. High-quality technical assistance and continuing consultation would have to be made available on terms that would assure that virtually every neighborhood that qualified under the definition of need could participate.

A host of important questions would have to be answered before such a proposal could enlist widespread support, including the difficult issue of what kind of local agencies could become recipients of these funds and who would be responsible for the requisite planning and coordination. In addressing such questions, the rich experience drawn from both successes and failures of attempts to improve outcomes among disadvantaged children during the last 25 years should prove invaluable, and could be expected to minimize the chances of repeating the mistakes of the past.

The significance of this proposal is not in its particulars. Rather, it should be seen as one among many attempts to find fresh answers to the agonizing question of how systems and institutions can be helped to meet the increasingly urgent needs of America's disadvantaged children, and thereby the needs of all Americans.

There is now increasing agreement about the high stakes as well as ample knowledge and experience on which successful interventions can be built. It is time to combine income supports, economic policy, and housing and community development with action to assure that the best schooling and health and social services the nation can provide will, at long last, reach the children and families who need them most. Then the children growing up without hope today will stand a real chance of becoming full participants in thriving American communities of tomorrow.

NOTES

1. Schorr, Lisbeth, with Schorr, Daniel, *Within Our Reach: Breaking the Cycle of Disadvantage*, New York: Doubleday, 1988.

2. Findings from longitudinal research on risk factors as well as the experience of practitioners suggest that a focus on the period between the mother's pregnancy and the child's entry into elementary school may be the most auspicious and economical time to intervene. I found a handful of risk factors that seemed susceptible to reduction or prevention through outside intervention. These included being born unwanted or to a teenager mother, low weight at birth, untreated childhood problems, failure to develop trusting relationships with reliable and protective adults early in life, and lack of language and coping skills at school entry.

3. Ginzberg, Eli. "Medical Care for the Poor: No Magic Bullets," *Journal of the American Medical Association*, June 10, 1988:259 (22), pp. 3309–3311.

4. Fossett, J. W., Perloff, J. D., Peterson, J. A., and Kletke, P. R., "Medicaid and the Underclass: The Case of Maternity Care in Chicago," paper presented at a Brookings Institution conference, Washington, DC, July 17, 1989.

MEDIA SCAN:
THE VIEW FROM OLYMPUS

The Medical Triangle: Physicians, Politicians, and the Public,
by Eli Ginzberg, Cambridge, Mass.:
Harvard University Press,
1990.

Hal Strelnick

For more than a dozen years of commuting to my practice in the Bronx, I have passed the Morningside Heights campus of Columbia University and the Washington Heights campus of its health sciences center. Only after reading Columbia Professor Eli Ginzberg's latest book, *The Medical Triangle: Physicians, Politicians, and the Public,* did I recognize the light-years that separate those Olympian heights from the Kingsbridge Heights and Morris Heights neighborhoods where I have served as a family physician and health advocate.

Professor Ginzberg brings an Olympian breadth and perspective to the health care system, covering topics from psychiatry before the year 2000 to rationing cancer care with a personal sense of much of our health system's postwar history. His Olympian perspective yields a distant "middle course" where, as he writes in his preface, he has tried "to focus on analysis, not ideology." What ultimately results, however, is a bound version of the highly ideological Conventional Wisdom.

How does one recognize the Conventional Wisdom (when not found in the *Newsweek* column of the same name)? In Ginzberg's book the Conventional Wisdom is regularly quoted: "The conventional wisdom about high-tech medicine is . . ." (p. 46); "the conventional wisdom views the Academic Health Center . . ." (p. 74); "the assumption prevailing throughout the first three post-World War II decades . . . is no longer conventional wisdom" (p. 121). Whether quoting or challenging its authority, Ginzberg seems to be sparring with the zeitgeist itself. Ginzberg speaks unself-consciously with the voice of authority: "The United States unequivocally rejected a comprehensive system of national health insurance" (p. 36); or, "In years of budgetary surpluses, there is nothing that politicians prefer more than appropriating additional money for good causes, such as biomedical research, which enjoy enthusiastic public support" (p. 43). In the Bronx our leading politicians are in federal prison, having made Wedtech, Reagan's favorite minority-owned business, a synonym for Abscam or Watergate. As far as the Conventional Wisdom is concerned, the gritty, streetwise, bloodied Bronx does not exist.

The Medical Triangle is a collection of essays written in 1985, yet the AIDS epidemic merits its first mention in the last paragraph of the chapter on New York City's health system, and drug abuse is mentioned only once in the entire book, in the description of the partitioning of the National Institute of Mental Health from the National Institutes of Health and the creation of the Alcohol, Drug Abuse, and Mental Health Administration. Equally neglected are the office-based private practitioners and community hospitals that account for the vast majority of the health services provided in the United States. Instead, Ginzberg concentrates on the interests of academic medical centers—medical education, foundations, privatization, physician supply, and high-tech medicine. To his credit, Ginzberg has chapters on both community health centers and medical care for the poor, both increasingly of interest to academic medical centers. What one chooses to analyze is ultimately ideological.

In his most interesting chapter, "The Politics of Physician Supply," Ginzberg shares his 30-year involvement with this issue by giving an overview that begins at the turn of the century and ends with the Conventional Wisdom's chimerical physician surplus. Here, and in his chapter on "The Reform of Medical Education," where his analysis leads to specific recommendations for change, Ginzberg is most critical of the Conventional Wisdom and the status quo. Both chapters are lively and controversial, yet neither convinced me that the author understood the need to correct the maldistribution of physicians in regard to specialty and geography. The view from Olympus bears a remarkable resemblance to the view from the Ivory Tower.

"The Medical Triangle" of the book's title alludes to the "Iron Triangle" —the recognition that the military-industrial complex thrived through its relationship with Congress. Ginzberg's triad—physicians, politicians, and the public—ignores the health care industry and its institutions (while his essay "American Medicine: The Power Shift" includes *ten* power centers). A more apt title might be *Medical Realpolitik: The Way Things Are Is the Way They Were Meant to Be*. Still, I am grateful to have learned where the Conventional Wisdom comes from and how it thrives without an agent or a publicist. It will probably come to the Bronx as graffiti or rap lyrics.

HARM REDUCTION: A NEW APPROACH TO DRUG SERVICES

Rod Sorge

Reaching the second floor of the Palacio de Congressos, the delegates to the Second International Conference on the Reduction of Drug Related Harm were greeted by the familiar registration desk and literature tables. On one of the tables stood a tall black metal box that I assumed was a weird-looking coffee urn. I pointed it out to one of my U.S. colleagues, joking about the hand-printed sign that someone had taped to the front of the box: "METHADONE DIS-PENSER." "That *is* a methadone dispenser," she said. This humane accommodation for those who were maintained on methadone exemplified the tone of the conference and indicated that representation by drug users was welcome, encouraged, expected, and that drug users were viewed as experts.

Sponsored by the Commission of the European Communities, the Plan Nacional sobre Drogas (Spain's National Plan on Drugs), the Generalitat of Catalonia, the city of Barcelona, and the *International Journal on Drug Policy*, the conference took place March 2 to 6, 1991, in Barcelona, Spain. Of about 260 attendees, nearly 100 were from the United Kingdom alone and almost 50 more were from the Netherlands—two leading countries involved in innovative drugs work and policy. Spain had the third largest representation, followed by Australia. Most of the rest of the delegates were from Western European countries, especially Germany and Italy. Only a handful of people came from Africa, Asia, South America, Eastern European countries, Canada, or Mexico. I was one of only 12 delegates from the United States.

People came from all over the world to learn about and discuss strategies for helping people who engage in an almost universally restricted or outlawed activity—using drugs—do so more safely. Some of the governments that make laws against drug use and possession even sponsored delegates at this conference to help them learn how to minimize drug-related harm that is often caused by these very laws.

Although many of the attendees believed that the decriminalization of drugs should form the basis of a coherent harm reduction program, it was not by any means the focus of the conference. A careful, realistic balance was struck between what we might like to have as drug policy in the best of all worlds and a pragmatism borne out of the necessity of working in our present situations. In this article I will not so much report on the conference, but will rather highlight some developments discussed there that are beginning to define a new era of drug services based on a harm reduction approach.

Principles of Harm Reduction

Most attendees came to the conference as believers in the notion of harm reduction, and the meeting came to be known colloquially as the harm reduction conference. The term "harm reduction" is commonplace in the vocabularies of drug outreach workers, social service workers, and policymakers in the United Kingdom and Australia, and increasingly in other Western nations including the United States. It describes the recent expansion of an exclusively abstinence-oriented service model to include the objective of helping users at any point on the continuum of drug-taking behaviors to manage their addiction and their health without necessarily requiring or expecting abstinence—what one advocate calls a "pragmatic acceptance of drug use."[1] Of course, for many, managing addiction might mean a movement toward abstinence, and drug treatment is certainly part of harm reduction. But abstinence in this view is one end of a continuum of behaviors—an end goal appropriate for some people in what is often a long and difficult process.

The emergence of HIV and the discovery that it is a blood-borne pathogen that can be transmitted by sharing injection equipment has been a major impetus for the acceptance and growth of the harm reduction paradigm over the past few years. Although harm reduction strategies have undoubtedly been practiced by individual social workers and drug treatment counselors for years, harm reduction is now becoming institutionalized by social service organizations in the area of drug work, and has even been adopted as government policy in some locales. One drug researcher posits that the advent of harm reduction thinking in the late 1980s will be "identified as a key period of crisis and transformation in the history of drugs policy."[2]

The concept of harm reduction is quite broad and demands different manifestations according to location, client demographics, the type of drug in question, the local legal and political milieus, and a host of other factors. Nevertheless, some general principles characterize harm reduction that unified most of the conference-goers and served as the basis for more complex and specific ideas and presentations.

One of the defining principles of harm reduction is that successful, relevant, and life-enhancing services can and must be designed for *active* drug users as well as for those individuals who are seeking to end their addiction (many of whom, of course, are also active users). Again, abstinence is not seen as the only clinically desirable endpoint or the only morally acceptable measure of success in providing care and services for drug users. The notion that drug-related problems are largely public health issues greatly influenced by the social environment has been officially adopted in Australian and British drug policy and has been put forth somewhat more tentatively by the World Health Organization.

In such an understanding, drug treatment's role in public health theory and practice is also reevaluated. The desired endpoint of treatment for many people might be total abstinence from drugs, but intermediate steps taken toward that endpoint are seen as valuable, and they could mean the difference between life and death. Relapse is not viewed as an utter failure by the client or the provider but recognized as a common feature of the process of working toward abstinence. In the United States, "getting off" drugs (what is called drug "treatment") and using drugs more safely (an intervention such as needle exchange) are conceptualized as separate and even contradictory strategies. Proponents of harm reduction see these as consistent strategies with the common goal of helping drug users reach and maintain physical and emotional health, regardless of where they are on the abuse-to-abstinence continuum. They recognize that between these two end-points there are a whole range of behaviors that can be ranked in terms of safety. Similarly, drug services must operate on a continuum in order to address the needs of all drug users. Most services that now exist are designed for those who seek treatment. Drug users who are unable to get into treatment, and those who are not interested in treatment are left without services.

Harm reduction focuses largely on the social and environmental aspects of drug taking, looking at the way that drug use is "produced," learned, experienced, organized, and controlled and then implementing interventions based on this information. The contexts and social networks of drug use are viewed as important vehicles for health information and interventions. Whereas before services were aimed at taking drug-using individuals out of their drug-using contexts, these contexts are now being seen as the very means by which services can be brought to people. Because most drug users do not have the luxury of leaving their drug-using circumstances behind after or even during treatment, interventions are focusing more and more on helping them make use of their contexts and communities to survive.

Viewing drug-related problems as a public health issue allows the drug user to be seen as a "rational actor who will respond to public health information."[3] While such a perspective puts responsibility on the individual drug taker, it recognizes that a drug user has an ability to make choices if presented with them, as well as the ability to stop or modify risky behaviors—in other words, that a drug user has agency. More and more data, much of it from studies about needle-related behaviors, corroborate this proposition. Finally, this perspective assumes that drug users have an ability and a right to represent themselves.

Harm reduction theory holds that if such change can occur on an individual level, it can also occur on the level of a street scene, of a social network, and even of the larger culture. To this end, research has concentrated on how, when, where, and with whom people use drugs. Ethnography has become indispensable to drug research, and the employment of former users in drug work and services has become routine, though not unchallenged.[4]

Normalization

"Normalization" is the name that has been given in Europe, particularly the Netherlands, to one component of harm reduction strategies: integrating drug users into mainstream culture to the extent that they can obtain services, medical care, and proper housing, to enable them to live in such a way as to greatly reduce the risks associated with drug use. At the conference, K. Schuller from Deutsch-AIDS Hilfe in Berlin presented information about experimental "shooting rooms" in Bremen and several German-speaking Swiss cities. Shooting rooms—literally a place where users go for the purpose of injecting—go one step further than some needle exchange programs by offering a safe, clean place in which to shoot up, as well as trained staff to deal with accidental overdoses and counseling on safer injection techniques and disease prevention.[5]

The practice in England and the Netherlands of general practitioners maintaining their drug-using patients on methadone (or in England, in some cases, on pharmaceutical heroin and other "hard" drugs) is another example of normalization. About 50 percent of Amsterdam's 400 general practitioners prescribe methadone for their patients. Drug maintenance is dealt with just like other health concerns—by doctors in a doctor's office. The atmosphere in the general practitioners' is far from that of the crowded, segregated methadone clinics of New York City, where users are frequently subjected to instant stigmatization by both the staff and the culture at large. Also, unlike programs in the United States, this health policy of normalized treatment fosters a continuity of services.

The syringe disposal system in Victoria and other Australian states also exemplifies normalization at work. Needle disposal chutes in public toilets offer users a safe and anonymous way of disposing of their used equipment, while obviously reducing the risk of accidental needle sticks from discarded needles.

Books like *Handy Hints*, published by the Australia I.V. League, are also part of a strategy of normalization. The I.V. League is the national umbrella organization for the community-based user groups in the various states. The book's opening credo speaks for itself about issues of drug users' self-representation:

Handy Hints was produced by users for users. *Handy Hints* is for all injecting drug users—no matter what you use, no matter how often you use it, and no matter how you use it. It is meant to be a current guide to using and staying alive in the 1990s. We hope it helps.[6]

Handy Hints is a comprehensive, easy-to-read, illustrated resource guide that fits in a pocket. It gives advice about everything from how to deal with the cops if arrested, why not to dissolve alkaline dope in lemon juice (it can cause fungal infections in the eye), to how to properly use a tourniquet, how to avoid vein collapse, how to have safer sex, and what to do if someone overdoses. The second part of the book gives a state-by-state breakdown of where to get injection equipment and drug treatment services, as well as details about laws relating to drug possession, same-sex sexual acts, sex work, HIV status, and the like. The cover of the book has no words. It is black except for a strip along the spine that shows a crowd of people, daring the reader to try and pick out the drug user.

Dr. Mary Hepburn, an obstetrician from the Glasgow Royal Maternity Hospital, illustrates how she fosters normalization and uses harm reduction strategies in her work with pregnant, drug-using women:

Abstinence is not the only acceptable objective and we recognise that the major problem is not drug use per se, but its effects on lifestyle. We therefore adopt no single approach, but tailor management to individual needs and wishes, with particular emphasis on long term support to maintain stability of lifestyle.[7]

Hepburn contends that from her experience in Glasgow, ''drug use and child care are not incompatible,'' and that drug-using women must have the right to make reproductive and drug treatment decisions.[8] The Glasgow Royal Maternity Hospital provides a range of nonjudgmental medical and social services at one site with the goal of helping each woman with her particular problems. This focus on helping the individual successfully negotiate and manage her life starkly contrasts with the movement in the United States to prosecute drug-using mothers. There have been about 35 such cases nationwide, often involving bizarre legal machinations, in which women have faced criminal charges for using drugs or alcohol while pregnant. For example, a woman in Michigan was charged with delivering cocaine to a minor during the time between the delivery of her baby and the clamping of her umbilical cord. A woman in Florida was *convicted* of the same charge.[9] In New York, most women have to choose between going into drug treatment or keeping custody of their children, and pregnant women are shunned by the drug treatment system, particularly if they are Medicaid recipients.[10]

The larger implications of harm reduction can be seen in Hepburn's work. Keeping women and their children together, in addition to being a therapeutic strategy, also has cumulative effects on the child welfare and criminal justice systems. Small interventions that affect people on an individual level, such as teaching someone how to inject safely or providing them with clean needles, create a ripple effect, affecting larger social, administrative, and bureaucratic systems—legal, judicial, health, child welfare, and social services of all kinds.

Harm reduction theory does not minimize the disability, morbidity, or mortality to which drug use can lead, but it does not see these conditions, particularly HIV infection, as the necessary outcomes of taking drugs. It cannot address every ramification of drug use, such as the legal problems often faced by drug users, the liver damage that can result from the prolonged use of toxins, or the abscesses or cellulitis that can occur even if one injects with sterile equipment. Not every drug user will make helpful decisions all the time. But a good outreach or education program based on harm reduction can, as the name suggests, *reduce* an array of health-related problems associated with unhygienic or dangerous drug use.

Outreach

With the conceptual shift that harm reduction theory represents comes a shift in the strategy in drug services. This new approach focuses on drug users who have no contact with helping systems—medical care, social services, drug treatment, or other institutionally structured services that are often irrelevant or traumatic to drug users. Outreach programs now occupy a central place in drugs services in Europe (and in HIV/AIDS prevention programs in the United States). They characteristically use an active, ''bottom-up'' method to meet people where they're at rather than a ''top-down'' approach to health education and services. This bottom-to-top approach starts with the basics—interventions that can be performed on the street—and then possibly moving upward, with the client's participation, to more institutionalized forms of care.[11] Of course, without significant changes in these institutional settings, they will remain unattractive and disempowering to users, and be under- or misutilized.

The health care and education delivered in outreach programs are different from that provided by hospitals or clinics. Very often, outreach teams operate as a collective and enjoy relative autonomy from the institutions that support them. They often employ workers indigenous to the targeted population and recognize a worker's life experience as part of his or her professional expertise. Outreach aims to empower individuals to act in some way, often by recognizing an expertise in its clients, sometimes by incorporating an overtly political component, since merely having information does not guarantee it will be used. Outreach schemes focus on the *process* of disseminating information to achieve a particular behavioral *outcome*. There is a distinction between "care" and "cure," but room for both.[12]

Harm Reduction and Law Enforcement

From the perspective of harm reduction, the United States' "war on drugs" approach to drug policy is misguided and outright harmful, especially as a singular strategy. For harm reduction advocates, US policies rely too readily on interdiction and criminalization and ignore the health and social issues involved in drug use.

In an attempt to fit law enforcement practices to a harm reduction theory, some countries have adopted an approach that is intended primarily to decrease the drug supply and *not* to punish drug use. Although this approach has inherent contradictions,[13] the distinction between users and dealers is becoming the new legal and moral dividing line.[14] In Australia and almost all Western European countries, needles and syringes can be bought over the counter, and there are no laws against needle possession. In Spain, drug taking goes completely unpenalized, and elsewhere in Europe, drug possession laws sometimes entitle people to carry quantities of drugs "for personal use" without fear of criminal prosecution. In Italy, drug *use* is still defined as "illicit," but entails no specific penalties, while drug *possession* is always punishable—either by administrative sanctions, such as the suspension of a driver's license if the amount is the allowed "average daily dose" (ADD) or less, or criminal sanctions if it is over the ADD. The ADD is a recent term that replaced a confusing and indeterminate category called "moderate amount," but the new ADDs have also come under fire for being too open to multiple interpretation and for favoring some drugs over others.[15]

Italy's new drug laws reflect the tension in many nations between trying to implement harm reduction policies aimed at improving the health and lives of users and reducing harm to society at large on the one hand or maintaining the more politically expedient drug war mentality founded on interdiction and prohibitionism on the other. Some countries, like Great Britain, have managed to strike a balance: England spends a lot of resources on stopping drug trafficking, but it also boasts over 150 needle exchange sites that were implemented and are now maintained with the cooperation of the police, the health service, and community-based agencies. The strong support for the conference from all levels of the Spanish government illustrates an increased willingness of governments to try to work within this contradiction. The participation of the Commission of the European Communities bodes well for possible coordination on drug policy among European nations in the future.

Harm Reduction in the US?

Harm reduction theory as it has been put into practice in Europe cannot be facilely transposed to the United States, especially given the vast differences between their health care systems, availability and quality of housing, and social welfare programs. The relative homogeneity of Western European culture and population in contrast to most parts of the United States is especially important to consider in attempting to implement harm reduction in this country, because any program that does not take into account the ethnic, racial, and cultural diversity of the United States will never succeed, particularly if a community-based approach is sought.

Concepts that have one manifestation in Europe will look different in the United States. The *junkiebond* or user's self-help organization, such as Germany's JES (Junkies, Ex-Junkies, and Substitute Drug Users), is a model that has been valuable in Europe. The *junkiebonden* emphasize drugs users' social networks as a means of disseminating information about HIV prevention and changing drug-using etiquette among users on a larger level. This emphasis has already become part of some U.S. needle exchange and bleach outreach programs, and other forms of organizing are being done on the street through illegal needle exchange programs, which are giving users an increased measure of control over their health and a new sense of entitlement. But drug users organizing drug users as a political force is not currently a conscious part of the organizing activity in this country.

JES has had success in working for the rights of users to self-representation, drug treatment, and AIDS services. Like the AIDS activist movement in the United States, the *junkiebonden* consist of people fighting for their survival. While a *junkiebond* per se will probably not appear in the United States anytime soon, some AIDS activist and service organizations, such as ACT UP (AIDS Coalition to Unleash Power) and ADAPT (Association for Drug Abuse Prevention and Treatment) in New York and Prevention Point in San Francisco, are becoming places where people can "come out" as current or former drug users and begin to advocate for their own services with the support of a larger group. In Europe and Australia, HIV intervention strategies aimed at drug users grew mostly out of *drug* treatment and service organizations—drug workers and CDTs, or community drugs teams, do AIDS prevention in England, for instance. In the United States, by contrast, such models have been produced mainly by AIDS organizations.[16]

It is clear that when the harm reduction approach begins to develop more fully in the United States, it will have to be different from the models established elsewhere. We can learn from those models, though, the importance of comprehensiveness and user friendliness, as well as the willingness to acknowledge that people do use drugs and that drug use is a complex social phenomenon involving a variety of behaviors, motivations, and contexts.

Harm reduction is an honest approach to drug use. One of the keys to harm reduction, however, is maintaining the honesty of one's approach. Methadone programs are essentially harm reduction programs—they were designed to reduce an individual's use of illicit drugs and trouble with the law while increasing his or her ability to be employed and otherwise function in society. Methadone maintenance is no longer thought of as a harm reduction model, however, but instead as a treatment approach that should work for all heroin addicts. Because its original purpose has become distorted, it is no longer seen as successful and is coming under fire. Methadone programs have not taken into consideration phenomena such as the cocaine epidemic of the 1980s, which had significant effects on opiate users; they have not adapted to changes in what people are using. Detoxification units have been similarly discredited (and largely defunded) because they were not helping people become abstinent. Detoxes helped many people to survive, to practice harm reduction, but because they were not getting people off of drugs, which they were not necessarily designed to do, they were not seen as useful any longer. If future harm reduction programs are to succeed in the United States, they must be seen and credited for what they are.

Conclusion

The Second International Conference on the Reduction of Drug Related Harm had an avowedly Western cultural perspective. Its organizers hope that the third conference, scheduled for 1992, will have a broader focus, including the economy of the "Golden Triangle" region of Southeast Asia from which much of the world's heroin comes. Its location in Melbourne, Australia, should make the conference more accessible to those from non-Western regions.

For me as a drug and AIDS worker in the United States, the Second International Conference on the Reduction of Drug Related Harm was inspiring for the possibilities it showed me, but disheartening, too, because it confirmed what I really already knew: that the United States is in the Dark Ages as far as providing services to drug users goes. Even more disheartening, this lag in drug services is based not on medical evidence or public health policy, but largely on ideological grounds that do not take a realistic account of the sources of and solutions to drug-related harm. Hopefully, it will not be too long before the United States follows the European example, declares a cease fire on the war on drug users, and treats drug use as the public health problem it really is.

NOTES

1. McDermott, Peter, "Drug Use and Drug Work: A Problematic Relationship," in Book of Abstracts, Second International Conference on the Reduction of Drug Related Harm, Barcelona, Spain, March 2–6, 1991.
2. Stimson, Gerry V., "Revising Policy and Practice: New Ideas About the Drugs Problem,"

in Strang, J., and Stimson, G.V., eds., *AIDS and Drug Misuse: The Challenge for Policy and Practice in the 1990s*, London: Routledge, 1990, p. 121.

3. Ibid., p. 127.

4. The practice of employing former drug users in outreach programs, although perhaps routine, is not entirely without problems. Relapses by such employees sometimes occur when they are in familiar drug-using situations. There is also a feeling that some former drug users toe a too harsh abstinence line for harm reduction programs. Yet the value of employing former users is clear for a variety of reasons, such as their ability to negotiate certain street scenes or to pick up on ethnographic subtleties non-users might miss. This question was addressed at the conference by McDermott, op cit.; see also Joyce Rivera-Beckman, et al., " 'Inside'-'Outside': Social Processes in Street Outreach," paper presented at the Second Annual NADR Meeting, Bethesda, MD, November 27–30, 1990.

5. See Schuller, K., "The Implementation of 'Shooting Rooms': A Step to the 'Normalisation' of the Living Conditions of Drug Users?" in Book of Abstracts, Second International Conference on the Reduction of Drug Related Harm, Barcelona, Spain, March 2–6, 1991.

6. *Handy Hints*, New South Wales: The Australian I.V. League, August 1990.

7. Hepburn, Mary, "Drug Use and Pregnancy—The Glasgow Experience," in Book of Abstracts, the Second International Conference on the Reduction of Drug Related Harm, Barcelona, Spain, March 2–6, 1991.

8. Hepburn, Mary, "Obstetrics, Women and Drug Use in the Context of HIV," in Henderson, Sheila, ed., *Women, HIV Drugs: Practical Issues*, London: Institute for the Study of Drug Dependence, 1990.

9. Lewin, Tamar, "Drug Use and Pregnancy: New Issues for the Courts," *New York Times*, February 5, 1990. For a definitive discussion and analysis of these cases, see Roberts, Dorothy E., "Punishing Drug Addicts Who Have Babies: Women of Color, Equality, and the Right of Privacy," *Harvard Law Review*, May 1991: 104(7).

10. Chavkin, Wendy, "Drug Addiction and Pregnancy: Policy Crossroads," *American Journal of Public Health*, April 1990: 80(4), pp. 483–487.

11. For a useful topology of outreach programs and evaluation methods, see Rhodes, T., Holland, J., Hartnoll, R., and Johnson, A., *HIV Outreach Health Education: National and International Perspectives*, London: Drug Indicators Project, Birbeck College, 1991.

12. Buning, Ernst, "The Role of Harm-Reduction Programmes in Curbing the Spread of HIV by Drug Injectors," in Strang and Stimson, eds., op. cit., p. 158.

13. For a good summary of the Dutch situation in this regard, see Engelsman, Eddy L., "Drug Misuse and the Dutch," *BMJ*, March 2, 1991:302.

14. This is certainly not a pure distinction, however, at least in an American context where many users are often dealers in order to support their habits. See Courtwright, D., Joseph, H., and Des Jarlais, D., *Addicts Who Survived: A History of Narcotics Use in America, 1923–1965*, Knoxville: University of Tennessee Press, 1989.

15. Arnao, Giancarlo, "New Italian Drug Laws," *International Journal on Drug Policy*, November/December 1990:2(3).

16. Sorge, Rod, "ACT UP Before You Shoot Up: Underground Needle Exchange in New York City," in Book of Abstracts, Second International Conference on the Reduction of Drug Related Harm, Barcelona, Spain, March 2–6, 1991.

BREATHING LIFE INTO OURSELVES: THE EVOLUTION OF THE NATIONAL BLACK WOMEN'S HEALTH PROJECT

Byllye Y. Avery

In July 1989, Byllye Y. Avery, founder of the National Black Women's Health Project, was named one of 29 people to receive a five-year grant from the MacArthur Foundation. Bestowed by an anonymous committee, the award can be used by recipients however they choose. It seems only fitting that Avery, a grassroots organizer who has never sought a personal spotlight, would receive such a prestigious award. Since 1981, she has worked tirelessly to help black women who are "sick and tired of being sick and tired" improve their mental and physical well-being through empowerment, healing, and self-love.

Through its community-based self-help programs, the NBWHP has created a safe place for black women to talk about the multitude of hurts that have kept us from living full and healthy lives. NBWHP conferences, weekend retreats, educational films and publications are widely acclaimed for dealing with black women's health concerns within the context of black culture. Under Avery's determined leadership, the National Black Women's Health Project has created a vital wellspring of black feminist activism that will have a significant social impact in the 1990s and beyond.

The following piece is an edited version of a talk Avery gave in Cambridge, Massachusetts, in July 1988.

I got involved in women's health in the 1970s around the issue of abortion. There were three of us at the University of Florida, in Gainesville, who just seemed to get picked out by women who needed abortions. They came to us. I didn't know anything about abortions. In my life that word couldn't even be mentioned without having somebody look at you crazy. Then someone's talking to me about abortion. It seemed unreal. But as more women came (and at first they were mostly white women), we found out this New York number we could give them, and they could catch a plane and go there for their abortions. But then a black woman came and we gave her the number, and she looked at us in awe: "I can't get to New York. . . ." We realized we needed a different plan of action, so in May 1974 we opened up the Gainesville Women's Health Center.

As we learned more about abortions and gynecological care, we immediately started to look at birth, and to realize that we are women with a total reproductive cycle. We might have to make different decisions about our lives, but whatever the decision, we deserved the best services available. So, in 1978, we opened up Birthplace, an alternative birthing center. It was exhilarating work; I assisted in probably around two hundred births. I understood life, and working in birth, I understood death, too. I certainly learned what's missing in prenatal care and why so many of our babies die.

Through my work at Birthplace, I learned the importance of being involved in our own health. We have to create environments that say "yes." Birthplace was a wonderful space. It was a big, old turn-of-the-century house that we decorated with antiques. We went to people's houses and, if we liked something, we begged for it—things off their walls, furniture, rugs. We fixed the place so that when women walked in, they would say, "Byllye, I was excited when I got up today because this was my day to come to Birthplace." That's how prenatal care needs to be given—so that people are excited when they come. It's about eight and a half or nine months that a woman comes on a continuous basis. That is the time to start affecting her life so that she can start making meaningful lifestyle changes. So you see, health provides us with all sorts of opportunities for empowerment.

Through Birthplace, I came to understand the importance of our attitudes about birthing. Many women don't get the exquisite care they deserve. They go to these large facilities, and they don't understand the importance of prenatal care. They ask, "Why is it so important for me to get in here and go through all this hassle?" We have to work around that.

Through the work of Birthplace, we have created a prenatal caring program that provides each woman who comes for care with a support group. She enters the group when she arrives, leaves the group to go for her physical checkup, and then returns to the group when she is finished. She doesn't sit in a waiting room for two hours. Most of these women have nobody to talk to. No one listens to them; no one helps them plan. They're asking: "Who's going to get me to the hospital if I go into labor in the middle of the night, or the middle of the day, for that matter? Who's going to help me get out of this abusive relationship? Who's going to make sure I have the food I need to eat?" Infant mortality is not a medical problem; it's a social problem.

One of the things that black women have started talking about regarding infant mortality is that many of us are like empty wells; we give a lot, but we don't get much back. We're asked to be strong. I have said, "If one more person says to me that black women are strong I'm going to scream in their face." I am so tired of that stuff. What are you going to do—just lay down and die? We have to do what's necessary to survive. It's just a part of living. But most of us are empty wells that never really get replenished. Most of us are dead inside. We are walking around dead. That's why we end up in relationships that reinforce that particular thought. So you're talking about a baby being alive inside of a dead person; it just won't work.

We need to stop letting doctors get away with piling up all this money, buying all these little machines. They can keep the tiniest little piece of protoplasm alive, and then it goes home and dies. All this foolishness with putting all this money back into their pockets on that end of the care and not on the other end has to stop. When are we going to wake up?

The National Black Women's Health Project

I left the birthing center around 1980 or 1981, mostly because we needed more midwives and I wasn't willing to go to nursing school. But an important thing had happened for me in 1979. I began looking at myself as a black woman. Before that I had been looking at myself as a woman. When I left the birthing center, I went to work in a Comprehensive Employment Training Program (CETA) job at a community college and it brought me face-to-face with my sisters and face-to-face with myself. Just by the nature of the program and the population that I worked with, I had, for the first time in my life, a chance to ask a 19-year-old why—please give me the reason why—you have four babies and you're only 19 years old. And I was able to listen, and bring these sisters together to talk about their lives. It was there that I started to understand the lives of black women and to realize that we live in a conspiracy of silence. It was hearing these women's stories that led me to start conceptualizing the National Black Women's Health Project.

First I wanted to do an hour-long presentation on black women's health issues, so I started doing research. I got all the books, and I was shocked at what I saw. I was angry—angry that the people who wrote these books didn't put it into a format that made sense to us, angry that nobody was saying anything to black women or to black men. I was so angry I threw one book across the room and it stayed there for three or four days, because I knew I had just seen the tip of the iceberg, but I also knew enough to know that I couldn't go back. I had opened my eyes, and I had to go on and look.

Instead of an hour-long presentation we had a conference. It didn't happen until 1983, but when it did, 2,000 women came. But I knew we couldn't just have a conference. From the health statistics I saw, I knew that there was a deeper problem. People needed to be able to work individually, and on a daily basis. So we got the idea of self-help groups. The first group we formed was in a rural area outside of Gainesville, with twenty-one women who were severely obese. I thought, "Oh this is a piece of cake. Obviously these sisters don't have any information. I'll go in there and talk to them about losing weight, talk to them about high blood pressure, talk to them about diabetes—it'll be easy."

Little did I know that when I got there, they would be able to tell me everything that went into a 1,200-calorie-a-day diet. They all had been to Weight Watchers at least five or six times; they all had blood-pressure-reading machines in their homes as well as medications they were on. And when we sat down to talk, they said, "We know all that information, but what we also know is that living in the world that we are in, we feel like we are absolutely nothing." One woman said to me, "I work for General Electric making batteries, and, from the stuff they suit me up in, I know it's killing me." She said, "My home life is not working. My old man is an alcoholic. My kids got babies. Things are not well with me. And the one thing I know I can do when I come home is cook me a pot of food and sit down in front of the TV and eat it. And you can't take that away from me until you're ready to give me something in its place."

So that made me start to think that there was some other piece to this health puzzle that had been missing, that it's not just about giving information; people need something else. We just spent a lot of time talking. And while we were talking, we were planning the 1983 conference, so I took the information back to the planning committee. Lillie Allen (a trainer who works with NBWHP) was there. We worked with her to understand that we are dying inside. That unless we are able to go inside of ourselves and touch and breathe fire, breathe life into ourselves, that, of course, we couldn't be healthy. Lillie started working on a workshop that we named "Black and Female: What Is the Reality?" This is a workshop that terrifies us all. And we are also terrified not to have it, because the conspiracy of silence is killing us.

Stopping Violence

As we started to talk, I looked at those health statistics in a new way. Now, I'm not saying that we are not suffering from the things we die from—that's what the statistics give us. But what causes all this sickness? Like cardiovascular disease—it's the number one killer. What causes all that heart pain? When sisters take their shoes off and start talking about what's happening, the first thing we cry about is violence. The violence in our lives. And if you look in statistics books, they mention violence in one paragraph. They don't even give numbers, because they can't count it: the violence is too pervasive.

The number one issue for most of our sisters is violence—battering, sexual abuse. Same thing for their daughters, whether they are 12 or 4. We have to look at how violence is used, how violence and sexism go hand in hand, and how it affects the sexual response of females. We have to stop it, because violence is the training ground for us.

When you talk to young people about being pregnant, you find out a lot of things. Number one is that most of these girls did not get pregnant by teenage boys; most of them got pregnant by their mother's boyfriends or their brothers or their daddies. We've been sitting on that. We can't just tell our daughters, "Just say no." What do they do about all those feelings running around their bodies? And we need to talk to our brothers. We need to tell them, the incest makes us crazy. It's something that stays on our minds all the time. We need the men to know that. And they need to know that when they hurt us, they hurt themselves. Because we are their mothers, their sisters, their wives; we are their allies on this planet. They can't just damage one part of it without damaging themselves. We need men to stop giving consent, by their silence, to rape, to sexual abuse, to violence. You need to talk to your boyfriends, your husbands, your sons, whatever males you have around you—talk to them about talking to other men. When they are sitting around womanizing, talking bad about women, make sure you have somebody stand up and be your ally and help stop this. For future generations, this has got to stop somewhere.

Mothers and Daughters

If violence is the number one thing women talk about, the next is being mothers too early and too long. We've developed a documentary called "On

Becoming a Woman: Mothers and Daughters Talking Together.'' It's 8 mothers and 8 daughters—16 ordinary people talking about extraordinary things.

The idea of the film came out of my own experience with my daughter. When Sonja turned 11, I started bemoaning that there were no rituals left; there was nothing to let a girl know that once you get your period your life can totally change, nothing to celebrate that something wonderful is happening. So I got a cake that said, ''Happy Birthday! Happy Menstruation!'' It had white icing with red writing. I talked about the importance of becoming a woman, and, out of that, I developed a workshop for mothers and daughters for the public schools. I did the workshops in Gainesville, and, when we came to Atlanta, I started doing them there. The film took ten years, from the first glimmer of an idea to completion.

The film is in three parts. In the first part all the mothers talk about when we got our periods. Then the daughters who have their periods talk about getting theirs, and the ones who are still waiting talk about that. The second part of the film deals with contraception, birth control, anatomy, and physiology. This part of the film is animated, so it keeps the kids' attention. It's funny. It shows all the anxiety: passing around condoms, hating it, saying, ''Oh no, we don't want to do this.''

The third part of the film is the hardest. We worked on communication with the mothers and daughters. We feel that the key to birth control and to controlling reproduction is the nature of the relationship between the parents and their young people. And what's happening is that everybody is willing to beat up on the young kids, asking, ''Why did you get pregnant? Why did you do this?'' No one is saying to the parents, ''Do you need some help with learning how to talk to your young person? Do you want someone to sit with you? Do you want to see what it feels like?'' We don't have all the answers. In this film, you see us struggling.

What we created, which was hard for the parents, is a safe space where everybody can say anything they need to say. And if you think about that, as parents, we have that relationship with our kids: we can ask them anything. But when we talk about sex, it's special to be in a space where the kids can ask *us*, ''Mama, what do you do when you start feeling funny all in your body?'' What the kids want to know is, what about lust? What do we do about it? And that's the very information that we don't want to give up. That's ''our business.'' But they want to hear it from us, because they can trust us. And we have to struggle with how we do that: How do we share that information? How do we deal with our feelings?

Realizing the Dream

The National Black Women's Health Project has 96 self-help groups in 22 states, 6 groups in Kenya, and a group in Barbados and in Belize. In addition, we were just funded by the W. K. Kellogg Foundation to do some work in three housing projects in Atlanta. We received $1,032,000 for a three-year period to set up three community centers. Our plan is to do health screening and referral for adolescents and women, and in addition to hook them up with whatever social services they need—to help cut through the red tape. There will be computerized learning programs and individualized tutorial programs to help young women get their General Equivalency Degrees (GED), along with a panel from the community who will be working on job readiness skills. And we'll be doing our self-help groups—talking about who we are, examining, looking at ourselves.

We hope this will be a model program that can be duplicated anywhere. And we're excited about it. Folks in Atlanta thought it was a big deal for a group of black women to get a million dollars. We thought it was pretty good, too. Our time is coming.

THE TROUBLESOME CRIPPLES OF ORLANDO: DISABILITY AND ACTIVISM

Jean Stewart

You're not supposed to cry when you do civil disobedience. It's gauche, like chewing gum during a violin recital. And it invites bad press. Count on it: The moment one errant tear creeps down your cheek every TV camera within a hundred miles will pick you out of the crowd and zoom in on your face. While your noble comrades, unnoticed by the media, are being shoved into paddy wagons, nary a tear soiling their proud defiant faces, you bawl your eyes out on the six o'clock news.

I tried not to cry in Orlando. I've been doing civil disobedience since 1967, which was the last time I cried. I do my job, the cops do theirs. Crying's not part of the gig.

But Orlando was different, on every level, from anything I've experienced. Orlando bumped up the disability rights movement beyond my farthest-fetched imaginings, or fears.

On October 4, 1991, I was among 250 people with disabilities who converged on Florida from across the United States. Not coincidentally, 3,500 nursing home owners and operators turned out for the same event, the American Health Care Association's (AHCA) annual convention. We—members of ADAPT, American Disabled for Attendant Programs today—had targeted AHCA to demand that 25 percent of the nearly 30 billion Medicaid dollars being poured down the bottomless gullet of this nation's nursing homes be channeled into attendant services, so that anywhere from 7.7 to 12,2 million disabled Americans who need assistance with everyday tasks such as eating or dressing might receive those nonmedical services in their homes, instead of being shunted into nursing homes. We pointed out that nearly 50 percent of these people have annual incomes of under $5,000. We cited statistics comparing the annual cost of maintaining someone in a nursing home—$30,000 is average—with the cost of attendant services: as little as $4,000 a year.

And we identified the reason for so appalling a form of involuntary incarceration: the profit motive. A powerful and corrupt lobby—AHCA represents 10,000 nursing homes nationwide—protects the interests of this vastly lucrative industry.

Many of the Orlando protesters were themselves nursing-home survivors. Some had to sue to get out. Perhaps a half dozen were nursing-home residents who'd managed to get passes for the week. Some feared reprisal if word got out what they'd been up to.

As for me, I've never been a nursing-home inmate. The closest I've come has been a weekly visit with my Uncle Donald in the "home" where he's been left to die and from which I am attempting to spring him. He's 77, has had a few strokes and is diabetic, but his mind is nimble and his use of language dazzling, if labored. Last time I visited he quoted Dante, at length. In Italian. He gets around reasonably well now that I've lent him my old wheelchair. With a little daily help—dressing, cooking, housekeeping—Donald could live peacefully in his own apartment, surrounded by his beloved books.

But Donald is destitute; if Medicaid won't pay for the attendant services that would allow him to live with dignity and independence, no one else will. It's Donald whose defeated face flashes before me just as I'm about to be arrested. It's Donald who starts me weeping.

We're wheeling, hundreds strong under blazing Florida sun, toward the posh Peabody Hotel where thousands of nursing-home owners are schmoozing over cocktails, devising ever more profitable ways to warehouse us. Media people are everywhere—we've alerted them—as are cops. *"Free our people now!"* we roar.

In a flash we arrive at police barricades, and in another flash we barge through to the hotel. Confronted by a long steep ramp, I hitch a ride with a quad from Texas, tattooed, earringed, his fierce features done in war paint, his power chair much stronger than my puny arms. Together we sail into the Peabody, to the astonishment of guests and security.

A few inches from the lobby doors we're apprehended. In those next few seconds first Donald and then the rest appear before me—Katherine, Isabel, Bob, the inmates of Greenwood, spectral visitants slumped in their wheelchairs, waiting. "This one's for you, Donald," I say aloud. As two deputy sheriffs seize my wheelchair sudden memories bombard me: my first visit to the nursing home, the smell of death, the look of abandonment in Donald's blue eyes, in all their eyes.

In the off-duty schoolbus that doubles as a lift-equipped paddy wagon, Sybil's wheelchair is positioned next to mine. Gentle, middle-aged, with silver curls and infinite patience, Sybil spent 21 years locked away in institutions. She remembers that when her muscles spasmed she was tied to her bed, or tied and left lying on the floor, alone. She remembers that bruises often covered her body, and that she received no formal education during all those 21 years, despite her age (15) at the time of admission.

When the cops anchor Sybil's wheelchair and go off to fetch someone else, I tell her the story of how my arresting officer, alone with me in the paddy wagon, removed the metal handcuffs,—he'd cuffed me violently behind my back at the time of my arrest—arranged my hands on my lap, and slapped a plastic cuff around my wrists. Ostentatiously, as if doing a favor, he adjusted the fit. "How's that?" "Fine," I said, whereupon he pulled the cuff tighter, paused as I yelped "You're hurting me!" and gave the cuff one last fierce jerk. The plastic dug into my skin, cutting off my circulation. I raged helplessly, trying to make out a name on his badge; but there was only a number, which I wasn't fast enough to read. He grinned and left.

We're unloaded and herded into a cavernous room. Hours pass, during which more cops, seated at a long table, fill out 73 reports. Turns out this makeshift booking center is the basement of the convention center where, starting tomorrow, AHCA festivities will commence. This is as close as we're likely to get to the proceedings; though ADAPT requested 45 minutes on the conference agenda to present our position, we were turned down.

The first thing I notice about Orange County Jail is the cold. Fifty degrees, someone says, which sounds about right. Having just come in from 95-degree Florida sun, we're wearing T-shirts and sandals; those of us whose disabilities don't easily adjust to temperature extremes instantly turn blue. A full day will pass before guards issue us prison sweatshirts. I'll pull on two—threadbare, stained, graffitied, cigarette-holed, reeking of disinfectant—but by this time the cold will have settled into my bones.

The second thing I notice is the fluorescent light—brilliant, like an interrogation chamber, like an operating room. Our eyes ache, our temples throb, we blink like moles just stumbled out of warm black soil. I start counting down the hours till bedtime, the sweet caress of dark.

No such luck: lights stay on round the clock. So do we. So do our headaches. In jail, night exists for us as a construct; we float in a state of no-time, the absence of time. Without watches (confiscated), without windows, without dark—our body clocks are jammed. Because we wear the same clothes day in day out, no change before bed or when we rise, the confusion's reinforced; we begin to lose the fine social distinction between night and day, with their respective behaviors. Sleep becomes an improbable memory, miraculous as lovemaking and equally remote. "Egg crates," thick foam rubber mats designed to aid circulation and prevent pressure sores, are not merely comforts but critical necessities for many of us. Though we ask for them repeatedly, only one is forthcoming; the mattresses we lie on feel indistinguishable from the metal bedframes. (On the undersurface of an upper bunkbed, scrawled in grayish black —a woman's name. "Fingerprint ink," Eleanor, who discovered it, murmurs, and we both stretch out our hands to touch the letters as if hoping to smudge our own fingers, in solidarity. It is our only contact with the regular inmate population.)

From the moment we arrive, guards from the men's side pass through our unit and leer at us every time we pee. Property confiscation being a serious matter to the Orange County Jail, authorities have taken everything, right down to the barrettes, rubber bands and pins that anchor my hair on my head. They've taken our address books, making it impossible to place a phone call to anyone whose number's not already memorized, since the collect-only telephones won't put through calls to information. (As for our lawyer, we place dozens of calls that are dutifully answered by a recorded message. He is, alas, unfamiliar to us, a name without a face; ADAPT's carefully cultivated nationwide legal support network somehow skipped Orlando.) They've taken our glasses; above all, they've taken our meds.

Medications. By the time we're actually behind bars—the paperwork takes forever—several of the women are overdue on their meds. Many people with severe disabilities follow daily regimens by means of which they control the effects of disability, including meds to manage pain, prevent bowel malfunction, etc. Lisa, for instance—postpolio, whose intelligent smile is what first draws attention—has had two surgeries for acute arthritis of the spinal column; she takes pain meds and muscle relaxers. Diminutive Cyndy's rare neuromuscular disorder visits upon her osteoporosis, which can result in stress fractures (her bones sometimes break while she's sitting motionless in her chair); circulatory problems; muscle contractions; and of course chronic pain. An M.A. in psychology and an articulate disability rights leader from the Boston area, she cannot function without pain killers and sleep meds. As for Sharon of the bonfire-red hair, she developed an abscess on her forearm where it chafed against the joystick of her brand-new power chair; she needs antibiotics to combat infection. And then there's Sybil, who takes five different meds a day to manage her cerebral palsy, including an antispasmodic, a stool softener, and a painkiller for her hip. Sybil, Cyndy, Lisa, and the others whose meds have been confiscated began expressing concern about potential problems as soon as they arrived in jail. "Don't worry," the guards reassured, "the nurse will take care of that."

To no one's surprise, the nurse doesn't. No night meds make the rounds. Sharon's arm is getting worse; Cassie from Philadelphia throws up all night long; Jennifer, a 20-year-old college student from Austin, Texas, tells the nurse she's getting a kidney infection. (Nurse: "Now how do you know that?" Jennifer: "Because I've lived in my body all my life!") By morning Sybil is beginning to spasm; the women who require painkillers are in pain; and the fifteen women who need egg crates to prevent skin breakdown have begun to deteriorate. The hunger strike we declared on arrival seems to be having little impact; while we slide into gaunt translucency, the conditions our strike is intended to address go unchecked.

At our first cellblock meeting we draw up a list of demands. The least consequential of these—that males be announced before they are permitted to pass through our wing—is obligingly honored. "*Man on the floor!*" will echo along the corridor, as if we were college dorm coeds. A more significant item on our list—presented to some suit-and-tie bureaucrat whose title we miss—is the cold. Elaborately he expounds: the temperature is maintained by an advanced technology that cannot be adjusted, nor can it be explained to us in terms we could possibly understand.

We're arrested Sunday. At our first court appearance on Monday, Judge José Rodriguez sets bail at $1,000 cash apiece and orders those of us who cannot pay—virtually all of us; we're a piss-poor lot, and those few with money have no intention of breaking rank—held until Friday, when the AHCA convention ends.

We stare at one another: held until Friday? With no meds, no egg crates, no attendant services? What about the women who are on bowel programs (suppositories and physical assistance provided by an attendant, without which many quads can't eliminate)? Sharon and Cyndy need to be seen by a doctor; several wheelchair batteries are running out of juice. And where is our attorney?

I shout these things at Judge Rodriguez in court. I shout because the judge is not in the room with us, is not in fact in the same building. Evidently he exists, for his black-robed image can be seen on a video screen mounted high on one wall of the small room into which we've been herded. Because of the room's size and because it's filled with desks that are bolted to the floor, there's hardly any space for our wheelchairs; so they shuttle eight or so of us at a time into the room, single file, while the rest form a long queue in the corridor and wait.

"Your Honor, we have a right to counsel! Where is our attorney?" I shout at the video screen.

"He's right here with me," the robe replies.

"Where? We want to see him!"

"He's here, to my right. See?" He mutters something off-mike and the torso of a young man in suit and tie tilts into a corner of the screen and waves at us.

At last I recover my senses. "I don't mean see. I mean we want to talk to him!"

Again the robe mutters off-mike; there's a brief scramble before the young suit-and-tie dances onto the screen and taps the mike, looking expectantly into the camera.

Endless silence. Finally it occurs to me that he's waiting for me to speak. "I don't mean *now*! I mean we want to *confer* with him. Privately!"

The robe mumbles off-mike to the suit and turns toward the camera. "I'm sure he'll be paying you a visit before your arraignment," he says primly.

"Your Honor," I explode, "some of us are in crisis! We need our meds . . . We need egg crates . . . We need attendant care . . ." I'm shouting as fast as I can, but the robe looks peevish, he's making motions to turn off the mike.

"These are matters," he raps, "you can discuss with your correctional officers. I'm sure every effort will be made to ensure your comfort—"

"*Comfort's not the issue!*" I shriek, but the guards are seizing our wheelchairs and shoving us out of the room. The video judge has disappeared. Back we go to our cells, and the next batch of eight is wheeled in.

Panic has begun to set in; the hunger strike is obviously causing our keepers neither worry nor shame. Our jailers won't feel compelled to stop depriving us of basic human rights without a public outcry; the public won't cry out if it doesn't know what's happening. But our efforts to contact the media and the legal community have so far been thwarted.

And what *is* happening to us? Lisa, in tears from extreme pain, has finally managed to get her meds by calling her mother collect, who called Lisa's doctor, whose secretary took a message and gave it to her boss, who called the Orange County jail nurse and dictated two prescriptions. The sullen nurse delayed Lisa's meds another hour by insisting on calling back the doctor "to confirm." Sybil likewise has succeeded in getting meds through her friend Cyndy, who understands Sybil's speech. Cyndy persuaded the nurse to call Sybil's doctor in Boston; when the nurse finally dispensed them she gave Sybil twelve antispasmodic pills. Sybil, whose doctor had already advised the nurse that her dosage totals *nine* in one day, was at that point in severe spasm and took all twelve, which will render her dopey for the rest of her time in jail.

We still have only one egg crate; the women who require them are doing poorly. As for the temperature, it remains unchanged. The suit-and-tie tries to convince us that he's turned down the air conditioner—having already told us the temperature's not adjustable—but we can discern no difference. Cyndy's disability in particular scares us; her old bone-breaks are extremely sensitive to cold. She too has finally been given her meds; they've been in her purse— confiscated, of course—all along. But by the time the nurse parcels out her first pills, she's missed some four doses, causing her pain to escalate out of control. The nurse refuses to administer any more than Cyndy's usual dosage; she also refuses to dispense the meds according to Cyndy's own long-established pain cycle (every three to four hours). All prisoners are expected to conform to Orange County Jail's schedule of meds at 6 A.M., noon, and 6 P.M. In sum, Cyndy is acutely undermedicated.

Over the course of our incarceration, a few guards evolve from adversary to ally. Like many ABs (able-bodied people), they seem at first terrified, as if we're aliens, as if our motley sizes and shapes embody some dark inchoate force that threatens their being. We're used to this reaction from the nondisabled world, but there's a difference in here: these women wield over us a measure of power that exists outside of prisons only in hospitals, mental asylums, and nursing homes.

My own personal pick of the guards is a sharpie I'll call Jill, whose pene- trating brown eyes signal an understanding of our issues beyond what she's able to say. She becomes our staunch defender; later she intercedes to save Cyndy's life.

I've been sitting on line, teeth chattering, waiting to be issued my uniform when Ellen, who hails from Texas and is one of my cellmates, appears at my side, looking panicked. "We've got to do something," she blurts, "Cyndy's getting worse, I don't know if she's going to make it." And she ushers me into the cell where Cyndy sits in her wheelchair.

Though no more than an hour has passed since I last saw her, I cringe. All color has drained from Cyndy, leaving her skin an oddly bleached white, like bones washed up on a beach. Her limbs are ice-cold, she's sweating profusely and starting to hallucinate. The expression on her face is unmistakable: the pain has passed beyond her threshhold.

I stare, catch my breath, ask what was the nurse's response to her last request to see a doctor. A numb ritual, this question, since the answer never varies: the nurse repeats that the doctor's not available, he's out making rounds. To Cyn- dy's request for an increase in pain med the nurse replies that it will not be possible without a doctor's prescription.

The fact is, severe pain interferes with Cyndy's breathing. Born with Werd- nig Hoffman Disease, Cyndy was not expected to live past the age of 2. Each day of Cyndy's 32 years has been a carefully managed miracle.

My eyes move from Ellen to Cyndy, back to Ellen. A kind of pressure is building in my chest, a constriction that quickly names itself: fear. Ellen's eyes are thick with it; Sybil, sitting on the other side of Cyndy, is glazed with it. There is a pause, a stillness, all of us staring at Cyndy's frozen weeping face, at one another.

What happens next unfolds in dream time, collapsing inward on itself, frame upon frame, a brittle technicolor nightmare. For what seems like hours our eyes remain locked together. Nothing I do, no sound I make over the next 10 minutes is volitional; "possession" comes closest to describing the deliberate mindless clarity that makes me reach for my aluminum crutches, walk into the cell across the corridor (too many wheelchairs blocking my path to get my own chair through, and too little time), and mumble some words to the women gathered there, I'm not sure what, something about not letting Cyndy die.

I walk back into the cell with Ellen and Cyndy and Sybil. Someone lifts a crutch high in the air and brings it down with dazzling force against the metal toilet. Someone roars, her voice unrecognizable, barely human, at horror-movie decibels: "*Doctor now!*" Crutch smashing again, metal on metal, and again the thunderous scream, again, louder than humans can scream: "*Doctor now!*" Rhythmic, incantatory. "*Doctor now!*"

Women rush into the cell: guards, prisoners. The room fills, everyone's staring at me. My crutch breaks, the bottom shearing off. Soon other voices join in, fists smashing on metal bunk beds, the metal sink, our voices a solid wall of sound, a steamroller, a tank.

Perched on her upper bunk, Ellen watches, transfixed. Later she'll describe the guards standing in our midst, gaping, stunned. Nothing in their experience or training has prepared them for this moment. They don't know what to do, their bodies, their faces immobilized with . . . Ellen will grope for the word: terror. The blond guard, the one whose boot-camp mentality we've found especially noxious, whose 10 pounds of makeup entirely obscure all human expression, is facing Ellen. Her rigid posture, the set of her head on its stem, seem suffused with anger until Ellen looks into the eyes and sees that they are full.

As the broken metal end piece of my crutch drops to the floor, a guard stoops, picks it up. Another guard gently reaches for what's left of the crutch, takes it from my hand. In that instant I crumple, my body slumps. Two guards take the broken crutch aside and without a word proceed to repair it, heads bent over their work. Still I pound my fists against the metal sink, still I scream, but by now the screams have given way to sobs. The guard whose arm encircles me is Jill, and she is weeping too. "*I won't let her die!*" I scream, "I *won't!*" still flailing at the sink.

"I won't let her die either," Jill says finally into the gathering quiet. "I'm going to get the doctor. I'll be back with him. Trust me."

When a distraught Cyndy returns from her three minutes with the doctor ("I told him I need to go to an emergency room and he said: 'I didn't get you in here and I'm not getting you out' "), Jill's lips pinch together. "Trust me," will become her watchword, and we do. None of us blames Jill when her efforts fail and Cyndy—who cannot bear to break rank—is forced to bond out if she wants to stay alive.

They release us on Tuesday (our lawyer finally cut a deal with the judge), one at a time. We wheel out into open air; it's dusk, the light a soft embrace, the temperature comforting, comfortable. Every time the door opens a cheer goes up. Someone in the crowd steps forward with a round ADAPT decal and presses it onto the chest of each just-freed prisoner. I am about to learn, in a frenzied round of story swapping with the men, that they were deprived of neither egg crates—some in fact went unused—nor meds. Glancing down at my gray prison sweatshirt with the cigarette hole between my breasts I see, arched like a rainbow: FREE OUR PEOPLE, and under it the little figure in its wheelchair, arms aloft, chains snapping from the wrists.

SECTION V

TOWARD ADEQUATE POLICY
IN HEALTH CARE DELIVERY

INTRODUCTION

Nancy F. McKenzie

To reform the health care system in the United States is to basically de-fund an industry. This industry is the sixth largest in the United States, ahead of the defense industry, and the third largest employer. If we are to go from a "sickness care system" to a "health care system" we must not only re-understand what health care delivery is and earmark our main providers and funders for new goals, we must confront issues of political control, about where care is to be provided and by whom, about local control of care with national financing. We must confront issues of for whom and upon whom research is financed and conducted. We must make basic decisions about the provision of basic health care across the board, about who reforms the model of care, as well as the blend of preventive, public, acute, and chronic care. But we must also confront issues of employment. Like "peace-time conversion," "health-time conversion" will require that literally millions of Americans find alternative jobs in health care delivery once the bureaucracies of health care finance and hospital dominance are dismantled. And we must speak to the training of providers that does not involve the over-specialization of our graduate medical education.

This section speaks to health care delivery issues and allows its authors to demand that the political issues become issues of health civil rights—issues to be decided by a "health-time conversion" constituency made up of all Americans.

It has been the presumption of this anthology that health care delivery—medical research, the configuration of care, the clinical priorities of practitioners, the social hierarchy, and the social attitudes of providers—has been so driven by the needs of providers and by the financial rewards and the political pressures of professional association as to be almost *irrelevant* to the health needs of the majority of individuals. The articles in our previous four sections have shown the fundamental disjunction between the needs of individuals and the health care they are offered or find impossible to obtain. It is in this section that we can begin to confront the mismatch between health needs and health care provision; a mismatch that cannot be remedied until health care in the United States is answerable to the people it serves. This is not a question of "accountability" —a bookkeeping term. It is one of responsibility that comes from an assumed responsiveness to human need. And it can occur only within the scope of a community-driven health care system that responds to the needs of individuals before it responds to the needs of providers, whether those needs be profit, research, gamesmanship, status, or power.

Health care reform cannot occur by pouring money into a medical procedures system. It cannot be dealt with by the elimination of third party insurance, and the mere setting up of a universal access system. Medical procedures will continue to dominate care, hospitals will continue to be the sole places of care, and without health prevention, health promotion, and local community input and control, acute, high-tech medicine will continue to be unresponsive to the needs of those most in need of health care.

There are some things that nations can always afford and never find too costly, constitutional guarantees and provision of the basics of everyday life that keep individuals from destitution: paid work, food, housing, and health care. Once a nation sacrifices one of these four for other national aims, public policy is deferred and the basics are no longer, in and of themselves, easily regained or smoothly provided.

It is not possible to speak of health care reform within present institutions. Health care has so long *not* been a priority of the American health care system, and individuals have so long been shut out of a role in informing health care that a social movement is now necessary. Where we wish to go—to rational health care delivery—is years and ideological eons away from where we are. Health care policy must be discussed in response to basic human needs for shelter, work, food, a clean environment. And that discussion must be among citizens.

The American medical care system is organized for treatment after the fact of illness, with only a small percentage of the national budget designed for preventive and public health. Not only is our health care system not designed for prevention, the logic of its development over the last thirty years has been to privilege medical intervention rather than medical support or medical care. The breakdown of health care delivery into bio/medical services, and, in turn, the reduction of bio/medical services to acute, bio/technological, largely in-hospital intervention has produced a medical care system that "produces" as many diseases as it treats. The medicalization of social problems, the power of medical professional associations, and the technology of medicine all produce medical categorization, rather than follow it.

And, ultimately, we must all wonder, as millions of Americans now do, how basic, everyday health care can be had and what it means to "treat" ailments if, as is often the case, the treatment so alienates the individual or the body that further repair is necessary and arbitrary.

For health care in the United States to be "adequate" it will be necessary that citizens control it. We have a right to our bodies! And those bodies must have input into how they are cared for by others. Without that, American citizens are victims, not patients. And health care delivery is an array of institutions that limits autonomy, defines roles and cuts each individual off from the basic right to self-determination.

Health care reform is the preeminent civil rights issue. Unless a social movement compels health care to be redefined by the needs of individuals, there is no chance that it will be adequate to our health care needs. The alternative to health care reform by citizens is health care reform by our present institutions

—by lobbyists, by professional associations, by financial boards, by strapped state agencies.

Our first article concerns a popular "health rationing" proposal—Oregon's Medicaid rationing plan, one that many legislators think should be adopted by all states. It is one that should truly frighten us and it should show us the ways in which health care must be tied to civil rights issues. This article is written from the position of the individuals most affected by what Oregon would eliminate in "medically necessary" procedures in favor of what they term "quality of life" priorities.

Bob Griss, co-chair of the Health Task Force of the Consortium for Citizens with Disabilities, puts his emphasis upon the fact that most of Oregon's eliminated categories (categories that the state wishes not to fund for treatment) are *exactly* the same categories that have protected classes of individuals under civil rights law: the Rehabilitation Act and Americans with Disabilities Act. Individuals with brain injuries, neurological impairment, and drug or alcohol addictions would be affected. And he points to the fact that Oregon's fundamental agenda is not health policy but the cutting of funding of medical services to those individuals most likely to be vulnerable, the most needy and the least able to fight on their own behalf. The fact that any state ever got to the point of "rationing" health care in the United States should be evidence enough that a health rights movement is necessary and urgent.

In a statement of general priorities for national health policy by the Consortium (see p. 514), the issue of affordability is one factor to be considered. The coalition points to the need for financial access, but it goes further to argue for a reconsideration of health care services that can include the needs of those least recognized by the present medical care system: the disabled, those in need of consistent and easily accessible rehabilitation, reproductive services for women, the chronically ill. The statement stresses comprehensive services, appropriateness, equality, and cost efficiency. Yet it still relies on a conception of medical services as items rather than processes. If we are to solve the issues of adequate health care delivery, we must begin discussions on a level that does not consider the present system to be adequate for anyone's health.

As Milton Terris points out in "The Components of Care" (p. 528) and as others have repeatedly pointed out, Britain offers a good example of what happens when medical services are accessible and equitable but the populations they serve are disparate in terms of wealth, employment, and physical and mental ability. In England, the mortality of the lowest classes has increased, rather than decreased, since the beginning of the National Health Service. At issue here is the fact that a truncated view of health policy predominates when policy is designed around disease but not its prevention. This is especially true in a country that has experimented with "free market" health care to such an extent that it is now witnessing unparalleled epidemics of infectious and environmental disease. As we deal with national health reform, it is important to see what Terris and his use of Sigerist can tell us about the neglect of "early" health care delivery—prevention and public health.

From a consideration of "early" health care, we turn to "late" health care delivery: the care that ensues once acute or traumatic episodes have subsided. This is a question that looms large for the United States since there is so little consideration given to rehabilitation medicine, to long-term care, to home care. And it is an issue that is stressed by both MADRE and the Consortium in their proposals. Health care should return people to as much autonomy as possible after illness or disability has occurred. Without rehabilitative medicine, without alternative strategies for recovery, home care, and long-term care (when living autonomously is no longer possible), one-third of the health needs of Americans is ignored.

In "A National Long-term Care Program for the United States" (p. 535) Charlene Harrington and the Working Group on Long-Term Care Design of Physicians for a National Health Program, speak to the need for the public coverage of all medically and socially necessary services for those who are disabled or too debilitated to care for themselves. As they call for substantial reform of long-term care in the United States so that it no longer privileges nursing homes, they show how biased current Medicaid payment is against independent living and how a public program could be federally financed but locally run and enhanced in quality by community input.

"In Search of a Solution" (p. 551) by Barbara Caress addresses what a new reliance on community health centers could do for the lopsidedness and inadequacy of health care delivery in terms of prevention, access to basic care and well-managed ambulatory and long-term care. The article offers specific recommendations for enhanced staffing, the development of community-based care, increasing the supply of physicians, enhanced mental health services and increasing the availability of long-term care.

In line with the theme of health civil rights, this section concludes with two articles that treat health care as a right and which envision health care as a community endeavor, one that should improve the quality of people's lives. Victor Sidel's "Health Care for a Nation in Need" (p. 559) offers a comprehensive set of principles that should explicitly underlie a national health care system. And Hal Strelnick, in "Another Kind of Bronx Cheer" (p. 574), offers a vivid history of a community-based clinic in New York that responded to evolving community needs and continually educated its health care providers.

━━━━━ HEALTH CARE: WE GOTTA HAVE IT!
A Set of Principles, MADRE, Women's Campaign and Congress for Universal Health Care

1. **Assessible quality health care for all on an equal basis. Single tier/Single class system.**
2. **All expenses paid by a single payor system.**
3. **Complete reproductive health and family planning services.**
4. **Pre- and post-natal care and care for the elderly.**

5. Substance abuse treatment and AIDS prevention and treatment.
6. Emphasis on prevention and education with increased research on women's health needs.
7. Support for community health care close to us, and in our own languages.

STATEMENT OF THE CONSORTIUM FOR CITIZENS WITH DISABILITIES HEALTH TASK FORCE "PRINCIPLES FOR HEALTH CARE REFORM FROM A DISABILITY PERSPECTIVE"

December 1991 (updated March 1992)

On behalf of:

AIDS Action Council
Alliance for Genetic Support Groups
American Academy of Physical Medicine and Rehabilitation
American Association for Counseling and Development
American Association of University Affiliated Programs
American Association on Mental Retardation
American Civil Liberties Union
American Congress of Rehabilitation Medicine
American Foundation for the Blind
American Occupational Therapy Association
American Physical Therapy Association
American Speech-Language-Hearing Association
The Arc, Association for Retarded Citizens of the United States
Epilepsy Foundation of America
Immune Deficiency Foundation
International Association of Psychosocial Rehabilitation Services
Learning Disabilities Association
National Alliance for the Mentally Ill
National Association of Developmental Disabilities Councils
National Association of Private Residential Resources
National Association of Protection and Advocacy Systems
National Association of Rehabilitation Facilities
National Association of State Mental Retardation Program Directors
National Council for Independent Living
National Easter Seal Society
National Head Injury Foundation
National Mental Health Association

National Multiple Sclerosis Society
National Organization for Rare Disorders
National Parent Network on Disabilities
National Recreation and Parks Association
National Rehabilitation Association
National Transplant Support Network
Spina Bifida Association of America
The Association for Persons with Severe Disabilities
United Cerebral Palsy Associations, Inc.

Principles

The CCD believes that any ultimate solution to the health care crisis must be based on the principle of **nondiscrimination** ensuring that people with disabilities of all ages and their families have the opportunity to fully participate. The CCD would define a successful health care system as one that offers a **comprehensive** array of health, rehabilitation, personal, and support services, as well as a system that ensures that these services are **appropriate** in that they are provided on the basis of each individual's need, personal choice, and situation. In addition, any truly effective solution must be **equitable**, ensuring that no group of individuals bears a disproportionate burden. Finally, the CCD asserts that an effective and accessible health care system must be **efficient**, ensuring that system resources are utilized to meet health care needs. The CCD strongly supports the right to health care for all persons regardless of income or health status.

Nondiscrimination: People with disabilities of all ages and their families must be able to fully participate in the nation's health care system.

People with disabilities are often discriminated against in the health insurance marketplace because they are presumed to be high health care users. In fact, most people with disabilities are not sick. Nevertheless, private insurers use medical underwriting practices which are designed to ensure that high users of health care are charged higher premiums, subjected to preexisting condition exclusions, or rejected totally as an "unacceptable risk." Discrimination occurs when a sizeable proportion of people with disabilities, who are actually low users of health care, are denied insurance or subjected to preexisting condition exclusions. Discrimination also occurs when high users of health care are denied adequate coverage because they cannot afford the premiums or are subjected to limitations on covered services. From a disability perspective, the very practice of experience-rating, which ensures that premiums are set on the basis of previous utilization, is a form of unfair discrimination against high users.

Access to health care for individuals with disabilities cannot be considered in a vacuum. Historically, discrimination on the basis of disability has limited opportunities in employment, education, housing, travel, and other aspects of daily life. Now, with rights guaranteed in so many of these areas by the passage of the Americans with Disabilities Act and other important civil rights legislation, there is a growing realization in the disability community that access to health care is a major barrier that threatens to interfere with the attainment of these rights. The CCD believes that the present inability of a substantial proportion of people with disabilities to participate in the nation's health care system at a level which meets their needs is a direct reflection of the continued misperception of both the skills and needs of people with disabilities. Nondiscrimination requires that the health care financing system:

- prohibits pre-existing condition exclusions;
- prohibits rating practices that discriminate against higher users of health care;
- ensures that all persons, regardless of income or health status, have access to the all-needed health-related services;
- provides access without regard to age, race, place of residence, or the characteristics of persons with whom one maintains family relationships;
- ensures continuity and portability of coverage.

Comprehensiveness: People with disabilities and their families must have access to a health care system that ensures a comprehensive array of health, rehabilitation, personal, and support services across all service categories and sites of service delivery.

The CCD asserts that an effective and comprehensive health care system, one that is responsive to the needs of people with disabilities, would provide a seamless array of lifelong health-related services. Comprehensiveness implies the broadest set of services that assist individuals with disabilities and their families to achieve and sustain optimum physical and mental function. The terms "health, rehabilitation, personal, and support services," used by the CCD, refers to a universe of services delivered by a range of practitioners in a variety of sites and illustrates the necessary breadth of a health care delivery system that is truly accessible to people with disabilities. Over the course of a lifetime, all people commonly require a broad array of health, rehabilitation, personal, and support services. However, access to the entire array of these services must be ensured for people with disabilities. Often it is the availability of these services that can determine their ability to live independent lives and fully participate in the community. Moreover, adequate access can prevent exacerbation of a small health problem into a larger, more costly health problem. People with disabilities would most benefit from a health care system that includes access to:

- preventive services, including services to prevent the worsening of a disability
- health promotion/education services
- diagnostic services
- inpatient and outpatient physician services
- hospital inpatient and outpatient care
- long- and short-term home and community-based services
- long-term care in medical facilities

- prescription drugs, biologicals, and medical foods
- mental health and counseling services
- habilitation services
- rehabilitation services, including audiology, occupational therapy, physical therapy, respiratory therapy, speech-language pathology services, cognitive, vision, and behavioral therapies, and therapeutic recreation
- personal assistance services and independent living services
- durable medical equipment and other assistive devices, equipment, and related services

Appropriateness: People with disabilities and their families must be assured that comprehensive health, rehabilitation, personal, and support services are provided on the basis of individual need, preference, and choice.

Particular attention must be placed on the appropriateness of available services. It is of critical importance to the disability community that full involvement of the "consumer" is assured in all decisions affecting the selection of service, service provider, service timing, and service setting. CCD is concerned that certain forms of managed care create an incentive for under-serving people with disabilities and often utilize gatekeepers who are not knowledgeable about the special health care needs of people with disabilities.

The issue of consumer choice and participation has a particular importance for persons with disabilities. While the present acute-care oriented health care system has a tendency to relegate all "consumers" to a dependent status embodied in the "sick role," this indignity is particularly disempowering to people with disabilities when their chronic health conditions are permanent. That is why the health-related services for persons with disabilities must be delivered in a way that minimizes interference with normal activities, and why health care financing policies which govern access to health care for persons with chronic conditions must be sensitive to issues of locus and control.

It is essential that decisions about health care services reflect personal preference and maximum benefit to the individual rather than provider and service setting availability, cost-containment goals, or coverage limits. CCD asserts that meaningful access to health care involves the right of the individual consumer to participate in the decision-making process regarding the provision of needed services and to be educated so appropriate self-care is possible.

In addition, CCD strongly believes that people with disabilities must be involved in policy decisions that will guide the nation's health care system. An appropriate health care system is one that:

- includes consumer participation;
- ensures consumer choice in relation to services and provider;
- ensures a range of service settings through an integrated delivery system;
- ensures appropriate amount, scope, and duration of services;
- ensures the availability of trained personnel.

Equity: People with disabilities and their families must be ensured equitable participation in the nation's health care system and not burdened with disproportionate costs.

The CCD asserts that equal access to health services will not be readily achievable unless payment for health, rehabilitation, personal, and support services is equitably distributed so that no individual or public or private sector interest is burdened with a disproportionate share of the cost. Because of cost issues, too often people with disabilities and their families have been required to make unfortunate choices between needed health services in appropriate settings and what they can afford. These types of choices obviously do not reflect the principles of nondiscrimination, comprehensiveness, and appropriateness of services. Health care reform must ensure that people have access to services based on health care need and not on their employment status or income level. As a group, people with disabilities have lower income than the general population and many adults with disabilities and families with members with disabilities devote a disproportionate share of their income to health care and disability-related services. An equitable health care system would be one that:

- limits out of pocket expenses and cost sharing requirements for participants;
- provides access to services based on health care need and not on income level or employment status;
- ensures adequate reimbursement for service providers.

Efficiency: People with disabilities and their families must have access to a health care system that provides a maximum of appropriate effective quality services with a minimum of administrative waste.

The CCD is concerned that the current fragmentary system has failed to achieve effective cost controls, or a rational allocation of health resources, and contributes to substantial administrative waste. It is estimated that more than 20 percent of health care expenditures are attributed to administrative costs as 1,500 private health insurers require different forms of provider documentation to trace every claim for reimbursement to the utilization by a specific individual with his or her own health insurance plan. In addition, the fragmentary system has contributed to the growth of excess capacity in the health care delivery system, inviting cost shifting, and undermining efforts to achieve effective cost controls. This has reinforced pressures for arbitrary cost containment by limiting coverage in ways that often adversely affect persons with disabilities.

Moreover, health care financing policy has not evolved much beyond acute care, failing to respond to the growing need for preventive care and for chronic health care management which could significantly reduce the growth of preventable diseases.

An efficient health care system is one that:

- reduces administrative complexity and minimizes administrative costs;
- allocates resources in a more balanced way between preventive services, acute care, rehabilitation, and chronic care management;
- ensures the delivery of effective services;
- maintains effective cost controls so that all people can get the health care services which they need.

Based on these "principles" from a disability perspective, CCD is reviewing all the health reform legislation before the Congress and submitting assessments of these bills as they are completed.

Conclusion

The disability community needs to be a major player in reexamining health care financing policy. People with disabilities are highly vulnerable to the limitations of both public and private systems as they are squeezed between a private system which is designed to charge accordingly to an assessment of risk and a public system which subsidizes health care according to age, poverty status, family structure, and an inability to work.

Private health insurance was developed and has remained a method for spreading risk of incurring excessive costs primarily for hospital and physician services. For individuals with disabilities, access to health care has been severely restricted because of preexisting conditions and the mistaken assumption that most people with disabilities need more hospital and physician care than the population as a whole. Health care reform needs to eliminate this restriction and assure access to needed hospital and physician services. Equally as important, the tradition of limiting covered services to hospital and physician services must be changed. Rehabilitation services, personal and support services, mental health services, and assistive technology must be recognized as essential components of health care.

Perhaps our greatest contribution will be in clarifying the principles which should guide our health care system. These include: 1) expanding the definition of "health" to include prevention services, rehabilitation therapies, assistive technology, and ongoing health-related maintenance services; 2) distributing all health-related expenses equitably throughout the population; and 3) restructuring our health care delivery system to more effectively support consumer-directed chronic care management.

For more information, please contact any of the CCD Health Task Force Co-chairs:

Bob Griss, United Cerebral Palsy Associations, 1522 K Street, N.W., Suite 1112, Washington, D.C. 20005, telephone: (202) 842–1266.

Kathy McGinley, The Arc, formerly the Association for Retarded Citizens of the United States, 1522 K Street, N.W., Suite 516, Washington, D.C. 20005, telephone: (202) 785–3388.

Janet O'Keefe, The American Psychological Association, 750 First Street, N.E., Washington, D.C. 20002, telephone: (202) 336–5934.

Bill Schmidt, Epilepsy Foundation of America, 4351 Garden City Drive, Landover, Maryland 20785, telephone: (301) 459–3700.

Steve White, American Speech-Language-Hearing Association, 10801 Rockville Pike, Rockville, Maryland 20852, telephone: (301) 897–5700.

CIVIL RIGHTS ISSUES UNDERLYING REJECTION OF OREGON MEDICAID RATIONING PLAN: ROUND ONE

Bob Griss

The Bush Administration has received much criticism from state health policymakers and political observers for rejecting the Oregon Medicaid rationing plan on the grounds that it violates the Americans with Disabilities Act by prioritizing health care services on the basis of presumed quality of life. This unexpected decision—far from being "politically expedient"—reflects President Bush's commitment to the Americans with Disabilities Act, and reminds policymakers at the state and federal levels that health care policy reforms cannot violate civil rights laws.

Oregon claims that its prioritization process was designed to eliminate ineffective medical treatments, but the prioritization list actually represents *subjective* judgments about how various treatments are expected to affect the "quality of life" of a person with a particular illness or disability. At the bottom of the list are treatments that are "valuable to certain individuals" but are expected to "cause minimal or no improvement in quality of life." The disability community is concerned that the prioritization process in the Oregon Medicaid rationing plan would legitimate discrimination on the basis of medical diagnosis. This would create a very dangerous precedent in the Medicaid program and in private health insurance. Federal approval of the Oregon Medicaid rationing plan would be the first time that the federal government would encourage states to move from a "medically necessary" standard to a "quality of life" standard in deciding what health services to cover.

Subjective Judgments About Quality of Life

Oregon's prioritization process was based on subjective judgments generated from:

1. a telephone survey of 1,001 Oregonians who were asked to rate various symptoms and functional limitations on a scale from zero (which is "as bad as death") to 100 (which represents "good health").
2. opinions expressed at community meetings (where 69 percent of the participants were health care professionals); the meetings were held after the disability community had been told that they would be exempt from the prioritization process.

3. questionable information collected from Oregon physicians (often at variance with the published literature or with the clinical judgments of physicians contracted by the US Congress's Office of Technology Assessment (OTA) to evaluate the prioritization process); and
4. subjective decisions made by the Oregon Health Services Commission (which changed 24 percent of the ratings at least 100 lines based on their view of what was "reasonable").

UCPA shares the concerns of the Bush Administration that a number of aspects of the ranking process reflect stereotypic assumptions that undervalued the quality of life of persons with disabilities.

Danger of Practicing Medicine by Diagnostic Category

Applying Oregon's subjective prioritization list—without regard to the characteristics of the individual that are most likely to affect medical outcomes—creates a dangerous precedent in medical practice. Oregon proposed to extend Medicaid coverage to all persons under 100 percent of the federal poverty level, but only to fund services above a fluctuating cut-off line based on the amount of money the state legislature decides it can afford to allocate to the Medicaid program in a particular year. That fluctuating cut-off line would determine what services Medicaid would pay for, and health care professionals would be exempt from "criminal prosecution, civil liability, or professional disciplinary action for failing to provide a service that the legislative assembly has not funded or has eliminated from its funding" in accordance with the prioritization list.

In addition, all Medicaid recipients would be served through capitated managed care providers, including HMOs. Thus there would be an incentive to underserve enrollees since providers and HMOs will receive a fixed prepayment that does not increase if more services are needed. There is a real danger that HMOs could engage in the practice of "down coding," by withholding medically necessary services from people who have conditions both above and below the cut-off line. Oregon chose to ignore the issue of co-morbidity in its prioritization list, even though age and co-morbidity (i.e., the presence of more than one medical condition) have the most significant impacts on expected outcomes.

In its evaluation of the prioritization plan, the Office of Technology Assessment speculated that Oregon avoided addressing the issue of how age and co-morbidity would be treated to avoid the appearance of discrimination.

Oregon has claimed that the prioritization list is based on medical effectiveness, and that the civil rights laws are being used to require them to cover medically ineffective services. This is patently false. Medicaid is not obligated to pay for any services that are not medically effective. Oregon's prioritization list ranks services not on the basis of medical effectiveness but on the basis of what is perceived to improve one's "quality of life." To the extent that the quality of life of persons with disabilities is viewed as lower than persons without disabilities, they are likely to be denied equal access to health care. This is in violation of civil rights laws.

History of Discrimination

The Americans with Disabilities Act acknowledges that persons with disabilities have been *"(S)ubjected to a history of purposeful unequal treatment"* in *"employment, housing, public accommodations, education, transportation, communication, recreation, institutionalization, health services, voting, and access to public services"* based on myths, stereotypes, and fears. As a result, individuals with disabilities have sought protection from "exclusionary qualification standards and criteria, segregation, and relegation to lesser services . . ." through the enactment of civil rights laws. What is not generally recognized is how persons without disabilities benefit from the protection of the civil rights of persons with disabilities.

Although the disability community has been accused rhetorically of blocking a rationing system that would enable Oregon to extend Medicaid coverage to all uninsured persons under 100 percent of poverty, we believe that raising these civil rights issues around access to health care for persons with disabilities will actually lead to greater health security for all Americans.

Fiscal Pressure Threatens to Raise the Cut-off Line

Oregon is already facing a budget shortfall of $1 billion for 1993–1995. When Oregon's Governor, Barbara Roberts, called a special legislative session in early July to consider her proposal for creating a state sales tax, the legislative session collapsed in disarray. Once the prioritization list is in place, the state can respond to the fiscal pressure by either raising taxes or raising the cut-off line on the prioritization list.

At the current proposed cut-off line of #587, 6 of the most common principal diagnoses, out of 25 for inpatient hospital care, would not be covered nor would 8 of the 25 most common diagnoses for physician visits. If the cut-off line is raised slightly, children born with spina bifida and hydrocephalus, the most common birth defect, who are now at #510, may find themselves below the cut-off line. This would result in the denial of the medically necessary services that could save their lives and permit them to live healthy and productive lives.

If Oregon is permitted to withhold medically effective services from persons whose conditions fall beneath the cut-off line, it is likely that other states will quickly seek to use this or other prioritization lists to try to achieve cost containment in their Medicaid programs. It is also likely that these quality of life standards will begin to be used by private health insurance companies.

Precedent for Private Insurance

Oregon has already passed legislation requiring employers by 1995 to provide health insurance to their employees and dependents that is substantially similar to the fluctuating benefit package in the Oregon Medicaid program. This may lead to persons with private health insurance being denied medically necessary services because their condition falls below the cut-off line on the Medicaid prioritization list.

In another example of discrimination on the basis of medical condition, in *McGann v. H & H Music Company*, the US Supreme Court is looking at an employee's challenge to the employer's right to reduce a lifetime cap on health insurance benefits from $1 million to $5,000 for AIDS-related services.

Violations of Civil Rights Laws

The prioritization of services on the basis of presumed quality of life has the potential to discriminate against people with disabilities in violation of the Americans with Disabilities Act (ADA), Section 504 of the Rehabilitation Act of 1973, and the federal Child Abuse ("Baby Doe") Amendments of 1984.

Title II of the ADA applies to state government programs and services such as Medicaid, and prohibits the denial of benefits of services and programs based on disability. **Many of the medical conditions on Oregon's prioritization list are actually "protected classes" under the Rehabilitation Act and the Americans with Disabilities Act because the conditions are disability groups**. This includes such conditions as traumatic brain injury (#684), myasthenia gravis (#593) or alcoholic cirrhosis of the liver (#690), which all fall beneath the cut-off line of #587 that Oregon has proposed to fund through its Medicaid program, at least for the first year. In an unmistakable example of discrimination on the basis of medical diagnosis, Oregon proposes to fund a liver transplant for a person with non-alcoholic liver failure (#366) but will not fund the same service for a person with alcoholic cirrhosis of the liver (#690), despite similar success rates, according to the OTA report.

While the Supreme Court has ruled in *Alexander v. Choate* [469 US. 287 (1985)] that states can use uniform limitations on health care services under the Medicaid program, even if the limitation disproportionately affects people with disabilities, a state cannot deny or limit access to care **based on disability or diagnostic category**.

The Oregon prioritization list also proposes to deny life supports to low birth weight premature infants born under 500 grams and under 23-week gestation (#708). However, the federal Child Abuse ("Baby Doe") laws prohibit the withholding of medically effective treatment from a child born with a disability that would be provided to a child born without a disability. Physicians are required to provide treatment to a medically fragile infant when it is the physician's reasonable medical judgment that the treatment "will be most likely to be effective in ameliorating or correcting" the infant's life-threatening conditions.

Based on these civil rights laws—which cannot be waived by a change in Medicaid requirements for Oregon's Medicaid rationing plan—**we cannot conceive how prioritizing services on the basis of presumed quality of life would not be inherently discriminatory**.

Fundamental vs. Technical Issue

The Bush Administration has communicated that it would like to approve Oregon's plan if it does not conflict with civil rights laws. Some have suggested that this can be easily accomplished by technical changes, such as eliminating information from the telephone survey that Oregon claims had only a minor impact on the ultimate prioritization ranking anyway. **But any prioritization based on quality of life would still violate civil rights laws by limiting medically necessary services on the basis of diagnostic categories.** Congressman Ron Wyden (OR), a staunch supporter of his state's proposed Medicaid rationing plan, was right when he was quoted in the *Congressional Quarterly*, August 8, 1992, as saying: **"The administration's objections really go right to the heart of the program . . . We may have to go back to the drawing board."**

Oregon continues to point out that *de facto* rationing is already condoned by the federal government since states are permitted to limit eligibility and services in their Medicaid programs for low-income persons, which Oregon rightly condemns as unfair and inefficient. But permitting these arbitrary limitations is very different from legitimating the process of *withholding* medically effective services on the basis of presumed quality of life.

Many in the disability community fear that rationing of health care on the basis of presumed quality of life would seriously erode the health security that all Americans deserve, and that America can afford. The United States pays at least 40 percent more for health care on a per capita basis than any other country, and yet continues to deny health insurance to 37 million Americans, provides inadequate health insurance to at least 60 million more, and continues to neglect prevention, rehabilitation, long-term and chronic care management. Some of these problems Oregon deserves some credit for trying to address, but it is unfortunate that they tried to finance some of these improvements by withholding medically effective services from people whose conditions are perceived as having a lower quality of life.

Uninsured Persons Already Contribute to Health Care System

Ironically, many of the 120,000 low-income uninsured persons in Oregon—who would have been covered by the extended Medicaid program—are already contributing to the over $800 billion that will be spent in the United States on health care in 1992. These hidden contributions take the form of:

- a 2.9 percent payroll tax that they and their employer pay on their earned income each year that goes to Medicare.
- their income taxes, a portion of which goes to Medicaid.
- the higher prices they pay for the products they purchase, which includes the inflated health insurance premiums for the employees who produced these products and their dependents.

- their own inflated health care expenses, like everyone's, which compensate for the excess capacity in the health care system, administrative waste, and failure to control for excess profits.

The challenge is to establish a system that not only ensures that everyone contributes, but also provides for all medically necessary health care.

Incomplete Victory

The disability community takes no satisfaction in the continuation of the status quo in Oregon or anywhere else where adequate health care is denied to any persons. What is more, we know that the health policy planners in Oregon have been trying to improve the health care system for everyone. Many persons with disabilities in Oregon are supportive of many of the proposed changes in the Medicaid program because it offered to expand services beyond acute care. These expansions included such important health-related services as dental care and physical rehabilitation, which are not covered in the existing Medicaid program. But while these changes can be viewed as welcomed improvements, the precedent of rationing health care on the basis of quality of life is viewed by many national disability organizations as creating a very dangerous precedent that threatens to erode health security for all citizens.

Rationing Is Inevitable in a System Out of Control

Oregon may be right that they have been more honest and open about the rationing process than have other states and the federal government. But that does not excuse a violation of civil rights. **Oregon felt compelled to ration health care because they sought to use the Medicaid program to compensate for the failure of private health insurance to cover all persons with an adequate and affordable health care plan**. Those who are concerned that rationing health care on the basis of quality of life violates civil rights laws had better advocate for a system of health care financing that ensures access to comprehensive health care and distributes those costs equitably throughout the population. It is not insignificant that every advocate for the Oregon Medicaid rationing plan began their testimony at the Congressional hearing held by Congressman Henry Waxman (CA) on September 16, 1991, by announcing that they really preferred a system of National Health Insurance. They only argued for rationing Medicaid dollars because that was the only solution they had the power to implement. Oregon is showing us what may be inevitable if health care priorities are set by what the Medicaid program can afford to pay for.

Conclusion

Prioritizing health care on the basis of presumed quality of life will create a "slippery slope" (that is getting steeper every day as the cost containment crisis intensifies) that will make it harder to ensure that all persons have access to medically effective treatment. **It is unconscionable for the United States to**

prioritize which medically effective health care services will be withheld from people in order to promote cost containment when our health care financing system encourages excess capacity, administrative waste, and excess profits that are driving the health care cost crisis.

The disability community is very aware of the arbitrary denials of access to health care in the existing system. We praise the state of Oregon for seeking ways to extend coverage to uninsured persons and to expand coverage of preventive services beyond acute health care. However, the disability community is sounding the alarm for all citizens that rationing health care on the basis of presumed quality of life must be regarded as a violation of civil rights and is neither a socially responsible nor an effective way to control health care costs. Instead we need national health policies which reduce excess capacity, administrative waste, and excess profits in the health care system in order to ensure that all persons can receive the medically necessary services that are needed to maintain health.

Current Status of Proposed Oregon Medicaid Rationing Plan

Representatives of the Department of Health and Human Services met with Oregon's Health Services Commission on August 26 to clarify how Oregon has to remove subjective quality of life information from the prioritization process. Their intent was to comply with the Americans with Disabilities Act and receive federal approval of their Medicaid waiver application.

For further information about the Oregon Medicaid rationing plan from a disability perspective, please contact Bob Griss, Senior Health Policy Researcher, United Cerebral Palsy Associations, 1522 K Street, N.W., Suite 1112, Washington, D.C. 20005; (202) 842-1266. Bob Griss is also Co-chair of the Health Task Force of the Consortium for Citizens with Disabilities that urged the Administration to reject the Oregon Medicaid rationing plan as a violation of ADA.

THE COMPONENTS OF CARE

Milton Terris

The writer contends that incorporating all the components of health, not only medical care, should be our goal as we strive for a comprehensive national system. In discussing the prospects for a national health program, Terris draws on the ideas and observations of Henry Sigerist, the noted medical historian who brilliantly analyzed the political preconditions for the establishment of national health insurance. Finally, he argues that the lessons of Canada offer progressives here a valuable point of departure.

Before discussing any proposal for a national health program, we must be certain to distinguish health care from medical care. One of the weaknesses of the medical care movement, to call it by its proper name, is the assumption that the two terms are identical, that creating a national medical care system is equivalent to establishing a national health program. The title of the June conference (''Rethinking a National Health Program'') bears unwitting witness to this misconception.

As Kristine Gebbie, Oregon's chief health officer, has so aptly remarked, ''It is regrettable that in a general discussion with the public, 'health care' is the euphemism for 'illness care' or 'treatment.' ''[1] The confusion results from a desire, conscious or unconscious, to sell the product to the public, to make the idea of such a system palatable. This is understandable, but hardly commendable, since the technique is strictly Madison Avenue, that is, the misusing of words to make things seem what they are not.

In the years preceding the establishment of the British National Health Service, progressives in Great Britain were much clearer on this point. The British Medical Association, for example, stated that ''greater attention should be paid to the economic, social and environmental determinants of health.'' And in 1934 the London Labour Party's Health Research Group, which included such notable members as Herbert Morrison and Somerville Hastings, declared that ''the three major causes of ill-health, in order of importance, were poverty, defective environment, and inadequate medical care.''[2]

The experience of the British and Canadian medical care systems has underlined the critical differences between true health care and medical care. Attempts in both countries to mitigate poverty have foundered on the rocks of increasingly unstable economic systems; unemployment rates of over 10 percent appear to have become permanent features of these societies. Nor have the British and Canadian health authorities paid serious attention to the prevention of disease; their entire focus has been on medical care. Scotland has the dubious honor of having replaced Finland as the nation with the highest rate of death from coronary heart disease, and England and Wales are not far behind. In Canada during the 1970s, the rate of death from lung cancer rose by 60 percent and from cirrhosis of the liver by 25 percent.[3] These are all preventable diseases—beyond the reach of medical care but ameliorable through a comprehensive national health program.

Furthermore, equity in access to medical care has failed dismally to assure equity in health. In England and Wales inequality in mortality between social classes has actually widened since the establishment of the National Health Service. The two highest social classes (I. professional and II. managerial) had a standardized mortality ratio (SMR) of 91 in 1951, 80 in 1961, and 80 in 1971. The two lowest classes (IV. semi-skilled and V. unskilled) had SMRs of 110 in 1951, 115 in 1961, and 121 in 1971. The difference in SMRs, therefore, rose from 19 to 35 to 41 during those years.[4]

Nor has the Canadian medical care system done much better. Georges Desrosiers, citing studies done in Quebec, concludes that the Canadian system "has not substantially reduced inequality in the face of sickness and death. The underprivileged social classes still pay a heavy tribute."[5]

Clearly, the achievement of equity in health status requires equity in socioeconomic status. Health workers have a primary obligation, therefore, to help achieve for all Americans: full employment and adequate income, decent housing, good nutrition, greater financial support for public education and the elimination of financial barriers to higher education, increased cultural and recreational opportunities, and affirmative action to end discrimination against minorities in all areas of our national life.

The most rapid and dramatic improvement in the health of the public will result from preventive measures. This was also true in the past; the conquest of infectious diseases resulted primarily from environmental control and immunization.

During the 1920s, 1930s, and 1940s, noninfectious diseases emerged as the main causes of death and disability. But medicine was powerless to combat them; their epidemiologies were unknown, and physicians clothed ignorance of them in such polysyllabic terms as "degenerative," "idiopathic," "essential," and "psychosomatic."

Unable to prevent the occurrence of these diseases, medicine retreated to a second line of defense, namely, early detection and treatment—so-called secondary prevention. But secondary prevention has—with few exceptions—proved disappointing; it cannot compare in effectiveness with measures for primary prevention. The periodic physical examination, the cancer detection center, multiphasic screening, and a host of variations have incurred enormous expenditures for relatively modest benefits. Once a patient contracts a disease for which no effective treatment is available, it is simply too late. Unfortunately, for most noninfectious diseases treatment is ineffective whether given early or late. Important exceptions include cancer of the cervix, for which early detection has proved dramatically effective, and, to a lesser extent, cancer of the breast, for which secondary prevention is still not feasible on a large scale because of the high cost of mammography and medical examination.

Beginning in 1950, dramatic breakthroughs occurred in the epidemiology of noninfectious diseases. During the next three decades, epidemiologists forged powerful weapons to combat most of the major causes of death. In doing so, they initiated a second epidemiological revolution which, if we act appropriately, will result in an enormous reduction in premature death and disability.

Heart disease, the leading cause of death, results, investigators discovered, from high levels of serum cholesterol caused by a diet rich in saturated fat, and from hypertension, cigarette smoking, and a lack of physical exercise. All of these are amenable to public-health programs.

Cancer is the second major cause of death in the United States. Etiologic agents have been discovered for some of the most important cancer sites; these include radiation as well as tobacco, alcohol, and many other chemical carcinogens. All of these are amenable to public health programs designed to establish epidemiological barriers between agent and host.

Cerebrovascular disease, the third leading cause of death, can be effectively prevented by treating hypertension, its major risk factor.

Accidents are the fourth leading cause of death, but rank first in the number of potentially productive years they take. Furthermore, accidents are not really so accidental—they are often avoidable; every accident results from the action of a specific agent or from environmental factors. Many of these can be eliminated through appropriate public health programs.

Chronic obstructive pulmonary disease, the sixth most frequent cause of death, results almost entirely from cigarette smoking, and is therefore preventable.

Chronic liver disease and cirrhosis, the eighth leading cause of death, is almost entirely a product of the consumption of alcohol, and is therefore preventable.

Given that most of the leading causes of death are in large part the result of human action, not of the agency of microorganisms, the highest priority in our national health program must be the prevention of heart disease, cancer, stroke, accidents, chronic obstructive pulmonary disease, and cirrhosis of the liver. Nor must we neglect the infectious diseases; our victories on this field are far from complete. Major respiratory, enteric, and venereal infections still elude effective control, and most will doubtless rely as heavily on public health measures as on benchtop research for their elimination. Furthermore, new epidemics arise as a result of technological and social changes which facilitate the growth and spread of microorganisms. Recent examples include legionellosis, the cause of which has been traced to the cooling towers used in large-scale air conditioning; genital herpes, whose spread can be ascribed to changes in sexual mores; and the most frightening of all modern plagues, acquired immunodeficiency syndrome, related to changes in sexual mores, widespread abuse of intravenous drugs, and the use of blood transfusions.

Humanity is threatened not only by microorganisms and other living agents, but by the products of its own making—both nuclear and chemical. Chernobyl and Bhopal were grim reminders of these new dangers, but both were acute incidents—sudden epidemics, as it were. The chronic effects of exposure to radiation and toxic chemicals are always with us in the form of cancer, birth defects, and other diseases. It is urgent that a national health program mobilize investigatory, epidemiologic, and other scientific resources to control and eliminate the occupational and environmental hazards resulting from industrial development.

We need also to strengthen greatly our programs for maternal and child health—diseases of infancy and childhood remain high among the causes of illness, disability, and death. The barriers to early prenatal care for all women must be removed; family planning programs need to be greatly strengthened; nutrition supplementation for women, infants, and children should be expanded to help prevent not only deficits in physical and mental development, but common illnesses, as well; immunization must include every last child; and childhood screening programs should be extended to the entire population to prevent the burdens of chronic illness and disability from being carried into adult life.

Faced with these challenges, we can no longer afford the luxury of spending many billions of dollars for medical care and only a pittance for prevention. The irony is that much of the vast sum spent for care goes for the treatment of diseases and injuries that could have been prevented in the first place.

Much of the current discussion of alternative medical care systems in the United States fails to recognize the political preconditions for their development. These were outlined more than 40 years ago by Henry E. Sigerist, the great medical historian, who considered three factors to be crucial to the emergence of national health insurance: 1) industrialization, with its attendant economic and social insecurity, 2) the emergence of new political parties representing the interests of the workers, and 3) the occurrence of a revolutionary threat to the established order. In 1943, Sigerist brilliantly and thoroughly analyzed the genesis of the first national health insurance legislation, enacted by Bismarck in 1884; he concluded that the three factors underlying this advance were the growth of German industry after the Franco-Prussian War, the development of a strong socialist party in Germany, and the alarming example of the French Commune which, in Sigerist's words, "had demonstrated that socialism was not an armchair philosophy but could become a very tangible reality."[6]

A similar constellation of events brought about national health insurance in Britain in 1911 when, as Sigerist noted, "the second industrial revolution was very strongly felt. The Labour Party entered parliament and from a two-party country England developed into a three-party country. The Russian Revolution of 1905 was suppressed to be sure, but seemed a dress rehearsal for other revolutions to follow. Social legislation was enacted not by the Socialists, but by Lloyd George and Churchill."[7]

Sigerist describes a third wave of health insurance legislation "following World War I when again the industries of every warfaring country were greatly expanded, when, as a result of the war, the Socialist parties grew stronger everywhere, and the Russian revolution of 1917 created a red scare from which many countries are still suffering. Again social security legislation was enacted in a number of countries."[8]

Canada, too, followed the pattern outlined by Sigerist; the emergence of a socialist party, the Cooperative Commonwealth Federation (later called the New Democratic Party) was the key factor in the development of the Canadian system of medical care. Unlike in Europe, the new socialist party itself pioneered the development of the Canadian system. The CCF enacted legislation in Saskatchewan mandating hospital insurance, later extending the system to cover physicians' services. The more conservative Canadian parties followed suit and instituted health insurance nationally in response to the growth of the CCF, just as Bismarck had acted to counter the German Social-Democratic Party and Lloyd George had responded to the emergence of the British Labour Party. As Sigerist stated, "every historical pattern we set up is to a certain extent artificial and history never repeats itself unaltered."[9]

What does this mean for the United States? For one thing, a nation which has not even achieved the political prerequisites for national health insurance can hardly be expected to muster the forces required to nationalize its health resources by creating a national health service. It took decades of Labour Party development, the devastation of World War II, and the election of a Labour government to bring about the nationalization of health in Great Britain. It took many decades of growth of the powerful socialist and communist parties of Italy before that country's conservative leadership undertook to develop a national health service. Most of the Social Democratic governments of Western Europe have not yet moved away from their mixed medical care systems, which combine salaried services and national health insurance, to establish a completely salaried national health service.

If a national health service must be considered politically unfeasible at this time, is this not also true for a national medical system based on payment to individual practitioners and facilities? This may well be the case: If one followed Sigerist's thesis to the letter, one would be forced to conclude that such a system will not come into being until after a new party arises to challenge the Republicans and Democrats—whether a labor party in the British tradition, a farmer-labor party in the CCF mold, a socialist party, as in Europe, or a new American variant which combines blacks and other minorities, labor unions, the aged, women, the peace movement, and environmentalists.

On the other hand, it is possible that the development of a broad coalition for a national medical care system may be one of the catalysts that bring about a fundamental restructuring of political forces in the United States. The need for such a realignment becomes increasingly evident as the Republican Party moves to the extreme right and the Democrats swing over to now-vacant conservative positions. A countervailing force is essential, and a citizens' coalition for a national health program—directed at prevention, care, and a raising of the standard of living—can help create it.

Any proposal for a national medical care system must take into account the unique features of the American situation. The United States is the only country in the world where capitalist development of the medical-care industry has been permitted to proceed to its logical conclusion: the increasing dominance of large-scale, profit-making corporations operating nationally. In other countries this development was halted at the level of the small producer, the practitioner for whom national health insurance meant economic stability and survival.

Given this situation we cannot blindly copy the Canadian system, since Canada is one of the countries to have solidified the role of the fee-for-service solo practitioner through national health insurance. Indeed, as John Hastings[10] and Theodore Goldberg[11] have pointed out, the Canadian system has, in one regard, played a retrogressive role; it has actually set back the movement for health-service organizations and community health centers in that country.

Nevertheless, we have a great deal to learn from the many positive features of the Canadian system; an American medical care system would do well to adopt them. Our system should cover the entire population; provide all needed services, including medical, dental, and long-term care, not excepting care in nursing homes; emphasize preventive services, home care, and rehabilitation; and fund all services without including deductibles, co-insurance, or extra charges. Finally, the program should be financed entirely through general tax revenue, rather than regressive social security taxes, and should calculate payments on the basis of a global budget, one that covers the full cost of efficient care by accounting for all services together.

We need to adapt the program, however, to take account of American experience and the specific features of the American situation. Payments to practitioners should be made only through organizations: community health centers (CHCs), group practice plans (HMOs), and individual practice associations (IPAs). These payments should be made on a capitated basis—a fixed amount per patient, with that sum reflecting the range of services provided by the organization in question. The capitation fees received by these organizations should be unaffected by their status as public or private, profit or non-profit. They should be allowed to pay their practitioners by any method they see fit: fee-for-service, salary, capitation, or any combination of these. The strengths and weaknesses of the several organizations and their methods of payment will be tested in the competition for subscribers; this will furnish the incentive, one hopes, for providing better and more attentive care.

There should also be higher capitation allotments for underserved rural and urban areas as incentives for physicians to move to those communities. Special assistance will be needed for construction of community health centers and other facilities in such areas, and for the affiliation of these local facilities with district and regional hospitals.

Administration of the national medical care system should be the responsibility of federal, state, and local health departments which would administer other health services as well, including programs for the prevention of disease, for environmental health, and for health research. All departments of health should be responsible to boards of health consisting of representatives drawn from all sections of the population. In addition, all providers, whether for-profit or non-profit, private or public, should be required to establish elected consumer councils to meet regularly with the directors of these institutions and which councils would have the right to appeal to the boards of health for investigation of and action on deficiencies in care.

Federal standards are essential to improving the quantity and quality of medical care and to assuring that an equal level of service is provided across the nation, but these standards must be developed in consultation with the state and local departments of health. Furthermore, there should not be one overarching federal program. Instead, the states should submit plans which meet the requirements of the national system, but should also have considerable latitude in devising ways to improve the basic program and tailor it to their needs. Such flexibility is necessary to prevent the solidification of existing patterns of service and administration.

A national health program should be able to garner the support of the growing number of citizens concerned with the need for effective disease prevention, an adequate standard of living, and government funding of medical care for the entire population. These concerns are shared by many groups—environmentalists, who see the EPA not only crippled, but setting standards that favor polluters; labor unions, whose members' health and safety are increasingly unprotected by OSHA; the unemployed, who have lost their health benefits; women, whose reproductive freedom is under attack and many of whose children suffer from sharp cutbacks in nutrition programs; families who have been dropped from Medicaid or who have had their benefits severely reduced; the aged, who see their inadequate Medicare benefits being further whittled away; and, indeed, everyone whose health protection has been undermined by the appalling escalation of medical-care costs, as well as by the decimation of public health programs by the Reagan Administration and its Republican and Democratic supporters in Congress.

Political leadership for a national health program will have the support of all these groups—in other words, of a majority of our nation. We must build a new movement, one that will provide this leadership and take the action necessary to make certain that health becomes a right, not a privilege, in the United States.

NOTES

1. Gebbie, K. "Impact of Cutbacks: Alternative Futures in Public Health Nursing," *J. Pub. Health Policy* 7 (1986): 21–27.

2. Fox, D. M. *Health Policies, Health Politics: The British and American Experience, 1911–1965.* Princeton, NJ: Princeton University Press, 1986, pp. 63–64.

3. Terris, M. "Newer Perspectives on the Health of Canadians: Beyond the Lalonde Report," *J. Pub. Health Policy* 5 (1984): 327–37.

4. Wilkinson, Richard G., ed. *Class and Health: Research and Longitudinal Data.* London and New York: Tavistock Publications, 1986, p. 14.

5. Desrosiers, G. "The Quebec Health Care System," *J. Pub. Health Policy* 7 (1986): 211–17.

6. Sigerist, H. E. "From Bismarck to Beveridge: Developments and Trends in Social Security Legislation," *Bull. Hist. Med.* 8 (1943): 365–88.

7. Sigerist, H. E. *Landmarks in the History of Hygiene.* London: Oxford Univ. Press, 1956, Chapter V.

8. Ibid.

9. Ibid.

10. Hastings, J. F. F. "Organized Ambulatory Care: Health Service Organizations and Community Health Centers," *J. Pub. Health Policy* 7 (1986): 239–47.

11. Goldberg, T. Review of Andreopoulos, S., ed., *National Health Insurance, Can We Learn from Canada?* in *J. Pub. Health Policy* 7 (1986) 405–14.

A NATIONAL LONG-TERM CARE PROGRAM FOR THE UNITED STATES: A CARING VISION

Charlene Harrington, R.N., Ph.D.;
Christine Cassel, M.D.; Carroll L.
Estes, Ph.D.; Steffie Woolhandler, M.D.,
M.P.H.; David U. Himmelstein, M.D.;
and the Working Group on Long-term Care
Program Design, Physicians for a
National Health Program

The financing and delivery of long-term care (LTC) need substantial reform. Many cannot afford essential services; age restrictions often arbitrarily limit access for the nonelderly, although more than a third of those needing care are under 65 years old; Medicaid, the principal third-party payer for LTC, is biased toward nursing home care and discourages independent living; informal care provided by relatives and friends, the only assistance used by 70 percent of those needing LTC, is neither supported nor encouraged; and insurance coverage often excludes critically important services that fall outside narrow definitions of medically necessary care. We describe an LTC program designed as an integral component of the national health program advanced by Physicians for a National Health Program. Everyone would be covered for all medically and socially necessary services under a single public plan, federally mandated and funded but administered locally. An LTC payment board in each state would contract directly with providers through a network of local public agencies responsible for eligibility determination and care coordination. Nursing homes, home care agencies, and other institutional providers would be paid a global budget to cover all operating costs and would not bill on a per-patient basis. Alternatively, integrated provider organizations could receive a capitation fee to cover a broad range of LTC and acute care services. Individual practitioners could continue to be paid on a fee-for-service basis or could receive salaries from institutional providers. Support for innovation, training of LTC personnel, and monitoring of the quality of care would be greatly augmented. For-profit providers would be compensated for past investments and phased out. Our program would add between $18 billion and $23.5 billion annually to current *spending on LTC. Polls indicate that a majority of Americans want such a program and are willing to pay earmarked taxes to support it.*

(JAMA. *1991;266:3023–3029*)

American medicine often cures but too rarely cares. Technical sophistication in therapy for acute illnesses coexists with neglect for many of the disabled. New hospitals that lie one-third empty house thousands of chronic-care patients because even the shabbiest nursing homes remain constantly full.[1] If the fabric of our acute care is marred by the stain of the uninsured and underinsured, the cloth of our long-term care (LTC) is a threadbare and tattered remnant.

For millions with disabilities, the assistance that would enable independent living is unobtainable. Nursing homes offered as alternatives to the fortunate few with Medicaid or savings are often little more than warehouses. In the home, relatives and friends labor unaided, uncompensated, and without respite. Geriatric training is woefully underfunded and carries little prestige.[2] Hence, too few physicians are well equipped to address remediable medical problems that contribute to disability,[3,4] while many are called on to assume responsibility for care that has more to do with personal maintenance and hygiene than with more familiar medical terrain; even when they know what should be done, the needed resources are often unavailable. The experts in providing care—nurses, homemakers, social workers, and the like—are locked in a hierarchy inappropriate for caring.

With the aging of the population and improved survival of disabled people of all ages, the need for a cogent LTC policy will become even more pressing. Yet policymakers have neglected LTC, for a number of reasons. 1) They have been unwilling to accept LTC as a federal responsibility in an era of cost containment. 2) Meeting routine living needs is a central feature of LTC, with biomedical issues often secondary. Hence, logic dictates that the system emphasize social services, not just medical ones, with social service and nursing personnel rather than physicians often coordinating care—a model that some physicians and policymakers may find threatening.[5] And, 3) LTC needs are largely invisible to policymakers because the majority of services for disabled people—of any age—are provided by "informal" (unpaid) care givers, mainly female family members, neighbors, or friends.

Long-term care services are those health, social, housing, transportation, and other supportive services needed by persons with physical, mental, or cognitive limitations sufficient to compromise independent living. The United States has a complicated and overlapping array of financing and service programs for LTC. Financing for LTC is largely independent of financing for acute care and varies depending on whether the need is intermittent or continuous, short or long term, posthospital or unrelated to hospitalization.[6–8] Private insurance companies have made only tentative efforts to market LTC insurance and currently insure less than 1 percent of Americans.[9] Insurance for LTC is unaffordable to most who need it and rarely covers all necessary services.[10–12] Thus, about half of the LTC expenses are paid out-of-pocket, with most of the remainder paid by Medicaid.

Presently the elderly spend 18 percent of their income for medical care, with out-of-pocket costs rising twice as fast as Social Security payments. Medical expenses cost the average elder 4.5 months of his or her Social Security checks.[13]

The financial burden for LTC falls most heavily on disabled people without Medicaid coverage.[14] To qualify for Medicaid, families must either be destitute or "spend down" their personal funds until they are impoverished. Furthermore, Medicaid is institutionally biased, funding nursing home care far more extensively than home- and community-based services.

Age restrictions on many LTC programs arbitrarily limit access, since about a third of the LTC population is not elderly.[9,15,16] Seventy-eight percent of the disabled who receive Social Security disability benefits, 14 percent of nursing home residents, and 34 percent of the non-institutionalized population reporting limitations on activity due to chronic conditions are under 65 years.[17,18] Children constitute 5 percent of the severely disabled, yet generally are not eligible for LTC under public programs unless they are poor.

Informal services are vital to millions but are neither supported nor encouraged by current programs. More than 70 percent of those receiving LTC (3.2 million people) rely exclusively on unpaid care givers.[19] Almost 22 percent use both formal and informal care, while 5 percent use only formal care.[19-22] Of the more than 7 million informal care givers, three fourths are women, 35 percent are themselves over 65 years old, a third are in poor health, 10 percent have given up paid employment to assume the care of their loved one, and 8 of 10 spend at least 4 hours every day providing care.[9] Such personal devotion can never be replaced by the assistance of even the kindest of strangers. It must be valued and supported, not supplanted by formal care.

We believe that a government-financed program will be required in order to ensure adequate LTC for most Americans. At most 40 percent, and perhaps as few as 6 percent, of older Americans could afford private LTC insurance.[9,10,23-25] The average nursing home costs of $20,000 to $40,000 per year would bankrupt the majority of Americans within 3 years.[26]

There is growing recognition that the crisis in LTC, as in acute care, calls for bold and fundamental change. We propose the incorporation of LTC into a publicly funded national health program (NHP). We borrow from the experience in the Canadian provinces of Manitoba and British Columbia,[27] where LTC is part of the basic health care entitlement regardless of age or income.[27] Case managers and specialists in needs assessment (largely nonphysicians) evaluate the need for LTC and authorize payment for services. This mechanism for directing appropriate services to those in need has allowed broad access to nursing home and community-based services without runaway inflation.

We also incorporate elements from several recent LTC proposals for the United States.[9,10,14,24,28-30] Most of these, however, have three important flaws: 1) they focus primarily on the aged and would exclude the 40 percent to 51 percent of those who need LTC but are under the age of 65 years[15,16]; 2) while most would expand Medicare, they would provide a major role for private insurers, perpetuating fragmented and inefficient financing mechanisms; and 3) they exclude nurses and social workers from certifying and prescribing nonmedical LTC services, inappropriately burdening physicians with responsibilities that are often outside their areas of interest and expertise.

Our proposal is designed as a major component of the NHP proposed by Physicians for a National Health Program.[31] The NHP would provide universal coverage for preventive, acute, and LTC services for all age groups through a public insurance program, pooling funds in existing public programs with new federal revenues raised through progressive taxation. This approach would improve access to the acute care that could ameliorate much disability, eliminate the costly substitution of acute care for LTC, prevent unnecessary nursing home placements, and provide a genuine safety net, both medical and financial, for people of all ages.

Goals for LTC

Nine principles are central to our proposal:

- Long-term care should be a *right* of all Americans, not a commodity available only to the wealthy and the destitute.
- Coverage should be universal, with access to services based on need rather than age, cause of disability, or income.
- Long-term care should provide a continuum of social and medical services aimed at maximizing functional independence.
- Medically and socially oriented LTC should be coordinated with acute inpatient and ambulatory care.
- The program should encourage the development of accessible, efficient, and innovative systems of health care delivery.
- The program should promote high-quality services and appropriate utilization, in the least restrictive environment possible.
- The financial risk should be spread across the entire population using a progressive financing system rather than compounding the misfortune of disability with the specter of financial ruin.
- The importance of "informal" care should be acknowledged, and support, financial and other, should be offered to assist rather than supplant home and community care givers.
- Consumers should have a range of choices and options for LTC that are culturally appropriate.

Coverage

Everyone would be covered for all medically and socially necessary services under a single public plan. Home- and community-based benefits would include nursing, therapy services, case management meals, information and referral, in-home support (homemaker and attendant) services, respite, transportation services, adult day health, social day care, psychiatric day care, hospice, community mental health, and other related services. Residential services would include foster care, board and care, assisted living, and residential care facilities. Institutional care would include nursing homes, chronic care hospitals, and rehabilitation facilities. Drug and alcohol treatment, outpatient rehabilitation, and independent living programs would also be covered. In special circumstances, other services might be covered such as supported employment and training, financial management, legal services, protective services, senior companions, and payment for informal care givers.

Preventive services would be covered in an effort to minimize avoidable deterioration in physical and mental functioning. The reluctance of some individuals to seek such preventive services requires sensitive outreach programs. Supportive housing environments, though essential for many who are frail and disabled, should be financed separately as part of housing rather than medical programs. Long-term care services would supplement and be integrated with the acute care services provided by the NHP, such as medical, dental, and nursing care; drugs and medical devices; and preventive services.[31]

The public program, with a single, uniform benefit package, would consolidate all current federal and state programs for LTC. At present, 80 federal programs finance LTC services, including Medicare, Medicaid, the Department of Veterans Affairs, the Older Americans Act, and Title XX Social Services.[21] Other public programs finance LTC for the developmentally disabled, the mentally disabled, substance abusers, and crippled children. State disability insurance programs also finance some LTC. This multiplicity of programs leaves enormous gaps in both access and coverage, confuses consumers attempting to gain access to the system, and drives up administrative costs. Furthermore, the system is grossly out of balance, biased toward acute and institutional care and away from community-based health and social services. In contrast, the proposed LTC program would be comprehensive, administratively spare, and "user friendly."

Comprehensive coverage permits use of the most appropriate services and may prevent unnecessary hospitalization or institutional placement. Since most individuals needing LTC prefer to remain at home,[24,26] services should promote independent living and support informal care givers, using nursing homes as the last resort rather than as the primary approach to LTC. Services must be culturally appropriate for special population groups including ethnic, cultural, and religious minorities; the oldest old; individuals who are mentally impaired or developmentally disabled; children; and young adults.

Administrative Structure and Eligibility for Care

With a federal mandate, each state would set up an LTC system with a state LTC Planning and Payment Board and a network of local public LTC agencies. These local agencies would employ specialized panels of social workers, nurses, therapists, and physicians responsible for assessing individuals' LTC needs, service planning, care coordination, provider certification, and, in some cases, provision of services. These agencies would serve as the entry points to LTC within local communities, certify eligibility for specific services, and assign a case manager when appropriate.

The LTC Planning and Payment Board and the local LTC agencies in each state would pay for the full continuum of covered LTC services. Each state's LTC operating budget would be allocated to the local LTC agencies based on population, the number of elderly and disabled, the economic status of the population, case-mix, and cost of living. Each local LTC agency would apportion the available budget to cover the operating costs of approved providers in its community—although the actual payment apparatus would be centralized in the state's LTC Planning and Payment Board to avoid duplication of administrative functions.

Each institutional provider, e.g., community agency, nursing home, home care agency, or social service organization, would negotiate a global operating budget with the local LTC agency. The budget would be based on past expenditures, financial and clinical performance, utilization, and projected changes in services, wages, and other related factors. Alternatively, institutional providers could contract to provide comprehensive LTC services (or integrated LTC and acute care services) on a capitated basis. No part of the operating budget or capitation fee could be used for expansion, profit, marketing, or major capital purchases or leases. Capital expenditures for new, expanded, or updated LTC facilities and programs would be allocated based on explicit health planning goals separately from operating budgets by the state LTC agency. For-profit providers would be paid a fixed return on existing equity, and new for-profit investment would be proscribed. As Physicians for a National Health Program has previously proposed,[31] physicians could be paid on a fee-for-service basis, or receive salaries from institutional providers. Physicians and other providers would be prohibited from referring patients to facilities or services in which they held a proprietary interest. Providers participating in the public program would be required to accept the public payments as payment in full and would not be allowed to charge patients directly for any covered service. Federal and state budget allocations for LTC services would be separate from those for acute care, as in Canada.

Coverage would extend to anyone, regardless of age or income, needing assistance with one or more activity of daily living (ADL) or instrumental activity of daily living (IADL). (ADLs are basic self-maintenance activities [i.e., bathing, dressing, going to the toilet, getting outside, walking, transferring from bed to chair, or eating]; IADLs relate to a person's ability to be independent [cooking, cleaning, shopping, taking medications, doing laundry, making telephone calls, or managing money].) High-risk patients not strictly meeting this definition would be eligible for services needed to prevent worsening disability and subsequent costly institutional care. Local panels would have the flexibility, within their defined budgets, to authorize a wide range of services, taking into account such social factors as the availability of informal care.

When case management or care coordination is needed, the local agencies would assume these tasks or delegate them to appropriate providers, e.g., capitated providers offering comprehensive services. Not all those needing LTC require case management.[32] Case managers and care coordinators would work with the client, family, and other care givers to assess adequacy and appropriateness of services, promote efficiency, and respond to changing needs. Progressive decline in function characterizes many chronic illnesses, while full recovery is possible in others. Thus, change in need is a nearly universal aspect of LTC and mandates frequent reevaluation and flexibility. In all cases, programs should encourage independence and minimize professional intrusion into daily life.

A universal need-based entitlement to LTC would replace the current irrational patchwork of public and private programs, each with its own eligibility criteria, by age, cause of disability, and income. All income groups would be covered without means testing, which is cumbersome and costly to administer, may increase costs in the long run by causing people to postpone needed care, creates a stigma against recipients, and narrows the base of political support for the program.[28] There are scant data on how to set simple eligibility standards that ensure coverage for all in need, while excluding those for whom LTC services are a luxury rather than a necessity. We have chosen an inclusive general criterion (one ADL or IADL) and have left fine tuning to local agencies able to individualize decisions.

In all, approximately 3.9 percent of the population (9.3 million people in 1985) would be eligible for covered LTC services. An estimated 3.6 percent (7.6 million persons) of the total noninstitutionalized population need assistance with ADLs or IADLs,[15] including only 8 percent of those aged 65 to 69 years but 46 percent of those aged 85 years and over.[15] Another 1.5 million people are in nursing homes and residential care facilities,[17] and 200,000 people are in psychiatric and long-stay hospitals.[33]

Utilization and Cost Controls

Removing financial barriers to LTC will increase demand for formal services. Long-term care insurance could legitimately result in a 20 percent increase in nursing home utilization and a 50 percent to 100 percent increase in use of community and home health care by the elderly.[9,24] Increases in utilization might be expected to level off after about 3 years, as occurred in Saskatchewan's LTC program.[27]

Our program would be financed entirely by tax revenues, without premiums, deductibles, co-payments, or co-insurance. However, people permanently residing in residential care would use part of their basic Social Security or Supplemental Security Income to contribute to "hotel" costs. Although other cost-sharing methods raise revenues and discourage utilization, these regressive financing mechanisms disproportionately burden the poor and the sick and reduce the use of preventive and other essential services.[28,34,35]

Although we eschew financial barriers to care, utilization controls are essential since many LTC services (e.g., "meals on wheels," homemakers) are desirable to people without disabilities. Several states' Medicaid programs have demonstrated that screening and utilization controls can both control costs and improve care by preventing unnecessary institutionalization, coordinating services, and ensuring the use of the most appropriate care.[35,36]

The local LTC agencies, each with a defined catchment area and budget, would apportion the finite resources for LTC among those in need. These local agencies, serving as the single point of entry for LTC service authorization, would work with clients and care givers to select and coordinate appropriate services from a comprehensive listing of providers. This approach relies on enforceable overall budgetary ceilings to contain costs. The local agencies would have strong incentives to support more cost-effective informal providers and community-based services that might forestall institutionalization.

Innovation in the Provision of LTC

Broad changes in the provision of LTC are essential.[37] The current system is fragmented among many acute care inpatient, ambulatory, and LTC providers. This fragmentation creates higher costs through the duplication of bureaucracy and the failure to achieve administrative economies of scale. More important, the lack of coordination compromises the quality of care. A unified financing system would foster the integration, or at least coordination, of acute care and LTC—an essential step, since virtually everyone needing LTC also needs acute care. Financing the full continuum of care from a common source might also enable a more rational targeting of resources, with emphasis on preventive services, early intervention, vigorous rehabilitation, and restorative care. Expanded community-based services would allow earlier discharge for many hospitalized patients and might forestall hospitalization for many others.

The goal of the national LTC program would be to support and assist informal care givers, not to replace them. However, informal care givers should not be expected to undertake an overwhelming burden of care and would be offered predictable respite care and other supportive services, such as counseling, training, and support groups.

The program would encourage the provision of LTC by multidisciplinary teams of social workers, nurses, therapists, physicians, attendants, transportation workers, and other providers. Collegial relationships and teamwork should be the rule, with leadership from nurses and social workers as well as from an expanded cadre of well-trained geriatricians, rather than the traditional hierarchical relationships between physicians and non-physicians.[38]

The availability of capitated funding would foster organizations providing consolidated and comprehensive LTC and acute care services. Two LTC demonstrations that have employed such a model are the social health maintenance organizations and the On Lok Senior Health Service in San Francisco, Calif. Both provide a full range of acute, ambulatory, and LTC services with a capitated financing system.[39,40]

Although such coordinated care may be optimal,[41] individual providers could continue to operate on a contractual or fee-for-service basis. In some cases, family members or other informal care givers could be approved as providers. However, in these situations responsibility for case management and care coordination would ordinarily rest with the local LTC agency.

Innovation would be supported by earmarked extra funding that the state LTC boards would award to local agencies offering the most promising proposals. While each local agency would be required to provide a standard set of services with uniform eligibility criteria and reimbursement rates, this supplemental funding would encourage state and local agencies to develop services beyond the basic level and to seek and reward innovation. This is particularly important for improving services to different age groups, disability categories, and cultural and racial minorities.

Finally, missteps are inevitable in the course of the major reform we envision. Funding for ongoing evaluation is essential to rapidly disclose problems and allow their timely correction. Particular attention should be focused on key policy questions where current expert opinion has not been fully tested by rigorous research. In what situations does case management improve outcomes or efficiency? What organizational framework best ensures appropriate attention to both medical and social needs? What, if any, preventive measures minimize deterioration in mental or physical function? Are categories such as ADLs and IADLs optimal for targeting care?

Quality of Care

No other segment of the health care system has as many documented quality of care problems as the nursing home industry, and concern is growing about the quality of home care.[42–44] As many as one third of all nursing homes are operating below the minimum federal standards.[45] Monitoring the quality of LTC has been hindered by variability in state regulatory programs and the lack of well-validated regulatory standards and procedures.[46]

Each LTC provider (including home care agencies) would be required to meet uniform national quality standards in order to be paid by the NHP. These standards would include structural measures (e.g., staffing levels, educational requirements), process measures (e.g., individualized planning and provision of care), and outcome measures (e.g., changes in functional or mental status, incontinence, mortality, and hospital admission rates). Earmarked funds from the federal LTC budget would support urgently needed research to validate and improve these standards and to develop new approaches to quality assurance.

Each LTC organization and agency would be required to establish a quality assurance program meeting national standards and a quality assurance committee with representatives of each category of service provider (e.g., social workers, homemakers, nurses, physicians, and so forth), clients and their family members or other care givers, and community representatives. The committee would meet regularly to review quality of care and to resolve problems and disputes, with unresolved issues reported to the public regulatory system discussed below.

All regulatory activities of the current licensing and certification agencies, peer review organizations, Medicare inspection of care, and other agencies that monitor LTC would be combined into a single program. This unified monitoring system would enforce regulations and have the power to sanction and decertify providers. This program would be administered at the federal and state levels, with input from the local LTC agencies and provider quality assurance committees. Consumer complaint systems and telephone hotlines for quality concerns would be mandated. The regulatory agency would be required to employ sufficient staff to conduct periodic surveys of each provider and to investigate complaints in a timely fashion. Providers would be required to disclose financial data and other management information such as staff turnover rates, incident rates, and patient outcome data.

Improving the training, wages, and morale of LTC workers is also crucial to improving the quality of care. Long-term care workers currently earn 15 percent to 45 percent less than comparable hospital employees (US Department of Health and Human Services, Division of Nursing, unpublished data, 1988), and 20 percent of nursing home workers have no health insurance.[47] Nursing homes are not currently required to provide around-the-clock registered nursing care, few have specialized staff such as geriatric nurse practitioners, and aides are often inadequately trained. Many home care agencies have no professional staff or consultants. Wages in LTC organizations receiving payment from the NHP would be regulated to achieve parity with the acute care sector, with funding for this increase phased in over 5 years.

Funding would also be allocated for training and inservice education of LTC professionals, paraprofessionals, and informal care givers. Formal providers would be required to meet minimum training and competency standards. Augmented training is particularly important for nurses and physicians, who often lack experience in working with the frail elderly, the disabled, and the mentally impaired and in working with multidisciplinary teams to develop community services. The development of a cadre of physicians and nurses with special training in gerontology and geriatrics is essential. These professionals would play key clinical and managerial roles in integrating LTC for the elderly with acute care, as in Great Britain and other countries.[48]

Consumer Choice

Consumer choice would be explicitly fostered by the national LTC program. Each individual eligible for LTC services would choose among the certified providers in his or her area. Individuals would select a primary provider organization and/or individual care provider, including a primary care physician, and could switch providers if they desired. An independent ombudsman would resolve consumer grievances over provider choice. Consumers and/or their delegated representatives would be encouraged to assume control over decisions regarding their care and would be given assurance that durable power of attorney and living will provisions would be honored.

Costs and Financing

Estimates of current expenditures for LTC are imprecise because of the diversity of payment sources. In 1990 an estimated $54.5 billion was spent for nursing homes, $14.1 billion for equipment and appliances, and $10.6 billion for home health services.[49] In addition, about 10 percent ($25 billion) of total hospital costs were spent on psychiatric, rehabilitative, and chronic care services.[49] Thus, the total LTC expenditures were at least $104 billion in 1990 (16 percent of total health spending), excluding informal LTC services. Public programs, primarily Medicaid, currently finance about half of formal LTC. Medicaid pays for 48 percent of nursing home care, Medicare for 2 percent, and other public payers for 3 percent.[50] Private insurance covers less than 2 percent of nursing home costs, while consumers pay 45 percent directly out-of-pocket.[50-53] Consumers pay out-of-pocket for 40 percent of home services in the United States.[54]

Our program would replace almost all of the $52 billion (all figures in 1990 dollars) currently spent each year on private LTC insurance and out-of-pocket costs with public expenditures. Additional funding would be needed, particularly in the first few years, to pay for the increased utilization of LTC for previously unmet needs. The expected utilization increases of 20 percent for nursing homes and 50 percent to 100 percent for home health care[9,24] would cost between $16 billion and $21.5 billion annually.

Further funding would be needed to improve quality through increased training, wages, and staffing levels. However, some of these costs would be off-set by reduced administrative costs and improved program efficiency. Additional savings may result from reductions in disability and inappropriate hospitalizations. Precise estimates of these costs and savings are impossible. For our estimates, we assume that the net increase needed for the quality improvement measures (after subtracting potential administrative and other savings) amounts to $2 billion per year.

Overall, a total of $70 to $75.5 billion in new tax revenues ($380 to $410 per adult) would be needed to finance our program. Of this total, $52 billion represents money that is currently spent privately that would be shifted onto the public ledger. In effect, a broad-based tax would replace payments by the chronically ill. Because LTC has been seriously underfunded, $18 to $23.5 billion in truly new spending ($100 to $130 per adult) would be needed to expand care and improve its quality. Since almost every family will use such services at some point, this seems a reasonable price for financial protection and improved services for the disabled and aged.

These revenues could be raised from several sources, including the Social Security system, general taxes, and estate taxes. Expanding Social Security payroll taxes that currently fund Medicare would build upon the existing tax system and ensure a broad tax base. For example, a 1 percent increase in payroll taxes for both employers and employees would raise about $50 billion.[10] Increasing the earned income tax credit for lower-income workers to lower their payroll tax and removing the current ceiling on Social Security taxes would generate about $49 billion in additional revenue, while making such taxes less regressive.[10,28] Federal estate taxes are another logical source of funds for LTC and would have little negative impact on low-income groups. A 10 percent surcharge on gifts and estates above $200,000 would raise $2 to $4 billion,[9,10] and taxing capital gains at death would raise about $5.5 billion.[10]

Comment

Our proposed LTC program would be integrated with the NHP, creating a single comprehensive and universal public program for acute care and LTC. The program would be federally mandated and funded but administered at the state and local levels. A single state board would contract directly with providers through a network of local public agencies responsible for LTC eligibility determination and for case management and/or care coordination. All payment would be channeled through the single payment agency in each state.

Single-source payment is key to controlling costs, streamlining administration, and minimizing inequalities in care.[31,55] Private insurance duplicating the public program would be eliminated in order to decrease administrative costs, prevent insurers from electing to cover only the healthiest (hence leaving only the most difficult and expensive tasks for the public sector), and guard against the emergence of two-class care.[30,56]

Prospective global budgeting for nursing homes and community-based services would simplify administration and virtually eliminate billing and eligibility determination. Prohibiting the use of operating funds for capital purchases or profit would minimize financial incentives both for skimping on care (as under the current per-diem nursing home payment system) and for excessive intervention (as under the fee-for-service payments received by many home care providers). The separate appropriation of capital funds would facilitate rational health planning.

Current capital spending largely determines future operating costs, as well as the distribution of facilities and programs. Combining operating and capital payments, as under the existing reimbursement system, allows prosperous providers to expand and modernize, whereas impoverished ones cannot, regardless of their quality or the needs of the population they serve. The NHP would replace this implicit mechanism for distributing capital with an explicit one. Capital funds would be allocated on the basis of a comprehensive planning process, with the involvement of health planners, community members, and providers. Priority would be given to underserved regions and populations and to the development of home- and community-based services, to correct the current bias toward institutional care. While funds for sheltered and supportive housing are more appropriately part of a housing rather than a medical care program, coordination in planning of housing and LTC is essential.

Issues of profit-making are particularly problematic in LTC, where 75 percent of the nursing homes and a growing proportion of home care agencies are proprietary.[17] There is ample documentation of LTC providers' skimping on basic services and staffing in order to maximize profits.[46,57] As previously proposed,[31] the NHP would pay owners of for-profit providers a reasonable fixed rate of return on existing equity. Since virtually all new capital investment would be funded by the NHP, it would not be included in calculating return on equity. The proprietary sector would gradually shrink because new for-profit investment would be proscribed.

We advocate fully public financing of LTC for four reasons: 1) single-source public funding facilitates cost containment through administrative streamlining and the ability to set and enforce an overall budget; 2) financial risk is spread across the entire population (who are all ultimately at risk for needing services) rather than falling only on the disabled and elderly; 3) few people today are covered by private LTC insurance, and there is little reason to believe that widespread private coverage is practicable; and 4) there is a need for clear public accountability.

Public insurance programs are far more efficient than private plans. Administration consumes 5 percent of total Medicaid spending[24] and only 2 percent of the Medicare budget. In contrast, in 1986 Blue Cross/Blue Shield and self-insured plans had overhead of 8 percent, prepaid plans averaged 11.7 percent, and commercial insurers averaged 18.9 percent.[52] Many Medicare supplemental policies (medigap insurance) have notoriously low payout ratios, 60 percent or less.[58] Payout rates for private LTC insurance are low[10] and virtually unregulated. According to the General Accounting Office, of the 33 states with minimum payout ratios for general health insurance, most do not report benefit and premium data separately for LTC insurance, only 20 states even monitor payout ratios, and 12 states have established minimum LTC insurance payout ratios.[13]

The multiplicity of public and private insurers in the United States results in exorbitant administrative costs. Health insurance overhead alone costs $106 per capita in the United States (0.66 percent of gross national product) compared with $15 per capita (0.11 percent of gross national product) in Canada.[59] Additional unnecessary administrative costs accrue to providers who must determine eligibility, attribute costs and charges to individual patients and insurers, and send and collect bills for myriad insurers and individual patients.[60] Overall, administration accounts for almost one fourth of US health spending, but only 11 percent in Canada.[60]

Finally, public opinion strongly supports public financing of LTC. Eighty-seven percent of Americans consider the absence of LTC financing a crisis, the majority prefer public over private funding, federal administration is favored over private insurance programs by a 3 to 2 margin, and two thirds believe that private insurance companies would undermine quality of care because of their emphasis on profits.[26] While respondents want a federally financed program, they support the administration of such a program at the state level.[26]

The oft-stated view that the public wants LTC coverage but is unwilling to pay for it is inaccurate.[61] The 1987 poll conducted by the American Association of Retired Persons and the Villers Foundation found that 86 percent of the sample supported government action for a universal LTC program that would finance care for all income groups, and not just the poor. Overall, 75 percent would agree to increased taxes for LTC.[26] A 1988 Harris poll reached virtually identical conclusions.[62]

Conclusions

In summary, we recommend that LTC be incorporated into a publicly financed NHP. We urge that a comprehensive public model be adopted as a single mandatory plan for the entire population and that new public revenues be combined with existing public program dollars. This approach would ensure universal access, comprehensive benefits, improved quality, and greater cost control. Most important, the financial costs would be spread across the entire population rather than borne by the disabled themselves. Our nation has the resources to provide better care for the disabled and elderly, and it has a responsibility to develop a reasonable system of LTC. The public supports this type of approach. Health and human services professionals and the makers of public policy need the vision and courage to implement such a system.

The reader is referred to the May 15, 1991, issue, which was dedicated to caring for the uninsured and underinsured.

This proposal was drafted by a 17-member Working Group, then reviewed and endorsed by 415 other physicians and other health professionals from virtually every state and medical specialty. Members of the Working Group were Charlene Harrington, R.N., Ph.D., San Francisco, Calif.; Christine Cassel, M.D.,

Chicago, Ill.; Carroll L. Estes, Ph.D., San Francisco, Calif.; Steffie Woolhandler, M.D., M.P.H., Cambridge, Mass.; and David U. Himmelstein, M.D., Cambridge, Mass., cochairs; and William H. Barker, M.D., Rochester, N.Y.; Kenneth R. Barney, M.D., Cambridge, Mass.; Thomas Bodenheimer, M.D., San Francisco, Calif.; Kenneth B. Frisof, M.D., Cleveland, Ohio; Judith B. Kaplan, M.S., Cambridge, Mass.; Peter D. Mott, M.D., Rochester, N.Y.; Robert J. Newcomer, Ph.D., San Francisco, Calif.; David C. Parish, M.D., M.P.H., Macon, Ga.; James H. Sanders, Jr, M.D., Brevard, N.C.; Lillian Rabinowitz, Berkeley, Calif.; and Howard Waitzkin, M.D., Ph.D., Anaheim, Calif.

NOTES

1. Holahan J., Dubay L.C., Kenney G., Welch W.P., Bishop C., Dor A. Should Medicare compensate hospitals for administratively necessary days? *Milbank Q.* 1989;67:137–167.

2. Hazzard W.R. A report card on academic geriatrics in 1991: a struggle for academic respectability. *Ann Intern Med.* 1991;115:229–230.

3. Rowe J.W., Drossman E., Bond E. Academic geriatrics for the year 2000: an Institute of Medicine report. *N Engl J Med.* 1987;316:1425–1428.

4. Kane R., Solomon D., Beck J., Keeler E., Kane R. The future need for geriatric manpower in the U.S. *N Engl J Med.* 1980;302:1327–1332.

5. Estes C.L., Binney E.A. The biomedicalization of aging: dangers and dilemmas. *Gerontologist.* 1989;29:587–596.

6. Kane R.A., Kane R.L. *Long-term Care: Principles, Programs, and Policies.* New York, NY: Springer Publishing Co Inc; 1987.

7. Estes C.L., Newcomer R.J., Benjamin A.E., et al. *Fiscal Austerity and Aging.* Beverly Hills, Calif: Sage Publications; 1983.

8. Harrington C., Newcomer R.J., Estes C.L., et al. *Long-term Care of the Elderly: Public Policy Issues.* Beverly Hills, Calif: Sage Publications; 1985.

9. *A Call for Action: Final Report.* Washington, DC: US Bipartisan Commission on Comprehensive Health Care; 1990.

10. Ball R.M., Bethell T.N., *Because We're All in This Together: The Case for a National Long-term Care Insurance Policy.* Washington, DC: Families U.S.A. Foundation; 1989.

11. Firman J., Weissert W., Wilson C.E. *Private Long-term Care Insurance: How Well Is It Meeting Consumer Needs and Public Policy Concerns?* Washington, DC: United Seniors Health Cooperative; 1988.

12. Estes C.L. *Long-term Care: Requiem for Commercial Private Insurance.* San Francisco, Calif; Institute for Health and Aging; 1990. Study prepared for the Annual Meeting of the Gray Panthers.

13. *Private Long-term Care Insurance: Unfit for Sale? A Report of the Chairman to the Subcommittee on Health and Long-term Care.* Washington, DC: US House Select Committee on Aging; 1989.

14. *InterStudy's Long-term Care Expansion Program: A Proposal for Reform.* Excelsior, Minn: InterStudy; 1988;1.

15. LaPlante M.P. *Data on Disability From the National Health Interview Survey, 1983–85.* Washington, DC: US Dept of Education; 1988. Prepared for the National Institute on Disability and Rehabilitation Research.

16. *Issues Concerning the Financing and Delivery of Long-term Care 1989.* Washington, DC: Employee Benefit Research Institute; 1989. No. 86.

17. National Center for Health Statistics, Hing E., Sekscenski E., Strahan G. The National Nursing Home Survey: 1985 summary for the United States. *Vital Health Stat [13].* 1987; No. 97. DHHS publication (PHS) 89-1758.

18. National Center for Health Statistics, Schoenborn CA, Marano M. Current estimates from the National Health Interview Survey: United States, 1987. *Vital Health Stat [10].* 1988; No. 166. DHHS publication (PHS) 88-1594.

19. Liu K., Manton K.G., Liu B.M. Home care expenses for the disabled elderly. *HCF Rev.* 1985;7:51–57.

20. Stone R., Cafferata G.L., Sangi J. Caregivers of the frail elderly: a national profile. *Gerontologist.* 1987;27:616–626.

21. *Developments in Aging: 1988: A Report of the Special Committee on Aging, United States Senate*. Washington, DC: US Senate; 1989;1–3.

22. Stone R. Aging in the eighties, age 65 years and over—use of community services: preliminary data from the supplement on aging to the National Health Interview Survey: United States January–June 1985. *NCHS Adv Data*. 1986;124.

23. Families USA Foundation calls for a FTC investigation of insurance industry abuse of frail elderly nursing home insurance buyers. Press release. Washington, DC: Families USA Foundation; February 26, 1990.

24. Rivlin A.M., Weiner J.M. *Caring for the Disabled Elderly: Who Will Pay*? Washington, DC: Brookings Institution; 1988.

25. *Source Book of Health Insurance Data: Update*. Washington, DC: Health Insurance Association of America; 1988.

26. *The American Public Views Long-term Care: A Survey Conducted for the American Association of Retired Persons and the Villers Foundation*. Princeton, NJ: R. L. Associates; October 1987.

27. Kane R.L., Kane R.A. *A Will and a Way: What the United States Can Learn From Canada About Care of the Elderly*. New York: NY: Columbia University Press; 1985.

28. Blumenthal D., Schlesinger M., Drumbeller P.B. *Renewing the Promise: Medicare and Its Reform*. New York, NY: Oxford University Press Inc; 1988.

29. *Long-term Care Conference*. Washington, DC: Villers Foundation; 1987.

30. *Draft Proposal Long-term Care Social Insurance Program Initiative*. Washington, DC: Lewin & Associates; 1987. Prepared for Advisory Committee on Long-term Care, sponsored by the American Association of Retired Persons, Older Women's League, and the Villers Foundation.

31. Himmelstein D.U., Woolhandler S., and the Writing Committee of the Working Group of Program Design of Physicians for a National Health Program. A national health program for the United States: a physician's proposal. *N Engl J Med*. 1989;320:102–108.

32. Callahan J.J. Case management for the elderly: a panacea? *J Aging Social Pol*. 1989;1: 181–195.

33. *Hospital Statistics: 1986 Edition*. Chicago, Ill: American Hospital Association; 1986.

34. Estes C.L. The United States: long-term care and federal policy. In: Reif L., Trager B., eds. *International Perspectives on Long-term Care*. New York, NY: The Haworth Press; 1985:315–328.

35. *InterStudy's Long-term Care Expansion Program: Issue Paper*. Excelsior, Minn: InterStudy; 1988;2.

36. Justice D. *State Long-term Care Reform: Development of Community Care Systems in Six States*. Washington, DC: National Governor's Association; 1988.

37. Kane R.L., Kane R.A. A nursing home in your future? *N Engl J Med*. 1991;324:627–629.

38. Freidson E. *Professional Dominance*. Chicago, Ill: Aldine Publishing Co; 1970.

39. Newcomer R.J., Harrington C., Friedlob A., et al. *Evaluation of the Social Health Maintenance Organization Demonstration*. Washington, DC: US Dept of Health and Human Services, Health Care Financing Administration; 1989. Publication 03283.

40. Zawadski R.T. The long-term care demonstration projects: what they are and why they came into being. *Home Health Care Services Q*. Fall/Winter 1983;4:3–19.

41. Campbell L.J., Cole K.D. Geriatric assessment teams. *Clin Geriatr Med*. 1987;3(1):99–117.

42. *Hearings Before the Special Committee on Aging of the US Senate*, 99th Cong, 2nd Sess (1986).

43. *Hearings Before the US House Committee on Ways and Means*, 99th Cong, 2nd Sess (1986).

44. Kusserow R.P. *Home Health Aide Services for Medicare Patients*. Washington, DC: US Dept of Health and Human Services; 1987. Unpublished report OA101-86-00010.

45. *Report to the Chairman, Subcommittee on Health and Long-term Care, Select Committee on Aging, US House of Representatives: Medicare and Medicaid: Stronger Enforcement of Nursing Home Requirements Needed*. Washington, DC: US General Accounting Office; 1987.

46. Institute of Medicine. *Improving the Quality of Care in Nursing Homes*. Washington, DC: National Academy Press; 1986.

47. Himmelstein D.U., Woolhandler S. Who cares for the care givers? lack of health insurance among health and insurance personnel. *JAMA*. 1991;266:399–401.

48. Barker Wh. *Adding Life to Years: Organized Geriatric Services in Great Britain and Implications for the United States*. Baltimore, Md: The Johns Hopkins University Press; 1987.

49. US Dept of Commerce, International Trade Administration. *Health and Medical Services: U.S. Industrial Outlook 1990*. Washington, DC: US Dept of Commerce; 1990.

50. *Hearings Before the Health Task Force Committee on the Budget, US House of Represen-*

tatives, 100th Cong, 2nd Sess (1987) (testimony of Nancy Gordon, assistant director for Human Resources and Community Dept).

51. Task Force on Long-term Care Policies. *Report to Congress and the Secretary: Long-term Health Care Policies*. Washington, DC: US Dept of Health and Human Services; 1987.

52. Division of National Cost Estimates, Office of the Actuary, Health Care Financing Administration. *National Health Expenditures, 1986–2000*. Washington, DC: Health Care Financing Administration; 1987;8:1–36.

53. Levit K.R., Freedland M.S. National medical care spending. *Health Aff*. 1988;7:124–136.

54. Price R.J., O'Shaughnessy C. *Long-term Care for the Elderly*. Washington, DC: The Library of Congress; 1990. Congressional Research Service Issue Brief.

55. Harrington C., Newcomer R.J., Friedlob A. Medicare beneficiary enrollment in S/HMO. In: *Social/Health Maintenance Organization Demonstration Evaluation: Report on the First Thirty Months*. Washington, DC: Health Care Financing Administration; 1987:chap 4. Contract HCFA 85-034/CP.

56. Bodenheimer T. Should we abolish the private health insurance industry? *Int J Health Serv*. 1990;20:199–220.

57. Hawes C., Phillips C.D. The changing structure of the nursing home industry and the impact of ownership on quality, cost, and access. In: Gray BH, McNerney WJ, eds. *For-Profit Enterprise in Health Care*. Washington, DC: Academy Press; 1986:492–538.

58. *Report to the Subcommittee on Health, Committee on Ways and Means, House of Representatives: Medigap Insurance Law Has Increased Protection Against Substandard and Overpriced Policies*. Washington, DC: US General Accounting Office; 1986.

59. Evans R.G., Lomas J., Barer M.L., et al. Controlling health expenditures—the Canadian reality. *N Engl J Med*. 1989;320:571–577.

60. Woolhandler S., Himmelstein D.U. The deteriorating administrative efficiency of the US health care system. *N Engl J Med*. 1991;324:1253–1258.

61. Blendon R.J. The public's view of the future of health care. *JAMA*. 1988;259:3587–3593.

62. Harris L. *Majorities Favor Passage of Long-term Health Care Legislation*. New York, NY: Louis Harris & Associates; 1988.

IN SEARCH OF A SOLUTION: THE NEED FOR COMMUNITY-BASED CARE

Barbara Caress

This article is based on proposals and suggestions made in a March 1989 report by Local 1199, Drug, Hospital and Health Care Employees Union, titled "Report to Governor Cuomo on New York's Health Care Crisis."

What must be done to break the gridlock that grips New York City's health care system? We must begin at the beginning. New York had an expensive and somewhat dysfunctional health care system even before the current crisis hit. With its excessive reliance on high technology and acute inpatient services to meet the health needs of the population, this system never provided adequate support for the types of services that would have averted the current crisis —primary, preventively oriented, well-managed ambulatory care. After-care resources—both institutional and community based—are similarly lacking. These are the services that can prevent hospitalizations and divert patients from the acute-care system.

The solution to New York City's health care crisis, then, lies in the creation—or re-creation—of community-based programs that can provide the services badly needed to relieve hospital overcrowding: primary care; prenatal services; preventive health care and education; substance abuse services; mental health services; early intervention with and management of chronic diseases, from arthritis to AIDS; and continuing aftercare.

For this effort to succeed, these services must be integrated and coordinated. If one provider or group of providers cannot furnish certain key services (such as drug abuse or mental health services), they must be tied into a service network that can. Creating isolated programs to deal with one set of problems without such a support network will prove both expensive, because some services will be duplicated, and ineffective, because many patients will not get the services they need. In time, creating a full and integrated network of services will prove cost-effective, but at the beginning it will require the pooling of existing resources and new investment.

Ultimately, this service network will be the salvation of that part of the state's Medicaid program that supports health services for the poor. Attempts to save the system by constraining utilization or cutting back on reimbursement to providers punishes recipients and will not improve care. Much of the perceived "overutilization" of health services by Medicaid patients simply results from the search to find care that will alleviate their pain. Once a network of truly responsive providers is established, penalties for overutilization can be imposed. Until then, they would be counterproductive.

We must alleviate the current crisis while creating the foundation for a re-configured health care system. Thus, we must address the problems in the hospitals where they are erupting, by taking steps to relieve the severe shortage of health care workers so that New York City's hospitals can provide more and better care. Simultaneously, we must relieve the pressure on our hospitals by providing alternatives to institutional care in the community. This means not only community-based primary care but also psychiatric services to relieve over-crowding of inpatient psychiatric services and long-term care facilities to remove the burden of non-acute care of the elderly and the chronically ill from the hospitals.

The proposals and suggestions presented here for discussion are intended for both the short and long term. We focus on the following areas: 1) reducing staff shortages, 2) community-based health care services, 3) increasing the supply of physicians, 4) reducing overcrowding in psychiatric services, and 5) increasing the number of nursing home beds.

Reducing Staff Shortages

The inability to recruit, train, and retain workers is at the heart of the hospital crisis. Upwards of 1,000 beds are unused because of staff shortages. Increasing both the supply and stability of the health care work force is an imperative. We must break into the vicious cycle at the point at which lack of adequate compensation creates the understaffing, which produces stress on the remaining workers, leading to greater turnover and continued staff shortages.

Health care workers are among the lowest paid of the state's unionized work force. In fact, the average wage of nonprofessional workers is about 20 percent below the hourly average reported for all workers in the state. Prior to negoti-ating a new industrywide contract, effective July 1, 1989, the majority of main-tenance and service workers were grossing just $320 a week, or $64 a day. That just isn't enough to support an individual or a family in New York City in 1989. No wonder, then, that the turnover among these workers is substantial. On any given day, fully 10 percent of the hospital workers represented by Local 1199, the Drug, Hospital and Health Care Employees Union, are still within their 60-day probationary period.

An additional effect of the hospital crisis and the precarious financial position of some hospitals is to put the workers' benefits in jeopardy. Among the 31 hospitals represented by Local 1199, 14 were more than two months behind in making payments to the health insurance fund. Two institutions were so far behind that the fund's trustees were forced to cut off health insurance benefits to over 2,000 workers.

Just throwing money at the related problems of staff shortages and high turnover among workers is no solution. The shortages among technical and professional workers have been long in the making. Enrollment in nursing schools is down 30 percent since 1980, according to the New York State De-partment of Health, and 14 percent fewer L.P.N.'s are being trained. The number of programs granting degrees in physical therapy declined 13 percent, and 20 percent fewer pharmacists graduated in 1985 than had in 1980. The list goes on and on—it's the same story for virtually every health profession.

The solution to the problems of both labor supply and stability lies in large part in creating real opportunities for people coming into the system as unskilled workers to become better-paid technicians and professionals. If most work were not dead-end, but rather a stepping stone to a career, more young people would be willing to suffer the rigors and unpleasantness of service and maintenance work. And, of course, no one should be asked to work for less than a living wage.

Specific recommendations to reduce the shortages and increase the stability of the work force include:

1. Increase wages and secure benefits.

2. Create a well-funded career ladder training program for current health care workers. Sufficient funds are needed to enable people to go to school full or part time while receiving full pay. A small add-on to the Medicaid and other third-party reimbursement formulas (0.5 percent) would provide enough resources to train upwards of 1,200 hospital, nursing home, and home care workers a year in New York State as nurses, lab technicians, X-ray technicians, and the like.

3. One of the most straightforward and effective ways to relieve the burdens of many health care workers' lives would be to provide day-care assistance.

4. An added inducement for people to consider hospital and nursing home work would be housing assistance. Institutions could use their tax-exempt status to purchase or construct housing at below-market costs for their employees.

5. To remove some of the inequities between well-heeled institutions and those serving primarily poor patients, facilities with severe staffing shortages should be entitled to additional reimbursement tied to recruitment and retention of people in shortage jobs.

Community-Based Health Care Services

Community-based health services are different than hospital-based care in that they are designed to meet specific needs of the patients or community. In the case of hospital-based services, ambulatory, mental health, and addiction services are all provided more or less grudgingly—they are never the main mission of the institution. At best, they are by-products of the training and research of residents. At worst, a hospital offers these services because the state health department has in some way coerced their creation.

Community-based services, on the other hand, must satisfy some community need, particularly if their income depends on patients using them. They are therefore more likely to be responsive to the particular problems of a community than hospital services.

Community-based services can be organized in a variety of ways under a number of auspices. They can be provided by community health and mental health centers and through small group practices. They may be run by local government, non-profit organizations, or independent practitioners.

Community health centers have a proven record of effectiveness and acceptance. But over the past 15 years, much of what made health centers unique— their community education and outreach activities—has been virtually wiped out by the stringent financial constraints imposed by federal and state funders. Still, and despite a multitude of self-inflicted problems, health centers are a major resource in many communities. In the Bronx, for example, upwards of 100,000 people depend on that borough's health centers for their care.

Even the best of health centers suffer from two basic problems—inadequate funding for treating uninsured patients and implementing capital projects, and insufficient management expertise. Both problems can be addressed through increased state and federal funding, channeled through regional or community development corporations.

Health centers and hospitals combined supply less than half the primary care received by people living in low-income communities. Even in the Bronx, where there are probably more health centers per capita and greater use of hospital clinics than anywhere else in the country, most people still depend on office-based practitioners. The problem is the quantity and quality of the doctors available to residents of low-income areas.

Few physicians choose to locate their practices in poor neighborhoods. Most who work in these communities are there because, as members of a minority group or as graduates of a foreign medical school, they haven't the funds to set up their own practice in a more affluent area, they can't get jobs in another practice elsewhere, and they haven't the academic credentials to join the clinical faculties of a medical school.

The most mercenary of these physicians know that few poor people are in a position to demand high-quality care and, as a scarce and needed resource, they can get away with ripping off their patients—working neither very hard nor very long hours. A 1988 survey by the New York City Community Service Society (CSS) of primary care physicians located in ten of the city's poorest neighborhoods found that over one-third of these physicians spent less than 15 hours a week in their offices and almost none had even an answering service to take calls outside of office hours. Less than 4 in 10 had admitting privileges at a hospital, and 80 percent had graduated from a foreign medical school. In fact, the survey, which located 701 physicians working among the 1.7 million people living in these areas, found that only 54 of them were graduates of one of New York State's 14 medical schools.

Yet some physicians are actively interested in establishing practices in poor and minority communities. The Health and Hospitals Corporation recently helped 10 young doctors to establish private offices in Queens and Brooklyn, and Presbyterian Hospital has opened three hospital-affiliated off-site centers employing 30 physicians in northern Manhattan. Neither had difficulty in recruiting doctors. The major obstacles to creating substantial numbers of similar private practices are obtaining funding for capital and start-up expenses and ensuring sufficient revenue from patient care. With Medicaid reimbursement set at $11 a visit, these doctors are otherwise tempted to resort to assemblyline and "ping-pong" style care to produce enough visits and procedures to generate adequate compensation.

Community mental health centers, another source of community-based care, are burdened with caring for the chronically mentally ill patients left out by decades of deinstitutionalization. There is rarely time or resources to do crisis intervention, preventive education, adolescent counseling, or community outreach. In fact, most community mental health centers can do nothing for someone with an immediate crisis or a serious addiction problem.

Perhaps the most direct solution to hospital gridlock is to provide community-based care through greater utilization of home care. But, although New York City's home health care system is probably the most extensive in the country, it is often hard pressed to find and train enough workers to meet the demand. In addition to the poor salaries and benefits home workers receive (particularly the lack of pensions), they are discouraged by the multiple licensing and certification processes imposed by the different state agencies that fund their patients' care. Frequently a worker must have three different licenses to care for the same patient because the patient's funding status changes as she or he depletes various entitlements.

The process of invigorating community-based care could begin with these specific recommendations:

1. Provide state and federal funding for regional community health center development corporations that would pool funds for capital investment and administer new allocations to pay for the uninsured.

2. Provide capital and start-up funds to qualified practitioners—physicians, midwives, physician assistants, and nurse practitioners—who are willing to establish practices in low-income communities, and raise their Medicaid reimbursement rate.

3. Refinance and expand funding for community mental health centers.

4. Improve wages and benefits of home care workers. Consolidate licensing under one authority.

Increasing the Supply of Physicians

Physicians tend to practice in communities similar to the ones they grew up in, and, by extension, minority physicians are more likely than others to practice in minority neighborhoods. But, far from encouraging those who would be likely to set up practice in New York's underserved low-income areas, its medical schools have a shameful record in educating minority physicians and an equally abysmal track record in producing primary care practitioners.

Of the 903 students entering one of New York City's seven medical schools in 1987, 63 were black and 30 were Latino, according to information gathered by the Association of American Medical Colleges. Only one in five came from a large city. Virtually all the rest came from the suburbs. True to form, very few planned to become primary care practitioners. Despite the fact that fully 15 percent of the nation's residents train in New York, fewer than 5 percent are enrolled in family practice programs. Even if we include general internal medicine, only 30 percent of the slots are allocated to primary care specialties—family practice, internal medicine, pediatrics, and obstetrics/gynecology.

Even fewer medical students, 14 percent, said they would be willing to locate their practices in a "deprived area." Still, these 125 or so students could potentially fill a big part of the gaping hole in New York City's supply of primary care providers in low-income communities. The deficit, according to the CSS survey of the 10 poorest areas, is a minimum of 550 to 650 full-time physicians. Unfortunately, after four years of New York City medical school and three to five years of residency training, these 125 will likely be reduced to no more than a handful.

Obviously, any hope of finding the people trained and willing to form the backbone of community-based care ultimately depends upon changing the admissions practice and educational philosophy of the medical schools and the structure of the residency programs.

The following recommendations are suggested to begin this process of transformation:

1. Limit reimbursement for the direct and indirect cost of medical education to training primary care physicians. Training of specialists can be financed entirely from patient care revenue. Provide a five-year phase-in during which the training institutions would be required to reverse the 30-to-70 ratio of primary care physicians to specialists.

2. Make state capitation assistance to medical schools contingent on implementation of affirmative action goals.

3. Establish and enforce affirmative action goals for residency training programs. Not even the hospitals of the city-run Health and Hospitals Corporation (HHC), whose patient population is 77 percent black and Latino, train many minority residents. Including graduates of foreign medical schools, only 12 percent of the 3,538 residents at HHC hospitals for whom ethnicity was reported in 1988 were either black or Latino.

Reducing Overcrowding in Psychiatric Services

Hospital psychiatric units are operating at 100 percent of capacity. On most days, hundreds of mentally ill patients are being held in emergency rooms or being discharged to non-therapeutic environments. But the outpatient mental health service system can't cope with the need for crisis care. People wait four to six weeks for even an intake appointment at community-based facilities.

The problem is obvious—the dearth of ambulatory intervention, drug addiction services, clinical after-care treatment, and residential placements for the mentally ill. With sufficient resources, many hospitalizations could be prevented or shortened. The revolving door of admission, discharge, and readmission could be slowed or stopped.

Acute-care hospital psychiatric bed capacity acts like a sponge that is never completely saturated. The moment a service is opened, it is filled. A large part of the problem is the lack of discharge alternatives. The experience of HHC is illustrative. Bed capacity was expanded 40 percent between 1982 and 1987, but the number of patients treated in the facilities was down 6 percent, because they were staying longer. The average length of stay increased from 12 to 26 days during the same period. Some of the increase was no doubt due to an increased number of people with complex psychiatric problems complicated by drug abuse. Most of it, however, was caused by the inability to find adequate supportive places to discharge patients to, particularly those with complex or drug-related problems. For example, almost none of the community-based agencies funded by the New York City Department of Mental Health will provide psychiatric or counseling services to people with drug abuse problems, not even those enrolled in detoxification or methadone programs.

The solutions are as obvious as the problems:

1. Establish more supportive residences in the community to provide discharge alternatives.

2. Convert some of the vacant space in state psychiatric facilities to residences and lease the facilities either to other providers, such as hospitals, or to community-based service organizations.

3. Establish relationships between inpatient and outpatient mental health providers. Most ambulatory mental health services, including hospital clinics, draw their patients from a relatively small catchment area; hospitals serve much larger geographic areas. There is almost never a relationship between the inpatient service and the various outpatient facilities, even in the same hospital.

4. Require publicly funded voluntary mental health agencies to provide services to hard-to-treat patients.

Increasing Nursing Home Beds

With nursing home occupancy also at nearly 100 percent of capacity, patients who might otherwise be released to the nonexistent long-term care beds continue to occupy acute-care hospital space. New York State's explicit and implicit policy of severely restricting construction of nursing home facilities is thus contributing to the gridlock in its hospitals. The facilities just aren't there to accommodate the needs of the rapidly increasing age group of those 85 and over. The city's fastest-growing population group, their number is expected to grow by 120 percent between 1980 and 2000.

Moreover, people with AIDS will increasingly be competing with the elderly and disabled for nursing home beds. In February 1989 there were 128 persons with AIDS in nursing homes in New York City. The New York City AIDS Task Force estimates that that number will increase tenfold this year and more than double again between the end of 1989 and the end of 1993. AIDS patients are thought to need more intensive medical services than the typical nursing home is prepared or willing to provide. Despite the establishment of very generous reimbursement rates for AIDS treatment in skilled nursing facilities, few nursing homes have stepped forward.

Clearly, an accelerated building program for nursing homes is needed. Some recommendations that would help speed the process include the following:

1. Lift the capital cap to encourage new construction. This ceiling on spending for nursing home construction is now set at $70,000 a bed, while realistic estimates of actual costs range from $90,000 to $120,000. Despite the recent authorization to approve applications for up to 2,000 additional beds in New York City, there have been virtually no takers.

2. Assist potential nursing home developers to assemble land parcels large enough to accommodate a facility in communities with the greatest need. The state or localities might create projects by assembling the property and then leasing it to the developer on a long-term basis.

3. Establish a central computer bank of available long-term care beds. Hospital social workers spend hours on the telephone trying to locate beds for patients who are ready to be discharged. It is not uncommon for them to make 50 telephone calls for one patient. To make such a system work, nursing homes would have to be required to list their beds on the system as a requirement for receipt of Medicaid reimbursement.

4. Lease unused beds from the Veterans Administration hospitals for long-term care of AIDS patients. Hospitals could become providers of long-term care for AIDS patients without converting any more acute-care beds and without major new construction by converting unused Veterans Administration space.

Enormous public pressure will be needed to compel the city and state to create community-based services capable of providing care to people where and when they need it. Continued attempts to "save the system" by discouraging the poor from using the few existing services available to them will only condemn our existing health care institutions to a crisis-ridden future.

HEALTH CARE FOR A NATION IN NEED

Victor W. Sidel

From a Socialist Perspective the Following Principles Should Underlie a Nation's Health Care System:

- Health care, like all other essential services, should be provided for improvement in the quality of people's lives rather than for profit. This precludes inducing people to use services they do not need or services more dangerous or more costly than necessary.
- Health care, like all other essential services, should be provided without exploitation of those who provide it. This requires distributing the limited resources for such services equitably among all health workers.
- Health care, like all other essential services, should be provided in ways that enlighten and empower people rather than cause mystification, alienation or increased dependency.
- Health care, like all other essential services, should be provided in ways that eliminate financial barriers at the time of need, permit the recipients to evaluate their care, to select among alternative services, and, where appropriate services do not exist, to insist that they be provided.

The Crises of Health Care and Medical Services

One of the most important failures in what is usually called the "US health care system" is its almost exclusive focus on medical services in contrast to health services. The most important determinants of the health of the vast majority of people in any society lie not in the quality of their medical services or even in the quality of their conventionally-defined health services but rather in the nature of their economic, social and cultural environment.

Care for the individual who has become ill—the usual definition of medical services—is of course important, but its importance almost always lies in the improvement of quality of life for individuals or their families. Medical services can make people's lives better through reduction in anxiety and amelioration of symptoms or of other consequences of illness. But medical services rarely have a major influence on the reduction of mortality rates for the population. The tasks of medical services are generally limited to binding up the wounds. These wounds have usually been made long before the patient arrives for medical services and often continue to be made, despite those services, in people's homes (or lack of them), workplaces (or lack of them) and communities.

Many physicians and other medical workers have attempted to respond to health needs through what is called preventive medicine. It is estimated, however, that in the US more than 20 times as much is spent on treatment than on prevention. Furthermore, this approach focuses on patients (people consulting a doctor or other providers of medical services) rather than on everyone in the community and, perhaps even more important, it usually focuses on the patient's individual lifestyle choices. Nonetheless such interventions can be useful and if physicians and other medical workers were better trained and better motivated in providing them, their patients would be better served.

But for most patients—and certainly for most people in the community—such techniques rarely scratch the surface in dealing with the determinants of poor health. Most of these determinants lie largely outside the control of individuals or of families. Nutrition and other elements of nurturing during the prenatal period, adequate diet and living conditions during infancy and childhood, good education, resistance to community pressures to use tobacco, alcohol, and other drugs, safety in the home and in the streets, and protection from environmental hazards are of critical importance in determining levels of health. Counseling individual patients and families on these issues, important as that counsel may at times be, usually ends up "blaming the victim" rather than accomplishing significant change in these determinants.

The ways in which people in the US are victimized are well-known: inadequate housing; high prevalence of hunger and of malnutrition; pressures to use harmful substances (such as cigarette ads) often focused on minority populations; and racism, sexism, and homophobia, which continue to deny equal opportunity and to increase the risks to those seen as different from the dominant group. Perhaps most important, poverty levels increased dramatically in the early part of this decade and remain high. We now have the greatest gap between rich and poor in the history of the collection of these statistics. One-fourth of all children under the age of 5 in the US live below the officially designated "poverty line" and one-half of all African American children under the age of 5 live below that arbitrary level. Furthermore, the "poverty line" is purposely set low and millions of children and adults who live just above it are also in terrible need. One of the problems of the US health care system is that these problems are rarely considered in medical care or even in conventionally defined health care.

Unequal Access to Medical Services

A fundamental problem in any medical service plan is placing limitations on the availability of specific services, which has been called "rationing." Limitations are necessary because no society can afford to pay for every medical procedure that physicians can provide or patients can demand. In the US rationing is now accomplished by limiting the coverage of public or private insurance programs that reimburse medical expenses in the private sector, or by failing to provide accessible or acceptable services in the public sector.

The result is that patients with sufficient private resources or insurance with comprehensive coverage can usually obtain the services they want, but access is limited for many middle-class and working-class people. Large groups, including many employed workers, students, and poor people not covered by Medicaid, are completely uninsured against the costs of medical care.

- Among people age 64 or younger, approximately 35 million (estimates range from 31 to 37 million), including some 12 million children, are not covered.
- The number of uninsured people has increased 30 percent since 1980.
- In 1980, two-thirds of the "poor" were enrolled in Medicaid; now less than 40 percent are enrolled. In 1981 alone federal budget cuts resulted in the elimination of 2 million people from the program.

Beyond those who are completely uncovered, another large group of people in the US are severely underinsured. Some 20 million people have medical insurance so inadequate that a major illness would mean financial ruin.

- People age 65 and older, covered by Medicare, now pay out-of-pocket more than 50 percent of their medical care expenses. This amounts, on the average, to 15 percent of income, although for many older people it is of course far higher. Even with massive governmental payments, these out-of-pocket payments constitute a higher percent of income paid for medical care than those age 65 and over paid before Medicare was established in the 1960s!
- For others, insurance is usually tied to employment. Large out-of-pocket co-payments are often required and the services covered by insurance are often less than comprehensive. Preventive and rehabilitative services are often omitted. Yet, in general, people don't understand the gaps in their coverage until they become ill.

Lack of insurance coverage is well-known to limit access, particularly to non-emergency care. For example, a recent study found that 50 percent of uninsured women were not screened by breast examination compared to 37 percent of insured women, and that 43 percent of uninsured women failed to receive a test for glaucoma compared to 28 percent of uninsured women.

Even for those who are insured, coverage may not make access equitable. For example, lower and slower reimbursements are given to providers by Medicaid than by Medicare or private insurers and many physicians and institutions therefore deny or limit access. Furthermore, some insurance mechanisms may lead to discharge of patients from hospitals "quicker and sicker" because incentives induce providers to do so. Other barriers include geographic maldistribution of personnel and facilities and difficulties in access associated with poverty, race, age, language, sexual orientation, and social conditions such as homelessness. For example, although they were all covered for costs by the End Stage Renal Disease Program, only 20 percent of African-American patients on dialysis received renal transplants in 1983 compared to 30 percent of white patients, only 21 percent of women compared to 31 percent of men, and only

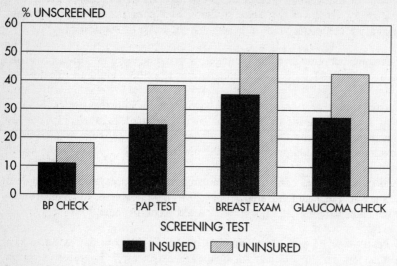

LACK OF PREVENTIVE CARE FOR
WOMEN 45–65: INSURED V. UNINSURED

Source:
Woolhandler and Himmelstein: *JAMA* 259:287

3 percent of those over age 55 compared to 85 percent of those aged 11 to 35.

Overall, a socialist perspective must recognize that the barriers to access to medical services not only consistently discriminate against the poor but are often also racist, sexist, ageist, and homophobic. Even the editor of the *Journal of the American Medical Association*, in a May 1991 editorial, points out that one of the major reasons for the lack of universal access to medical care in the US (along with South Africa) is "long-standing, systematic, institutionalized, racial discrimination."

The Quality Crisis

The costs to providers for billing and collection from patients and insurers are immense, constituting a major part of US physician and hospital expenses. Some 30 percent of hospital and physician overhead is devoted to billing, attributing costs for supplies to individual patients, bad debt service and dealing with 1500 different insurance carriers. The costs to insurers for payment and audit are also extraordinary. Private insurance firms in the US have an average overhead of 12 percent compared to two percent overhead in Canada and 3.5 percent in the US Medicare and Medicaid programs. Such administrative expenses of course divert resources from patient care.

Along with its failure to provide needed services, the United States relies on a fee-for-individual-service reimbursement system that provides hard-to-resist incentives to supply unneeded services to those who are insured or who can pay for them. Furthermore, the threat of malpractice litigation has led many physicians to practice "defensive medicine," performing tests or procedures to protect themselves from suits rather than because they are truly needed. Such unneeded services are not only costly to patient and/or insurer but are often dangerous.

Despite our huge medical education system, medical care in the US is often characterized by inadequate training and supervision. Medical licensure in the US is regulated on a state-by-state basis and most states are extraordinarily lax or inefficient in regulating and monitoring medical practice. Because of duplication of services, many doctors and institutions perform too few procedures for maintenance of needed skills. Conversely, because of control of licensure and financing by medical professionals there is often limited access to alternative services such as acupuncture, community support groups, or culturally-based medical care for specific groups such as Latinos/as and Native Americans.

Overall, a socialist perspective must recognize that the failure to maintain a consistent high quality of medical services predominantly affects the poor, racial and ethnic minorities, women, children, the elderly, and the socially or medically stigmatized—in short those who cannot protect themselves against the system.

Out of Control Costs

The cost of the U.S. medical care system is the highest in the world (currently over 12 percent of GNP, approximately $2500 annually per person) and growing rapidly—far faster than inflation. It has been estimated that the cost will reach 15 percent of the GNP by the year 2000. In theory, this cost should not be worrisome; it is preferable that these resources be used for medical and health care than, say, for military purposes. But when one examines how the money is currently distributed within the "health industry," when one contemplates who currently pays the cost (e.g., worker-paid premiums for family health insurance rose 70 percent since 1987), and when one considers how public funds pouring into the industry are being diverted from public education, public housing, reconstruction of our infrastructure and other urgent needs, the cost of the medical care system is indeed a troubling issue. According to the National Association of State Budget Officers, medical costs account for almost 12 percent of state budgets—the second largest expenditure after elementary and secondary education.

A major problem with the huge amount of resources flowing into the medical care system is that only a selected few benefit from it. There are large differences among incomes of doctors in different specialties, an even larger gap between doctors' incomes and incomes of other health workers, and enormous profits being made by drug companies and other medical suppliers. A widely-discussed reason for high physician incomes is the disproportionately high costs for education and training. Less widely discussed is the failure of our society to compensate family members or others (almost invariably women) adequately for the time they spend helping sick people in the home or in other settings.

Overall, a socialist perspective must recognize that the vast resources used by the medical care system represent theft from other vitally needed public services such as education and child care, and that the wealth pouring into medical care selectively benefits the haves at the expense of the have-nots.

Demanding Change

Every poll shows large majorities of the public calling for substantial change in the medical care system. Even among physicians, despite the widely publicized fears of many of them, 56 percent in a 1986 poll favored some form of national health insurance. Yet, because American Medical Association lobbying is so powerful, 74 percent of these physician respondents thought the majority of doctors were opposed to such a change.

Despite the obvious needs and the public demand, opposition to effective change persists. The AMA and other physician groups fear loss of physician power and income. Insurance carriers and medical suppliers fear loss of vast profits. Medical care institutions fear loss of control of resources. Medical schools fear changes of emphasis in physician education. Lawyers fear loss of income from medical tort cases. Government officials resist any demand for higher taxes to provide services. Management (except for managers of specific industries such as the auto industry, which is already paying high medical costs for its workers through agreements reached in collective bargaining) fears higher medical care costs to their firms. Some leaders of organized labor fear dismantling of their union benefit and insurance programs, which provide them with income and power. Nonetheless the increasing demand for change in the health care system may now begin to produce effective action.

The Scope of Changes Needed in Health Care

Dealing effectively with the vast problems that require attention but whose solution lies outside the conventionally defined health care system is virtually impossible for doctors or other health workers acting alone, however well-informed and well-motivated they are. It is only through political action—by health workers together, and in conjunction with others—that there is any hope of meeting these urgent needs in the community and in the workplace. Rudolf Virchow, a famed Berlin pathologist, was asked by the Prussian government in 1848 to investigate a raging epidemic in Upper Silesia. The underlying causes of the epidemic, he reported, were oppression, poverty, religious exploitation, illiteracy, and government neglect. Virchow taught that it was as much a part of the physician's role to work for social change in the interest of health as to treat individual patients.

In addition to increased attention by the health care system to community-based and workplace-based problems, part of the care of individual patients and families must include increased attention to "preventive medicine," such as immunization and counseling to stop smoking or wear seat belts. There is little or no incentive under current insurance programs to provide such care. A special area of concern is the area of occupational health, which is almost universally neglected in US medical education and medical practice. All physicians should be trained in counseling patients on occupational hazards and on recognition and care for occupational illness in its early stages. Furthermore larger numbers of physicians and other health workers need to be trained in specialized work in this field and given greater incentives to work on behalf of workers and labor unions rather than on behalf of management.

Principles For Medical Care

The specific problems of access, quality, and cost of medical care have attracted most of the attention of those seeking solutions to the problems of the US health care system. The following principles are based on those that have been proposed by the Coalition for a National Health System:

1. *Universal Coverage.* Access to care must be universal and cover all residents in the system in order to avoid a "two-class" system of care.

2. *Comprehensive, High-quality Care.* Coverage should include prevention, treatment, and rehabilitative services. Freedom of choice in choosing providers of these services in all disciplines of the medical and healing arts should be guaranteed to all.

3. *Local Control.* Communities should control their own health and medical services, which should be accountable to democratically elected boards representative of the people served by the program and of those who work in it.

4. *Rational Organization.* A network of services should be developed that are easily accessible and available to all. The quality and availability of services must be of a uniform high standard in all parts of the country, with integrated quality assurance.

5. *Equitable Financing.* The system should be funded through progressive federal taxation methods. All jurisdictions would receive proportionate funding based on population and special needs, through a centralized funding process.

6. *Elimination of Financial Barriers.* Out-of-pocket payments and other charges made at the point of service delivery should be totally eliminated because they are barriers to access that are inequitable, unrelated to the need for care, and administratively unwieldy and unnecessary. Financial incentives that interfere with the exercise of professional judgment, potentially leading to overcare or undercare, should be closely regulated or eliminated.

7. *Sensitivity to the Particular Health Needs of All.* Services should be designed to address the specific health needs of the community, particularly to hitherto underserved and oppressed populations, to bring all communities up to national health standards. Affirmative action provisions should ensure equitable opportunity to all groups in both receiving and providing care.

8. *Efficiency in Containing Costs.* The system should be publicly owned and administered locally with all personnel salaried. Rational and efficient expenditure of funds based on priority of needs will be the guiding principle in policy development.

9. *Integration of Research and Training.* Health services training and research must be an integral part of the system. The cost of education should

not bar any entrant into health care work nor leave debt that would discourage public service.

Unfortunately, almost all the "viable" proposals that have been advanced for changing the US medical care system simply attempt to fill in some of the gaps in insurance coverage and to control costs in the public sector. Most proposals do little or nothing to change the structure of the system.

Since it has been difficult to achieve a comprehensive federal program, activists in many parts of the United States are supporting state-based alternatives. The problem with state-based programs, of course, is that (1) the states are severely limited in their tax-based resources and may feel they cannot raise taxes to rates higher than those of other states and (2) there is little to prevent people in need of medical services who live in states with poor coverage from moving into states with better coverage. On the other hand, there may be value in supporting the best of these efforts in order to increase pressure on the federal government and because a federal program will undoubtedly require administration at the state or local level.

Most of those who advocate changes that would approach the principles set forth here favor federal action. However, national program proposals range from those that would do almost nothing to change the system except expand coverage on a retrogressive financing basis, to proposals that would establish an adequate national health program. Some of these proposals are:

A National Health System for America, proposed by the Heritage Foundation.

Would require consumers to pay for health insurance directly from insurance companies, rather than through their employers. Consumers would receive across-the-board tax credit for insurance and out-of-pocket medical expenses. An expanded Medicaid program would cover the long-term unemployed and the very poor.

Health Access America, proposed by the American Medical Association.

Would require employers to provide health insurance for full-time employees and their dependents, combined with the expansion of Medicaid to cover all below the poverty line.

Universal Health Care For All Americans Act (H.R. 8), introduced by Representative Mary Rose Oakar.

Would require all states to enroll their citizens in a qualified state health plan meeting certain minimum federal standards, jointly financed.

Recommendations to Congress on Health Care by the U.S. Bipartisan Commission on Comprehensive Health Care (Pepper Commission).

Would broaden the current job-based and public coverage system. All employers would be required to either provide insurance for employees or contribute to a public plan. The program would also cover the unemployed and self-employed. In addition, it would call for government-sponsored long-term care, including home- and community-based services.

HealthAmerica Sponsored by Senators Kennedy, Mitchell, Riegle, Rockefeller.

Would require employers to provide basic health insurance to employees and their families or pay an amount equal to 8 percent of their payroll to fund AMERICARE, an expansion of Medicaid, which would also cover the unemployed. A basic set of benefits, including hospital and physician services, prenatal and well-baby care would be mandated, but it would permit co-payments and deductibles. A commission would seek voluntary compliance with cost controls by hospitals, physicians, drug companies, and medical suppliers.

The Kerrey Bill.

Currently being drafted, it would be similar to the Russo Bill (below) in its use of progressive taxation and a single-payer system but would differ in its methods for payment to hospitals and medical group practices.

The Russo Bill (H.R. 1300).

Similar to the PNHP proposal (see below) in many ways. It would, however, allow for-profit hospitals, nursing homes, and HMOs to continue to operate if the states so choose, would cover only "legal" residents of the US, would severely limit reimbursement for psychiatric and long-term care, and would permit private insurance companies to act as "fiscal intermediaries." On the positive side, the plan would be financed by progressive taxes, would be a single-payer plan and would eliminate co-payments and deductibles for covered services. Introduced by Representative Marty Russo with strong support from many progressive organizations, including Citizen Action, PNHP, and a large number of labor unions.

Proposal by the Physicians for a National Health Program.

Modeled on the single-payer medical care reimbursement system in Canada. Calls for the federal government to finance medical care for all, with state-level administration, global budgeting for hospitals and negotiated fee schedules for practitioners.

Proposal by the National Association of Social Workers.

A federal single-payer program administered by states under a National Health Board. Provides universal, comprehensive benefits, including medical services, hospitalization, long-term care, dental and vision coverage, financed by a combination of progressive payroll and personal income taxes, with limitations for small businesses and additional taxes on polluters. The Board would establish global budgeting and negotiate fee schedules. Expected to be introduced by Senator Inouye.

Progressive Proposal for a National Medical Care System, proposed by the Council on Medical Care, National Association for Public Health Policy.

Recommends fundamental changes in the financing and structure of the medical care system and urges that 6 percent of all medical care expenditures be devoted to public health measures.

US Health Service Act (H.R. 2500), introduced by Representative Ronald Dellums.

Would establish a National Health Service with responsibility for all medical and health care for the entire population. Currently being redrafted.

The first few proposals would do little or nothing to change the US medical system in the direction of the CNHS principles and would not even approach the socialist principles listed at the beginning of this report. Proposals near the end of the list would be more effective. The proposal of the PNHP, now for the most part introduced as the Russo Bill, goes much further in changing the reimbursement system but fails to address many of the remaining structural problems. Nonetheless it has attracted the support of many of the progressive forces concerned about US health care. The proposal that in many ways comes closest to meeting the socialist principles is the bill introduced into Congress by DSA Vice Chair Ronald Dellums, but it is still incomplete and has essentially no chance of enactment in its current form.

The most important difference between the proposals at the beginning and at the end of the list is that the ones near the end would control costs by limiting the supply of medical services and providing rational methods for equitable distribution of available services. Proposals near the beginning of the list would place no limit on supply but would control costs by placing limitations on what individual patients covered by public funds could obtain. The principles on which the proposals near the end of the list are based are similar to those of countries with health care services based on socialist principles and incorporate many of the principles set out at the beginning of this report; the proposals near the beginning of the list are much more likely to be based on ability to pay and to leave unchanged the current inequitable and costly medical care system, therefore preserving the worst capitalist principles on which the current system is based.

Paying for It All

Where is the money for such ambitious programs to come from? For the medical services portion of the program, reorganization that markedly reduces the extraordinarily high administrative expenses of the current medical system, eliminates duplication of services, curbs excess physician income and private sector profits, rationalizes the malpractice tort system, and reduces the provision of unneeded services, would permit large sums to be shifted to the provision of needed care. These might be sufficient, given adequate controls on cost inflation and technological expansion of the system, to meet the needs of new patients who would now be able to use medical services. For the health services ("preventive medicine") portion, additional sums might be needed, but these would not be overwhelming. On the other hand large additional funding would be required in any realistic attempts to reduce the societal causes of illness through community services and social change.

Some of these additional funds could be recaptured from the military—the so-called "peace dividend"—but we are unlikely to see a great deal of these resources in the immediate future. The other source, of course, is progressive taxation. At this point approximately 35 percent of our national wealth is owned by the top 1 percent of our population—very similar to the situation in 1929. There was then a fall, to 23 percent of wealth owned by the top 1 percent. Now, as a result of tax breaks and other economic advantages for the rich, our obscene and dangerous maldistribution of wealth has returned to the 1929 level. Higher taxes on the wealthy and on corporations is the only just response to this maldistribution, and would also provide a source of funding to meet our need for publicly financed services.

Sweden, which many of its progressive leaders believe may now demand too much in taxes, collects them at a level of 57 percent of its Gross Domestic Product (GDP) at the national, provincial, and local level. Sweden is followed in descending order of percent of GDP collected in taxes by Denmark (51), the Netherlands (46), Norway (46), Belgium (45), France (44), Luxembourg (43), Austria (41), Ireland (39), Italy (38), West Germany (38), Great Britain (37), Greece (36), Portugal (35), Finland (35), Spain (34), Canada (33), Switzerland (32), Iceland (32), Japan (31), Australia (31), and the United States, which collects only 30 percent of its GDP in taxes. To meet the needs of our people and to conform to principles of justice, the U.S. will have to move from its current tax levels to the levels of Western Europe, from 30 percent to 35 or even 40 percent of GDP, with the burden falling appropriately on the rich through steeply progressive tax rates.

CHANGES IN AVERAGE FAMILY INCOMES, 1979–1989
(BEFORE TAX, IN 1989 DOLLARS)

National income category	1979	1989	change: 1979–89 ($)	(%)
Poorest fifth	$ 9,990	$ 9,431	$ −599	−5.6%
Next poorest fifth	22,040	22,018	−22	−0.1
Middle fifth	33,287	34,206	919	2.8
Next richest fifth	45,837	49,213	3,376	7.4
Richest fifth	79,425	92,663	13,238	16.7
Richest five percent	$120,253	$148,438	$28,185	23.4%

Center on Budget and Policy Priorities

Source:

US Census Bureau

DISTRIBUTION OF TOTAL
FAMILY INCOME IN 1989

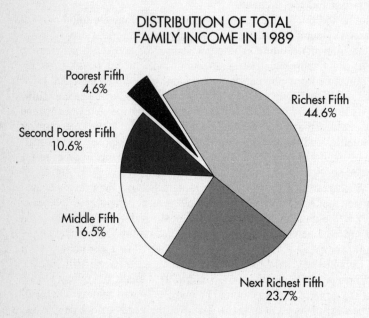

Poorest Fifth
4.6%

Second Poorest Fifth
10.6%

Middle Fifth
16.5%

Richest Fifth
44.6%

Next Richest Fifth
23.7%

Center on Budget and Policy Priorities

Source:

U.S. Census Bureau

INSURANCE OVERHEAD
UNITED STATES & CANADA, 1987

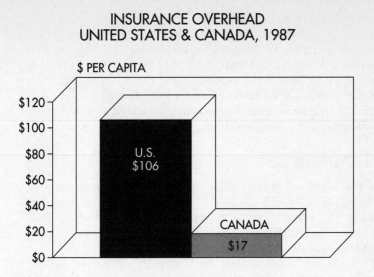

$ PER CAPITA

U.S.
$106

CANADA
$17

Source:
NCHS and HLTH and Welfare Canada

PERCENT OF PEOPLE AVOIDING CARE
BECAUSE OF COST, 1981 AND 1987

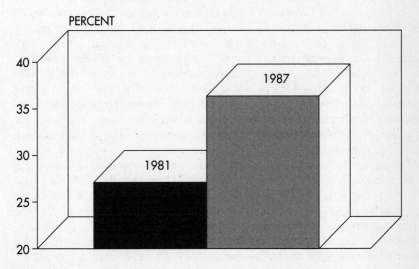

PERCENT

1987

1981

Source:
HLTH AF 1989;8(1):111

How then can the rich be prevented from distorting the system by buying whatever services they want? The answer lies in an almost exclusively public system, as in Sweden and in the United Kingdom before Thatcher. If a ''one-class'' system is to be approached, those who want private services must pay the true costs of the facilities, the education of the professionals, and the opportunity denials to others. The true cost is likely to be so high that only a tiny percentage can afford the non-covered private services and, if they do, they will contribute substantially to funding good care for everyone else.

What Can Activists Do?

It is clear that significant change in the US medical care system is coming, and coming soon. The editor of the *Journal of the American Medical Association* entitled his May 1991 editorial, which we referred to earlier, ''National Health Reform: An Aura of Inevitability Is Upon Us.'' The issue is not whether change will come but the shape of that change.

The best way to fight for change in the US health care system so that it meets the goals we have set forth to any large degree is within the broader struggle for democratic socialism to change the socioeconomic principles on which US society is based. Yet societies such as Sweden teach us that it is possible within a basically capitalist society to operate on socialist principles that bring health services and many other social programs closer to our model. Even lacking such principles in the general society, it is possible politically, I believe, to begin to restructure the US health care system in ways that bring it closer to our desired principles and even bring our society closer to a just and decent one.

Our struggle for national health care must address both the crisis of access and the crisis of quality. We should fight for community-based answers to health problems, providing care that focuses on individuals and families and on the social and physical environment in which we live. For example, a health care system based on a socialist perspective will make certain that: adequate nutrition and other elements of nurturing are available during the prenatal period; adequate diet and living conditions are available especially during infancy and childhood; effective education is provided for all; resistance is strengthened to community pressures to use tobacco, alcohol, and other drugs; measures are introduced to increase safety in the home, workplace and streets; and that there is adequate protection from environmental hazards.

Having the support of labor unions, which were instrumental in forcing the development of excellent health care programs in Europe and Canada, is a vital first step. Convincing the skeptics among organized labor that it will be in labor's interest to join in the effort for a significant change in the health care system will have to be a large part of the struggle. There are also some large industries, such as the auto industry, that may be supportive because of their current large outlays for insurance—outlays they would not have to make if the medical care system were rationalized and financed from progressive tax revenues. But the real support for change will have to come from the users of the system, middle and working class as well as poor people, who would have to be convinced that with the new system they would receive better care without significant added cost.

Democratic socialists have a special role to play in the struggle for national health care. Because of their exhaustive critique of the U.S. economic and political system and participation in a broad range of progressive efforts, democratic socialists are able to make important links among all of the issues affecting the health of our country. A demand for reorganization of our national health care system consistent with the principles set forth here will not only enhance the debate but will also improve the chances for success.

ANOTHER KIND OF BRONX CHEER: COMMUNITY-ORIENTED PRIMARY CARE AT THE MONTEFIORE FAMILY HEALTH CENTER

Hal Strelnick and Richard Younge

Fordham Road is the main east-west commercial strip in the Bronx, passing not only the now-closed original Alexander's Department Store; but Dick Gidron Cadillac, the largest black-owned business in New York City; Tremont Savings and Loan, for many years the tallest building in the Bronx; Sears and Roebuck; and the Rose Hill campus of Fordham University. Just east of the University, Fordham Road divides the world-famous Bronx Zoo from its equally famous New York Botanical Gardens. During the 1970s and 1980s Fordham Road also served as the northern boundary, both geographically and sociologically, of the South Bronx and its epidemic of fires and abandoned buildings, the symbol of urban poverty.

This section of Fordham Road has seen many businesses come and go: Crazy Eddie's, the discount electronics chain that terrorized the airwaves with their "insane" commercials before going bankrupt; Jahn's, the century-old ice cream parlor that closed after a fire; and Loehman's, the discount women's clothing chain that began here and recently moved its Bronx store to a former ice skating rink on Broadway. Fordham Road also passes the University parking lot where Fordham Hospital once stood and until 1977 served this community's health care needs.

To secure the health and economic viability of Fordham Road, New York State's Urban Development Corporation built a wedding cake–shaped, salmon-colored, tinted-glass office building halfway between Alexander's and Dick Gidron Cadillac, next door to Theodore Roosevelt High School and across the street from the university. The office building's construction was delayed for many years by a conflict with the US Postal Service over the relocation of its local branch office, one block south.

In the mid-1970s Paul Brandt, a Jesuit priest, Fordham faculty member, and student of Saul Alinsky, began organizing community groups to prevent the spread of the arson and abandonment of the South Bronx to this Fordham neighborhood. Each based in a local church, neighborhood organizations were formed in Morris Heights, Kingsbridge, University Heights, South Fordham, Fordham-Bedford, and Mosholu-Woodlawn, focused on issues ranging from youth to garbage collection, antiarson to antiredlining. Together they formed the North-west Bronx Community and Clergy Coalition. By the mid-1980s the coalition had such a strong reputation for effective action that in 1985 then-Mayor Edward Koch asked its grandmotherly president to appear in one of his reelection commercials. She declined.

Health care had been on the coalition's agenda beginning in the early 1970s. Paul Brandt had led demonstrations outside many of the storefront clinics that had proliferated in the Fordham and Morris Heights neighborhoods in what were officially called "shared health facilities," but colloquially were known as "Medicaid mills." These clinics were frequently owned by entrepreneurs who hired physicians paid on a piecework basis that only could survive financially through high-volume, brief-visit medicine. The demonstrations followed several incidents of poor patient care. Many of the picketed clinics closed. Others just moved a few blocks away.

An antiquated physical plant doomed Fordham Hospital, which served the Fordham and Belmont neighborhoods. A site for the "new Fordham Hospital" was razed in the Crotona section of the Bronx, just a few blocks south and east, but the city's fiscal crisis ended those plans. Then in 1977 Fordham Hospital was closed by New York City's Health and Hospital Corporation, as clinical services were consolidated from Morrisania Hospital in the West Bronx and Fordham in the Central Bronx in a new facility, North Central Bronx Hospital, which stands next door to Montefiore Medical Center on land donated by Montefiore to the city. The coalition organized efforts to "Save Fordham Hospital," but the fiscal crisis prevailed. Paul Brandt was reassigned to Chicago.

Meanwhile, Montefiore's Residency Program in Social Medicine was looking for a new site for its family practice program. The Residency Program was begun in 1970 at the Dr. Martin Luther King, Jr., Health Center (MLK) when its founders could not find primary care physicians who could work collaboratively in health teams with community activists and family health workers. Family practice was added in 1973 when Dr. Frances Siegel, a long time Bronx family doctor, was recruited as its first director. Family practice residents saw patients at the Bathgate Satellite of MLK, but as the housing stock disappeared in that neighborhood, there were not enough patients to support the training program. In 1977 most of the family practice residency moved to North Central Bronx Hospital, but this arrangement was not community-based and the health-team model conflicted with the hierarchial structures of the hospital. The family practice program began looking for a new home.

With the help of the Montefiore Planning Department under Vice President Mo Katz, several Bronx neighborhoods were studied to see if their demographics (e.g., the percentage of the population covered by insurance, mostly Medicaid) could support the family practice program. Several closed hospitals, including University and Bronx Eye and Ear hospitals, were studied as potential office sites. Finally, a site one block north of Fordham Road was identified in the hotel workers union health center, which had fallen into disuse as its membership dispersed throughout the metropolitan area and took indemnity insurance with it.

The Carter administration was sponsoring an Urban Health Initiative, designed to integrate the Community Health Centers and National Health Service

Corps, so that federal grants were available to start small health centers in medically underserved urban areas. One of the family practice residents (Hal Strelnick) had worked with MLK on its Urban Health Initiative grants in Morris Heights and in Crotona. Through pure serendipity he met the community organizers from the Coalition, Bill Frey and Joyce Kettner of the South Fordham Organization based at Our Lady of Mercy Roman Catholic Church on Marion Avenue one block south of Fordham Road, and Lois Harr and Arthur Marsh of the Fordham-Bedford Organization based at Our Lady of Refuge Roman Catholic Church. Meetings including the RPSM administrator, Eddie Fried, at Our Lady of Mercy began in the winter of 1978 to explore how the Urban Health Initiative might meet some of the neighborhood health needs created by the closing of Fordham Hospital.

In order to maintain accreditation of its family practice program Montefiore needed to create a full department with a chairman who would have the same authority as chiefs of medicine or surgery. After a national search Dr. Robert Massad, who had served as the chief of family medicine at San Francisco General Hospital and the University of Iowa's network of family practice residencies, was identified for the position. In order to recruit Dr. Massad, the president of Montefiore, Dr. David Kindig, had to commit the medical center to developing a community-based health center to house the residency program. With Dr. Massad's arrival at Montefiore in the summer of 1978 all of the key elements in the creation of the Montefiore Family Health Center were in place.

The Montefiore Family Health Center was originally conceived as a network of small Urban Health Initiative centers that shared administrative, social, mental health, and outreach services. The residency training center would consist of two such centers on separate floors in the old union health center. Dr. Massad secured funding support to develop the network from the Robert Wood Johnson Foundation. The foundation was working in ten cities to develop such networks with the federal government. Jack O'Connor and Anne Umemoto were recruited to continue the work with the South Fordham and Fordham-Bedford organizations and to develop and open the Family Health Center.

In November 1980 the Montefiore Family Health Center (FHC) opened its doors to its first patient, memorialized in a blown-up photograph of the neighborhood children coming in its entrance. The photo decorates the entire wall behind the third-floor reception desk. In November 1980 Ronald Reagan was elected President. His first budget in 1981 cut all community health centers by 25 percent. Many closed, and plans for all ten urban networks were scrapped.

The FHC was organized around four health teams, two on each floor, one on each hallway, originally to draw their patients from distinct neighborhoods around it. Both Massad and O'Connor sought to learn from more than a decade's experience in the Bronx with community health centers to prepare for a leaner and meaner 1980s. Many of the FHC staff were recruited from the Dr. Martin Luther King Health Center that Montefiore had helped start in the 1960s, where the RPSM began. Career ladders were developed for medical assistants and receptionists in lieu of MLK's extensive training programs. In place of the family health workers Ambulatory Care Assistants were graded, with the senior ACA III responsible for triage, outreach, and referrals. Family nurse practitioners, family physicians, and family medicine residents from Montefiore provide the primary care services. Leadership for the center's governing community board came from among the neighborhood activists from the South Fordham and Fordham-Bedford organizations.

In the summer of 1981 under the guidance of Dr. Vincent Esposito a community survey of hypertension was being conducted by medical students and ACA IIIs, door-to-door in the six-story apartment buildings that surround the FHC. Drs. Sidney and Emily Kark, who had pioneered the concept of "community-oriented primary care" (COPC) in South Africa and Israel, were coming to New York City for a sabbatical with Dr. Jack Geiger at the Sophie Davis Biomedical Program at City College-CUNY and would be teaching a faculty seminar on COPC at Montefiore. Dr. Esposito wanted to prepare with the community surveys that the Karks' books describe.

In the building across 193rd Street from the FHC a medical student and ACA III making their way door-to-door encountered an apartment with several children who spoke neither Spanish nor English. When an adult arrived, they discovered that the family was Khmer, recently arrived from Cambodia via the refugee camps in Thailand and the Philippines. After some investigation other Khmer families were found in the same building. Investigation revealed that in the closing days of the Carter administration, the process was set in motion to resettle almost 800 Khmer families in the Bronx. The resettlement agencies, of course, had arranged for the refugees' health care at hospitals near their offices in midtown Manhattan!

When looking for hypertension, the FHC outreach team had found displaced refugees with a myriad of health problems brought with them from Southeast Asia: intestinal parasites, tuberculosis, post-traumatic stress disorders, and depression. First, the Cambodians came for medical care with family members who could translate; then doctors and patients would pass a telephone back and forth while a translator at the resettlement agency interpreted. Soon, a couple of English-speaking Cambodians were hired as translators. Then the health center was alerted to Vietnamese refugees in the Bronx; long-time enemies of the Khmer, their medical care was organized on a separate floor and their own translator hired.

The refugees' problems began to reflect the stresses of their new environment: children with lead poisoning and adults with psychosis and post-traumatic stress disorders, and depression. A group of family practice residents during their orientation to the Bronx and the FHC went to a meeting of angry and confused tenants in the building across 193rd Street where the first Cambodian family was discovered. The mix of Spanish, English, and Khmer created chaos. They had problems of heat, hot water, security, and children suffering from lead poisoning. The family practice residents called in a community organizer from the coalition who helped the tenants fight the landlord for heat and hot water, new paint, and a secure front door. The iron grate door with the half moon design on 357 East 193rd Street stands as a reminder today of their organizing success.

The mental health problems of the refugees continued to grow more apparent. One middle-aged Khmer woman who spoke no English had a psychotic break on the subway when she became lost. The FHC's social worker, Renee Shanker, began exploring better ways than medications and hospitalizations to help her patients cope. When she learned that their traditional healing practices relied upon their Buddhist priests, she called in people from Montefiore's non-profit housing and economic development agency, the Mosholu Preservation Corporation. Working together with members of the Cambodian community, a house on Marion Avenue was secured, and their first Buddhist temple created. Today, the FHC's first translator has become a social worker and his successor a registered nurse; the temple on Marion Avenue still houses an active Buddhist temple. Grants have been secured to continue mental health services. The days of collecting used clothing for the refugees is past. A second wave of refugees, Amerasian children and their families, has arrived from Vietnam, while a new generation is being born after receiving prenatal care at the center.

In 1982 the New York State Department of Health decided to redirect the monies from the Reagan block grant for Maternal and Child Health that had traditionally gone to the major teaching hospitals for children and youth programs and to support community health centers. Dr. Michael Fisher with help from the FHC's first medical director, Dr. Richard Younge, responded with a proposal to establish a low birth weight prevention team that would do extensive outreach to encourage early prenatal care, as well as recruit a staff obstetrician to help increase the quality and intensity of prenatal care at the health center.

In the South Bronx with its many young families prenatal care should be among the highest priorities of a community-oriented primary care practice (COPC). Prenatal care works: The components of good prenatal care have been well described; they are inexpensive, and save lots of money.

Many studies have shown that women who enter prenatal care early in pregnancy have better birth outcomes than those who receive late or no prenatal care at all. Clinicians disagree about what components of prenatal care are most important for healthier newborns, but none deny that some prenatal care is better than none at all. To make care even more attractive, women at highest risk for problems benefit the most from good prenatal care.

Few aspects of medical care have been described and studied as well as prenatal care. Extensive, well-documented protocols provide guidance about what constitutes quality prenatal services. The American College of Obstetrics and Gynecology and the Institute of Medicine have produced comprehensive monographs that outline in detail what should be done at each stage during pregnancy. These guidelines address medical issues, such as the appropriate use of laboratory tests, ultrasound, and the physical examination. Psychological, social, and familial aspects of care and patient education and childbirth preparation are covered as well.

Compared to what other services the health care dollar can buy, prenatal care can be delivered fairly inexpensively. Nothing about prenatal care is particularly "high tech." The important screening laboratory tests are not complicated and readily available. The fanciest equipment needed to care for all but the most complicated pregnancies are fetal monitors and ultrasound, now made portable for doctors' offices. Good pregnancy care probably costs from $900 to $1500.

The $900 to $1500 spent on prenatal care can potentially save up to 100 times that amount. The costs of supporting a premature, low birth weight infant in a neonatal intensive care unit can run into the tens of thousands of dollars. If the tiny premie survives, the costs of aftercare, rehabilitation, special education, and other supportive services must also be considered.

Despite the fact that prenatal care works, that it is well-described, inexpensive, and cost-effective, supported rhetorically by politicians and opinion polls like "motherhood" of the cliché, clearly not every woman who wants or needs care has access to quality maternity care. In 1980 almost one-third of women in the FHC's neighborhood received late or no prenatal care. This lack of adequate maternity care and the availability of state funds for community health centers inspired the FHC to make prenatal care a central part of its mission in 1983.

The Low Birthweight Prevention Program (now called "Perinatal Services") at the FHC encourages women to register early for prenatal care, screens all pregnant women for pre-existing and developing pregnancy risk factors from hypertension to drug abuse. The LBW prevention team is staffed by a family nurse practitioner, a women's health nurse practitioner, a community outreach worker, a social worker, and one or two consultant obstetrician-gynecologists. The team works with the FHC primary care clinicians to develop and implement treatment plans for all women receiving maternity services at the FHC.

The team social worker addresses concrete service needs of patients regarding income and shelter. Helping to decrease stress about food, housing, and family relationships may play a role in preventing premature labor—the most common cause of low birth weight infants. The nurse practitioners teach individuals and groups of patients about diet, smoking, drugs, and recognizing preterm labor, as well as more traditional childbirth preparation classes in English and Spanish. They also review charts to help the primary care clinicians anticipate and respond to patients' biomedical and psychosocial needs. The community health worker coordinates patient follow-up and encourages women who have dropped out of care to return to the FHC. In the earliest days of the program she also promoted prenatal care as a community issue at local churches and community agencies.

Women who have medical problems at the beginning of pregnancy or who develop problems during pregnancy continue to receive their care from their usual family physician or family nurse practitioner, rather than being referred to a "high-risk" clinic at the backup hospital. This makes the FHC LBW prevention project unique. The patient's primary provider instead consults with the FHC's obstetrician-gynecologist on site as needed. Bringing the expertise to the patient, rather than sending the patient to an unfamiliar environment, has proven to be very effective, especially in maintaining continuity with high-risk women.

The LBW prevention program has succeeded. The FHC cared for about 350 pregnant women in 1983 and 650 in 1990 (see Chart 1). Close to 55 percent of the women entering prenatal care at the FHC came during their first trimester in 1990, compared to 30 percent in 1984 (see Chart 2). The women continue to be largely high-risk (see Chart 3).

The project may have had a more far-reaching effect in improving birth outcomes in the community. In 1987, the FHC provided prenatal care for about

14 percent of the 4,383 live births in its target area. Between 1980 and 1987, the low birth weight rate in this neighborhood declined from 10.5 percent of live births to 10.24 percent, a 2.8 percent reduction in the low birth weight rate. During the same period, the low birth weight rate for all of the Bronx grew from 10.3 percent to 10.76 percent of live births—a 4.5 percent increase. Similarly, between 1980 and 1987 infant mortality in the target community declined from 20.6 to 11.86 per 1000 live births, a 42.5 percent reduction, while the Bronx as a whole experienced only a 22 percent decline from 17.3 to 13.4 per 1000 live births. (See Chart 4.) Similar relative improvements can be found in neonatal and post-neonatal mortality for the target community compared to both the Bronx and New York City as a whole.

The relative improvement in perinatal outcomes for the FHC's catchment area compared to the rest of the Bronx could be due to a number of changes that occurred between 1980 and 1987, among them the LBW prevention program. Other changes in the community, such as decreased poverty, increased education levels, or other demographic changes, may be the cause for these trends. A more complete analysis of the contribution of the FHC's efforts to reduce adverse birth outcomes community-wide will be completed when the 1990 census data are available.

The FHC continues to look for ways to improve its maternity care and other community-oriented services. Recently, a number of FHC clinicians have become concerned about the increasing prevalence of substance use among child-bearing women due to the crack and cocaine epidemic. Substance use during pregnancy is underdiagnosed, even at the FHC, in spite of the continuity of care and emphasis that is placed on exploring psychosocial issues with patients. Acting Medical Director Dr. Joseph Lurio published the discrepancy he found between medical histories and anonymous urine drug screens in identifying substance use in the *New England Journal of Medicine*. When substance use is diagnosed, few drug treatment facilities are willing to treat a pregnant woman with a drug problem. The FHC has developed linkages with a program that treats addicted pregnant adolescents and its Health Care for the Homeless Outreach team has provided prenatal care to such women in welfare hotels and shelters. The FHC has begun enhancing its capacity to counsel addicted patients and plans to expand its capacity to serve addicted mothers through grant funding specifically targeted for chemically dependent women.

Prenatal care and services for Southeast Asian refugees are not the FHC's only community-oriented services. Special enhanced services are provided by an outreach team to the homeless and a team dedicated to HIV-related illness. The FHC works with adolescent group homes and a residential drug-free treatment program and has conducted employment-based hypertension surveillance and treatment, parenting and adolescent groups. A self-help network of Latina women in their mid-life transition based at the FHC recently celebrated its tenth anniversary of empowerment and advocacy. A satellite WIC office was opened on the ground floor in space once occupied by the X-ray viewing office.

The FHC faces the challenges of being at the epicenter of the urban epidemics of poverty, homelessness, HIV, and drugs. Space inside the FHC is at a premium, and outside realtors are speculating on the recovery of the business

CHART 1
PRENATAL ENROLLMENT MONTEFIORE FAMILY HEALTH
CENTER, 1982—1987

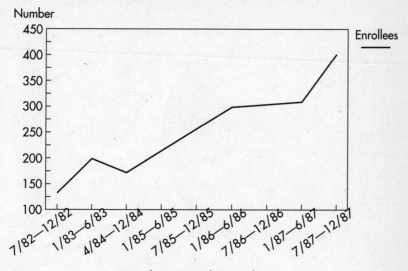

Time by Six-Month Intervals

district from the success of Fordham Plaza, whose primary tenants are the financial and administrative ''back office'' staff of Montefiore Medical Center. Recruiting young family physicians to the South Bronx from outside New York City swims against a tide of debt and Me-Generation values. Federal and state grant dollars become more precious and knotted in red tape and paperwork every year.

This Christmas (1991), despite the recession, the physicians and nurse practitioners at the FHC were bestowed with more gifts from their patients than any year in memory: ties, cologne, handkerchiefs, souvenirs from Puerto Rico and the Dominican Republic. Simple yet elegant ways of demonstrating how important a role the Family Health Center plays in their lives.

CHART 2
PRENATAL RISK STATUS 1987
FOR 629 PATIENTS

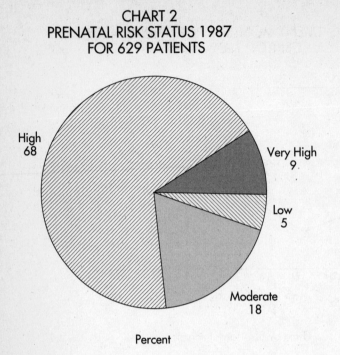

High
68

Very High
9

Low
5

Moderate
18

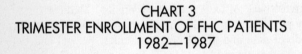

Percent

CHART 3
TRIMESTER ENROLLMENT OF FHC PATIENTS
1982—1987

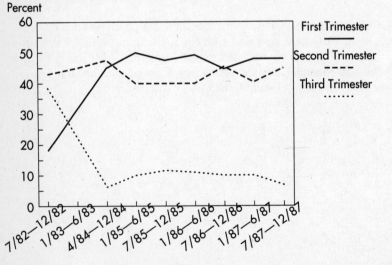

First Trimester

Second Trimester

Third Trimester

Time by Six-Month Intervals

CHART 4
COMPARATIVE PERINATAL BIRTH STATISTICS
MONTEFIORE FAMILY HEALTH CENTER, THE BRONX,
AND NEW YORK CITY, 1980–1985

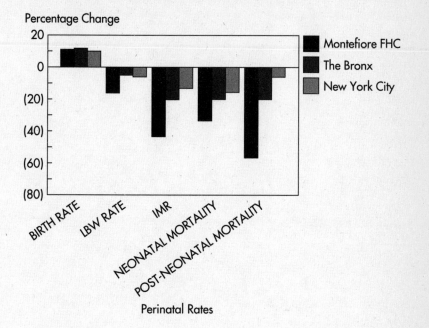

Percentage Change

Legend:
- Montefiore FHC
- The Bronx
- New York City

Perinatal Rates

SECTION VI

PROPOSALS FOR A NATIONAL AGENDA

INTRODUCTION

Arthur Levin

The national debate over whether and how to go about reforming our ailing health care system began to heat up in 1991 during local election campaigns and presidential primaries. After the Harris Wofford victory in Pennsylvania was taken as a divine sign that the nation's health care "crisis" was indeed an important political issue, the media seized upon the crisis, raised it up for consideration by the American public, covered it in *Time* and *Newsweek*, and filmed countless network and PBS television specials. For some health activists who had been on the scene for many decades it was a breath of new life for their lingering hope that health care reform would someday be a reality. For the more skeptical, it was yet another reoccurring cycle of several years of concern followed by years of neglect that has stymied enactment of a national health care plan for almost a century.

The placing of health care reform on the national political agenda dates back to the early 1900s. Teddy Roosevelt, in his campaign against Woodrow Wilson, argued that "the hazards of sickness and accident, as well as old age, should be provided for through insurance." Some two decades later another President Roosevelt, Franklin Delano Roosevelt, also made the case for a national program to deal with illness, but the idea of including medical benefits as part of the new Social Security program was scuttled to ensure passage. It likely is no coincidence that both Roosevelts were well acquainted with the human costs of serious illness and disability, even when money was no concern.

A decade and one world war later, President Harry Truman sent Congress a bill that included a commitment to the idea that medical care was a right. Organized medicine, playing to America's roiling storm of anti-communist hysteria, fought back, warning that the notion of medical care as a right was the left-led prelude to "socialized medicine." It wasn't until the 1960s, during the Great Society era of Lyndon Johnson, that the federal government finally made a commitment to meeting the medical care needs of at least some of its citizens through the passage of Medicare and Medicaid in 1965. Medicare was seen by some activists as a hopeful sign that meaningful, albeit limited, change was possible. The program was a single-payer, universal access plan for the elderly, a group that had been discovered in the 1960s to be sliding into poverty. (Medicare was expanded in 1972 to include coverage of the disabled.)

In the early 1970s, during Richard Nixon's administration, the debate about a national health plan re-emerged with new intensity. No less than 22 health care reform bills, most proposing some sort of national health insurance, were introduced in Congress. The discussion appeared not to be about whether America would finally adopt a plan, but which one progressive health care advocates and planners should support. The most progressive reform effort was introduced by Congressman Ron Dellums (D-Calif.). As Leonard S. Rodberg argues in his "Anatomy of a National Health Program," (p. 610) the Dellums bill (updated and reintroduced as H.R. 3229) is still seen by many as the only model advocating meaningful reform. But despite the optimism of more than a few that reform was close at hand, differences over the various proposals delayed action until the moment passed. The national attention soon refocused on matters other than health care reform, including Watergate and the resignation of Nixon.

In 1980 the federal government, led by Ronald Reagan, began in earnest its long march away from responsibility and concern for the social well-being of its citizens and residents. Social programs that had begun so hopefully in the Great Depression fifty years before, and that had been reaffirmed with such fervor in the 1960s, were seen as terrible mistakes and as the root of all the country's problems. Now, a dozen years have passed since the conservatives cynically began to punish those without wealth for having benefited by the emergence in 1932 of both a federal social conscience and tax policies that attempted to redress the gross maldistribution of wealth. In the 1990s the confluence of federal abandonment; the impoverishment resulting from severe national, state, and local recession; social epidemics of homelessness, drugs, violence, and HIV; and the ever-present inflation of medical costs have produced an American health care system that appears to most observers to be on the ropes, waiting for the knockout punch.

Harry Sultz, a professor of social and preventive medicine, writing in the *American Journal of Public Health*, delivered a stunning indictment of the decade that was the 1980s:

Nothing in the history of the United States revealed that public duplicity in such bold relief as our health-related conduct during the decade of the 80s. It was a period of national fantasy, an escape from reality. Directed by a president who believed that "homeless people live on the street because they want to," the scenario called for more money for weaponry of questionable utility at the expense of services to the hungry, homeless, disabled, poor, women, children, and others. Decades of public health advances were rescinded in a few years and there was hardly a whisper of outrage. The American people, their elected representatives, their professional organizations, and their leaders of every kind let it happen.[1]

Although, as H. Jack Geiger points out in "Taking Stock and Turning Corners," (p. 603) potential responses to federal neglect had begun to be discussed during the late 1980s, the 1990s has seen a much more active and broadly based national debate about the need for and content of health care reform. There can be little doubt that the major catalyst for this cycle of concern is the perception of a health care sector with costs spinning out of control against the ominous background of severe recession and global economy performance anxiety.

The dimension of the inflationary problem is so large as to seem almost unreal. According to the Health Care Financing Administration (HCFA), 1980 health care costs were $250 billion, 9.2 percent of the gross national product (GNP), and $1,063 per capita. By 1990 they were $662 billion, 12.2 percent of the GNP, and $2,566 per capita. If nothing else changes, HCFA predicts that in the year 2000, costs will be $1.6 trillion, 16.4 percent of the gross national product, and $5,712 per capita.

Health care reform has rocketed to the top of the national list of concerns because a varied group of institutions and interests have come to believe that the country cannot continue to afford a health care sector of such magnitude, especially when tens of millions are uninsured or underinsured and go without needed care. Thus the crisis in health care financing has brought reform back to the political fore. And the slide of the middle class from health coverage comfort to health coverage jeopardy has helped make reform a more acceptable public policy issue.

Even in the chilling political climate created by the right (health care not as a social good, but an economic one) it is again "okay" for politicians to talk about problems of access to health services. Since the problem of affordability now impacts on far more people than just the very poor, the political debate can be steered away from issues of social justice for the poor and minorities. With the health care industry poised to inhale whatever "peace dividend" becomes available for its own marketplace purposes, and as the prospects for national economic recovery remain dim, health care access is, perhaps more than ever before, defined as a middle-class economic concern—and thus it becomes a concern that is "acceptable" for public policy debate. That worry about health care access has spread into mainstream America is clear from the results of an August 1991 poll in which the public, when asked whether they thought there was a health care crisis, answered "yes" 91 percent of the time (*Los Angeles Times*-Gallup poll, August 1991).

It should come as no surprise, therefore, that almost without exception, current proposals to address health care reform focus on financing and the majority feature employment-based, middle-class solutions for affordable access. Prior to President Clinton's inauguration, at least 6 major bills were in the Congress. Waiting in the wings were other nationally proposed plans ranging from the meager tax-incentive and tort-reform package of then-President George Bush to a full blown, Canadian single-payer model put forward by Physicians for a National Health Program and supported by a growing national coalition of grass-roots organizations.

Proposals like that of PNHP and the American Health Security Act (S. 491, H.R. 1220) are generally considered to be examples of the most promising reforms, but not as far-reaching as the Dellums bill. There is a lot that is attractive about the Canadian system and PNHP makes a compelling argument on its behalf in "Liberal Benefits, Conservative Spending" (p. 666). However, as Samuel Wolfe points out in his essays, the social and historical context out of which the Canadian system emerges is very different from that of the United States, and universal access does not automatically confer social equity.

Many of the current proposals for reform deal with the financing issue through one or another version of employer-mandated health insurance. At its most basic, this approach has a required role for some or all employers to subsidize insurance for their employees and usually proposes expanded public sector coverage to insure others. A popular variation of the employer mandate is the so-called "pay or play" approach designed to deal with problems in insuring low-wage or part-time employees and reducing the perceived burden of "pay or play" for small businesses. This plan usually allows certain categories of employers the option of paying a tax instead of offering insurance to their employees. The Pepper Commission Health Access and Reform Act (H.R. 2535-Henry Waxman) and the Mitchell-Kennedy bill are versions of "pay or play." Since one criticism of "pay or play" has been that it does nothing to contain costs, other variations have been developed that do introduce cost control measures such as managed care or single rate-setter options.

Since January 1993 President Clinton's Health Care Taskforce, led by Hillary Rodham Clinton and consisting of hundreds of "experts," has been struggling to come up with a plan for reform. Originally promised for May 1, 1993, the Taskforce plan has so far been thrice delayed, and considering President Clinton's current political misfortunes, it is not at all clear when it will finally be made public. Despite the importance of the Taskforce's cause and the enormity of their effort, the relative secrecy under which they have worked has provided little opportunity for public debate over the principles and substance of reform. Instead, the American people have been left to watch and wait and to ponder the meaning of snippets of often contradictory health care reform proposals that are "leaked" to the national press almost daily.

To help foster a more democratic debate, Health/PAC published a special report entitled "Managed Competition" in the spring of 1993. Included here are several articles from that report. Ronda Kotelchuck guides readers through the "thicket" of managed competition proposals which include both the "Jackson Hole" original conception and a more progressive version known as the "Garamendi Plan" championed by Paul Starr. Nancy F. McKenzie, in her reasoned critique of managed competition, suggests that unless proposals for reform are based on health rights and the needs of individuals and communities, we will waste the country's hopes for reform. Ken Frisof, interim convener of the Universal Health Care Action Network (UHCAN), describes the reality and rationale behind the grassroots movement for single-payer reform. Frisof maintains that building a strong grassroots movement is the necessary condition for achieving meaningful reform in the face of politics as usual. An outline of the *American Health Security Act of 1993* introduced by Senator Paul Wellstone and Representatives Jim McDermott and John Conyers along with 54 other representatives as a version of single-payer health care reform concludes this section.

What are we to make of all this activity? While it is difficult to predict the future, many observers continue to believe that President Clinton, having told the country that "America cannot afford not to have a national health care plan . . . cannot afford not to provide universal coverage . . ." during his campaign, must bring a meaningful proposal to the 102nd Congress, who in turn must take some action before January 1995. The reform measures that are enacted will likely focus primarily on the financing of health care and will not attempt to change the organization and content of those services in any meaningful way.

Should we support this reform? A number of progressive advocates argue that any reform that provides universal access to basic health care services establishes a measure of social equity worthy of our support. And, they say, reform has failed in the past because differences among advocates have allowed the moment of political opportunity to slip away.

But what of those who still have questions, not about the form but the substance of reform? Past experience suggests that the medical/industrial sector will not brook much interference in the ways in which it chooses to do business, and after all, health in America is a very big business indeed. The past also tells us that while the industry may initially oppose reforms that grant increased access (Medicare, for example) it quickly figures out how to ''game'' the system for its own advantage, and opposition disappears. Therefore, I worry whether a ''halfway'' solution, even one that provides universal access, might present more risk than benefit.

As long as there is profit and power to be derived from the provision of health care services, the provider agenda will be directed by self-interest. And, unfortunately, provider self-interest often is the polar opposite of the interests of people needing care, especially the most vulnerable among us: the poor, people of color, women and children, drug users, and people affected by the new epidemics. Because it is politically impossible to excise profit from the system, we must look to reforms that change the locus of power, the control of the system, from providers to those that they serve. Unless there is a strong national will to tie reform of financing to both structural reform and democratic community control, there will continue to be a health care ''crisis'' in America.

NOTES

1. Sultz, Harry D.D.S., M.P.H., ''Health Policy: If You Don't Know Where You're Going, Any Road Will Do.'' *American Journal of Public Health* 4 (1991):418–420.

WHAT'S BLOCKING HEALTH CARE REFORM?

Vicki Kemper and Viveca Novak

For all his decrying of the health care crisis, Pennsylvania Democrat Harris Wofford can say one good thing has come of it: It fueled his unexpected Senate victory over former Attorney General Richard Thornburgh last fall.

Early in the campaign, underdog Wofford discovered that voters were obsessed with the skyrocketing costs of health care, their difficulties in obtaining health insurance, and Washington's seeming indifference to the problem. He devoted five television ads to health care, saying that "if criminals have a right to a lawyer," sick Americans should have the right to see a doctor.

Pennsylvania voters responded; post-election polls suggested that one of every three votes for Wofford was cast solely for his position on health care. Wofford campaign manager Paul Begala may have put it best: "This issue is strong enough to turn goat spit into gasoline."

Wofford's surprising victory over Thornburgh guarantees that health care reform will be a hot-button issue in this year's congressional and presidential elections. Opinion polls indicate that 90 percent of Americans believe the nation's health care system needs "fundamental change" or a "complete rebuilding."

In December, Wofford and three other Democratic senators—Majority Leader George Mitchell of Maine, Jay Rockefeller of West Virginia, and Bob Graham of Florida—toured hospitals and held health care hearings in five states. On January 14 Democratic members of Congress held some 285 town meetings across the country focusing on the issue. Democratic presidential candidates are formulating their own proposals and talking up reform in stump speeches— knowing that with 34.7 million people uninsured and health costs growing at twice the rate of the sluggish GNP, millions of Americans have concluded only government intervention can remedy the nation's ailing health care system.

For much of the past year reform proposals—calling for everything from minor treatment to major surgery—have been pouring out of medical associations, insurance companies, labor unions, businesses, grassroots organizations, and ad hoc coalitions. Even the American Medical Association (AMA), which has used money and hardball politics to fight government-sponsored health care programs since the early part of this century, has its own limited prescription for universal coverage. Dozens of reform bills are pending in Congress.

But whether electioneering and political rhetoric will translate into concrete action is another question. Given the obvious need for change, who or what is standing in the way?

For starters, Democrats point to the White House, where President George Bush and his advisers have met repeatedly with industry leaders since Wofford's win. In December, after two and a half years of study, an administration advisory panel rejected calls for a systemic overhaul and instead suggested only limited reforms, including an emphasis on "healthier lifestyles." Panel chair Deborah Steelman, a key Bush adviser on health care issues, is a lobbyist who represents the Pharmaceutical Manufacturers Association, Aetna Life & Casualty, and other companies that oppose broad reforms.

Bush laid out his opposition to major change in his January 28 State of the Union message, proposing only a tax credit for low-income individuals who buy health insurance and promising more details in February. After a last-minute rebellion by congressional Republicans, the administration stopped the presses and stripped further, though modest, proposals—including taxing wealthy Americans' employer-provided health benefits as income—from its 1993 budget request presented the day after the President's message.

Congress has not done much better. Many Democrats want comprehensive reform but can't agree on what kind. A Senate Republican task force, after months of caucusing, produced a proposal that leaves the current system essentially intact, and a group of House Republicans met weekly for more than six months without introducing a bill.

Meanwhile, doctors blame lawyers and the government for the current mess. Health care purchasers point to insurance companies that cover only the healthy, while insurers single out greedy doctors and hospitals and unrealistic consumers. Outside analysts frame the problem as a lack of consensus; public interest groups define it as a lack of political courage; and everybody talks about how complicated the issue is.

For all this finger-pointing, few in Washington are willing to blame what may be the biggest culprit of all: the political influence of special interest groups with a vested interest in the status quo. The same insurance companies, doctors, hospitals and drug manufacturers that live off the $700 billion-a-year health care industry are battling comprehensive reform on Capitol Hill and at the White House.

"If the elected officials listen to the public, there are some pretty clear messages," says Stephen McConnell, senior vice president of the Alzheimer's Association. "But if they listen to the organized lobbyists," he adds, "it's a stalemate."

"The people with stakes in the issue who have the most to lose are very well organized, very vocal, and very well-heeled," says a high-ranking congressional aide.

What Really Ails Us

Throwing money at the process are more than 200 political action committees—representing everything from the legendary AMA to the obscure

Philippine Physicians in America, from the pharmaceutical giant Pfizer to something called the Health Care Committee for Political Responsibility. Together these medical, pharmaceutical, and insurance industry PACs contributed more than $60 million to congressional candidates between 1980 and the first half of 1991. PAC contributions from the health care industry have increased far more than gifts from most other special interests: 140 percent over the last decade, compared with 90 percent for all PACs.

Almost half the contributions from the health industry to current members of Congress came from physicians, dentists, nurses, and other health professionals; health insurance companies contributed nearly one-third of the total; and the remainder came from pharmaceutical companies, hospitals, nursing homes, and other health care providers. The money was carefully targeted: More than $18 million—or 42 percent—of the contributions went to members of the four congressional committees that have jurisdiction over health-related legislation.

The top recipients of health-related PAC money all hold powerful committee positions: Rep. Pete Stark (D-Calif.), who receives contributions from almost every health-related PAC except the AMAs, is chair of the Ways and Means health subcommittee. Sen. David Durenberger (R-Minn.), a favorite of the hospital lobby, is the ranking Republican on the Senate's Medicare subcommittee. The campaign coffers of Senate Finance Committee Chair Lloyd Bentsen (D-Texas) are brimming with insurance-industry money; doctors and insurance companies are heavy contributors to Sen. Max Baucus (D-Mont.), a high-ranking member of the Finance Committee; and the AMA and other medical associations give generously to Rep. Henry Waxman (D-Calif.), chair of the Energy and Commerce health subcommittee. (Both Stark and Waxman have introduced comprehensive reform bills, while Bentsen has sponsored a more limited approach.)

Twelve of the 21 senators who received more than $200,000 from medical industry PACs serve on the Finance Committee, which has jurisdiction over Medicare and other health-related matters, as well as tax policy. All of the top 25 House recipients of medical industry PAC money serve in House leadership positions or on the key Ways and Means or Energy and Commerce committees.

Some industry players also distribute so-called "soft money" to the Republican and Democratic parties. In 1991—the first year the Federal Election Commission (FEC) required disclosure of soft money contributions—Aetna, Warner-Lambert, Chubb, the American Dental Association's PAC, and the Humana hospital chain each gave $20,000 to the GOP; Blue Cross and Blue Shield gave $29,000 to the Republicans and almost $17,000 to the Democrats; Upjohn gave $25,500 to the Democrats and $23,000 to the GOP; and the pharmaceutical company Glaxo gave $50,000 to the Democrats.

All that medical industry money hasn't bought better health care—but that's not what it's for. What it has bought is access in Washington for physicians, hospitals, and insurance and pharmaceutical interests, along with inaction on the issue of health care reform.

"We spend our money on those members . . . most interested in maintaining the current system," says Tom Goodwin, public affairs director of the Federation of American Health Systems. The federation, which represents some 1,400 for-profit hospitals, has contributed $934,709 to congressional campaigns since 1980, making it the eleventh-biggest giver among health-related PACs.

Like other PACs, those in the medical industry exist to protect their own interests. Consider the primary mission of foot doctors: to make sure that "whatever does transpire, there will be parity and equity for doctors of podiatry," says John Carson, director of governmental affairs for the American Podiatric Medical Association, which has contributed more than $1.1 million to congressional campaigns since 1980. "The PAC has helped us tremendously," Carson says. "I would hate to have been without it for the past almost 20 years."

Or take ophthalmologists, whose primary interests include increased Medicare coverage of cataract surgery and beating back the efforts of optometrists —who also have a very active PAC—to "encroach into their bailiwick." While ophthalmologists make up only 3 percent of the nation's physicians, they are "a very vocal group," acknowledges Cynthia Moran, director of government relations for the American Academy of Ophthalmology. The fourth-largest giver, the academy's PAC has contributed more than $1.9 million to congressional candidates since 1980.

The stream of health-related PAC money into Washington has swelled at a time when U.S. spending on health care has shot past other economic indicators. Health care spending now accounts for 13 percent of the country's GNP—the highest proportion in the world—and it will consume 37 percent by the year 2030 if costs continue to increase at their current rate, according to Richard Darman, director of the Office of Management and Budget.

The average cost of corporate health plans rose 85 percent between 1985 and 1990. Most companies passed along some of the expense to their employees in the form of higher insurance co-payments and deductibles. Health care costs have also raised the prices of American-made products. Chrysler says that some $600 of the cost of every car it makes in the United States goes into the nation's health care system. The comparable amount in Germany is $337 and in Japan, $246—one reason why American auto manufacturers support comprehensive change.

Washington has done little over the years to contain health care costs—at least in part, many believe, because of the PAC contributions that have bought political access for physicians, hospitals, and insurance and pharmaceutical firms. "The monied interests have caused gridlock," says Dr. Robert Berenson, a Washington, D.C., physician who served on President Jimmy Carter's domestic policy staff.

Insurance companies represent one huge obstacle. "They are actually against doing anything, because they realize that any kind of reform is going to involve some federal regulation of the insurance industry," says Robert Blendon, chair of the department of health policy and management at the Harvard University School of Public Health.

Most Americans dislike insurance companies, but few politicians are willing to take the industry on. Insurance PACs have contributed $19 million to congressional candidates since 1980, and 7 of the top 20 medical industry PACs are affiliated with insurance companies or associations. The National Association of Life Underwriters ranks second, with $5.5 million in contributions to congressional races since 1980. The group's counsel, David Hebert, says candidates who support comprehensive reform are less likely to get its PAC dollars.

Insurance companies such as Prudential, Metropolitan, and Travelers, along with the small-business community and a number of health care providers, helped launch a powerful anti-reform coalition in October, the Healthcare Equity Action League, or HEAL. "We are willing to support . . . incremental, market-oriented changes" that leave the current system essentially intact, says John Motley, co-chair of HEAL's legislative committee and a lobbyist with the National Federation of Independent Business. In an effort to influence the "public relations game," Motley says, HEAL sent advance teams to meet with reporters in the cities where Mitchell and other Democrats held hearings in December.

Some observers doubt whether public opinion is forceful or cohesive enough to overcome the money, connections and political savvy of these groups. "There are a lot of interests at risk," says a staff member of the House Energy and Commerce Committee. "Without some clear political constituency that politicians can see and hear and touch and feel"—the kind that materialized for Wofford's campaign—"it's going to be very hard for them to say they have a clear mandate to move forward on reform."

House Calls

Health care reform has never fared well politically in the United States, and for most of the twentieth century there has been one enduring reason: the intractable opposition of the AMA. By the 1920s nearly all western European countries had some form of national health insurance, but when President Calvin Coolidge called for massive increases in federal spending on health care—which then represented 3 percent of the GNP—the AMA spearheaded opposition to the plan, calling it a "socialist" and "German" invention.

AMA resistance persuaded Franklin Roosevelt to leave health care out of the New Deal, and when President Harry Truman promoted a plan for national health insurance, AMA members wrote him angry letters on pink paper labeling the plan a "communist plot." The organization spent a phenomenal $1.3 million in nine months—$7.1 million in today's dollars—to defeat Truman's plan.

John Kennedy made federally guaranteed health care for older Americans a key element of his 1960 presidential campaign platform. But even Medicare, a boon for tens of millions of the elderly—not to mention doctors and hospitals —was enacted over the strident opposition of the AMA. Calling it "socialized medicine," the AMA enlisted a Hollywood actor named Ronald Reagan to help block the program on Capitol Hill. "If you and I don't stop" Medicare, Reagan warned on a phonograph record the AMA sent to doctors' wives, "we'll spend our sunset years telling our children and children's children what it was like in America when men were free."

The passage of Medicare and Medicaid were the last significant government actions to help large numbers of Americans gain access to affordable health care. In the 1970s, politics and interest-group opposition defeated numerous initiatives for further reform, and for the Reagan administration health care reform wasn't even a blip on the screen.

Meanwhile the AMA and its state affiliates' PACs have contributed more than $11.9 million to congressional campaigns since 1980—along with some $3 million in "independent expenditures" made on behalf of certain candidates. That's more than double the amount of contributions made by any other health-related PAC.

And political participation by physicians extends beyond the AMA PAC; FEC records indicate that individuals identifying themselves as doctors made at least $7.48 million in direct contributions to congressional races from 1981 through 1990.

Has all this physician involvement in the political process made a difference? "Let's face it," says Princeton University political economist Uwe Reinhardt, when it comes to influencing politicians in Washington, "what the head of the AMA thinks in the shower in the morning is so much more important than the aspirations of 10 million Americans."

Still, times have changed even for the powerful, anti-government AMA. The group issued its own health care reform proposal in March 1990. "The doctors have been very smart on this," says Harvard's Blendon. "After 50 years of saying 'do nothing,' they come out and say they're for universal coverage." By plunging into the debate with its own proposal, the AMA has "positioned itself to play a big role," he adds.

But there's a catch: The AMA wants to make sure Congress protects doctors from malpractice suits and doesn't hit them with cost controls, and its proposal reflects those concerns. Likewise, reform proposals pushed by insurance companies, hospitals, drug manufacturers, and other interest groups emphasize their varying and self-serving priorities.

Band-Aids or Surgery?

Nowhere is the lack of consensus more pronounced than in the nation's capital, where the high-stakes battle to determine the nature of reform has begun in earnest. Neither the Democrats nor the Republicans have been able to agree among themselves—much less with each other—on what course to take.

House Speaker Tom Foley (D-Wash.) opened three days of Ways and Means Committee hearings on health care reform in October warning that "many interest groups will have to hold the good of the whole above their own." Committee members then spent most of two and a half days listening to pitches from such vested interests as the insurance industry, hospitals and various medical professions.

For all their differences, most reform bills fall into one of three major categories. The most limited approach seeks to make health insurance more affordable. In an effort to help small businesses and the self-employed buy insurance, supporters propose tax breaks and limited regulation of insurance premiums.

A second approach would expand the nation's current employment-based health insurance system. Employers would be required to either "pay" the gov-

See a Specialist

The intensifying debate over health care reform could be big business for some Washingtonians. Among them are a number of lawyers and lobbyists who used to work on Capitol Hill or in the executive branch and today labor on behalf of such medical industry clients as the American Medical Association, American Dental Association, and the Health Insurance Association of America.

Identified recently in the industry lineup were:

	THEN	NOW
FRANK MCLAUGHLIN	Aide to former house Speaker Tip O'Neill	Head of American Dental Association's PAC
JOHN SALMON	Aide to House Ways and Means Committee Chair Dan Rostenkowski	Lobbies for Federation of American Health Systems
KENNETH BOWLER	Staff director of House Ways and Means	Lobbies for Pfizer
JOHN JONAS	Tax counsel for House Ways and Means	Lobbies for Metropolitan Life, Massachusetts Mutual Life, and National Association of Life Underwriters
RICHARD VERVILLE	Assistant secretary of HEW	Lobbies for Academy of Physical Medicine and Rehabilitation, Medical Group Management, and Joint Council on Allergy and Immunology
DAWSON MATHIS	Member of Congress	Lobbies for Metropolitan Life and Massachusetts Mutual
GORDON WHEELER	Congressional liaison, Office of Management and Budget (OMB); assistant to President Bush	Political affairs director. Health Insurance Association of America
DEBORAH STEELMAN	Domestic policy adviser to Bush transition team; OMB official	Bush health care adviser and medical industry lobbyist
MARTIN GOLD	Counsel to former Senate Majority Leader Howard Baker	Lobbies for the American Pathologists

ernment to enroll their employees in a new public health program or "play" by providing their employees with a minimum package of private health insurance benefits. The third, most far-reaching, group of proposals would create a public, government-financed health insurance program that would cover every American.

In the first category, Sen. Bentsen and Rep. Dan Rostenkowski (D-Ill.)—heads of the Senate and House tax-writing committees—have sponsored legislation that would make a standard benefits package available to all small-business employees, control premiums for small-group plans and prohibit insurance companies from denying coverage to employees with "preexisting conditions." Their proposals would also allow self-employed persons to deduct all health insurance costs from their income taxes. Rostenkowski says he hopes these limited reforms would meet the health care needs of many Americans until more comprehensive reform is passed—something he believes is a long way off.

Senate Republicans offered a similar proposal after Democrat Wofford's upset victory. Sen. John Chafee (R-R.I.) introduced legislation that would provide health insurance tax credits for some; more affordable premiums for small businesses; malpractice law reform; increased funding for community health centers; and greater reliance on "managed care" health programs that limit such things as doctor visits.

The "pay-or-play" reform model is embodied in the "Health America" plan introduced by Democratic Sens. Mitchell, Edward Kennedy (Mass.), Rockefeller and Donald Riegle (Mich.), and in House bills authored by Reps. Waxman and Rostenkowski.

This approach expands on the current system, which already provides some health insurance to 83 percent of all Americans under age 65. Tax incentives and insurance reforms for small businesses, along with an expanded government medical program to replace Medicaid, would provide insurance for persons not covered through the workplace. Because a pay-or-play plan would keep intact much of the current system, supporters believe it might survive politically. For those who seek more sweeping reform, pay-or-play is a good first step, they say.

Others believe that nothing short of a radical overhaul will do. They support a "single-payer" program similar to the national health care system in Canada. There citizens choose their own doctors and receive care in private clinics and hospitals, but the government imposes strict cost controls and functions as the nation's insurance company, reimbursing doctors, hospitals, and other health care providers for their services.

The single-payer proposal introduced by Rep. Marty Russo (D-Ill.) has garnered more cosponsors than any other reform bill. Democratic Sen. Paul Wellstone (Minn.) and Reps. Stark, Mary Rose Oakar (Ohio), John Dingell (Mich.), and Sam Gibbons (Fla.) have also introduced single-payer bills, and presidential candidate Sen. Bob Kerrey (D-Neb.) has proposed a variation of the single-payer system.

No Easy Cure

Of course, health care reform won't come cheap. Even the limited proposals offered by Bentsen and Rostenkowski carry estimated price tags of $10 billion over five years. For the more sweeping reform proposals, there are widely varying cost estimates—and while sponsors prescribe different methods for paying for universal coverage, almost all would require tax hikes of some kind.

Financing a single-payer system would be the most costly, in a direct sense, for the government and would require increases in corporate and personal income taxes. But supporters say the taxes would replace insurance premiums as well as a host of indirect costs that employers and employees now pay. In a Gallup poll conducted last July for the Employee Benefits Research Institute, roughly half of those questioned said they would be willing to pay more in taxes for guaranteed health coverage.

The GAO estimates that a single-payer system would save $67 billion in administrative costs—which, according to the agency, consumed 12 cents of every health insurance dollar in 1987. A study by the American Federation of State, County and Municipal Employees (AFSCME), Public Citizen and Physicians for a National Health Program concluded that a single-payer system would save state and local governments—whose budgets are being crippled by increasing health costs—up to $30 billion a year.

A key sticking point is how to control health care costs. Limited reform proposals would merely control access to health care services. More direct cost-control provisions range from the Kennedy-Mitchell bill's recommended spending targets to the strict health care budgeting contained in Rostenkowski's pay-or-play proposal and Russo's single-payer plan.

Naturally, doctors and hospital administrators strongly oppose efforts to regulate their fees. "We would have problems with any reform based on global budgeting and mandatory cost controls," says Richard Davidson, president of the American Hospital Association (AHA). The AHA, which represents some 5,500 not-for-profit hospitals, reinforces its position with six well-connected lobbyists as well as PAC contributions—nearly $1.8 million to congressional races since 1980.

The Federation of American Health Systems—the for-profit hospital people—is also worried about cost controls, "even if they're voluntary," says public affairs director Tom Goodwin. "The bottom line is rate-setting for hospitals. They are anathema, and we will oppose them as vigorously as we possibly can."

Russo's more far-reaching, single-payer proposal—which calls for strict cost controls—has been endorsed by numerous liberal organizations and labor unions. But few believe such a comprehensive reform proposal can withstand interest-group opposition.

Bitter Medicine

Significant movement on the issue would require overcoming the insurance companies and small businesses that oppose all but the mildest reform proposals. A single-payer system would do away with the need for most private health insurance, and insurance executives worry that a pay-or-play system would give employers more incentive to pay into the public program than to provide their employees with private insurance. "We oppose that strenuously, and are working to see that it is not enacted," says David Hebert of the National Association of Life Underwriters.

The Health Insurance Association of America (HIAA), which represents 300 commercial insurance companies that cover some 95 million Americans, "strongly opposes" both pay-or-play and single-payer proposals, says spokesperson Donald White.

To strengthen its hand against federal action, HIAA plans to spend at least $4 million on lobbying, public relations, and legal work in 15 "target states." What HIAA does support are "bare-bones" policies for small businesses, provisions that allow workers to keep their insurance when changing jobs and curbs on the denial of coverage due to preexisting conditions.

The wealth and power of the insurance industry are hard to overstate. "The health insurance industry . . . has tons of money and they love to spend it to get their way on Capitol Hill," says Public Citizen spokesperson Robert Dreyfuss. "In this case they're fighting for their lives." Last fall, congressional aides say, insurance companies and trade associations were doing more lobbying than any of the other interest groups.

In addition to the National Association of Life Underwriters, top insurance interests with PACs include the American Family Corp., Travelers, Prudential, Metropolitan Life, Torchmark Corp., CIGNA, HIAA, and Blue Cross and Blue Shield. Sen. Bentsen is one of the top recipients of insurance-industry money, and his bill has been endorsed by many in the industry, as well as other members of the anti-reform coalition HEAL.

Small business also wields big clout. With premiums 25 percent to 40 percent higher than those for larger firms, the cost of health insurance is the "No. 1 problem" of some 500,000 small-business owners, according to the National Federation of Independent Business (NFIB). As a result, many don't provide coverage and don't want to be forced to. They favor tax breaks and lower premiums such as those contained in the more limited reform proposals.

The wealthy pharmaceutical companies have so far been relatively quiet. But should a viable reform plan include coverage and cost controls on prescription drugs, "the drug companies will go crazy" and deploy their lobbyists to defeat it, warns Harvard's Blendon.

That leaves the AMA at the forefront, where doctors will retain their traditional activist role. "You underestimate the AMA's influence at your peril. They have truly awesome power," says AMA member Dr. Quentin Young, a Chicago physician who heads the 4,000-member Physicians for a National Health Program. It supports a Canadian-style, single-payer system.

Referring to the influence of the AMA PAC, spokesperson James Stacey says modestly, "We support a large number of congressional candidates. We don't expect that we are buying their minds, their hearts or anything else. Yet we hope that we will have some access to them. The bigger issue is to get physicians involved in the political process."

Prognosis Doubtful

In the absence of federal action, several states, overwhelmed by skyrocketing Medicaid costs, have undertaken their own health care reform programs. Through a combination of mandated employer-provided coverage, insurance reforms, Medicare, and Medicaid, Hawaii provides basic coverage for virtually all its residents at premium rates roughly 50 percent lower than those in California. Massachusetts and Oregon have passed, but not yet implemented, pay-or-play programs, and single-payer legislation is being considered in Michigan, California, and other states. On the other hand, cash-strapped Maryland recently stopped paying hospital bills for some 29,000 of its poorest residents.

Many would like to see comprehensive reform efforts confined to the state level—at least for now. The administration's advisory panel recommended a federal outlay of $3 billion for state-level experiments. But others say that's not enough.

"A Band-Aid approach won't stop the hemorrhaging of the system," says John Ball, executive vice president of the American College of Physicians.

Backers of major reform have organized grassroots campaigns and formed coalitions, with strategies that range from public relations and street-smart politics to policy analysis. In New Hampshire 180 organizations sponsored a media and advertising campaign designed to force all presidential candidates to deal with the issue.

In November the National Leadership Coalition on Health Care Reform proposed a variation on the pay-or-play theme that has won endorsements from a couple of dozen corporations, unions and associations, including Chrysler and the United Steelworkers, and former presidents Jimmy Carter and Gerald Ford.

During this key election year, grassroots activity is likely to intensify as the health insurance dilemma worsens for individuals and families of all income levels. A new Public Citizen study shows that the number of Americans without insurance increased by 1.3 million between 1989 and 1990, with 74 percent of the new uninsured earning more than $25,000 a year. With the economy mired in recession and large-scale layoffs a daily occurrence, workers increasingly worry as much about losing their health benefits as their paychecks.

All of this misery may force Congress to enact some type of reform soon. "The issue of the uninsured is not enough to move the process," says one congressional aide. "But as the problem becomes worse for the middle class, for working people, and people who vote, people will begin to say that this is not acceptable."

TAKING STOCK AND
TURNING CORNERS

H. Jack Geiger

Tracing the complex changes that have taken place in the nation's health-care system over the last eight years, Geiger points out why opportunities are now ripe for change. If progress is to be made towards establishing a national health-care program, he argues, we must shift the terms of the debate away from fiscal and technical details and return it to the arena of public concern and social responsibility.

The central premise of the Health/PAC conference on national health was that we are on the threshold of change. Some of us glimpse not just a change in the health-care system but a massive shift away from the regressive thrust of the past eight years. We know, in broad terms, the outcomes we want. We must discuss, now, how we get from here to there.

Let's begin, in that context, by looking at how we got to where we are, by examining what was on the nation's mind with regard to health care in the 1960s and early 1970s, what happened, and why. It was a time, first of all, of industrial growth, rising expectations, and an expanding economic pie. The middle class was doing well. It was the beginning, furthermore, of one of those periodic cyclic swings that Arthur Schlesinger and others have described: every thirty years or so Americans turn liberal, egalitarian, and, rediscovering poverty and inequity and their consequences in our society, palliate these problems up to the point where such reform threatens a real redistribution of resources.

Despite its relative comfort, the middle class did have one big problem back then: its growing difficulty in paying for the medical care of its aging parents. What was on our national mind in the early 1960s, therefore, was the cost of care for the elderly. Then, with the rediscovery of "the other America"—the underprivileged—a broader dilemma came forward. The nation began to focus on inequity in health care, specifically on lack of access, on the financial, geographic, racial, and cultural barriers to decent health care particular to certain communities. We talked about fragmentation of care, the particular lack of primary care, and the lack of participation and influence—let alone control—by consumers. The times seemed ripe for major change.

Because of the larger political climate, the dramatic swing to the Left, we were able to introduce certain health-care innovations that stood outside the established system, notably the attempt to create a network of neighborhood health centers, primary-care institutions that were community-based and consumer-controlled. Underlying this development was a concern for the health status of populations, not just of individuals, and an attempt to integrate self-care, preventive and curative, with the classic approaches of public health. We even dreamt that such new health-care institutions would be instruments of empowerment and vehicles to broader economic, political, and social change.

Our own progressive efforts (I'll call them that, rather than merely liberal) reached their apotheosis in the 1970s with the Dellums Bill, which called for a unified health care system, integrated and budgeted nationally but controlled by communities, prepaid, oriented toward prevention, and focused on primary care. This was a direct challenge to the mainstream, to a "private" sector that was driven by profit, centered on continually expanding hospitals and, although supported essentially by public funds, rather poorly regulated.

But the conception of pluralism upon which the system built its ideological framework is deeply grounded in American values and traditions—and its beneficiaries have deep pockets from which to fund public relations and lobbying. The Dellums Bill, as we know, went nowhere.

What Congress gave us, instead, was Medicare and Medicaid, with their underlying premise of "mainstreaming," which does not seek to change the system, but gets the old, the poor, and minorities into the system by removing financial barriers which stand in the way of individual members of these groups.

Some of us did understand, then—and it is inescapably clear in retrospect —that a bargain had been struck with the medical establishment: access to the health-care system would be expanded, but only on that establishment's terms, without structural change. The inevitable consequences followed—a huge increase in costs as a result not merely of the number of new people in the mainstream but also of the built-in incentives to provide more care than necessary. The system, with an underfunded, second-tier "public" system for the poor and unwanted now existing beneath the "private" sector, remained fragmented, chaotic, and elitist—wholly unsuited as an instrument for improving the nation's health.

At the same time the nation embarked on a massive expansion of the physician pool and a substantial increase in the number of hospital beds. Few paid attention to the fact that medical care costs were already rising at a rate higher than inflation—from $185 per capita in 1960 to $229 per capita in 1965; that is from 5.3 to 5.9 percent of the Gross National Product. If anything, people thought the share of the GNP devoted to health care should be higher. Nor did anyone worry very much about another force whose effects were already evident: our national attraction to ever more sophisticated and more expensive technology.

Meanwhile, the larger political climate was itself changing. As medical care costs rose, so did the costs of the Vietnam War, the political costs even more than the financial. Meanwhile, the economy was slowing (even before the oil crunch of 1973), and the reforms of the Great Society had not turned out to be so great. In 1970 Nixon warned the nation that it faced a crisis because health-care expenditures totalled $75 billion—7.5 percent of the GNP or $292 per capita.

What followed, inevitably, was not deep reform, but an endless series of attempts to regulate costs. All these measures failed. Health Maintenance Organizations (HMOs) were developed with federal support and heralded as obviating any need for more fundamental restructuring. Their own architects now concede their inadequacy. Attempts were made to cap or limit capital expenditures, with only partial success.

What was failing—and being desperately propped up—was a free-market system of health care. But the public perceived the failure as the government's—as that of "social welfare policy"—because the government was paying so much of the bill of this supposedly free enterprise. And that, ironically, contributed to the larger shift in the nation's political mood, which assured Reagan's election in 1980. This, in turn, buttressed the Right's ongoing attempt to redefine health care as a commodity, rather than as a social responsibility, as something best handled by, that's right, a free-market model.

Other, more general trends are exacerbating the crisis in our health care. The United States is growing grayer, and the demands of the elderly cannot be ignored, for senior citizens are organizing themselves ever better; the American Association of Retired Persons now boasts more than 23 million members.

Our economy is undergoing a major and permanent shift from manufacturing industries to services. One result of this is a decrease in the number, membership, and power of unions, and in their ability to negotiate effectively for health benefits. We are experiencing an almost unprecedented widening of the gap between rich and poor, a steady increase in the number of people who are downwardly mobile, and a revolution of shrinking expectations. Their corollaries are a further disintegration of the inner city, an increase in rural poverty, chronically high unemployment and underemployment, and a devastating impact on the nation's children, more than 25 percent of whom now live in poverty. Finally, of particular relevance to the health care system, we are plagued with the AIDS epidemic.

With all this, the past seven years has seen a change in the very identification of the fundamental problem of our health-care system. Where once people worried about access, equity, and health status, now the public and its representatives are most concerned with cost. (There are some good reasons for this: in 1987, Americans will spend approximately $500 billion on health care—a record 11.4 percent of the GNP. That works out, after the figures are adjusted to account for inflation, to a per-capita increase of 143 percent since 1960.)

And so now we face, above all, soaring costs, a function not merely of the irrationality of the present system but also a consequence of the increased use and technological intensity of its services. Furthermore, this problem has overwhelmed all others; we have moved from considering health a policy issue to considering it a budget issue. We have, for almost eight years, moved from a definition of health care as a public and social responsibility toward its definition as a function of the market, a problem to be solved by "competition," "entrepreneurial efficiency," and the great engines of private-sector investment and innovation (and never mind that government is still paying most of the bill!).

The consequences are known to all of us. We are immersed in attempts to control cost and utilization, essentially by restricting eligibility and coverage—that is, by removing people and services from the system. Yet these attempts are failing spectacularly to control costs, to limit the Medicare bill, the Medicaid bill, the total national health-care bill, and the extent to which medical-care costs rise faster than our very modest general inflation. We confront a huge increase in the number of uninsured, which now stands at 35 million, not counting the possibly 20 million who are deeply underinsured. Seventy percent of these people work full-time or are members of families which include two people who hold part-time jobs.

This last calamity has, in turn, created an impending crisis for hospitals, which no longer can lay the costs of the uninsured on others. The crisis is so severe that even for-profit hospitals are clamoring for publicly funded coverage for such patients. Hospitals and governments are now attempting to shift these burdens to the individual patient, increasing his or her costs, while eliminating peripheral services and reducing access to the services that remain. The messages from the health-care establishment have become: don't come into the system; if you're in, get out as fast as possible; and if you're in a hospital bed, get out even faster! DRGs—so many hundred dollars for this disease, so many hundred for that, the ultimate commodification—are part of this attempt to limit the availability of health care. Yet these mechanisms are neither controlling costs nor preserving the financial viability of providers, as witnessed, for example, by the growing tendency of HMOs to abandon certain populations, such as the elderly, and simply renege on their contracts.

These financial failures have also come to characterize the large chains, both for-profit and nonprofit, despite increasingly frenzied marketing on their part. The proprietary corporations are getting out of acute care hospitals and into medical supplies, home health care, rehabilitation and psychiatric hospitals. This comes on top of their expansion into sports medicine, substance-abuse treatment, wellness clinics, weight-reduction centers, and other forms of middle-class health care. Meanwhile, the aging population presents us with an impending crisis in our ability to provide long-term care.

Physicians are facing simultaneous threats to their autonomy and income. There is growing public unease and suspicion, moreover, about their incentives, motivation, and loyalties. Perception influences interpretation. When medicine is primarily patient-oriented, a gatekeeper is a guide and helper. When medicine is seen as a business, especially in prepaid or capped plans, a gatekeeper may be seen as a barrier to care.

On all providers, finally, there is enormous pressure to minimize risk, avoid the sick, the poor, the elderly. The one exception is the public hospital system, and—as part of the abandonment of public responsibility—that is being slowly destroyed. (A sad and ludicrous attempt is now under way by the federal government to ''recover'' 10 hospitals of the Public Health Service that were sold, abandoned, or given away in the last decade, in order to turn them into a national network of pesthouses for AIDS patients.) We already have, in consequence, a system of at least three tiers. The indigent and uninsured, together with the poor on Medicare and Medicaid, make up 99 percent of the patients in public hospitals. The middle-class sick go to the nonprofits. The for-profits look for plastic-surgery cases.

That is what's happening now. As we consider this and plan for the future, there are some informed predictions that we should keep high in our minds. Eli Ginzberg, in a recent issue of the *New England Journal of Medicine* (April 2, 1987), identified the following four pillars of the efforts at cost containment and predicted that all of them would crumble.

1. *Prospective financing for Medicare hospitalizations.* This is ultimately doomed to fail because of population growth, continuing advances in technology, the need to increase salaries of hospital workers, and continued resistance to closing hospitals or scaling back some of their operations despite chronically lower rates of occupancy.

2. *HMOs, Prospective Payment Organizations (PPOs), and other forms of prepaid health-care delivery.* These are failing because of their inability to capture more than a limited share of the market, due in part to their inability to provide employers with the savings they promised; the steeply growing costs of marketing; the difficulties of structuring and managing large prepaid plans; and the growing insistence of employers and consumers on mechanisms of quality control.

3. *The abundant supply of physicians.* This will continue to increase, given the large number of students already being trained. But even though an increase in the number of physicians tends to depress the income of each individual doctor, such an increase would actually make total health care costs rise. For one thing, expenditures for physicians' incomes would remain constant. For another, utilization of services increases with the number of physicians—that is, more treatment takes place when there are more doctors around. Finally, as a doctor's income falls, he or she will tend to order more procedures in order to prop up his or her income.

4. *For-profit enterprises.* These are not quite failing yet, but there is also no evidence that for-profit hospitals provide equivalent care for less money than non-profit hospitals. As I have already noted, several chains have moved from the acquisition of hospitals to their divestiture, and those they still retain show rates of occupancy many percentage points below those of non-profit hospitals.

These failures, if they continue, will steadily increase the cost of health care. They may also help convince the middle class that the policies of the last eight years—indeed, the whole structure of the health care system—doesn't work. And they will, simultaneously, both hurt the middle class and cost it a great deal. In that same issue of the *New England Journal of Medicine*, Victor Fuchs lists these and other factors—among them concern about the physician-patient relationship, concern about quality, and the fears of health care workers—as contributing to a counterrevolution in health care financing, a return to the belief that the federal government must act, and widespread support for a system that mandates coverage for everyone and emphasizes equity.

When this happens, a strategy of coalition building, of forging common interests between the poor and the middle class, will seem anything but absurd, despite what people think of such a possibility now. But Fuchs warns that we will not be able to avoid the problem of cost. Merely addressing the issues of access and equity will not be enough. And much will depend on the timing of the next change in the political climate and the overall state of the economy.

These are things we need to keep in mind as we rethink a national health program. It is vital that we consider not merely the mechanics of a plan, and not only its political and philosophical underpinnings, but also the ways in which we can use the contradictions and failures of the present system, as they become increasingly evident, to build political support, incrementally, across class and race and regional lines for whatever system we propose. In other words, even after we have defined our plan, we will still face the problem of getting from here to there.

This realization gives special urgency to the formulation of such a national health program. The 1988 election campaign has already begun. Congress still seems committed both to piecemeal initiatives and to evermore regressive types of coverage, to a continuing shift from entitlement to means testing. The changes in health care I have briefly described will keep happening with us or without us.

There are many specific and technical topics to be addressed in our planning for a national health program: the organization of care, the development of new models of primary care, the problems of equitable financing, the huge problem of costs. They must be addressed, but, as we prepare to do so, I want to add an urgent warning.

To the extent that we present the provision of health care as a primarily technical problem, a matter of organizational mechanics and financial mechanisms, the progressive cause will suffer. For almost two decades now, we have permitted the problems of the health care system to be presented as technical. Yet, for most Americans, the choice of a health care system for the nation is a values-based choice, and we must say so over and over again. For here there is room for optimism. Americans do still believe deeply in the right of everyone to health care, in fairness, and in equity. They continue to believe in the social responsibility of government. They want more, not less, done about housing and hunger and homelessness.

Indeed, polls show quite clearly that, despite the (until recently) high personal popularity of President Reagan, the American people have never adopted his fundamentalist, right-wing ideology; there has been no great ideological shift in the last decade. What has occurred, instead, is a disillusionment with what are perceived as formulaic ''liberal'' or ''social-welfare'' proposals as routes to the democratic and equitable solutions that are still deeply desired.

That imposes on us the responsibility to question the values that underlie any proposal for a national health program, not only its organizational and technical details. In so doing we take the issue out of the hands of marketplace technicians—the ''saviors'' of the past decade, now failing—and return it to the arena of public concern and social responsibility.

By making that effort, finally, we will help make the national debate on the health care system part of a broader movement for social and political change.

I mention this because we are unlikely to achieve fundamental or structural change in one single sector of the political economy, health care, without simultaneous change in other parts of the system. We want a rational and decent national health program. We want a more just and equitable society. The two are inseparable.

ANATOMY OF A NATIONAL HEALTH PROGRAM: RECONSIDERING THE DELLUMS BILL AFTER 10 YEARS

Leonard S. Rodberg

Ten years ago Representative Ronald Dellums (D-Calif.) introduced his Health Service Act in Congress. Despite the continuing failure of his colleagues to take up serious discussion of the bill, Dellums has reintroduced the legislation every two years, with the convening of each Congress.

With the exception of his stubborn persistence in making the case for national health, progressive health politics has virtually shut down in Washington. Now, however, with the approaching end of the Dark Age of Reagan, many of us anticipate a resurgence of progressive health activism. To help us prepare for this coming period of struggle around national health policy, I would like to review the objectives of the Dellums bill, and the reasoning behind its design. Since the issues we addressed in the mid-1970s remain the most critical problems facing health care today, the design put forward then is a valuable guide to a renewed progressive approach to health policy.

The Dellums bill was the first legislation ever introduced into Congress to create a national health service. Although those who participated in its development were charged with being utopian, we were under no illusion that the bill would be enacted quickly, or even that it would soon be widely debated in the media. Our objective at that stage was not to pass legislation, but to create a vehicle for educating the public on the need for a new way of organizing and delivering health services.

There were other reasons, too, why the charge of utopianism was mistaken. The Dellums bill did not spring from the heads of a few off-beat ideologues, but was an outgrowth of the progressive movements of the 1960s and early 1970s. When Dellums decided to prepare such legislation in 1972, he asked the Medical Committee on Human Rights, an organization of health workers allied with the civil rights movement, to prepare a draft of the principles that should underlie a national health program. That draft became the basis for the Health Service Act.

As the legislation evolved, many other groups, representing the elderly, minorities, women, social workers, trade unionists, public health professionals, and health policy analysts, became involved in its preparation and gave it their support. The bill was backed by the American Public Health Association, the National Association of Social Workers, the Gray Panthers, and the United Electrical Workers, among others. The experiences of these groups, and the specific improvements they sought in health services, were reflected in many provisions of the Dellums bill.

This support made it clear that the concepts which underlie the Dellums bill had a significant constituency. It was not a constituency that counted for much in American politics, but it was substantial and it was broad. Polling data indicated that, if the bill's provisions could be made widely known, they would gain the support of a much wider part of the population; when the public is asked its views on the nation's health system, between 30 and 40 percent consistently say they favor making the government responsible for providing health care.

Pragmatism in Service of Ideals

Finally, the Dellums bill was realistic because it proposed a system which could actually solve the problems it addressed. Those of us who supported a national health service found that our principal debate was with the advocates of national health insurance. (Those who opposed a significant government role in health care refused to engage either of us in debate!) In our view, the supporters of NHI were the utopians, but because of well-publicized proposals like the Kennedy bill, the general public now identifies national health with NHI. It is therefore important to differentiate between such a scheme and a true national health program.

National health insurance would not offer significant benefits to more than the 15–20 percent of the population which now lacks insurance or is underinsured. While these people surely need help, they lack health insurance precisely because they have no political power. Are they likely to generate the political power needed to achieve passage of national health insurance? Our opposition to NHI was thus a matter not only of ideals but of realpolitik, as well; only if the system had something in it for everyone—not just for the poor and uninsured—would it garner the kind of political backing needed for adequate funding and longevity.

We felt the system had to be designed to serve everyone and be available to all, regardless of income or citizenship. Under our plan, health care would be the right of every resident. This country had been the first to establish the idea that education is a basic human right; it would now catch up with the rest of the industrialized world by assuring access to health care for everyone.

The Dragon of Cost

The three primary issues we sought to address in designing the Health Service Act were cost, access, and democratic control.

First came the issue of cost, not because it was central to our concerns, but because it was the primary issue in health care 10 years ago, as it is today. Upon assuming power, the Carter administration set up a 40-member task force to develop a national health plan; one member was a physician, 39 were economists. Recognizing that most policymakers, and the mass media, believed the problem with American medical care to be simply one of expense, we made sure to propose a plan that would not add fuel to the inflation of medical costs.

It is instructive to recall how others were addressing this problem 10 years ago. The liberal solution was to impose some regulatory mechanism that would constrain cost increases without tampering with the organization of health care. Conservative economists, ironically, agreed with us that such a strategy was futile, and that the problem of cost was deeply embedded in the structure of American medical care. That structure married fee-for-service payment, in which payment is made on the basis of the type and quantity of service delivered, to third-party insurance coverage. This mix of an entrepreneurial market with third-party reimbursement inevitably touched off an explosion of costs.

The conservative solution was to retain fee-for-service and make "consumers" (as patients have come to be called) responsible for holding down costs. Whether by accepting higher deductibles and co-payments, paying taxes on health-related fringe benefits, choosing the least expensive providers, or discontinuing high-cost in-patient services when their DRGs are used up, patients would shoulder the burden of costs.

Our alternative was to replace fee-for-service with a budgeted plan. It made no sense to continue to act as if medicine were still a cottage industry. The massive institutions which today dominate medical care require a constant stream of capital to remain stable; payment has to be assured in advance. The growing popularity of prepaid health plans attests to the recognition of this on the part of both consumers and many members of the health care industry.

Fee-for-service payment, moreover, arose when medicine was oriented toward acute, curative care. This may have been appropriate practice a century ago, or even 25 years ago, when infectious and viral diseases were the principal threats to health. As Milton Terris has forcefully shown, however, the principal illnesses we face today—cancer, heart disease, stroke—require long-term preventive action aimed at both the individual and society (*Health/PAC Bulletin*, Vol. 17, No. 5). We need a reorganization of the health care system that emphasizes prevention as well as cure while providing the financial stability that health-care institutions require.

Although circumstances forced us to focus first on the problem of cost, no less central to our concern was the severe maldistribution of medical resources. Large numbers of people in this country lack access to adequate health care. According to the federal government, 50 million people—nearly a quarter of our population—live in medically underserved areas. This problem was, in fact, the principal one for the constituencies most responsive to the proposal we developed.

We felt, too, that the medical care system needed a dose of democracy. It was not being run with the participation of the people who used it or worked in it. Hospital boards did not represent the people who use hospitals, and physicians behaved as private entrepreneurs. We needed a process that would assure democratic control over the health care system, that would make the system more responsive and accountable to the people who worked in it and the communities which it served.

Applying Federalism to Health Care

The bill calls for the creation of a community-based national health service. Our intention was to design a national system without creating a giant bureaucracy. (Neither we nor anyone else wanted a large and unaccountable agency running our medical care system.) Instead, the Dellums bill seeks to apply federalism, the principle of involving each level of government in an appropriate way, to the health care system. While the proposed health service would be funded nationally and mandated by the federal government, it would rest on a network of community-based prepaid health plans coordinated at the regional level.

The system would be funded nationally so that economic inequality would not be a barrier to the equitable provision of health services. It would be mandated federally to guarantee access to residents of every community. Regional coordination would ensure that both general and specialized services would be available to every region on a rational and equitable basis. A firm basis in the community would provide the core of democratic control we believed to be essential. Finally, the network would be built on a prepaid health program, to replace the obsolete and inflationary fee-for-service system with one that would be prospectively budgeted and oriented to prevention.

Under the Dellums bill, health care would be funded through federal tax revenues. Funds would be disbursed on a per-capita basis, so that low- and middle-income communities would have the same access to quality medical services as would wealthier communities. Money would not be distributed, as it is in an insurance system, based on the fees institutions charge, but on the number of people served. A supplementary fund would be provided for the elderly and the poor, whose more extensive needs would require more funds per capita than the national average. Service would be provided by salaried workers, although the bill would not attempt to eliminate private practice. Funds would be made available through annual budgets for capital and operating expenses, placing the establishment and provision of medical services on a secure financial footing.

From the Bottom Up

The geographic organization of the system would follow the rationale espoused by nearly every health planner. Primary care would be offered through community-based facilities, making it accessible to people in the localities where they live and work. General inpatient services would be provided on a somewhat broader level, and specialized services on a still-broader, regional level. Strategic planning and basic research would be conducted at the national level.

The plan envisions, then, a four-tiered structure beginning with what we called the Community, an area of between 25,000 and 50,000 people where primary care would be provided. Our inspiration for this arrangement was the community health center, of which there are now hundreds throughout the country, mostly in low-income areas. The plan does not require each community to build a physical structure called the "community health center." Instead, it views the community health system as a network of primary-care providers integrated so that people can find their way through it without the kind of turmoil and confusion that patients experience today.

The second level of organization would be the District, serving approximately a quarter of a million people with general inpatient hospital services. Above the District would be the Region, serving a metropolitan-sized area with specialized inpatient services (e.g., trauma services, organ transplants). Regions would also be responsible for the education of health workers. The national level would establish standards for the provision of care and priorities for research.

Medical schools, nursing schools, and other training programs would be integrated into this national health system. A community-based, prevention-oriented approach would inform the education of health care workers. Much of their training would take place in primary-care settings, rather than in tertiary-care facilities providing specialty services. The legislation also provides for ladders of training, through which health workers could progressively expand their skills and acquire broader responsibilities. In an attempt to deal with the current dominance of medical care by physicians, the bill envisions teams of health care workers, in which the supervision of patient care would be a collective responsibility.

Assuring Accountability

Democratic control of this system would be provided by a governing structure operating in parallel with the medical care structure. Each community would elect a health board, in the same way school boards and the boards of community health centers are presently chosen. Voting would coincide with congressional elections in order to maximize participation. Boards would be composed of representatives of users of the system and representatives of those who work in it, with the former outnumbering the latter by two to one.

The Community Health Board would not only administer local health facilities, it would act as a "health advocate" for the community. Because the entire system rests on the belief that the health problems facing us are best dealt with through prevention, a primary responsibility of the community health boards would be to press local governments to take action to eliminate health risks.

District health boards would be composed of representatives from the community health boards, regional boards of representatives of districts, and the National Health Board of regional representatives. These boards would be responsible for allocating funds to the institutions under their respective supervision. Control would therefore run from the bottom up, and those who use the system, and those who work in it, would be represented at every level.

The Dellums Health Service Act was devised as a vehicle for education, using concepts that had been developed in the civil rights movement and in other progressive movements. The Act has been used across the country to show a different, progressive vision of how medical care can be organized. The Act remains relevant in spite of the changes that have occurred in health care since its preparation. The problems it addresses—escalating cost, maldistribution of resources, lack of emphasis on prevention, absence of democratic control—are with us still, exacerbated by the growth of the corporate, for-profit medical industry. The Dellums bill still describes the kind of health care system progressives ought to want. If it is, in fact, what we want, we should organize to get it.

MANAGED COMPETITION

A Guide to the Thicket

Ronda Kotelchuck

A not-so-funny thing happened on the way to a national health plan. The chariot seems to have detoured, at least temporarily, into a thicket of proposals known as "managed competition."

Whether this is a temporary detour or the final destination depends on the success of those trying to build a groundswell for a broader solution. And there are reasons for hope. The period is a politically fluid one. Against Bill Clinton and his affinity for the Jackson Hole Group, there is Hillary Rodham Clinton and her roots in the Children's Defense Fund. "Single-payer" solutions have actually made it onto the political map, exceeding the wildest hopes of many. The stakes are high and the larger prize worth the fight.

Should this struggle fail, however, advocates may have to struggle within the thicket. There are many reasons to curse the thicket, and many have already spelled them out. This article does something different. It attempts instead to guide the reader through the thicket of managed competition, identify the forks in the road, and provide the ammunition that may be needed (or, more accurately, to identify the targets) should this be the place of struggle.

This article attempts to make understandable (if not interesting) the four key elements of managed competition proposals: 1) the standard benefit package, 2) tax reform, 3) health insurance purchasing cooperatives (the now-famous HIPCs), and 4) health plans. It seeks to identify the issues and the options available within each component, and to examine the progressive and regressive potentials within each.

Managed competition proposals range on the political spectrum from the laissez-faire, market-oriented right to roughly the center. In a right-to-left progression, the major proposals include those authored by the Heritage Foundation (an extreme free-market proposal that will not be considered further here), the Jackson Hole Group, Jim Cooper (D-Tenn.) (which was already introduced in Congress), and the Progressive Policy Institute (think-tank of Bill Clinton's Democratic Leadership Council), and a state proposal offered by California Insurance Commissioner John Garamendi and widely touted on a national basis by Princeton sociologist Paul Starr.

Standard Benefit Package

Every health insurance plan, existing or proposed, defines a package of health services for which it will pay. The differences in existing health benefit packages are endless, ranging from the most comprehensive to the most spare, depending on what the purchaser wants and is willing to pay (or, more frequently, what the bargaining unit can exact).

Managed competition would standardize this package. Consumers could purchase broader or richer benefits, but the standard package would set a floor beneath what is available (hopefully) for all. This package would be determined either legislatively or by a specially appointed national commission, depending on the proposal adopted. Most frequently referenced is the package of benefits required of federally qualified HMOs.

A standardized benefit package serves several purposes under managed competition. It provides a basis for "portability," so that benefits do not change as a person moves from place to place or job to job, contributing to problems of "job lock." The standard benefit package is also fundamental to tax reform (as is explained in the following section). Finally, it allows comparison of the cost and effectiveness of different plans and providers, key ingredients for "perfecting the market mechanism," as envisioned under managed competition.

The first dilemma to be faced in defining a standard benefit package is an ethically and strategically complex one. Realistically, in an environment of limited resources, in which 37 million Americans lack any health insurance coverage whatsoever, comprehensiveness of benefits will be traded off against universality of coverage. Should a comprehensive package of benefits be offered to fewer persons or a bare-bones package be made available to more? The importance of expanding any form of access is incontrovertible. Yet the comprehensiveness of the benefit package will shape America's future health system, as it has that of the present. This will occur in at least two fundamental ways.

The first is known as "You-get-what-you-pay-for," not only in health benefits, but in the resulting shape of the health delivery system. Benefit packages in the past have paid handsomely for very expensive and rarely needed acute, emergency, and specialty care. Highly effective and routinely needed primary and preventive care has most frequently been uninsured, underinsured, or the object of co-payments, presumably because it is relatively inexpensive. It is also one of the few kinds of care that can be considered "discretionary" for the consumer.

This pattern is consistent with the medium of American health coverage, the insurance model, which deals well with risk but poorly with certainty. The need for quadruple bypass surgery is a risk; the need for immunizations or prenatal care a certainty. Not coincidentally, this pattern also supports and is consistent with the priorities and array of powerful forces in the American health care system.

The fruit of this insurance model is the current "inverted pyramid" of the health care delivery system, in which tertiary services form the base and primary and preventive care the tip. The outcome is also a system that cannot control cost or meet need because it has only the most expensive, least appropriate care to offer. And misguided attempts to control spending by imposing more and more out-of-pocket costs on primary and preventive care simply exacerbate the cost problem.

The standard benefit package will also shape American health care in a second way. It will help determine the extent to which the resulting health system continues to be a two-class system. At issue is the adequacy of the package. To the extent that essential services are missing, Americans will pay for them out of pocket. Access to the resulting care will be available to those with means and unavailable to those without. At issue is inclusion not only of primary and preventive services, but of benefits frequently omitted altogether from current packages, such as prescription drugs, dental care, mental health and substance abuse services, durable medical equipment, home care, respite care, and rehabilitation services.

Finally, in benefit packages, one size does not fit all. A richer package of benefits is required to effectively care for low-income and medically needy populations. This frequently includes, for example, social services, transportation, interpreters, and more extensive mental health and substance abuse services. The Medicaid benefit package reflects this fact. A narrowly defined medical model of benefits will neither do the job nor be cost effective for some populations.

Tax Reform

The second major element of virtually all managed competition proposals is tax reform. Currently, health benefits are virtually free of taxation or totally tax deductible. Employers pay no payroll tax on their contributions, nor are health benefits considered part of the employee's wage and thus are not subject to income tax.

Managed competition partisans argue that because health benefits are tax deductible to employers and not taxed for employees, while wages are taxed, employers and unions have an incentive to invest in health benefits rather than wages—to "overinsure" their employees. Moreover, the argument goes, such "overinsurance" encourages consumers to overutilize the health care system by insulating them from cost. They also argue, with cause, that total tax deductibility is socially regressive, giving larger tax breaks to workers who receive generous benefits rather than subsidizing those most in need.

Under managed competition, only the standard benefit package would be tax deductible. Its dollar value would be set at the cost of the least expensive benefit package available in the region. Any benefits beyond the cost of the minimum package would have to be purchased by the consumer and would be paid for with after-tax dollars.

This reform would have several effects: It would discourage "overinsurance" by "leveling the playing field" in the trade-off between wages and health benefits. It would make consumers "cost conscious" in their choice of benefits and plans. It would force plans to compete based on price. And last, but not least, it would create a new revenue source to fund expanded coverage of the currently uninsured (or, in the worst case, to reduce the federal deficit).

Managed competition purists believe fervently that reform of tax incentives is critical to the success of managed competition. The President's fervor on this issue has recently lagged, probably in contemplating how he will sell the labor movement on the loss of hard-fought benefits and the middle class on tax increases as the first step in health care reform. Interestingly, the health insurance industry has decided to accept increased taxes on its product if this is the price of staying in the game.

Health Insurance Purchasing Cooperatives

The third element common to all managed competition proposals is a new entity known as a health insurance purchasing cooperative, or "HIPC" (pronounced "hippic," not "hiccup"). The HIPC would be the source of health insurance for many, if not all, purchasers of health coverage, offering them a menu of approved health plans providing the standard benefit package. (See discussion of health plans in the following section.)

HIPCs could be either private, non-profit, or public entities and would be established on a statewide or regional basis. Broader proposals suggest that only one HIPC could operate in a region, while the more laissez-faire proposals would allow as many as the market would bear. Under most proposals employers and individuals would purchase coverage through a HIPC.

The broadest proposal (Garamendi/Starr) has several distinguishing features. The HIPC would replace the current employer-based system entirely. The traditional employer and employee contributions for health insurance would be replaced by a 7 percent payroll tax and a 1 percent income tax. These would fund the HIPC directly, and everyone would obtain coverage through the HIPC.

Because HIPCs would create an important new "market" of customers looking for health insurance, health plans would compete for their business. The HIPC would pay plans a fixed rate per individual (capitation), adjusted for risk, for the standard package of services, and contracting plans would be required to provide all needed services, regardless of cost. The rate would be set at the level of the lowest-cost acceptable plan in a region.

In the managed competition schema, HIPCs become the key agent for "managing" competition or making it work in the health sector. They would do this in a variety of ways:

• HIPCs would consolidate the purchasing power of consumers into a force that could advocate and effectively bargain on behalf of consumer interests.

• They would collect, analyze, and provide information on cost, quality, and effectiveness of different plans and services. Such information is now lacking, depriving consumers of the ability to make meaningful health care choices, as is required by a market mechanism.

• Finally, HIPCs would be instrumental in reforming the insurance market. Plans would be prohibited from engaging in "bad forms" of competition. The most rampant "bad form" now is avoiding high-risk enrollees, using such techniques as medical underwriting, redlining, skimming, excluding pre-existing conditions, retroactive denials of benefits, and refusing to renew policies (see Donald Light, "Excluding More, Covering Less: The Health Insurance Industry in the U.S.," Spring 1992 issue, *Health/PAC Bulletin*). Instead, health plans would be forced into "good forms" of competition, on the basis of quality and cost.

HIPCs would be responsible for enforcing this insurance reform. In the broader managed competition proposals, HIPCs, and not health plans them-

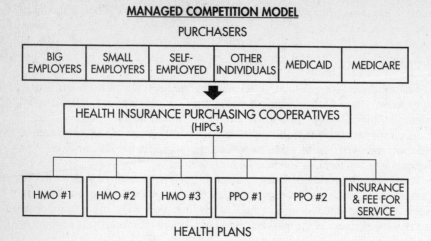

MANAGED COMPETITION MODEL
PURCHASERS

BIG EMPLOYERS	SMALL EMPLOYERS	SELF-EMPLOYED	OTHER INDIVIDUALS	MEDICAID	MEDICARE

HEALTH INSURANCE PURCHASING COOPERATIVES
(HIPCs)

HMO #1	HMO #2	HMO #3	PPO #1	PPO #2	INSURANCE & FEE FOR SERVICE

HEALTH PLANS

selves, would conduct the actual marketing and enrollment functions. Their enrollees would form a "broad risk pool," including the full spectrum of high- and low-risk members. Plans would be forced to accept any enrollee sent to them from the HIPC.

Managed competition is supposed to enhance the sovereignty of "consumer choice." And while consumers will be able to choose more knowledgeably among plans, the choice they care about most—selecting their own physician —will be limited to those available through a particular plan (see diagram).

The importance of the HIPC under a managed competition system raises a host of critical issues. Perhaps the most important is whether the HIPC will be the source of coverage for everyone, or only for particular (and usually unin-surable) segments of the population.

In the broadest proposals (such as Garamendi/Starr), HIPCs constitute the "single source" from which everyone obtains their coverage. The more con-servative proposals (Jackson Hole, Progressive Policy Institute) allow large em-ployers, who are presumed to have sufficient bargaining power, to continue purchasing coverage directly from plans or insurance companies.

HIPCs would be available for those who lack similar clout and find them-selves squeezed out of the current market—small employers, individual pur-chasers, and the uninsured, many of whom will be subsidized to purchase coverage. Most proposals would eventually incorporate Medicaid and Medicare beneficiaries into the HIPC.

The decision on whether HIPCs will serve everyone or only normally un-insurable populations is another key, along with the adequacy of the benefit package, to whether managed competition will be a one- or two-class system. Small employers, individual purchasers, and the uninsured lack access to the current insurance market precisely because they present higher risk and are less profitable to insure than the clientele of large employers.

Splitting the source of coverage for these two groups would not only create two tracks of care, it would also undercut the ability of HIPCs to "manage" competition. If they served only the uninsurable, HIPCs could not maintain a broad risk pool. Their ability to force health plans to compete on the basis of price and quality, control discriminatory practices, or exact vital information on costs and outcomes would be severely compromised. Their ability to set rates, rather than being comprehensive, would be limited only to the high-risk portion of the population. These problems would be even worse if more than one HIPC were allowed to function in a region.

Another major issue regarding HIPCs is the extent to which they will be able to prevent health plans from discriminating against high-risk consumers. Will all plans offered on the HIPC menu be required to provide the standard benefit package for the same fixed rate? Or will only a few plans offer the "economy model," while others sport more attractive amenities and richer services at higher prices, available only to those who can pay? The answer determines whether "consumer choice" applies to all consumers or only to those of means.

To eliminate financial grounds for discrimination, HIPCs must "risk-adjust" rates (that is, pay more for higher-risk populations) to assure that plans treating high-risk populations are paid adequately and not penalized. Risk adjustment, however, is not a highly developed art. Will HIPCs be able to control the many and subtle practices by which plans encourage some consumers to enroll and not others (such as the third-floor walk-up syndrome, which clearly discourages the less-than-healthy from signing up)? The answer is doubtful, at best.

Finally, the performance of HIPCs raises another important set of questions. With such a potential concentration of power in HIPCs, how will they avoid dominance by special interests in the health system, such as hospitals and insurance companies, instead of representing consumer interests? How will they be regulated and governed? How will good performance be ensured, and what are the consequences of indifferent or bad performance? Will they not simply add an entirely new and expensive layer of administration, bureaucracy, and other nonproductive costs?

HIPCs offer some positive potential (such as a single source for obtaining coverage and tax-based rather than employment-based options) depending on how these key issues are addressed. The stakes are very high and the cumulative probabilities of success small, however, for such an untried venture.

Health Plans

The fourth major element of managed competition—the health plan—will be the fundamental building block of the new health system. Health plans will contract with HIPCs for enrollees and will actually produce and be responsible for care. Health plans will be certified or approved for contracting under managed competition by the HIPC or state or federal government.

HIPCs will pay plans a capitated rate (a fixed rate per capita for a package of services). It is this unit of payment, capitation, that creates the financial incentives fundamental to managed care and competition and the cost savings upon which they are predicated (see "Medicaid Managed Care: A Mixed Review," Fall 1992 issue, *Health/PAC Bulletin*).

Unlike the traditional fee-for-service payment arrangement, in which the provider is rewarded for producing more services, capitation rewards providers for producing less. Contracting plans will be obligated to provide all the services needed under that package, regardless of cost. Thus, plans are placed "at risk." If the enrollee uses few services, the plan profits. If the enrollee uses many and costly services, the plan must absorb the loss.

Plans can respond to this incentive by providing ample primary and preventive care to keep the enrollee well, or they can use more insidious means to simply avoid providing the needed service altogether (for example, long waits, busy telephone lines, and refusing to refer patients for tests and to specialty services). As noted, managed competition will attempt to prohibit the past practice of avoiding or excluding high-risk enrollees.

Capitation, the unit of payment, not only establishes new financial incentives, but it will also paint a new health care landscape. The entity receiving capitation must offer all covered services—inpatient, outpatient, emergency, primary, and specialty care. Gone will be the days of individual, autonomous providers such as private practitioners, to be replaced by the "network" or "plan."

For the first time, the basic unit of the system—the plan or network—will integrate the traditional functions of both insurer and provider, a precondition of efficiency and cost savings. This is the distinguishing feature of managed care entities such as health maintenance organizations (HMOs), which case manage services to the enrollee, and preferred provider organizations (PPOs), which simply limit the consumer to using a network of discount providers. Conceivably HIPCs could also contract with traditional insurers that pay providers on a fee-for-service basis. Because they will be forced to compete based on cost, however, it is assumed that plans using fee-for-service payment will be at a competitive disadvantage compared to capitation plans and will eventually be squeezed out.

The most important issue with health plans, as noted earlier, is whether high-risk enrollees will have access to all plans, or whether they will be concentrated in a few—a sure setup for a two-class system. This will depend on a variety of factors: whether all plans offer the standard benefit package at a fixed rate, or whether some plans offer Chevrolets (or worse, bicycles) while others sell only Cadillacs; whether out-of-pocket augmentation of the standard benefit package is limited or unlimited; whether a variety of plans is accessible to underserved areas; and whether HIPCs successfully risk adjust rates and enforce non-discriminatory enrollment.

Other issues of concern: Competition will presumably limit the number of plans available. After the non-competitive plans have been shaken out and only a few big ones remain, how will competition based on cost and quality be maintained? Once health plans are certified, what will ensure their continued quality performance? And how will the system deal with unsatisfactory performance, since termination of a plan will be difficult, if not virtually impossible?

Universality of Coverage

Under managed competition, universal coverage is not simply a laudable social objective, it is a necessary condition of successful competition, since it is assumed that everyone must receive some form of care, and institutions cannot be competitive if some must absorb the cost of uncompensated care. The dilemmas of how to achieve and how to finance universal coverage are not particularly unique to managed competition.

Three fundamentally different approaches exist to achieving universal coverage, and these are also represented in different managed care proposals:

1. Remove health insurance from its current employer base and create a universal system financed through taxation (the Garamendi/Starr approach).

2. Patch up the current system. Mandate that all employers cover their employees and dependents. Consider subsidizing small employers to ease the financial pain. Fill in the gaps by offering a graduated subsidy to the low-income uninsured. Clinton, who started out advocating employer mandates and backed away early in his campaign, now seems to be reconsidering this approach.

3. Laissez faire: Let competition reduce the cost to affordable levels, and more employers and individuals will choose to buy. Assist the low-income uninsured by providing vouchers or tax credits.

Proposals vary by whether they recommend folding Medicaid and Medicare into a unitary system or preserving and expanding them in an attempt to reduce gaps in the current system.

Clearly, the single most important issue in achieving universal coverage is whether coverage will be mandatory or voluntary. A voluntary system would be neither universal nor a system. Large numbers of Americans will "choose" to be uninsured because they find other financial needs more pressing. Yet they will continue to need care. Will the system cover undocumented workers? Difficult to manage populations, such as substance abusers or the homeless?

The second major issue is how to pay for the cost of covering the uninsured, estimated at $60 to $90 billion. The "T-word" (tax) is still off-limits, although it appears slightly more acceptable when linked to sin (as in additional taxes on health-destroying substances such as tobacco). Some also argue that the Garamendi proposal, which would replace current employer and employee contributions for health insurance with payroll and income taxes, can be sold to employers as being cheaper, easier, and more appealing than the current system.

Currently three new sources of revenue are mentioned: (1) use new revenues produced by reducing the tax deductibility of health benefits. This will produce roughly $10 to $20 billion. (2) Redirect funds currently subsidizing care of the poor and uninsured, especially those reimbursements under Medicare and Medicaid, known as indirect medical education and disproportionate share reimbursement, for extra expenses to hospitals serving large numbers of poor. The viability of America's "safety net" institutions depends upon these funds, however, and cannot be jeopardized as long as that safety net is still needed. (3) Wait for cost controls to take effect and phase in expanded coverage using the savings achieved. Given the conflicting interests of major power blocks and their past record on cost control, this could be a very long wait, indeed.

Summary Chart of Managed Competition Proposals

BASIC ELEMENTS/KEY ISSUES	JACKSON HOLE
Minimum Benefit Package **Key Issues:** * Does it include essential services? * Do enrollees have to pay out of pocket? * Does package include supplemental benefits needed by poor?	* Minimum benefit package to be determined by National Health Board. * Benefits in excess of minimum package and additional amenities may be purchased privately with after-tax dollars. No limitation on private purchase.
Tax Policy	* Only minimum benefit package tax deductible. * Value set at price of lowest-cost package in state. * Deductibility available only for benefits provided by accountable health plans (APHs).
HIPCs **Key Issues:** * Is HIPC source of coverage for everyone or only hard-to-insure groups? * Is all marketing and enrollment done by the HIPC (and not plans)? * Is more than one HIPC allowed to operate in a region? * Is HIPC public or private? How is it governed?	* HIPC contracts with competing AHPs for minimum benefit package. * Serves small employers, individual enrollees only; big employers negotiate directly with AHPs. * Purchase through HIPC required for small employers to obtain tax deductibility. * Conducts all enrollment. * Governed by contracting employers.

COOPER BILL	GARAMENDI/STARR	PROGRESSIVE POLICY INSTITUTE
* Minimum benefit package to be established by National Health Board. * Includes cost sharing by enrollee. * Some Medicaid benefits not included in benefit package (prescription drugs, glasses, hearing aids).	* Benefit package the same as that required of federally qualified HMOs. * Benefits in excess of minimum package, additional amenities may be purchased privately with after-tax dollars. Private purchase limited to 150% of minimum.	* Minimum benefit package to be established by National Health Board. * Benefits in excess of minimum package and additional amenities may be purchased privately with after-tax dollars. No limit on private purchase.
* Employers pay excise tax of 34% unless: —Premium goes to AHP or HIPC. —Premiums exceed reference rate. —Employer contribution cannot vary by plan. * For self-employed, deduction increases from 25% to 100%.	* Only minimum benefit package tax deductible. * Additional benefits and amenities may be purchased privately with after-tax dollars.	* Deductibility on minimum package only: —Premiums deductible if employer offers employee two AHP options. —Deductible set at lowest-cost AHP in region. —Employer contribution becomes taxable income to employee; but household receives tax credit if it subscribes to AHP.
* HIPC contracts with competing AHPs for minimum benefit package. * Serves small employers; other employers required to offer AHPs to employees. * Enroll individuals into AHPs. * Federal legislation establishes state as HIPC; state may designate smaller area.	* HIPC acts as "single sponsor" or purchaser of coverage in each region. * Contracts with health plans for minimum benefit package. * Conducts all marketing and enrollment. * Pays plan a uniform, risk-adjusted rate. * Provider payment by plans is negotiated; HIPC does not regulate. * Board includes employers, consumers.	* Whether all groups obtain coverage through HIPC is unspecified. * HIPC contracts with competing health plans to offer minimum benefit package. * HIPC is sole point of marketing and enrollment. * Could be quasi-public or non-profit agencies. * HIPC requirements (size, governance, solvency) defined by federal legislation.

Summary Chart of Managed Competition Proposals (*cont.*)

BASIC ELEMENTS/KEY ISSUES	JACKSON HOLE
Health Plans **Key Issues:** * Is minimum benefit package available without out-of-pocket costs to all enrollees? * Are private payments in excess of minimum benefit package limited? * Must plans accept all enrollees? * Are risk-avoidance practices (waiting periods, pre-existing condition exclusions, redlining, skimming) prohibited? * Must plans accept fixed, community rate for standard benefit package?	* Will be registered with National Health Board based on: —Health outcomes reporting. —Insurance practices. —Scope of coverage. —Accountability for quality of care. * No requirement that minimum package be available at minimum price from all AHPs. * No limitation on private payment. * Plans must accept all enrollees. * Plans must accept community rating; risk-avoidance practices prohibited.
Universality/Finance **Key Issues:** * Is participation mandatory or voluntary? * How is universal coverage to be achieved? Financed?	* Universal coverage required; some gaps possible (e.g., homeless). —Full-time employees: employers required to buy minimum coverage at rate of lowest-price benefit package. —Part-time employees/non-poor: charged payroll tax. —Poor/near poor: subsidy for purchase of coverage. —Medicaid, Medicare to be integrated.

COOPER BILL	GARAMENDI/STARR	PROGRESSIVE POLICY INSTITUTE
* Health plan must be certified as "accountable health plan" in order to participate: —Minimum benefit package. —Reporting requirements. —Financial solvency. —Nondiscriminatory practices. —Effective grievance procedure. * AHPs allowed to exclude pre-existing conditions for up to 6 months. * Can be open or closed, based on size (open AHPs can establish standard premiums, contract with HIPCs). * Can offer additional benefits. Lower cost sharing separate from minimum benefit package. * No limit on private payment.	* Can offer additional amenities and flexibility at extra cost to enrollees. Extra costs are limited to 150% of premium. * Plan receives a fixed premium, based on price of lowest-cost plan. * Plan must accept all enrollees. * Risk-avoidance practices prohibited. * Must meet data-reporting requirements.	* Health plan must be certified as "accountable health plan" in order to participate. * Must meet federal reporting requirements (cost, outcomes, patient satisfaction). * Federal law to: —Prohibit risk avoidance practices. —Require health plans to charge same rate for all HIPC enrollees (actuarial adjustment possible). * Insurers, plans selling supplemental coverage could not experience rate. * HIPCs to experiment with reinsurance, risk adjustment to assure risk-sharing.
* Employer participation is mandatory: —Small employers must contract with HIPC. —Large employers must offer AHPs. * Individual participation not specified. * Abolishes Medicaid, offers subsidy to poor: —Full payment for those under 100% of poverty level. —Sliding-scale premiums, cost sharing.	* Participation is mandatory. * Everyone obtains coverage through HIPC. * Premium contributions are funded through tax assessments (small adjustment for small firms, low-income workers). —Employers pay 6.75% payroll tax. —Employees pay 1% tax on wages. —Self-employed pay through income tax. * Medicare, Medicaid to be integrated later.	* Universal coverage is required; means is left to state option. * Medicaid is abolished and fund used to subsidize purchase of coverage through HIPC. * Medicare to be integrated later.

Summary Chart of Managed Competition Proposals (*cont.*)

BASIC ELEMENTS/KEY ISSUES	JACKSON HOLE
Cost Control	* Competition only.
Federal/State Role	Federal role: * National Health Board (public): * Adopts, revises minimum benefit package. —Sets tax-deductibility cap. —Registers AHPs, HIPCs. —Oversees transition. * Health Standards Board (private): Advises on minimum benefit package. * Outcomes Management Standards Board (private): adopts data collection and reporting standards. * Health Insurance Standards Board: sets standards for insurance practices (rating practices, risk adjustment). State role: * Selects HIPCs.

It's the Infrastructure, Stupid!

Universal coverage does not ensure access to care. Neither does a broad benefit package. This is especially true for those living in America's underserved urban and rural areas, where providers and services simply do not exist. No reform proposal, no matter how visionary, will ensure access to health care unless it addresses critical gaps in the infrastructure of health services.

The most critical gap, discussed earlier, is the lack of primary and preventive care in underserved communities. Without this missing link in the health care infrastructure, little can be done. Managed competition cannot be implemented; health care needs cannot be addressed; use of the system cannot be rationalized; costs cannot be saved without critical compromises; and access will never be expanded.

Health care reform could easily create another gap. Currently a network of public and inner-city hospitals and health services provide a safety net for those who would otherwise have no access to care by virtue of their poverty, lack of insurance, lack of legal residence, social problems, or complexity of illness.

COOPER BILL	GARAMENDI/STARR	PROGRESSIVE POLICY INSTITUTE
* Competition only.	* Global budget: revenue to plans is limited to amount collected through taxes.	* Competition only.
Federal role: * National Health Board: —Establishes uniform benefit package. —Establishes cost-sharing requirements. —Registers AHPs. —Establishes reporting standards. * Establish advisory boards: —Health Benefits and Data Standards Board. —Health Plan Standards Board.	* Competition: consumer choice of plans based on cost, quality. * Administrative savings: —No brokers fees. —No billing costs. —Consolidates health insurance, workers compensation, auto insurance into single coverage.	Federal role: * Legislation defines HIPC requirements (size, governance, solvency). * Defines reporting requirements for AHPs. * Legislation sets standards for state health insurance regulation; bans risk-avoidance practices. State role: * Required to guarantee universal coverage (can be employer-based, single-payer with competing private insurers, or tax credit). * Implements prohibition on risk-avoidance practices.

Many of these safety net institutions are the sole providers available in underserved communities. In addition to local tax support, these providers also depend heavily on indirect medical education and disproportionate share reimbursement under Medicaid and Medicare.

To the extent that managed competition leaves gaps in covered services or covered populations, either permanently or in transition, America's safety net will continue to be needed. Health care reform cannot cut away support from the only health care infrastructure now serving the nation's poor and uninsured. In fact, it must reinvest in these facilities, especially if they are to survive under competition.

The Historic Moment

Managed competition is hardly the vision for which health activists have struggled over the decades. It is not our idea of how to address the problems of cost, quality, or access that are unraveling America's health care system.

Overlaying the current system with the new layers of administrative costs entailed in HIPCs and health plans, building and maintaining complex and costly information systems and review functions, while reducing the actual health care rendered, hardly suggests effective or responsible cost control or utilization of resources. The fee-for-service system embodies an inflationary incentive that will not withstand the imperatives of cost control. The reverse incentive built into managed care—the incentive *not* to provide services—is even more troubling, however, in its ability to undermine access and quality.

Competition has rarely been a friend of social justice, and its suitability as a tool for addressing the needs of the poor and the very ill is deeply suspect. The odds of managed competition succumbing to the multiple opportunities to create a two-class system are overwhelming.

And finally, the odds that America's health care problems will be solved by a system so complex, so opaque and so largely untried seems unlikely.

Yet health care progressives cannot lose sight of the historic moment. For the first time in recent memory, change appears to be possible. The system is unraveling, and the powerful forces that have held the American health system hostage to the status quo are beginning to shift and split up.

That change may take a course different from that anticipated is perhaps less significant than the fact that it is possible at all. In struggling for their vision, advocates cannot underestimate, or in their disappointment defend by default, the evil of a status quo that daily denies care to vast segments of the American public.

Perhaps the most important goal for the moment is assuring the breakup of the powerful forces of the status quo. And perhaps the standard that should be applied to whatever change occurs is not whether it achieves the vision, but whether it at least charts the right direction.

Thus, if we are forced into the thicket of managed competition, important achievements are still possible. Simply to establish that all Americans have a right to health care is incalculable social progress, even if progress toward this right is faltering. The possibility that all Americans will obtain coverage from a single source is progress. The possibility that cooperative organizations could work on behalf of the consumer would be progress. The possibility that the system could be tax based is progress.

Unfortunately for the weary, it is unlikely that progressive health care reform will arrive in a fell swoop. Instead, it is likely to arrive in fits and starts, the fruit of continued struggle over decades to come.

ACHIEVING EFFECTIVE COST CONTROL IN COMPREHENSIVE HEALTH CARE REFORM

The Jackson Hole "Managed Care Managed Competition" Approach

Alain Enthoven

The managed competition approach was originated by Alain Enthoven, a professor at the Stanford University Graduate School of Business, in the late 1970s, and has since been refined by Enthoven and a group of colleagues meeting in Jackson Hole, Wyoming. This outline was presented by Enthoven at hearings on cost control in health care reform held by Senator Edward Kennedy (D-MA) in December 1992.

I. The Jackson Hole "Managed Care Managed Competition" model is built on the integration of five main ideas:

1. Universal coverage.
2. A pro-competitive regulatory framework.
3. Health Plan Purchasing Cooperatives to pool small employers and individuals.
4. Managed competition: and
5. Accountable Health Plans that integrate financing and delivery and are publicly accountable for quality and cost.

II. Accountable Health Plans

Much of the economic failure of our health care system can be ascribed to the traditional model of fee-for-service, solo practice, "free choice," and remote third-party payment.

- The incentives are mostly wrong.
- There is no effective accountability for quality or per capita cost.

We must convert to integrated financing and delivery systems—HMOs and new partnerships among insurers, doctors, and hospitals—with per capita prepayment (i.e., global budgets set in advance in the marketplace), providers at risk for the costs of care and costs of poor quality, so that they are rewarded for improving quality and cutting cost.

There is much such organizations can do to improve quality and cut costs.

- Evaluate practice patterns and choose cost-effective ways of caring for patients.
- Match numbers/types of doctors and other resources (beds, CT scanners, etc.) to needs of enrolled population.
- Regional concentration of costly, complex services.
- Total Quality Management and continuous improvement in productivity and quality.

Many different systems and styles of care can fit into this model, including individual practice, networks of small multispecialty groups, and large multispecialty groups. They do not all have to look like Harvard Community Health Plan.

With the advent of modern information technologies, we are seeing development of information system-based "HMOs without walls" that can grow fast, use familiar practice styles and locations, and adapt to the requirements of less populated areas. They channel the business to the providers who offer the best "value for money."

III. Managed Competition

Most employers today pay all or most of the premium or cost of an open-ended, fee-for-service coverage, and the premium of HMOs as long as they do not exceed the cost of the fee-for-service plan. As a result, there is little or no value for money competition among managed care plans.

Employers have not given managed care plans a strong incentive to hold down cost. This is worsened by the open-ended exclusion of employer contributions from the taxable incomes of employees—which works as a very heavy tax on cost containment.

Managed competition is a purchaser strategy based on informed, premium price-conscious consumer choice designed to reward with more subscribers those organizations that do the best job of improving quality and cutting cost.

Managed competition depends on sponsors, i.e., large, active, well-informed collective purchasing agents that contract with health plans on behalf of insured people. Examples of sponsors are the federal office of Personnel Management, CALPERS, large employers, and HCFA. In managed competition, the sponsor's roles are:

1. Through contracts, establish and enforce principles of equitable behavior such as coverage of all eligible persons, continuity of coverage, commu-

nity rating within the sponsored group, no exclusions or limitations on coverage for pre-existing conditions.

2. Select participating plans.
3. Manage the enrollment process.
4. Create price-elastic demand.
- Employer contributions and tax-free amounts must not exceed the price of the lowest-priced plan.
- Standardize the coverage contract.
- Provide quality-related information.
- Offer choice of plan at the individual level.

5. Manage risk selection to take the reward out of selecting risks.
- Single point of entry.
- Standardize coverage.
- Risk-adjust premiums (e.g., Medicare AAPCC).
- Monitor voluntary disenrollments.
- Monitor specialty and tertiary care arrangements.

A limit on tax-free employer contributions at an amount that does not exceed the (risk-adjusted) price of the low-priced plan is a key part of this.

The combination of (1) per capita prepayment with providers at risk and (2) health plans in "value for money competition," facing price-elastic demand represents a powerful reversal of the financial incentives of the past 50 years.

IV. Health Plan Purchasing Cooperatives

Small employers of up to 100 or even 1,000 (in varying degrees) are too small to:

1. Spread risks.
2. Achieve economies of scale in administration.
3. Acquire needed information and expertise.
4. Manage competition.
5. Offer multiple choice of plan to the individual subscriber.

Such employment groups—and individuals—should be pooled through the creation of a national system of Health Plan Purchasing Cooperatives (HPPCs) that would function as sponsors on behalf of all small employers and individuals in a geographic area. Each HPPC would accept all qualifying employment groups in its area. They would not be allowed to exclude employment groups or individuals because of health status.

Each HPPC would:

- contract with several accountable health plans;
- contract with participating employers (and the state for state-sponsored groups);

- spread risks and costs widely;
- relieve employer of COBRA and other administrative burdens.

An excellent example of an HPPC in the public sector is CALPERS [California Public Employees' Retirement System], which covers over 870,000 people, employees, retirees and dependents of over 760 employers, through 23 HMOs and 5 Preferred Provider Insurance plans.

A key issue in creation of a HPPC is the need for a powerful incentive to cause the groups and individuals with good health risks to want to join. The Jackson Hole Initiative proposes making buying through the HPPC a condition for receiving the tax exclusion in the case of small employers.

V. Pro-competitive Regulatory Framework for Technology Decisions, Outcomes Reporting, and Underwriting Practices

- An authoritative science and value-based process—a Health Standards Board—a kind of "Supreme Court of Medical Technology" to define "uniform effective health benefits" eligible for tax-favored treatment.
- An outcomes Management Standards Board to set data collection and reporting standards for patient outcomes and other quality measures.
- A Health Insurance Standards Board to set standards for insurance practices (e.g., approved rating practices and risk adjustment methods).

VI. Universal Coverage

Millions of Americans not covered, millions more "pseudo covered," has many destructive consequences including: financial hardship, disease and disability that could have been prevented, costly late care in costly settings, uncovered people putting providers in a moral bind, closed emergency departments, and cost shifting.

Everybody should be covered.

Employers and employees should have to buy coverage for full-time employees.

A reformed market makes this a much more bearable requirement.

A payroll tax on part-timers.

A tax or "individual mandate" on non-poor non-employed (unemployed, early retired).

Subsidies for the poor and near poor, a main source of which is federal and state budget savings accruing from the limit on tax-free employer contributions.

VII. Concluding Comments

1. This model relies on incentives and rational organization in decentralized and pluralistic private market rather than centralized command and control regulation by government.
2. This approach respects American cultural preferences for limited government, voluntary action, decentralized decision-making, individual choice, multiple competing approaches, pluralism, and personal and local responsibility.
3. What about quality? Far more often than not, in medical care quality and economy go hand-in-hand. The correct diagnosis made promptly, the appropriate procedure done proficiently are best for the patient and the payer. Mistakes cost money. This model would give purchasers and consumers far better quality-related information than they have had before.
4. How can we know this will work?

   We know some types of managed care can cut cost substantially. RAND found Group Health Cooperative of Puget Sound cut cost 28 percent compared to fee-for-service, and they did it without competition or cost-conscious buyers. Their medical director has stated they could have cut costs much more if there had been incentives to do so. Many other non-experimental comparisons show similar savings.

   We know there are wide variations in costs for many procedures; for example, four-fold variations in the price of open-heart surgery. The best producers have the lowest costs. In managed competition, health plans would have powerful incentives to pick the high-quality low-cost providers.

   We know that when given responsible choices, people choose value for money.

   We know HPPC-like arrangements work well.

   All the pieces of a managed care/managed competition model are in actual practice somewhere. The challenge is to put ''best practice'' together in one complete managed competition system.

   The rest is extrapolation based on generally accepted principles of rational economic behavior.

   All reform proposals must rely on similar extrapolation.

CALIFORNIA HEALTH CARE IN THE 21ST CENTURY

A Vision for Reform

John Garamendi

California Insurance Commissioner John Garamendi's proposal for revamping the state's health care system is considered by many to be an improvement on Alain Enthoven's version of managed competition because it separates insurance from employment and includes budgets and a single source of financing. Princeton sociologist Paul Starr, a prominent member of the National Health Care Taskforce, is a proponent of a similar plan on a national basis. This is an excerpt from the Executive Summary of the plan; in 1992 the California legislature approved a commission to study the proposal, only to have it vetoed by Governor Pete Wilson.

California Health Care in the 21st Century proposes a unified health care system to which all would contribute and upon which all would depend.

- The health care system would be managed by a private/public partnership of government, employers, and consumers.
- The delivery of health care would remain in private hands, and would be provided by many of the same private organizations that provide health care today. Health care would be publicly guaranteed, but privately delivered.
- Consumers would be able to choose from among competing health care plans, all of which would be providing the same state-guaranteed benefit package. There would be no pre-existing condition exclusions, no waiting periods, and no extra charges due to health status or age and sex.
- The health care components of all private insurance policies—workers compensation, auto, and health—would be consolidated into a single health care system. Individuals would receive the same protection and the same care regardless of when, where, or why an injury or illness occurred.
- The proposal would blend the best of regulatory and competitive features of health care reform approaches. It does not make a final determination of the appropriate blend, instead allowing the mix to vary over time and across regions.
- The proposal would keep California's strongest economic players in one health care system, providing the impetus for them to make it work for everyone.

Built-In Mechanisms for Controlling Costs

- An overall health care budget would provide restraint. Public costs would not increase faster than wages unless the state increased employer/employee premium rates, always a difficult political act.
- Placing greater choice in the hands of consumers would encourage them to spend dollars more wisely.
- Inefficient insurers that now compete on the basis of their ability to avoid high-risk individuals would be forced to compete on the basis of the value they offer to consumers.
- Much of the administrative waste in the current system would be eliminated:
    - Employers would no longer need to buy insurance, a particularly important consideration for small businesses.
    - Managed care plans—which generally have lower administrative costs than traditional insurers—would be promoted. Inefficient insurers would be unable to compete.
    - With a Health Insurance Purchasing Corporation providing consumers with better information and direct access to health plans, the overhead costs of insurance broker commissions would be unnecessary.
    - It is expected that competition would drive health plans to become more integrated (i.e., that they would form networks of physicians, hospitals, and other providers). Through such integrated arrangements, hospital and physician billing costs would be reduced.

Twenty-four-Hour Care: The Consolidation of Health Coverage

- The health care components of all private insurance policies—workers compensation, auto, and health—would be consolidated into a single health care system.
- Consolidation would reduce the cost of coverage for employers and consumers, as well as reduce the administrative costs involved in fighting over who pays when someone gets sick or injured.
- Employers would see substantial savings—an estimated 20 percent—in their workers compensation premiums, and the employer health care premiums of 6.75 percent of payroll would cover the increased costs in the health care system.
- A portion of the savings would be used to increase California's disability benefits under workers compensation.

Access to Quality Health Care for All Californians

- All Californians would be guaranteed access to comprehensive health care benefits.

- The benefits would be comparable to those now covered by HMOs, providing comprehensive medically necessary care (inpatient care, primary care, prescription drugs, etc.). Modest co-payments would be required for some services, though they would be waived for low-income individuals. There would be no deductibles.
- Cost-effective preventive care would be encouraged and would be provided with no co-payments.
- The public/private managers of the system would assure that all health plans met quality-of-care standards.

Expanded Consumer Choice

- All consumers would be able to choose from among all of the private health plans certified in a region. Health plans would include many of those providing coverage today (e.g., HMOs and insurance companies).
- A standard premium payment of 6.75 percent of payroll for employers and 1.0 percent of wages for employees would guarantee all Californians access to the comprehensive benefits. At least two health plans in each region would offer the guaranteed benefits at no additional charge. Individuals could choose to enroll in plans that charged an additional amount for more amenities or flexibility (e.g., wider choice of providers).
- All health plans would be required to accept any individual regardless of health status. There would be no pre-existing condition exclusions, no waiting periods, and no extra charges due to health status or age and sex. Health plans would not be allowed to compete by avoiding risk.
- The system would be managed by a private/public sponsor—regional Health Insurance Purchasing Corporations (HIPCs). Each purchasing corporation would ensure that all plans deliver quality care and assist individuals in choosing among plans by providing consumer information (e.g., complaints against plans, waiting times, etc.).
- Consumer choice and continuity of care would be enhanced by removing the link between health coverage and a job. Changing jobs—or becoming unemployed—would not mean a loss of coverage or even having to switch to a different health plan or doctor.

MANAGED COMPETITION AND PUBLIC HEALTH

Let's Do the Right Thing

Nancy F. McKenzie

Managed competition is reputed to be health care reform as substantial as the programs of the New Deal. While managed competition will in some ways reconfigure the economic players shaping our eighth largest industry, it is hardly health care *reform*. But this is difficult to discern, given that over the last 12 years politicians have spoken of health care reform when they meant essentially cuts in service. Moreover, the debate over health care reform has been so specialized that hardly anyone not attached to an affected industry or agency can understand what is at issue. To cut through the verbal fog, we need not only to critique managed competition, but to remind ourselves of what we mean when we talk of health care policy and reform.

Managed Competition: More of the Same

Like the "cost-containment" strategies of the Reagan/Bush years, managed competition is so particulate in the financial issues it addresses, so complicated, so technical, and so parochial, as to be entirely opaque to everyone except the designated players. It is unclear whether a health care system based upon managed competition, once presented *in toto*, will be understandable or of interest to the American public, who so desperately need true health care reform. The fact that managed competition is so intellectually inaccessible does not bode well for the hope of its making health care more, and not less, available to 250 million Americans.

Were it not for the fanfare of the Clinton Health Care Taskforce and the novelty of the new distributor of health care—HIPCs, the regional business collectives known as health insurance purchasing cooperatives—we could perhaps live with health care business practices that are in essence simply more of the same. But the offering of health care *reform* makes us expect more, and filtered through those expectations, managed competition looks progressive. Many will be disappointed, as a quick reading of history indicates.

The first proponents of Alain Enthoven's managed competition theory in the federal government were not the Clintons or even the Jackson Hole Group. Rather, they were David Stockman and Richard Gephardt, as part of the "trickle-down," "let'em eat ketchup," school of economics. Enthoven offered a market-based health care plan to the Reagan administration precisely to deregulate health care and shake providers loose from any public oversight. His Jackson Hole colleagues are not health planners, but corporate designers from the insurance and pharmaceutical industries, and their recommendations may be called policy, rather than economics, but they offer about as much health policy and reform as Dan Quayle's Council on Economic Competitiveness offered environmental policy and reform.

Managed competition continues the Bush/Reagan tradition. It concentrates on business players, favoring certain financial arrangements that take federal subsidies and financial incentives from Peter (academic medical centers and fee-for-service doctors—the old health care "empires") and gives them to Paul (insurance-owned health maintenance organization "empires"). Under managed competition, profits from the delivery of medical services will accrue to new insurance-based owners of prospective payment plans (HMOs) contracted by HIPCs, rather than to a wide assortment of physicians and hospitals as under the current system (hence the current outcry from the American Medical Association). More patients will be served in more cost-contained franchises, but health care reform this is not.

In the name of universality—health insurance coverage for everyone—managed competition will probably end Medicaid and Medicare as we know them. While many have been ill-served by a greatly flawed and discriminatory federal health safety net, many have benefited. The importance of these programs as a public commitment to health care cannot be overemphasized. Managed competition will replace these somewhat meager public programs with an "integrated system" of basic, purchasable medical services for the currently insured and the uninsured. But this will not give us a system of health care. Given the way that managed competition views the uninsured, public programs, and the underinsured, it is clear that it will maintain our current alternative tier of poor medicine (hence, the phrase "integrated system").

If the new managed competition system is to be *forced* to care for the sick —which it can't be under a strictly "competition" system—it must be through still more economic incentives. Imagine how complicated the strategies must be to garner profits from our "wholesale poor" and underserved! There is nothing in the logic of managed competition or in the parts of the plan leaked so far from the task force that will stop the current practices of disinformation, skimming, and intentional strategies to keep the sickest individuals from the doors to care.

Managed competition will make well-endowed, healthy individuals happy with their health care. There will probably be streamlined billing; less cost for a few years to some individuals, to employers, and to unions; secure coverage; and risk shared by diverse markets. But those who are or will become more marginal—the one-third of Americans who work part time, who are unemployed, or who are disabled or too sick to work—will find the worst of primary care tied to the worst of micro-management and the worst of provider "gate-keeping," all linked together in a "basic benefits package." This package is beginning to look suspiciously like what we in New York know as the vastly inferior Medicaid Managed Care. Under managed competition, the poor and the very sick will, more than ever, be the economic ''outlier'' (those who cannot bring a profit margin for providers).

Whether the ''integrated system'' will lower health care costs is anyone's guess, since no non-medical industry study has shown that managed care saves money or that cost containment in health care comes from competition. Even Clinton's preliminary work plan for the Interagency Health Care Taskforce admits that little evidence exists that managed care produces cost efficiencies except through ''perverse behaviors (e.g., risk selection, claims denials).'' Most of us in health policy have seen the highly critical analyses of managed care by the Congressional Budget Office and the General Accounting Office, the scandals of HealthPass of Philadelphia (Medicaid Managed Care in Pennsylvania), and the predictable opportunism of private companies in Medicaid Managed Care in other states, notably California. So have the members of the Health Care Taskforce. Reputable economists know that health ''goods'' don't operate like other ''consumer items.'' After all, a person who's ill with cancer can't choose to forgo expensive medical treatment in favor of another item—say, a refrigerator—that's cheaper. It is obvious that the health marketplace is a fiction of deregulation advocates.

Health Reform and Public Health

While the nation has debated for more than two decades the relative merits of national health care, universal coverage, national health insurance, and managed competition, our public health care infrastructure has continued to be defunded, dismantled, and abandoned. At this point in our history, if a ''basic benefits package'' were premised on need, it would have to be an emergency package, and it would require an Emergency Infrastructure Administration— similar to the Social Security Administration of the 1930s. Because the health infrastructure is the true issue of American health care reform, the EIA would have to be in effect for as long as it took to bring individuals into the health care system and to find the many ways that their environments, their neighborhoods, their lack of geographical accessibility to routine care, the overemphasis on acute health care without preventive care or adequate treatment of chronic disease are directly jeopardizing their health.

The HIV epidemic taught America that getting a fatal chronic disease can change one's class status, as can cancer, kidney disease, or any other disabling condition. One has only to look at our elderly sick, our housing policy, our mental health policy, our disability medicine, our tuberculosis programs, our drug treatment programs to see that poverty begets disease, and disease begets poverty, and both serve to stigmatize individuals and keep them from care. Any health care reform, no matter how dressed up in consumer language, that neglects these individuals and focuses on the acute problems of usually healthy people will be a transparent slap in the face of the American public.

As the truncated debate about managed competition attests, the economic development of American medicine has affected our popular conception of health care, its access, and its distribution, and it has substituted health care financing for health care as the priority. But it is still obvious to most Americans that while the framers of national health care policy act as if we all lived in Geneva, Switzerland, increasing millions of us live in the conditions of Sao Paulo, Brazil. When progressives have spoken directly to this divergence of meaning between the health care debate and the health care reality, the Reagan/ Bush retort was to point to a duality in the client—the ''deserving sick'' versus the ''undeserving sick.'' Ordinary citizens know a shell game when they see it—when health emergencies get defined as financial emergencies, so that health policy can be designed by corporate managers. The cost-benefit craze may have fooled the lobbyist and perverted health discourse, but the people still feel the loss in reasonableness, in humaneness, in decency.

While we do not know definitively what will finally be included in ''managed competition,'' most clues indicate that there is no true provision for long-term care; nor are there structures or strategies for emphasizing chronic disease over acute care, for responding to the crushing public health needs of AIDS, tuberculosis, measles, and lack of housing or to the colossal institutionalized disparities in the quality of health care delivery that now confront the United States. No matter how inclusive the HIPCs are, managed competition is designed to solidify services at the level of the status quo. Under that status, according to Ira Magaziner, manager of the Health Care Taskforce, delivery of care to the very sick will be designed as ''supplements to vulnerable populations.'' Yet those vulnerable populations—poor women and children, people with terminal illness, people disabled and in need of special support services and rehabilitative medicine, people in need of home care, people sick from exposure, from mental illness, from alcohol and drug addiction, from trauma and violence, from stress and chronic disease—make up more than a third of the American population.

The Health Premise for Health Reform

Having come this far in the national awareness of the health care industry's greed, of self-interest and self-promotion by health corporations; having come this far with an overwhelming public demand for health care reform, one would expect real discussion of health policy. Yet this is more urgently needed than ever. After 12 years of Republican aggression against health care access and public health, it is obvious that more ''competition'' will only exacerbate the main perversity of our system: *In the United States, those who need health care the least have the most access to it and the greatest assurance of quality care, and those who need it most have the least.*

Nor is this illogical state of affairs only a health policy issue. It is also an issue of democracy. It points to a breakdown of the social contract: between government and individuals; between providers and patients; between citizen and citzen. Bill Clinton was elected to heal this rent in our social pact with one another. The Clinton administration will not have credibility if it designs a new ''competitive'' health care distribution on the basis of this status quo.

If the Clintons are really intent on health care reform, they will begin with common sense premises and jettison the model they inherited from the history of the American health care system. The financial model is based on the assumption that a health care system should be designed around acute and extraordinary delivery of care to otherwise healthy individuals. If this consumer premise were replaced with a health premise, and health need became the orienting principle of our national agenda, we would have true health care reform.

In that reform, the "basic benefits package" would form the wide base of a narrowing pyramid of benefits, replacing the current inverted pyramid. Basic health care would be very wide, indeed, defined by reference to those most in need of health care. It would include early, preventive care and after care for everyone leaving a hospital with a continuing health need. Health benefits would narrow as individuals were either more healthy or better off economically, socially, and psychologically. Such a reversal of premises—away from business priorities and toward health policy—would, of course, require a realistic and honest appraisal of the health and social service interventions that individuals, caught in the jaws of early debilitation and death now so much a part of poverty in the United States, would respond to. Such an appraisal would not only save health dollars but would be welcomed with relief by a concerned public.

The Future of Health Reform Debate

Perhaps discussing and then building a health care system is not simple, but, at the risk of going against the canon, I believe that adequate health care is not complex. Principled premises lead to principled argument, clarity, simplicity. If the issue were education reform, and 78 percent of the American people asked for substantial change, it would be possible to come up with a model that was designed for everyone and that guaranteed access to services based on need. This reform would not allow "the market" to set up enterprise zones or to set the educational standard so low in one tier of the system that it amounted to "reads well enough to fill out a driver's license application" and so high in the other tier that every student had to get into Harvard. Such reform would not refer to both tiers collectively as "a system," as offering "equal access," as "one benefits package." It would be understood that an educational system must guarantee the basics that are of public urgency and allow "competition" at higher, *less* essential levels.

Clinton seems to be clear sighted about what "remedial and emergency" measures are needed to "jump start" individuals back into occupational and economic health in our country, but he doesn't apply the same premises to health. It may be that the task force believes that healthy, middle-income individuals will find managed competition user-friendly, and that everyone else will be pretty much morally invisible. I don't think so. The individual American will think it ludicrous to talk of health care reform and not talk of people without housing, about our aged sick, our poor, our epidemics, our broken, heartless health care delivery infrastructure. And they will view it as perverse to have no discussion on policies for public health, for long-term care, for rehabilitative medicine.

Hundreds of thousands of individuals are organizing around health care as a moral issue [see "Change the Health Care System? How UHCAN!" on p. 645 and "Organizations for Health Care Reform" on p. 655]. Those who go

644 PROPOSALS FOR A NATIONAL AGENDA

along with managed competition for political expediency and do not base their arguments on the moral necessity for health care to every individual will have done no more good than add "a little more" to "more of the same." And the harm will be great. Support for managed competition will have given our important voice, with much hypocritical fanfare, to the solidification of a two-tiered, and, finally, immoral health care system.

Most of us know that health policy or the public right to health care cannot come from corporate health care. As Faust knew, false premises lead to false outcomes. Rights will never emerge from financial arguments. They can only emerge from a declaration of rights.

Can we have health care reform without challenging the premise that health care is about financing? Can we have health care delivery without basing that delivery on the needs of individuals? I don't think so. And I don't think that the American people, schooled on profit and denied health policy for the last decade, think so either. They want a rational health care system. Right now, they believe that the Clinton task force is about health care reform, about the right to health care.

If we are going to go to the trouble to have laws that change the policies of our health care system, shouldn't they be based on health rights and health care premises? If we are going to fight to get change, shouldn't we support appropriateness, rationality, and, ultimately, simplicity? Otherwise, besides missing the point, aren't we wasting a nation's hope and idealism?

Perhaps the task force will come to its senses and, by the time it comes to writing legislation, will join the American public in supporting true health care reform.

CHANGE THE HEALTH CARE SYSTEM?

How UHCAN!

Ken Frisof

Who decides how America's health care system runs?

A) Special interest groups.
B) Policy experts.
C) The American people.

If you picked (A), you'd be right most of the time. If you picked (B), you'd be right some of the time. If you picked (C), you'd be right only a little of the time, but that time just might be now.

Throughout most of the recent history of the American health care system we have witnessed only minor changes, usually undertaken at the behest of some of health care's "stakeholders." But the current period may be one of those few exciting times of major change, resulting from action by ordinary people and consequently reflecting their needs.

There have been two other decades in the twentieth century when the voice of the people made a difference in American social policy. In the 1930s, mass action with a Democratic president in office led to a strengthening of economic rights—unions for workers, social security for retirees. In the 1960s, popular turmoil with Democratic presidents in office led to expansion of civil rights and women's rights. In the 1990s, health care reform has the potential to galvanize a popular struggle for human rights, for the triumph of need over greed.

This is not the first attempt to win systemic health care reform. As Ted Marmor recently wrote in the Winter 1993 *American Prospect*, "Reformers in the Progressive Era and the New Deal, under President Truman and during the early 1970s thought universal health insurance was imminent and were bitterly disappointed. Now, as then, entrenched interests try to block change by skillfully manipulating our deepest fears and beliefs to maintain their privileges" (p. 53). As in the past, this will also be ultimately a battle over "our deepest fears and beliefs."

Health/PAC heralded the beginning of the current era of the struggle for health care reform when it held a conference in June 1987 entitled "Health Care in the Post-Reagan Era." Eighteen months later, in January 1989, the *New England Journal of Medicine* published a pair of articles that defined the debate we are having today: the single-payer vision as described by Physicians for a National Health Program versus the managed competition model created by business professor Alain Enthoven. The importance of this academic debate was underscored the following month, when a Harris Poll revealed that 90 percent of Americans thought our health care system needed a major overhaul.

George Bush's election in 1988 extended the Reagan era, guaranteeing that no meaningful federal health care legislation would pass in the next four years. In the face of political gridlock in Washington, health activists developed a largely state-level legislative strategy and a national educational strategy. The first state single-payer bill was introduced in Ohio in April 1989. Since then, nearly half the states in the union have introduced similar legislation, and a version has passed houses in both New York and California legislatures. At the federal level, the Russo Bill was the main legislative single-payer vehicle. Introduced in March 1991, it garnered 75 sponsors before dying at the end of the last congressional session. Other important pieces of legislation that fall generally in the single-payer camp were introduced by John Conyers, Bob Kerrey, and Paul Wellstone.

With no chance of short-term national victories, our goal since the late 1980s has been to show the public that a politically acceptable, reasonable alternative to profit-oriented health care could be easily constructed using the principles of our northern neighbor, Canada. This beginning education and activation was to serve as the warmup for the significant popular mobilization that would ultimately be needed to make fundamental reform happen.

At the same time, some of us hoped that a growing part of the business community would see that their enlightened self-interest lay in the single-payer model's use of an aggregate health budget to control health care costs. (In managed competition, companies worry only about their narrow self-interest—the cost of health benefits for current workers and some retirees.) However, there has been little progress on this front over the last four years. Business leaders have apparently decided that they dislike government more than avaricious physicians and inefficient insurance companies, and most have cast their lot with Enthoven and the managed competition camp.

What Kind of Change?

The 1992 election was a choice between George Bush's "stay the course" and change of some sort or other. When you add Perot and Clinton's vote, Americans overwhelmingly voted for change. But what kind?

During the campaign, the leaders of the business and media establishments put forth a heavy propaganda onslaught for managed competition. They declared victory when Clinton announced that the framework for his health reform proposal would be "managed competition" rather than "pay or play."

Where does this leave progressives who have been working for a people-oriented health care system, for the single-payer vision? As a system that "puts people first," single payer has much more moral logic than managed competition, a model that forthrightly states that its main focus is cost containment. The challenge for activists is to create the momentum that makes the political logic of the single-payer system as compelling as its moral logic.

At this point in the political road, there will naturally be splits and realignments. There is, after all, a spectrum of positions that fit the rubric of "managed competition," ranging from the pure quality competition embodied in Kerrey's legislation and the Catholic Health Association's "Working Proposal for Systemic Health Care Reform," through California Insurance Commissioner John Garamendi and Paul Starr's blended versions, to the abysmal price competition approach that Enthoven himself champions. Some well-meaning progressives are taking the position that since the battle is over the definition of "competition," that is where they need to put their energies.

Most single-payer activists are, however, staying with their vision. But we have a difficult task in front of us. How do we maintain momentum in the face of the imminent release of a proposal that ignores our basic principles by a president whose party controls Congress? The answer is to be *radical*, to go back to our roots: the people.

A new organization to facilitate this was created immediately after the election: UHCAN!—the Universal Health Care Action Network. The Northeast Ohio Coalition for National Health Care, a five-year-old regional grassroots coalition that had spearheaded the drive for the first state-level single-payer bill, coordinated two national conferences in 1992. The hastily organized first conference drew 100 participants from 25 states in early March. The second, the Universal Health Care Strategies Conference, held immediately after the election and right before the American Public Health Association convention, brought together over 250 people from 34 states. The conference participants included activists with close ties to progressive national organizations active in the fight for a single-payer system, such as unions and Citizen Action. But the vast majority of attendees were grassroots activists whose major organizational affiliation was a local or state health coalition, religious network, or disability advocacy group. At the final plenary, the conference overwhelmingly voted to create a new national network to coordinate their activities—UHCAN!

Some activists with national organizational connections were angry at the creation of yet another organization, seeing this as a typical case of fragmentation on the left. But UHCAN! activists see it another way. For many, health care is the *only* focus of their political lives. Organizations with multiple agendas and priorities may compromise on the health care issue to obtain success on other fronts. UHCAN! benefits from attracting individual activists and organizations who are passionately engaged by our health care debacle.

Danger and Opportunity

The Chinese character for crisis combines symbols for danger and opportunity. The election of Bill Clinton can be seen as such a crisis for the health movement. Hillary Rodham Clinton's task force will come up with a compromise proposal this spring, and strong pressure will be put on liberal politicians and organizations to go along so that the administration can chalk up a victory. The danger of rapid passage of flawed reform is great. On the other hand, the Clinton victory has begun to open people's eyes and hearts after the 12 years of Reagan-Bush psychological and economic depression. The rising expectations of the grassroots could force reform to go further than the elite intend—if the health care movement can learn quickly how to get its messages out rapidly and effectively.

We need to think beyond the small organizing steps of the 1980s. The first month of UHCAN! demonstrates why. When the November Universal Health Care Strategies Conference was being planned, none of its organizers was thinking of any specific campaigns in the immediate future. In response to a question at Saturday's lunchtime keynote address, Rep. Marty Russo, the congressional standard-bearer for a single-payer system of the previous two years, suggested that health activists go to Little Rock to publicly press the case for a single-payer system during the transition period. Within hours, an ad hoc task force had met, chosen a date, and done preliminary planning. The proposal was overwhelmingly approved at a plenary session 24 hours later. A California Neighbor to Neighbor organizer used "revival style" fundraising to raise $5,000 in ten minutes from the assembled audience.

The People's Health Care-a-van descended on Little Rock barely one month later, on December 12, 1992—1,000 people strong from 32 states. It had been organized with UHCAN! handling the North and Midwest and Georgians for a Common Sense Health Plan working in the South. The original plan was to have a town meeting to share our stories and teach the incoming administration. But, when it became clear that neither the administration nor the media would pay us any attention if we were squirreled away in a Little Rock hotel, the participants spontaneously decided to march to the state Capitol to meet the president-elect. The march was a beautiful sight, stretching over a quarter of a mile, led by activists in wheelchairs, peopled by the young and old, black and white, northern and southern, employed and unemployed, sick and well, professionals and laborers, grandparents and grandchildren, veterans of many campaigns and newcomers to political action. After a long wait, and a lot of repetitions of the old Civil Rights Movement anthem, "We Shall Not Be Moved," Bill and Hillary Clinton finally came out and talked to people in the crowd.

The event vividly brought home to those present the potential for building a strong grassroots movement again. Yet the fact that this extraordinary effort on the part of 1,000 ordinary Americans received almost no media coverage in this era of managed news also made us painfully aware of the challenges we face.

UHCAN! sees its special contribution to the health care reform movement as stemming from its commitment to promote grassroots activism through education and empowerment. It is truly a network of like-minded organizations; UHCAN! exists to enhance their ability to communicate and collaborate. It puts organized groups from different constituencies in contact with one another for sharing and inspiration. It aims to translate the complex jargon of health care reform to the simple language of social values that leads ordinary people to meaningful political action.

THE AMERICAN HEALTH SECURITY ACT OF 1993

The American Health Security Act (S 491, HR 1200) was introduced in the U.S. Senate by Paul Wellstone (D-Minn.) and in the House of Representatives by John Conyers (D-Mich.) and Jim McDermott (D-Wash.), along with 54 co-sponsors. The legislation, which replaces and strengthens the 1992 bill proposed by former Rep. Marty Russo and Sen. Wellstone, presents a single-payer alternative to managed competition proposals. This summary is excerpted from material provided by Sen. Wellstone's office.

Benefits and Eligibility

Health insurance would be provided for all citizens and legal residents of the United States. Everyone would receive a health insurance card entitling him or her to benefits covered under the American Health Security Program. The National Board can also cover undocumented workers, or states can do so at their own expense.

The covered benefits include:

- Primary and preventive services, including screening exams, well-child care, immunizations, and reproductive health care.
- Prenatal, postnatal, and well-baby care.
- Services of health care professionals who are authorized to provide such services under state law.
- Inpatient and outpatient hospital care.
- Diagnostic tests.
- Prescription drugs and biologicals.
- Nursing facility services.
- Home care and community-based services for individuals unable to perform at least two activities of daily living (ADLs).
- Hospice care.
- Mental health and substance abuse services, subject to coordination of care, and to regulated utilization review after 15 days of inpatient care and 20 outpatient visits a year.
- Expanded services by community clinics and migrant health centers.
- Other medical or health care items or services as the National Health Board determines to be appropriate.

Consumers would be free to choose their own health providers.

Over the counter drugs (aspirin, cold medicine), surgery performed only for cosmetic purposes, physicals for purposes of litigation or obtaining life insurance would not be covered under the plan.

Cost Containment

The program would contain costs in a variety of ways. It would reduce administrative waste, cap provider payments by global budgets and negotiated fees, continue consumer-oriented managed care plans, reshape the service delivery system to emphasize primary care, control prescription drug prices, set separate budgets for costly new equipment, and control fraud and abuse.

No Cost Sharing

There would be no coinsurance, deductibles, or co-payments for benefits covered under the American Health Security Plan.

High-Quality Care

The bill would improve the quality and efficiency of the service delivery system.

It would promote and expand the use of outcomes research and practice guidelines, including research on primary and preventive care, and encourage the integration of public health principles and services to improve the community's health.

Within five years, 50 percent of doctors in training would have to be in primary care programs, compared to the current 20 percent, and an advisory council would set goals for training more mid-level practitioners and non-professionals such as outreach workers.

It would encourage training programs and practices that include multi-disciplinary teams, an important feature of high-quality group practices such as the Mayo Clinic. Accountable managed care systems, called Community Health Service Organizations (CHSOs), could compete based on the quality of their integrated services.

States could concentrate specialty care in centers of excellence to promote better outcomes while containing costs.

States would control health care fraud and abuse, assisted by a national data base.

Underserved Rural and Inner-City Areas

The bill would double funding for community clinics and migrant health centers and greatly increase funding through public health block grants for services such as maternal and child health care and care for people with AIDS under the Ryan White Act.

It would also expand funding for the National Health Service Corps, which sends doctors and midlevel practitioners into underserved areas for two years in exchange for help with educational expenses.

States could plan how to distribute services on a local or regional basis, to address current inequities.

Payments to Providers

Hospitals and nursing homes would be paid based on global budgets established annually through negotiations with the designated state agency and reviewed by the state advisory boards.

Community Health Service Organizations (CHSOs) could offer comprehensive, integrated services for an annual, capitated rate.

Other facility-based services, including hospice care, outpatient services, and home, school-based, and community-based services would be paid through one of the following options:

- Annual operating budgets.
- Fee schedules.
- A capitation payment.
- An alternative prospective payment method.

A professional board would classify prescription drugs into categories, as a basis for the Board to negotiate prices for similarly classified drugs. The Board would establish price limits.

Health care professionals would be reimbursed according to fee schedules negotiated at the state level.

Payments for capital items, such as new buildings and equipment, would be budgeted and allocated separately.

The payments from the states to providers would constitute the payment in full for covered benefits. No additional payments or charges would be permitted.

Administration and Budgets

The American Health Security Standards Board would implement guidelines for national benefits and national and state budgets. The budget could not increase more than the annual percentage increase in Gross Domestic Product.

Each state would administer the program at the state level.

The budget would act as an expenditure target, so that if the budget for a service were exceeded, the state and the Board could lower payments for that service the following year.

Each state and national budget would include an amount for total expenditures for capital-related items, operating expenses, health professional education, and administration.

The state health budgets would be determined based solely on the following factors:

- The population of the state.
- Reasonable differences in the prices for goods and services.

- Any special social, environmental, or other condition affecting health status or the need for health care services.
- The geographic distribution of the state's population, particularly the proportion of the population residing in rural or medically underserved areas.

THE GROUPS WORKING TO ENACT THE AMERICAN HEALTH SECURITY ACT INCLUDE:

Actors Equity
Amalgamated Clothing and Textile Workers Union
American Federation of State, County and Municipal Employees
American Medical Students Association
Americans for Democratic Action
American Public Health Association
Church Women United
Citizen Action
Communication Workers of America
Consumer Federation of America
Consumers Union
Graphics Artists Guild
International Brotherhood of Teamsters
International Union of Electronics and Electrical Workers (IUE)
International Ladies' Garment Workers Union
International Association of Machinists
National Association of Social Workers
National Council of Senior Citizens
National Family Farm Coalition
Neighbor to Neighbor
Oil, Chemical and Atomic Workers Union
Older Women's League
Screen Actors Guild
United Auto Workers International Union
United Electrical, Radio and Machine Workers Union (UE)
U.S. Public Interest Research Group

The state could enter into a contract with a fiscal intermediary to process claims. Only one contract would be allowed for each state.

Advisory boards representing both consumers and health care providers would advise on the implementation of the program at the local, state, and federal levels.

Financing

All revenues collected for health care would be placed into an American Health Security Trust Fund and could only be used for health care expenses.

The program would be financed by collecting at the federal level all funds currently spent on health care.

The national insurance program would be financed through a 7.9 percent payroll tax on employers, increasing the existing 1.45 percent Medicare payroll tax by 6.45 percent; an increase in corporate income tax from 34 percent to 38 percent for businesses with more than $75,000 in profits; increases in the personal income tax from 15-28-31 percent to 15-30-34 percent, with a top rate of 38 percent for families with incomes over $200,000, and a health premium equal to about 0.5 percent of income (or 7.5 percent of income taxes paid); reforms to close loopholes in the tax code; a long-term care premium equal to the Medicare Part B premium plus $25 a month for the elderly above 120 percent of poverty; an increase in the amount of Social Security benefits included as taxable income from 50 to 85 percent. State and federal spending will remain the same as current health care payments, with increases limited to growth in the Gross Domestic Product.

Questions and Answers

How does this plan compare with managed competition?

Unlike many managed competition proposals, the American Health Security Act would base eligibility for services on residency rather than place of employment. Also, it suggests many other proven service delivery strategies for controlling costs in addition to the use of managed care plans, many of which have not actually saved money. Managed care plans are also not practical in many rural and underserved areas. It calls on providers to compete based on quality, not on the price of their services, which under the current system has led to two-tier services. Finally, it removes insurance companies from making decisions about who may receive which health services, though they may still play a role in administration of state plans and covering services not covered by the plan. It shares similar features with some managed competition proposals that would rely on global budgets, universal coverage, and competition among providers based on quality.

How is this bill different from the Russo/Wellstone bill?

The bills, introduced by Rep. Marty Russo in 1991 as HR 1300, and by Sen. Paul Wellstone in 1992 as S 2320, proposed a financing and payment structure for the health care system that is very similar to the current legislation.

This bill explains in greater detail how a single-payer system would be implemented and clarifies and strengthens some of the provisions that relate to cost containment and the health care service delivery system. In particular:

- States play a stronger role. They administer the program and may encourage innovations in paying and planning for care that would control costs, improve the quality of care, and distribute services more fairly.
- The federal American Health Security Program is administered by a seven-member Board appointed by the President.
- The bill emphasizes primary and preventive care by setting goals for training more doctors and mid-level practitioners in primary and preventive care, and encourages primary care services and research that use public health indicators.
- The bill greatly expands services to underserved rural and inner-city communities, by doubling funding for community-based primary care services and public health block grants.
- It spells out the role and structure of consumer-oriented managed care plans, called Community Health Service Organizations.
- As a publicly financed and administered system, the program was always designed to be accountable to consumers. In addition, this bill specifies consumer representation on key decision-making bodies and advisory boards.
- A broad range of mental health and substance abuse services are provided through a system of coordination of care and utilization review.
- Prescription drug prices are controlled by state negotiations for similarly classified drugs.
- State administrative expenses are capped at 3 percent.
- 1 percent of each state budget could be spent to assist health insurance administrative workers who may be displaced from their jobs.
- Strong anti-fraud provisions have been added to reduce loss of revenue from unscrupulous health care providers.
- Clarifies that there are no changes to the Veterans Administration health system, or to the Indian Health Service. Veterans retain their current benefits and are also eligible for benefits under this act.

ORGANIZATIONS FOR HEALTH CARE REFORM

The following list is meant as a resource for grassroots organizing for health care reform. Many organizations are stepping up their efforts in response to the imminent announcement of the Clinton administration's health care reform proposals. There are three major national organizations working for the same goals in support of a single-payer system: Universal Health Care Action Network (UHCAN!), a network of health care reform groups with a national clearinghouse in Cleveland, Ohio; Citizen Action, with affiliates in more than 30 states; and Physicians for a National Health Program (PNHP), centered in Cambridge and Chicago and with local chapters in various states. There is also a national organization, Campaign for Health Security, working in support of the American Health Security Act of 1993 (S. 491 and HR 1200), the Wellstone-Conyers-McDermott single-payer bill. Many states have health care campaigns supporting a single-payer system, as do many progressive unions.

National Organizations

Universal Health Care Action Network (UHCAN!)
1800 Euclid Avenue #318
Cleveland, Ohio 44115
(216) 241-8422
(216) 566-8100 Diane Lardie
Fax (216) 566-8153

Citizen Action
1120 19th Street, NW, Suite 630
Washington, DC 20036
Ed Rothschild
(202) 775-1580
Fax: (202) 296-4054

Physicians for a National Health Program
332 South Michigan Avenue, Suite 500
Chicago, Illinois 60604
Ida Hellender, Director
(312) 554-0382
Fax: (312) 554-0383

Center for National Health Program Studies
(Education Division of PNHP)
Macht Building, Room 401
1493 Cambridge Street
Cambridge, Massachusetts 02139
(617) 661-1064
Fax: (617) 498-1671

Campaign for Health Security
1120 19th Street, NW, Suite 630
Washington, DC 20036
(800) 555-1234

Alabama

HEAL (Health Education & Action League)
P.O. Box 4474
Huntsville, Alabama 35815
Walker Townsend, Sr.
(205) 881-2118

California

Neighbor to Neighbor Action Fund
2601 Mission Street, Suite 400
San Francisco, California 94110
(415) 824-3555

Health Access
1535 Mission Street
San Francisco, California 94103
(415) 431-3430

People for a National Health Program—Leisure World
P.O. Box 2902
Laguna Hills, California 92654
Ted Rosenbaum, Vice President

Florida

Florida Health Care Campaign
(800) 421-7292

Georgia

Georgians for a Common Sense Health Plan
c/o Nancy Moulton
486 Stovall Street, SE
Atlanta, Georgia 30316
(404) 622-0707

Send material in print and in IBM compatible form.
Disk format allows accessibility for visually impaired.

Idaho

Citizens Coalition for Universal Health Care
2813 Jerome
Pocatello, Idaho 83201
Carl Martinez, Chairman
(208) 237-9562

Louisiana

Louisiana Health Care Campaign
P.O. Box 2228
Baton Rouge, Louisiana 70281-2228
(504) 383-8518

Maryland

White Lung Association
P.O. Box 1483
Baltimore, Maryland 21203
Jim Fite
(410) 243-5864

Montana

Montana Senior Citizens Association
1618 Sherwood
Missoula, Montana 59802
Doug Cambell, President

New England

Citizens for Participation in Political Action (CPPAX)
25 West Street
Boston, Massachusetts 02111
Dick Mason
(617) 426-3040

New Jersey

Citizen Action Health Committee
Communications Workers of America, Local 1034
321 West State Street
Trenton, New Jersey 08618
Joy Shulman, Staff Representative
(609) 394-1967

New Mexico

Network of Health Professionals for a National Health Program
1201 Calle de Ranchero NE
Albuquerque, New Mexico 87106
(505) 841-4112

New York

Coalition of Mental Health Professionals and Consumers
P.O. Box 438
Commack, New York 11725-0438
Joyce Edwards, Karen Shore, Paul Miller, co-chairs
(516) 424-5232

Health Care Policy Network
National Association of Social Workers
New York City Chapter
545 Eighth Avenue, 6th floor
New York, New York 10018
(212) 947-5000
(212) 452-7112 (Terry Mizrahi)

Jobs with Justice Health Care Campaign
80 Pine Street
New York, New York 10005
Gene Carroll
(212) 344-2515

Nassau Coalition for a National Health Plan
P.O. Box 4227
Great Neck, New York 11023
Donna Kass, Co-Chair
(516) 829-1225

New York State Health Care Campaign
Community Service Society
105 East 22nd Street
New York, New York 10010
Anjean Carter

United for AIDS Action
175 Fifth Avenue, Suite 2179
New York, New York 10010
(212) 337-1227
Fax: (212) 337-1220

Women Organize for National Health Care
Health Care: We Gotta Have It!
121 West 27th Street, Room 1202A
New York, New York 10001
Meredith Kolodner
(212) 366-6700
Fax: (212) 229-2557

Ohio

Northeast Ohio Coalition for National Health Care
c/o United Labor Agency
1800 Euclid Avenue, Suite 318
Cleveland, Ohio 44115
(216) 566-8100
Fax: (216) 566-8153

Vermont

Physicians for a National Health Program
Vermont Chapter
219 Western Avenue
Brattleboro, Vermont 05301
Lee Emerson, Coordinator
(802) 254-5251

Wyoming

Consumer Task Force on Health Care Education
Wyoming Governor's Planning Council on
Developmental Disabilities
122 West/25th Street
Herschler Building, 4th floor, East
East Cheyenne, Wyoming 82002
Rose Kor
(307) 777-7230

Note: If there is no agency listed in your area, you can contact UHCAN! to find out about local organizing efforts.

UNIVERSAL HEALTH INSURANCE: WHO SHOULD BE THE SINGLE PAYER?

Thomas Bodenheimer

Over the past two years, the single-payer concept has become a serious contender for the universal health insurance model that can solve the United States' health crisis. "Single payer" means that one institution in each geographical area receives virtually all money spent on health care and pays hospitals, physicians, health maintenance organizations (HMOs), and other health providers.[1] Business executives, labor leaders, politicians, and health analysts are interested in the single-payer model because of its international track record in solving simultaneously the problems of health access and health cost inflation. A number of single-payer bills have been proposed in Congress and in various state legislatures.[2] Polls taken in 1988 and 1990 indicate that over 60 percent of the American public is sympathetic to the single-payer concept.[3]

Two political drawbacks reduce the attractiveness of the single-payer approach, however: first, the need to raise taxes to finance universal health insurance under a single payer (which has been considered elsewhere[4]), and second, a deep-seated distrust of government. This distrust is manifest in such frequently heard responses to the suggestion of a single-payer system as "Government made a mess of Medicaid, it created a complex and inadequate program for Medicare, and the Veterans Administration hospitals are a disaster. If government has done such a terrible job of running health programs, why do you want to give it even more power? If you like the Post Office, you'll love the single-payer health system."

In part, the distrust of government is misguided and promoted by the dominant conservative ideology in the United States.[5] Each governmental program has its own history and its own peculiar failures that should not be attributed to an all-encompassing notion that "whatever government touches is bad." Moreover, a number of government programs *are* successful. Social Security is highly popular, and Medicare, in spite of its difficulties, in fact commands strong public support as well.[6] The administrative costs of the Medicare and Medicaid programs are far lower than those of private health insurers.[7]

On the other hand, the public's distrust of government is amply justified by the unethical and illegal activities of some government officials, as in the recent savings and loan scandals, as well as by government coverups of unpopular activities ranging from the Vietnam War to the Watergate scandal to the Iran-Contra affair.

For reformers who support the single-payer concept, the response to such public distrust of government must be twofold: on the one hand, the government is not quite as bad as that; but on the other hand, it could be a lot better, and we'd better look for some creative approaches that could minimize governmental ineptitude. Supporters of the single-payer approach must seriously ask themselves: Do we want to cede control of the entire health system to the federal or state governments? If so, why? And if not, then who should be the single payer? Before confronting these questions, let us review why we favor a single payer at all.

Why Do We Want a Single Payer, Anyway?

Health care reformers working for universal health insurance have one overriding goal: to efficiently insure everyone in the United States, on an equal basis, for a comprehensive array of health care services of the highest quality, with reasonable control over costs. The single-payer mechanism is seen as the means to this goal; it is not the goal itself.

Four major reasons can be cited to explain why the single-payer structure can best realize this goal: 1) Only with everyone in a single insurance system is there a chance to achieve equality in medical care; 2) international experience demonstrates that only a single payer (or closely coordinated payers acting together, the equivalent of a single payer) can control medical cost inflation;[8] 3) only a single payer can achieve the administrative efficiencies that allow the nation to extend comprehensive health insurance to everyone without incurring burdensome new costs;[9] 4) a single payer provides the potential for greater public input into major health care decisions—for example, the proportion of the GNP to be dedicated to health care or the priorities given to low-cost preventive and primary care versus high-cost interventions in late or end-stage disease processes.

In order to best achieve these goals, while addressing the widespread distrust of government control, who, then, should be the single payer? We will assume that the single payer resides at the state level; to promote equality among states, a proportion of the funds could be collected at the federal level and transferred to states according to formula.

Some Single Payer Candidates

1. A private company. This option would utilize the public utility model, in which an industry with a natural tendency toward monopoly (such as telephone, gas and electricity, or transportation) is given monopoly status by the government and in return is regulated more tightly than competitive private enterprise. Public utilities are private businesses regarded as "so impressed with peculiar public interest as to justify intensive government regulation of practically every detail of their activities."[10]

The public utility model would eliminate the argument that too much control of the single-payer health system resides in government. On the other hand, accountability to the public would be lowered, because the management's primary loyalty would be to the company's stockholders or other financial interests, rather than to the public. Because they are monopolies, public utilities have enormous clout and can often evade strict regulation by government agencies. In health care, the major candidates for public utility status as single payers would be the largest private insurers and HMOs in a given region. Overall, considerable risk is involved in placing so much power in the hands of one private company.

An alternative method for utilizing a private company in the single-payer apparatus is the fiscal intermediary concept currently functioning in the Medicare and Medicaid programs. In the early years of these programs, however, some fiscal intermediaries, who tended to be Blue Cross or Blue Shield plans, engaged in some questionable practices.[11] The use of fiscal intermediaries is also likely to increase administrative costs.

2. A governmental department. The structure farthest removed from the public utility approach is the Canadian method of placing the single payer directly within a government department. Such an option runs directly into the political problem of big government, and means a complex and cumbersome decision-making apparatus involving the governor, the legislature with its committees, plus political and technocratic departmental personnel. It also bogs the single payer down in the quagmires of the state budget, which are increasingly contentious and paralyzing.

3. A government commission. Keeping the single payer within government but separating it from the departmental apparatus of the executive branch is another option. A commission that would include members representing interests involved in health care—both provider and consumer—could be appointed or elected. Depending on how commissioners are chosen, this option could afford some measure of public accountability. But the commission concept does not circumvent the problem of tying health financing to the legislative tax and budgetary process and thereby linking the fiscal fate of health care to the vagaries of government revenue–expenditure–deficit politics. The budgetary difficulty might be overcome by earmarking revenues for the health insurance system and guaranteeing certain revenue increases each year according to formula.

4. A public fund with decentralization of decisions to smaller regions. One mechanism for diffusing the mistrust of big government is to decentralize the financing of health care. A statewide fund could be established that would collect all health revenues, but would hold no decision-making authority. The statewide fund would distribute its money to different regions of the state according to a strict formula; these regional funds would become the actual single payer for each geographic area.

Alternatively, the statewide fund might collect only some of the health revenues, while other funds are collected directly by the regions, in a fashion similar to the process used by Canada's federal and provincial governments. California, for example, has a district hospital law which allows voters in a geographic area to tax themselves in order to operate a hospital for their community. However, any mechanism that allows regional financing all but guarantees inequities, as wealthier regions tend to tax themselves at a greater rate to obtain a higher level of health resources than do poorer regions. On the other hand, the decentralized model would bring decision-making closer to the people and might be more acceptable than a centralized payer, particularly in more populous states. An additional drawback would be the administrative problem created when people living in one region obtain care in another region.

5. A public enterprise. One institution that might be capable of allowing public accountability while separating the health system from state government is the public enterprise or public corporation. The public enterprise is a business that is controlled in full or in part by the government, but exists as an autonomous corporate entity with separate finances. Like any corporation, the public enterprise must be financially viable and must therefore operate as a business. On the other hand, the public enterprise has overriding social goals other than financial viability, such as promoting the health of the public. Whereas the "enterprise" concept in a public enterprise means keeping the institution financially viable, the "public" notion requires public decision making and prohibits profits (net income) from accruing to private individuals.

The synthesis between the public and enterprise concepts is a delicate balance. If it tilts too far in one direction it becomes a non-public enterprise; if it goes too far the other way, it turns into a public nonenterprise. Public decision making is often at variance with financial viability.[12] For example, the enterprise-as-business might wish to raise prices in order to meet costs, but the social goal of access to health care might argue against such price increases. Other issues that might create tension between the public and the enterprise concepts are whether or not to have high co-payments and whether to have people with higher incomes subsidize lower income people and the elderly.

In a public enterprise, decision making is diffused among the government agency that created the public enterprise, the board of directors of the enterprise, its management, and its clients. The methods of choosing the board of directors could be any combination of election at-large; election from districts; appointment by the governor, with or without approval by a legislative body; and appointment (or election) by constituent organizations, such as medical societies and business, labor, and consumer groups.

A number of public enterprises exist in the United States, some with positive, some with negative popular ratings. Perhaps the most troublesome in terms of image is the US Postal Service. Given the Postal Service's proximity to the federal government and its absence of direct public representation, it is not an ideal model for a potentially more democratic, state-level public enterprise that might serve as a single payer of health services. Other examples of public enterprises are the US Government Printing Office, the Tennessee Valley Authority, the Pennsylvania Turnpike (tolls pay for the operating expenses and service the debt), state liquor stores, the New York City Transit Authority and transit systems in about 50 other municipalities, municipal gas and electric power companies throughout the country, and the Port of New York Authority established by the states of New York and New Jersey.[13]

The public enterprise and the governmental commission are not entirely distinct entities, but can be seen as a spectrum of institutions that are closer to or farther from the parent government. The purest form of public enterprise operates on user fees and does not require a budgetary allocation from the government. Those public enterprises that do rely heavily on fiscal assistance from their parent government—for example, the New York City Health and Hospitals Corporation—are closer to the commission concept in the sense that they are heavily dependent on the legislative budgetary process.

6. A cooperative. A cooperative is a democratic association of persons who voluntarily organize to furnish themselves an economic or social service under a plan that seeks to eliminate entrepreneur profit and that strives for substantial equality in ownership and control. Cooperatives are owned by members who are their users, as distinguished from corporations, whose owners are primarily investors. Cooperatives are organized on democratic principles: boards of directors are elected by the rule of one member, one vote. Membership is voluntary; people can join or leave as they please. Generally, members share the risks, financial obligations, and benefits in proportion to the use they make of the organization. If a cooperative makes a profit, the surplus is distributed to the members according to how much they use the cooperative; in a cooperative food store, for example, the distribution would depend on how much food an individual or family purchased during that year.[14]

For over 150 years, producer cooperatives have thrived in the field of agriculture, bringing together farmers to market their products. Consumer co-ops also exist as retail stores, and service co-ops provide insurance, banking, transportation, and telephone service. In health care, two prominent co-ops are Group Health in Washington, D.C., and Group Health Cooperative of Puget Sound in Washington State.

In order to function as the basis of a single payer of universal health insurance, the cooperative principle would have to be modified to allow compulsory, rather than the usual voluntary membership; otherwise, the services provided would not be universal.

7. A coordinated multiple payer system. Can multiple payers join together to form the equivalent of a single payer? The most frequently cited model is the payment structure of the West German health system during the 1980s, in which all payers and providers came together in a body called Concerted Action in Health Care to negotiate payments and implement controls on expenditures.[15] Although this coordinated multiple payer has slowed the West German rate of health care inflation, it has disadvantages compared with a strict single payer in the areas of administrative efficiency and equity.[16] The German example is of questionable relevance to the United States, however, because the multiple payers in Germany (sickness funds) are generally quasi-public institutions without the long history of economic competition that marks the American private health insurance industry. It is unlikely that US health insurance companies and HMOs, with their growing competitive practice of skimming desirable health risks in order to increase profitability, could truly cooperate in a coordinated multi-payer system.

We Must Experiment

The single-payer form of organization for universal health insurance has the potential to provide equality, cost control, administrative efficiency, and democracy in health care. All seven single-payer options outlined here have the potential to control health costs. The first six are also capable of ensuring equality and efficiency. The major difference among these options revolves around the issue of democracy: How much voice can the health provider community and the general public have in such critical decisions as the total size and overall priorities of the health budget, in contrast to the current image of the government as an immovable, unfeeling bureaucracy that pays no attention to the people it is designed to serve?

Can one or another of these single-payer options solve the fundamental American dilemma of an undemocratic democracy? It is difficult to predict which might work the best. Perhaps the best answer to the question of who should be the single payer is to try different versions of these options in different states. Only real-life experiments will provide the answer.

NOTES

1. Grumbach, Kevin, Bodenheimer, Thomas, Himmelstein, David U., and Woolhandler, Steffie, "Liberal Benefits, Conservative Spending: The Physicians for a National Health Program Proposal," *Journal of the American Medical Association*, 1991:265, pp. 2549–2554.

2. Frieden, J., "Many Roads Lead to Health System Reform," *Business and Health*, 1991: 9(11), pp. 38–66.

3. Blendon, R. J., Leitman, R., Morrison, I., and Donelan, K., "Satisfaction with Health Systems in Ten Nations," *Health Affairs*, 1990:9(2), pp. 185–192.

4. Bodenheimer, Thomas, and Grumbach, Kevin, "Funding Universal Health Insurance: Taxes, Premiums and the Lessons of Social Insurance," *Journal of Health Politics, Policy and Law*, Fall 1992, in press.

5. Blumenthal, S., *The Rise of the Counter-Establishment*, New York: Times Books, 1986.

6. Navarro, Vicente, "The 1980 and 1984 U.S. Elections and the New Deal," *International Journal of Health Services*, 1985:15, pp. 359–394.

7. Woolhandler, Steffie, and Himmelstein, David U., "The Deteriorating Administrative Efficiency of the U.S. Health Care System," *New England Journal of Medicine*, 1991:324, pp. 1253–1258.

8. Evans, R. G., "Tension, Compression, and Shear: Directions, Stresses, and Outcomes of Health Care Cost Control," *Journal of Health Politics, Policy and Law*, 1990:15, pp. 101–128.

9. Woolhandler and Himmelstein, op. cit.

10. Koontz, H., and Gable, R. W., *Public Control of Economic Enterprise*, New York: McGraw-Hill, 1956.

11. Bodenheimer, op. cit.

12. Ramandadham, V. V., *The Nature of Public Enterprise*, London: Croom Helm, 1984.

13. Ginzberg, E., Hiestand, D. L., and Reubens, B. G., *The Pluralistic Economy*, New York: McGraw-Hill, 1965.

14. Abrahamsen, M. A., *Cooperative Business Enterprise*, New York: McGraw-Hill, 1976.

15. Kirkman-Liff, B. L., "Physician Payment Methods and Cost Containment Strategies in the Federal Republic of Germany: A Source of Ideas for Medicare Reform," *Journal of Health Politics, Policy and Law*, 1990:15, pp. 69–99.

16. Navarro, Vicente, "The West German Health System: A Critique," *International Journal of Health Services*, 1991:21, pp. 565–571.

LIBERAL BENEFITS, CONSERVATIVE SPENDING: THE PHYSICIANS FOR A NATIONAL HEALTH PROGRAM PROPOSAL

Kevin Grumbach, M.D.;
Thomas Bodenheimer, M.D., M.P.H.;
David U. Himmelstein, M.D.;
Steffie Woolhandler, M.D., M.P.H.

The Physicians for a National Health Program proposes to cover all Americans under a single, comprehensive public insurance program without co-payments or deductibles and with free choice of provider. Such a national health program could reap tens of billions of dollars in administrative savings in the initial years, enough to fund generous increases in health care services not only for the uninsured, but for the underinsured as well. We delineate a transitional national health program budget that would hold overall health spending at current levels while accommodating increases in hospital and physician utilization. Future national health program spending would be indexed to the growth in gross national product adjusted for demographic, epidemiologic, and technologic shifts. Financing for the national health program would transfer funds into the public program without disrupting the general pattern of current revenue sources. We suggest a funding package that would augment existing government health spending with earmarked health care taxes. Because these new taxes would replace employer-employee insurance premiums and substantial portions of current out-of-pocket expenditures, they would not increase health costs for the average American.

(*JAMA.* 1991;265:2549–2554)

The American approach to financing health care has gone awry. From physicians to patients, from The Heritage Foundation to the AFL-CIO, there is agreement that the system needs reform. But what kind of reform? Although all concur that the system is ailing, proposals diverge in their therapeutic approach. Many advocate adjustments of familiar regimens: larger doses of employment-based insurance and greater infusions of public funds to expand Medicaid or to subsidize risk pools for the uninsured.[1-4] Because such measures do not confront the interdependent problems of rising costs and declining access, they cannot ensure health services to all at a cost the nation can afford. A lasting remedy requires basic restructuring of the way we pay for care.[5,6]

The Physicians for a National Health Program plan would cover all Americans under a publicly administered, tax-financed national health program (NHP). A single public payer would replace the present array of more than 1,500 private insurers, Medicaid, and Medicare. A unitary program could initially pay for expanded care out of administrative savings without adding new costs to the overall health care budget and would establish effective mechanisms for long-term cost control. Although consolidation of purchasing power in a public agency may cause apprehension among some physicians, the program could free them from the myriad administrative intrusions that currently plague the practice of medicine.

Structure of the NHP

We have previously described the design of the NHP in some detail.[7,8] It would create a single insurer in each state, locally controlled but subject to stringent national standards. States could experiment with the precise structure of the single insurer. Some may place it within a government agency, while others may choose a commission elected by the citizens or appointed by provider and consumer interests.

Everyone would be fully insured for all medically necessary services including prescription drugs and long-term care. Private insurance duplicating NHP coverage would be proscribed, as would patient co-payments and deductibles. Physicians and hospitals would not bill patients directly for covered services. Hospitals, nursing homes, and clinics would receive a global budget to cover operating expenses, annually negotiated with the state health plan—based on past expenditures, previous financial and clinical performance, projected changes in cost and use, and proposed new and innovative programs. Itemized patient-specific hospital bills would become an extinct species. No part of the operating budget could be diverted for hospital expansion, profit, marketing, or major capital acquisitions. Capital expenditures approved by a local planning process would be funded through appropriations distinct from operating budgets.

Fee-for-service practitioners would submit all claims to the state health plan. Physician representatives (probably state medical societies) and state plans would negotiate a fee schedule for physician services. The effort and expense of billing would be trivial: stamp the patient's NHP card on a billing form, check a diagnosis and procedure code, send in all bills once a week, and receive full payment for virtually all services—with an extra payment for any bill not paid within 30 days. Gone would be the massive accounts receivables and the elaborate billing apparatus that now beleaguer private physicians. Alternatively, physicians could elect to work on a salaried basis for globally budgeted hospitals or clinics, or in health maintenance organizations capitated for all nonhospital services.

Table 1
Personal Health Care Costs for 1991, Excluding Nursing Home Care, With and Without a National Health Program (NHP), in Billions of Dollars*

	NHP	Current Policies
"Baseline" conditions	567	567
New costs for previously uninsured	12	...
Discount for 11.2% hospital administrative savings	(31)	...
Discount for 6.25% physician administrative savings	(9)	...
Subtotal: Personal Health Care	**539**	**567**
Insurance administration and profits	8†	35‡
Total Personal Health Care Plus Insurance Overhead	**547**	**602**

* This assumes Canadian-level administrative efficiency and changes in utilization only among the previously insured.
† 1.4% of personal health care expenditures.
‡ This is the amount estimated by the Health Care Financing Administration.[9]

Costs of the NHP

To estimate total costs, we start by using the Health Care Financing Administration's projection of 1991 costs under current policies as our "baseline" figure. The Health Care Financing Administration estimates that $567 billion will be spent on personal health care services and products in 1991, excluding nursing home costs and insurance overhead and profits (Table 1).[9] (Although long-term care is covered by the NHP, we have omitted these costs to permit comparison with other acute care proposals.)

Universal coverage should increase the use of health services by the uninsured. According to the Lewin/ICF Health Benefits Simulation Model, approximately $36 billion of the $567 billion in 1991 spending projected under current policies will be accounted for by care for the uninsured, including free care at public hospitals, uncompensated care at private facilities cross-subsidized by insurance revenues, and services purchased out-of-pocket. The Lewin/ICF model estimates that an additional $12.2 billion would be required to increase the utilization by the uninsured to levels commensurate with those of the insured (Needleman et al[10] and J. Sheils, oral communication, October 1990).

The NHP will not only assist the uninsured, but will also cover services (e.g., preventive) and payments (e.g., deductibles) that many insurers currently exclude. Would this more extensive coverage "induce" a surge of utilization among those currently insured? The RAND Health Insurance Experiment found that costs for persons assigned to a plan with no cost sharing were approximately 15 percent higher than the age-adjusted, per capita health care expenditures for the United States as a whole.[11] However, a more natural experiment, a study before and after the implementation of an NHP in Quebec, failed to detect the overall utilization surge predicted by the RAND experiment.[12,13] Although the use of physician services in Quebec rose among those with lower incomes, the increase was counterbalanced by a decrease in utilization among the affluent. The net effect was convergence of utilization rates (adjusted for health status) among income groups, with no change in the overall rate.

Would an across-the-board increase in utilization be desirable? In the RAND experiment, lower-income patients with medical problems who received free care had better outcomes than those in cost-sharing plans.[14] At the same time, many medical services currently provided are of no or of extremely marginal benefit,[15–17] and it is not the intent of the NHP to inject an additional bolus of such unnecessary care into the health care system.

All these factors make it difficult to predict the level of overall utilization that would result from the NHP. For this analysis, we have added on the full $12.2 billion cost of bringing utilization rates of the uninsured up to those of the insured. We will discuss in the "Budgeting Under the NHP" section below how the NHP budget could also accommodate increases in utilization among the currently insured.

Savings of the NHP

The administrative efficiencies of a single-payer NHP offer the opportunity for large savings during the implementation of the program.[18] Providers would be relieved of much of the expense of screening for eligibility, preparing detailed bills for multiple payers, responding to cumbersome utilization review procedures, and marketing their services. In 1987, California hospitals devoted 20.2 percent of revenues to administrative functions,[19] in contrast to 9.0 percent spent by Canadian hospitals (L. Raymer, Health and Welfare Canada, written communication, April 1990). (These figures exclude malpractice premium costs and administrative personnel in clinical departments such as nursing.) The 11.2 percent difference is attributable to Canada's simplified hospital payment method, a method we propose for the United States.

Determining the potential administrative savings in physician expenditures is more difficult. Although practice expenses are 49 percent of physician gross income in the United States and only 36 percent in Canada,[20,21] it is uncertain how much of this difference is due to billing costs. Malpractice costs for US physicians, for example, are higher than those in Canada. We therefore extrapolated billing cost data from a recent American Medical Association survey to project minimum expected administrative savings in physician expenditures.[22] The average physician spent approximately $14,500 in 1988 billing Medicare and Blue Shield alone, representing 5.5 percent of gross physician income. In addition, physicians spent approximately 2.75 percent of their own professional time on billing-related activities for these claims. (The survey did not measure the costs of billing other third parties or patients and therefore yields a low estimate of physician billing costs.) We liberally estimate that physician billing expenses in Canada are 1 percent of physician costs and that Canadian physicians spend at the most 1 percent of their time on billing (D. Peachey, M.D., Ontario Medical Association, written communication, June 1990). In sum, US billing costs for physician time and practice expenses are at least 8.25 percent of total physician expenditures in contrast to at most 2 percent of Canadian physician costs. An NHP functioning at Canadian-level administrative efficiency could save at least 6.25 percent of physician costs. Most of these savings can be realized rapidly. In the private practice of one of the authors (T. B.), for example, the change to a single payer would allow an immediate reduction in office payroll of 18 percent.

Administrative savings to hospitals and physicians function as price discounts when calculating costs. For example, if physicians could lower their overhead by 6.25 percent of gross income by trimming billing expenses, fees could be lowered by 6.25 percent and physicians would still earn the same net income for the same volume of services. We therefore estimated the minimum potential administrative savings in hospital and physician expenditures to be $40 billion by discounting projected hospital and physician costs by 11.2 percent and 6.25 percent, respectively (Table 1).

Additional savings accrue from the reduced administrative "load factor" of a public plan. In 1987, the cost of public and private insurance overhead and profits expressed as a percent of personal health care expenditures was 5.9 percent in the United States and only 1.4 percent in Canada.[9,23] If our NHP operated with the efficiency of Canada's, the administration of health insurance would cost $8 billion, less than one quarter the $35 billion projected by the Health Care Financing Administration in 1991.

As indicated in Table 1, the net cost of personal health care and insurance overhead for universal coverage under the NHP, including expanded services for the previously uninsured, would be at most $547 billion if the system operated with the administrative efficiency of the Canadian system. This is $55 billion less than the $602 billion that will be spent in 1991 under current policies that exclude approximately 35 million Americans.

Budgeting Under the NHP

We do not propose reducing the health care budget by $55 billion under the NHP. As noted above, we are uncertain how utilization patterns might respond to universal, first-dollar insurance coverage. Nor can we be completely confident that hospitals and physicians will immediately shed their excess administrative poundage and assume the leaner proportions possible under a simplified payment system. We therefore propose the following budgetary strategy for the NHP: We would set the overall health care budget for the NHP's initial year at the amount projected under current policies ($602 billion if implemented in 1991). To keep expenditures within this target, we would rely on the ability of a single payer to allocate and enforce prospective budgets for physician and hospital services. These budgets would challenge providers to extract administrative savings and redirect resources into patient care for the underserved. The budget would allow a range of utilization responses among patients and physicians.

For example, the NHP could set total hospital operating budgets at the Health Care Financing Administration projected "baseline" 1991 level of $273 billion (Table 2), though some individual hospitals' budgets might be adjusted to reflect past underfunding or large operating surpluses. On average, a hospital able to achieve full administrative savings would have 11.2 percent of its budget to devote to more or better clinical services. Billing personnel could be transferred to clinical departments to perform clerical duties, freeing up nurses for bedside care. Hospitals unable to realize immediate administrative savings would not be penalized in the short run. However, in the longer run, the single payer within each state would evaluate hospitals' clinical performance and efficiency and modify budgets, taking account of these hospital quality measures as well as community needs. The Canadian experience demonstrates that such a budgeting process need not be cumbersome or expensive, consuming less than $2 per capita in British Columbia (D. Cunningham, British Columbia Ministry of Health, written communication, July 1990).

Prospective budgeting of physician services under fee-for-service methods would require expenditure targets or caps. On average, fees would be set at 6.25 percent below current levels, reflecting expected administrative savings to physicians. The expenditure target, however, could be set at $154 billion, 6 percent above the "baseline" projected level for 1991 (Table 2). This would allow physician payments to accommodate a net utilization increase of up to 12.25 percent, sufficient to satisfy increased demand by the uninsured and underinsured, while allowing a net increase in physician income of 6 percent. A utilization increase above 12.25 percent would trigger a compensatory decrease in fees to keep expenditures within the budget target. Such a plan allows for control of costs with a minimum of the administrative waste or encumbrances of our current utilization review mechanisms.[24]

Summing the aggregate hospital operating budget of $273 billion, the physician budget of $154 billion, and the other categories of personal health care spending and administration would still leave total expenditures $18 billion below our proposed $602 billion budget (Table 2). The $18 billion balance could be used for start-up costs for the NHP, job training and placement programs for displaced administrative personnel, improved long-term care, and revitalized public health programs.

Financing the NHP

Health insurance proposals are frequently shipwrecked on the shoals of their financing; any serious proposal must specify a revenue package. Although the NHP would not result in a net increase in total health care expenditures, it would produce a major shift in payment sources toward government and away from private insurance and out-of-pocket payments. We emphasize that the average individual and business would not pay more for health care under the NHP but would pay taxes that take the place of, but do not exceed, current premium payments and out-of-pocket costs. Moreover, with the single payer's capacity to control inflation, individuals and businesses should soon enjoy reductions in the rate of increase of their health care costs.

What principle should underlie the choice of revenue sources? Health care is only one factor—sometimes a minor one—in the promotion and preservation of health. Poverty, racial oppression, substance abuse, lack of education, lack of exercise, overnutrition and undernutrition, and occupational and environmen-

Table 2
National Health Program (NHP) Budget, by Category of Expenditure, in Billions of Dollars

Category	NHP	Current Policies*
Hospital	273	273
Physician	154	145
Other†	149	149
Insurance administration and profits	8	35
Subtotal	**584**	**602**
New health initiatives and transition costs	18	0
Total Budget	**602**	**602**

* These are Health Care Financing Administration projections.[9]
† "Other" includes drugs, dental and other professional services, and so forth.

tal hazards all damage health. Some of these factors can be influenced by society's revenue-generating mechanisms. For example, raising excise taxes on cigarettes and alcohol reduces their consumption and thereby improves health, particularly among teenagers and the poor.[25] On the other hand, burdening low-income families with high payments (whether taxes, premiums, or out-of-pocket dollars) reduces their disposable income and amplifies the ill effects of poverty. In contrast, a system of taxes and other payments that reduces the burden on low-income families without impeding job formation may ameliorate poverty's health consequences. Thus, funding mechanisms can be "healthy" or "unhealthy."

Health care financing in the United States is markedly regressive and hence unhealthy. The bottom income decile receives 1.3 percent of total income but pays 3.9 percent of health costs, while the top income decile receives 33.8 percent of income and pays only 21.7 percent of health costs. By comparison, in Britain the bottom decile receives 2.3 percent of income and pays 1.7 percent of health costs, while the top decile receives 24.9 percent of income and pays 25.6 percent of costs.[26] Any departure from the existing configuration of US health care funding should reverse the current unhealthy pattern.

We estimate that public expenditures will account for 85 percent of health spending under the NHP, requiring $509 billion in revenues for 1991 (Table 3). We will discuss these revenues in three categories: payroll taxes, general government revenues, and payments by individuals (see chart).

Payroll Taxes

Employer-employee payments for group health insurance (31 percent of personal health expenditures [excluding nursing-home care][27]) are, in essence, a payroll tax,[28] with the money going to an insurance company or a self-insured fund rather than to the government. Social Security payments for Medicare (12

Table 3
Public Plan's Share of 1991 Personal Health Care Expenditures Under National Health Program (NHP), in Billions of Dollars

Service	Total Cost	% Covered by NHP	NHP Cost
Hospital	273	96*	262
Physician	154	91*	140
	149	55†	82
New health initiatives and transition costs	18	100	18
Administration	8	85†	7
Total	602	85	509‡

* These figures are based on the public share of spending for these services in Canada. The shares are less than 100% because certain services, such as cosmetic surgery, life insurance examinations, and private room surcharges, are not covered benefits.[24]
† These figures are based on our "best guess" estimate, since the NHP will provide more extensive coverage of nonhospital and nonphysician services than do the Canadian provincial plans. Non-prescription drugs are an example of a product in the "other" category that will not be covered.
‡ A total of $93 billion of personal health care expenditures uncovered by the NHP remain as out-of-pocket and individual private insurance premium costs.

percent of health expenditures[27,29]) are also a payroll tax. It is logical to combine these two sources of financing, which together account for 43 percent of health expenditures. To minimize economic disruption, we propose that a similar proportion of the NHP be funded by payroll tax.

The regressive nature of a payroll tax makes it a less-than-healthy revenue source; the employer share is often shifted to employees as lower wages or to consumers as higher prices.[30] It should be made more progressive by reducing the employee share for lower-wage employees, by raising the employee share for high-income employees (e.g., eliminating the current Social Security cap), and by reducing the employer share for small business. Employers and employees currently pay almost 2 percent of total payroll for Medicare-related Social Security taxes and approximately 10 percent for private health insurance—a combined health-related payroll tax of 13 percent.[29,31,32] Using Department of Commerce figures, we project that under the NHP, an average tax rate of 9 percent for medium and large employers, with an average 2 percent rate for employees, and half these rates for businesses with fewer than 20 employees, would raise $228 billion in revenues.[33] These precise tax rates are only initial suggestions and must be negotiated with the affected parties.

General Government Revenues

Twenty-six percent of personal health expenditures (excluding nursing-home care) comes from non-Social Security governmental revenues at the federal, state, and local levels.[27,29] Of this total, 51 percent comes from individual income

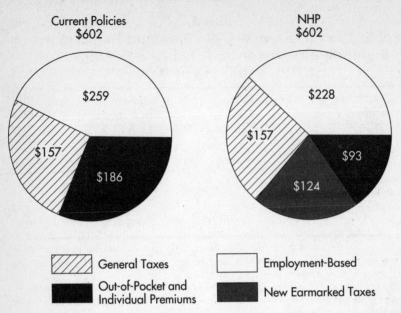

Current Policies
$602

$259

$157

$186

NHP
$602

$228

$157

$93

$124

General Taxes

Out-of-Pocket and
Individual Premiums

Employment-Based

New Earmarked Taxes

Revenue sources. Figures are in billions of 1991 dollars. NHP indicates national health program.

taxes, 12 percent from property taxes, 12 percent from sales taxes, 12 percent from corporation income taxes, 5 percent from gasoline, tobacco, and alcohol taxes, and 8 percent from other sources.[34] Although some of these revenue sources are unhealthy, we propose leaving them intact, adhering to the principle that implementing the NHP should not demand radical economic restructuring. These revenues would generate $157 billion for the NHP in 1991.[9,29]

Payments by Individuals

The third major source of health financing consists of payments by individuals; these payments currently account for 31 percent of health expenditures (5 percent in individual insurance premiums, 24 percent in out-of-pocket payments, 1 percent in Medicare premiums, and 1 percent in other private funds).[27,29] They are the least healthy revenues because they burden lower-income families far more than they do the affluent. To the extent that they pay for services covered under the NHP, they will disappear.

We propose replacing the majority of individual payments with "healthier" revenues—taxes that reduce income disparities and discourage the use of harmful and polluting substances. The following measures, according to a Congressional Budget Office study,[35] would generate $124 billion per year and could be considered as NHP tax revenue sources: 1) a new federal income tax bracket of 38 percent for families with income higher than $170,000, 2) a cap on mortgage interest deductions for luxury homes, 3) a 0.5 percent tax on transfer of securities, 4) an increase in energy taxes to encourage energy conservation and reduce pollution, 5) an increase in excise taxes on cigarettes to 32 cents per pack and on alcohol to 25 cents per ounce, 6) an excise tax on sources of air and water pollutants, and 7) a tax on fossil fuels to reduce carbon dioxide emissions. Although some of these taxes are regressive, their overall effects are health promoting.

To summarize, the NHP would fund approximately 38 percent of health expenditures from a payroll tax similar to current payroll expenses for Medicare and health insurance premiums; 26 percent from existing federal, state, and local revenues; and 21 percent from new, healthy federal tax revenues that would largely supplant current out-of-pocket expenditures. Fifteen percent of expenditures would remain out-of-pocket (See chart).

A majority of Americans would accept this type of tax package if it were earmarked for health care and placed in a health care trust fund. A 1990 poll found that 72 percent would support an NHP even if it required a tax increase; however, only 22 percent would pay more than $200 extra per year.[36] Our proposal would not increase the sums paid for health care by low- and middle-income groups. It is designed to minimize winners and losers, aside from the private health insurance industry.

Two additional principles should be incorporated in NHP funding. Per capita health spending should be equalized throughout the nation, with federal funds transferred to states under formulas adjusted for age, income levels, health status, wage, and other input costs. Finally, to protect the NHP from annual budgetary debacles in Washington, DC, it must be an entitlement program with a statutory expenditure floor as well as a ceiling. In contrast to entitlement programs restricted to poor families, the NHP would embrace the entire population and could thus command the level of support enjoyed by Social Security. Adequate increases in NHP funding (based on such factors as aging of the population, epidemics, advances in medical technology, and inflation) must be mandated by law. As suggested in our original NHP proposal,[7] an expanded program of technology assessment would help guide budgetary allocations.

Comment

In health insurance, as in many things in life, simplicity is a virtue. The NHP's approach to universal access is simple: Every American automatically qualifies for equal, comprehensive health insurance under a unitary public plan. The economic premises of the NHP are also simple: Funnel all third-party payments through a single payer, thereby saving billions of dollars in administrative costs and achieving cost containment through global controls rather than minute bureaucratic scrutiny.

The administrative cost reductions during the NHP's initial phase are not, as some have argued, only a one-time saving.[37] Whether in Canada or New Zealand, Sweden or Britain, single-payer systems have stabilized costs in the past decade, while US health care inflation has been impervious to the most earnest attempts to control costs.[38-40] Economist Robert Evans[41] has concluded that "universality of coverage and sole-source funding are, as far as we know now, preconditions for cost control."

Global expenditure control can also enhance clinical freedom. Under the micromanagement model of cost containment, each of the multiple payers, lacking global budgetary levers, resorts to intrusive patient-by-patient utilization review.[24] Such day-to-day interference in medical practice is minimized in single-payer systems.[40] As John Wennberg[16] recently observed:

> The key to the preservation of fee-for-service markets, as the Canadians seem to recognize, is not the micromanagement of the doctor-patient relationship but the management of capacity and budget. The American problem is to find the will to set the supply thermostat somewhere within reason.

The NHP would benefit most Americans, though a few powerful interest groups would suffer. It would virtually eliminate financial barriers to care for those who are currently uninsured and underinsured, ensure patients a free choice of providers, ensure physicians a free choice of practice settings, diminish bureaucratic interference in clinical decision making, stabilize health spending, and reduce the growing burden of health care costs for many individuals and employers. Small-business owners who do not currently cover their employees would face modest cost increases, though far less than mandated by most alternative proposals. The health insurance industry would feel the greatest impact. Indeed, most of the extra funds needed to expand care would come from eliminating the overhead and profits of insurance companies and from abolishing the billing apparatus necessary to apportion costs among the various plans. Job retraining programs for displaced administrative and clerical personnel would be essential.

Although few dispute the ability of the NHP to provide universal coverage and control costs, critics have raised the specter of rationing, pointing to queues for some high technology services in Canada.[42] We do not advocate cutting US health spending to Canadian levels. Even with a slower rate of growth under the NHP, US health expenditures will remain well above those of any other nation. Deploying our greater resources with Canadian efficiency would permit increases in utilization and improvements in technology without skyrocketing costs. Compared with Americans, Canadians do, in fact, get more health care for their health care dollar. About half of the cost differential between the two nations is squandered on insurance overhead and paper pushing.[18,43] Stanford economist Victor Fuchs[44] has concluded that "the quantity of [physician] services per capita is much higher in Canada than in the United States . . . the data firmly reject the view that Canadians save money by delivering fewer services."

Health financing reforms unable to extract administrative savings inevitably impose added costs for expanded services. Employer mandate proposals (e.g., the Pepper Commission Plan,[1] the American Medical Association's Health Access America plan,[3] the National Leadership Commission's proposal,[2] and Massachusetts' Universal Health Care Law [*New York Times.* April 11, 1991:A1]) would leave existing insurance in place while expanding public programs for the unemployed and requiring employers to insure their workers. None of these plans offer improved coverage for those currently insured, nor do they offer new cost control mechanisms. Hence high initial costs presage continuing inflation or far more stringent and intrusive micromanagement—probably both. Modifications of the employer mandate approach (eg, the UNYCare proposal in New York State)[45] that attempt to meld the cost containment features of a single-payer system with a continuing role for private insurance also eschew most administrative savings, compromising the ability of such measures to expand access without raising costs.

There is slim evidence that Enthoven and Kronick's[46] "managed competition" plan—featuring competing managed care insurers and higher patient co-payments—can hold costs in check.[47] Does forcing consumers to bear premium costs for higher-priced plans hold down overall costs or simply segregate the market based on ability to pay? Do low-cost plans provide care more efficiently or simply market themselves more effectively to lower-risk subscribers? Is the rubric "Consumer Choice Health Plan" appropriate for a system likely to lock the vast majority of patients and physicians into closed panel health maintenance organizations run by insurance companies? The ultimate vision of managed competition—a landscape dominated by a limited number of huge health maintenance organizations managing salaried physicians—is a more radical departure from the current health care scene than the NHP.

The objectives of the NHP are simple: (1) to minimize financial barriers to appropriate medical care, (2) to distribute costs fairly, and (3) to contain costs at a reasonable level. Once a structure is in place for meeting these basic concerns, the medical profession and society as a whole can move on to the more complicated questions: Which health services truly improve the quality of life? What share of our human and material resources should we devote to health care? How shall we reduce the toll now extracted by poverty, ignorance, and addictions? By implementing a national health program, we can turn and face the challenges ahead.

NOTES

1. US Bipartisan Commission on Comprehensive Health Care. *A Call for Action*. Washington, DC: The Pepper Commission on Comprehensive Health Care; 1990.

2. National Leadership Commission on Health Care. *For the Health of a Nation*. Ann Arbor, Mich: Health Administration Press; 1989.

3. *Health Access America*. Chicago, Ill: American Medical Association; 1990.

4. Kennedy E. Senate Bill S.768. November 20, 1989.

5. Woolhandler S, Himmelstein DU. Resolving the cost/access conflict: the case for a national health program. *J Gen Intern Med*. 1989;4:54–60.

6. Grumbach K. National health insurance in America: can we practice with it? can we practice without it? *West J Med*. 1989;151:210–216.

7. Himmelstein DU, Woolhandler S. A national health program for the United States: a physician's proposal. *N Engl J Med*. 1989;320:102–108.

8. Woolhandler S, Himmelstein DU. A national health program: a northern light at the end of the tunnel. *JAMA*. 1989;262:2136–2137.

9. Health Care Financing Administration. National health expenditures: 1986–2000. *Health Care Financing Rev*. 1987;8(4):1–36.

10. Needleman J, Arnold J, Sheils J, Lewin LS. *The Health Care Financing System and the Uninsured*. Washington, DC: Lewin/ICF; 1990.

11. Newhouse JP, Manning WG, Morris CN, et al. Some interim results from a controlled trial of cost sharing in health insurance. *N Engl J Med*. 1981;305:1501–1507.

12. Enterline PE, Salter V, McDonald AD, McDonald JC. The distribution of medical services before and after 'free' medical care: the Quebec experience. *N Engl J Med.* 1973;289:1174–1178.

13. McDonald AD, McDonald JC, Salter V, Enterline P. Effects of Quebec Medicare on physician consultation for selected symptoms. *N Engl J Med.* 1974;291:649–652.

14. Brook RH, Ware JE Jr, Rogers WH, et al. Does free care improve adults' health? results from a randomized controlled trial. *N Engl J Med.* 1983;309:1426–1434.

15. Eisenberg JM. *Doctors' Decisions and the Cost of Medical Care.* Ann Arbor, Mich: Health Administration Press; 1986.

16. Wennberg J. Outcomes research, cost containment, and the fear of health care rationing. *N Engl J Med.* 1990;323:1202–1204.

17. Chassin MR, Kosecoff J, Park RE, et al. Does inappropriate use explain geographic variations in the use of health care services? *JAMA.* 1987;258:2533–2537.

18. Himmelstein D, Woolhandler S. Cost without benefit: administrative waste in US health care. *N Engl J Med.* 1986;314:441–445.

19. *Aggregate Hospital Financial Data for California: Report Periods Ending June 30, 1987–June 29, 1988.* Sacramento: California Health Facilities Commission; 1989.

20. Gonzalez ML, Emmons DW. *Socioeconomic Characteristics of Medical Practice.* Chicago, Ill: American Medical Association; 1988.

21. Iglehart J. Canada's health system faces its problems. *N Engl J Med.* 1990;322:562–568.

22. American Medical Association. The administrative burden of health insurance on physicians. *Socioeconomic Monitoring Survey Rep.* 1989;3:2–4.

23. *National Health Expenditures.* Ottawa, Ontario: Health and Welfare Canada; 1990.

24. Grumbach K, Bodenheimer T. Reins or fences? a physician's view of cost containment. *Health Aff.* 1990;9(4):120–126.

25. Last JM. Controlling the smoking epidemic. *Am J Prev Med.* 1985;1:1–3.

26. Wagstaff A, Van Doorslaer E, Paci P. Equity in the finance and delivery of health care: some tentative cross-country comparisons. *Oxford Rev Econ Policy.* 1989;5:89–112.

27. Levit KR, Freeland MS, Waldo DR. National health care spending trends: 1988. *Health Aff.* 1990;9(2):171–184.

28. Reinhardt UE. Health insurance for the nation's poor. *Health Aff.* 1987;6(1):101–112.

29. Levit KR, Freeland MS, Waldo DR. Health spending and ability to pay: business, individuals, and government. *Health Care Financing Rev.* 1989;10(3):1–11.

30. Pechman JA. *Federal Tax Policy.* Washington, DC: The Brookings Institution; 1987.

31. Bergthold LA. *Purchasing Power in Health.* New Brunswick, NJ: Rutgers University Press; 1990.

32. DiCarlo S, Gabel J. Conventional health insurance: a decade later. *Health Care Financing Rev.* 1989;10(3):77–89.

33. Bureau of the Census. Statistical abstract of the United States 1990. Washington, DC: US Dept of Commerce; 1990.

34. Bureau of the Census. *Quarterly Summary of Federal, State, and Local Tax Revenue, July–September 1989.* Washington, DC: US Dept of Commerce; 1990.

35. Congressional Budget Office. *Reducing the Deficit: Spending and Revenue Options.* Washington, DC: The Congress of the United States; 1990.

36. Blendon RJ, Donelan K. The public and the emerging debate over national health insurance. *N Engl J Med.* 1990;323:208–212.

37. Aaron H, Schwartz WG. Rationing health care: the choice before us. *Science.* 1990;247:418–422.

38. International comparisons of health care financing and delivery: data and perspectives. *Health Care Financing Rev.* 1989;10(suppl):1–196.

39. Pfaff M. Differences in health care spending across countries: statistical evidence. *J Health Polit Policy Law.* 1990;15:1–24.

40. Evans RG, Lomas J, Barer ML, et al. Controlling health expenditures: the Canadian reality. *N Engl J Med.* 1989;320:571–577.

41. Evans RG. Accessible, acceptable, and affordable: financing health care in Canada. In: *The 1990 Richard and Hinda Rosenthal Lectures.* Washington, DC: Institute of Medicine; 1990:7–47.

42. Board of Trustees, American Medical Association. *Study of the Canadian Health Care System.* Chicago, Ill: American Medical Association; 1989. Report V(A-89).

43. Evans RG. Split vision: interpreting cross-border differences in health spending. *Health Aff.* 1988;7(4):17–24.

44. Fuchs VR, Hahn JS. How does Canada do it? a comparison of expenditures for physicians' services in the United States and Canada. *N Engl J Med.* 1990;323:884–890.

45. Beauchamp DE, Rouse RL. Universal New York Health Care: a single-payer strategy linking cost control and universal access. *N Engl J Med.* 1990;323:640–644.

46. Enthoven A, Kronick R. A consumer choice health plan for the 1990s: universal health insurance in a system designed to promote quality and economy. *N Engl J Med*. 1989;320:29–37, 94–101.

47. Jones SB. Can multiple choice be managed to constrain health care costs? *Health Aff*. 1989; 8(3):51–59.

IMPORTING HEALTH CARE REFORM? ISSUES IN TRANSPOSING CANADA'S HEALTH CARE SYSTEM TO THE UNITED STATES

Samuel Wolfe

We are especially pleased to be publishing this article by Samuel Wolfe, a Canadian who has spent a majority of his professional life in the United States. Before coming south of the border, Wolfe helped preside over the implementation of North America's first universal publicly funded medical care insurance program in Saskatchewan province. This program was to serve as the prototype for national health insurance in Canada—a scheme that a growing number of experts advocate for the United States.

Having survived (but not unscathed) the famed Saskatchewan doctors' strike and the battles over consumer-controlled community clinics, Wolfe went to the United States, finally coming to rest at Columbia University School of Public Health. He served there as Division Chair of Health Administration until 1980 and then as professor until his retirement this past spring. Given his varied professional experiences on both sides of the border—including practice as a rural family physician, additional training in psychiatry, and then a career encompassing public health practice, governance, and research—Wolfe is able to provide especially unique insights into why Canada's health care system may neither be as readily transferable to the United States as some would hope, nor as trouble free as some would have us believe.

Many of us have known Sam Wolfe in at least one or more of his roles as teacher, advocate, analyst, researcher, mentor, loyal supporter of Health/PAC, and friend. As he gets ready to depart for British Columbia, we want to publicly thank him for his untiring dedication over many decades to the struggle for social justice and health care for all and to let him know he will be missed.

—Arthur Levin

In discussing the Canadian health care system, I start with the assumption that even though Canada and the United States share an unarmed and generally friendly border, Canadians don't know much about the United States, and U.S. citizens don't know much about Canada. This applies with special emphasis in the fields of politics and health care, because even though we share democratic systems and parallel systems of medical education, medical practice, and hospitals (although not of financing), the differences are great. So, I'm going to describe the Canadian system of health care, with special reference to financing, emphasize what makes it different from the experience in the United States, and conclude with issues to be faced if attempts are made to transpose the Canadian system to the United States.

The Canadian Difference

A headline in *The New York Times* Week in Review section for March 25, 1990, read, "Canada, Where Officers Halt All Cars and Drivers Cheer." The article describes flying roadblocks, where groups of police officers halt every car, shine their lights inside, and have brief conversations with the drivers to find the slightest signs of impairment. The campaign is highly popular in Canada, and few drivers complain, but such roadblocks would have been illegal in the United States (at least until the recent Supreme Court decision). It illustrates the difference between the Canadian emphasis on the group and the emphasis in the United States on the individual. The Canadian courts ruled that brief roadside stops by police officers who were looking for drunken drivers were not an invasion of the rights of all the non-drinking drivers. In the United States, authorities needed a probable cause, a reason to be suspicious about a particular car. In Canada, the momentary inconvenience is weighed against the safety of the larger society. Similarly, Canadians wait in line more willingly than do Americans, and it is illegal in Canada to carry handguns. We are by and large a Royal Canadian Mounted Police law-and-order society.

Canada is a parliamentary, not a republican, democracy, and there is no sharp separation of powers between the executive and the legislative branches of government. The prime minister is elected only by the voters in his own geographic district and holds his position by virtue of the fact that he is the leader of the party that holds the majority of the seats in the House of Commons in the Canadian parliament. In the parliamentary democracies, elected members rarely vote against their own party platform. This means that if the party with a majority proposes a major piece of legislation, it is almost certain to become the law of the land.

Furthermore, since the 1930s Canada has had a major third force, a social democratic party that has played a significant role in the Canadian parliament and has held at various times the majority power in Saskatchewan, in Manitoba, and in British Columbia. Thus, there has been some pressure from the left as a Canadian reality for over 50 years, and in this respect, Canada is much more like Britain or Scandinavia than like the United States.

Participation in or partial ownership of natural monopolies such as radio, television, railways, airlines, telephones, and electric power by the federal or provincial government is accepted as normal by most Canadians. Canadians appear more trusting of these arrangements, and of government in general, than do Americans.

Pioneering Provinces

In Canada, the provinces and not the federal government in Ottawa have most powers relating to health, education, and welfare. Federal participation involves agreements between the ten provinces and two territories and Ottawa. The responsibility for and administration of health insurance plans in Canada are therefore at the provincial level, with federal participation in planning, development, and financing. The pattern has been that individual provinces develop and implement plans, these are picked up by other provinces, and then Ottawa passes legislation spelling out the conditions under which the federal government will participate in federal-provincial sharing arrangements, including financing.[1]

As of July 1990, it has been 43 years since Saskatchewan, a Canadian prairie province with less than a million people in an area of about 250,000 square miles, implemented acute care hospital insurance for all residents. By the end of 1990, it will have been 29 years that *all* residents of Canada have been protected against the costs of acute care in hospitals, as well as for the costs of outpatient ancillary services. Again, as of July, it has been 28 years since Saskatchewan once again pioneered with its medical care insurance plan, under which all physician services and certain other services were paid for universally through the public purse. By the end of this year, all Canadians will have been covered by medical care insurance for 19 years. Both the hospital and medical care plans are operated and administered by the provinces with federal-provincial cost-sharing arrangements.

We Canadians cannot be accused of being too hasty. It took from 1919, when it was first a major plank in the platform of a political party, to 1961— 42 years—to achieve universal entitlement to acute-care hospital insurance, and 52 years, until 1971, to achieve universal entitlement to medical care insurance. These two programs are the centerpieces of the Canadian national health insurance system.

The Canadian System

To get federal dollars, the provincial plans must provide universal access to care with equal terms and conditions for all, must cover all services determined medically necessary by physicians, must provide province-to-province portability benefits and must be publicly administered on a nonprofit basis. Insured hospital services include all inpatient services provided at a standard ward level and all necessary drugs, biologicals, supplies, and diagnostic tests, as well as a broad range of outpatient services. The services of psychiatrists and mental hospitals are fully covered. There are no upper limits to the care provided, as long as it is medically necessary.

The insured services of physicians, who by and large are paid on a fee-for-service basis, include all medically required services provided by licensed medical practitioners, regardless of whether they are provided in hospitals, clinics, doctors' offices, or elsewhere. Fees are negotiated by each province with its provincial medical association.

Acute care hospitals are paid on a prospective payment system based on global budgeting. At a given time of year, each hospital negotiates its global budget for the coming year with the provincial government, based on historical trends and actual use and cost data for the most recent full year. Once the overall budget is set, the hospital, starting on January 1, receives 1/26th of its budget every two weeks, thus assuring an adequate cash flow. It is unheard of for a Canadian hospital to declare bankruptcy. This is a prospective payment system, but without the use of diagnosis-related groups (DRGs). Once the global budget is set, the hospital cannot exceed it unless there are very extenuating circumstances. But a hospital can change categories within its budget, thus giving it a small measure of flexibility. Capital costs for hospitals are borne in general by the provinces and not shared by Ottawa.

Residency training is built into the global budgeting. I might point out that 52 percent of Canadian doctors are family doctors (compared to about 30 percent in the United States, including general internists, general pediatricians, and family practitioners), and that all Canadian teaching hospitals and many community hospitals have major training programs in family medicine. In Canada we have a large and growing supply of family doctors serving people of all ages in the population. Remember also that Canadian medical school tuition averages about $1,500, so graduates are not faced with the mountains of debt that US medical school graduates confront.

Blue Cross and Blue Shield as well as other commercial insurers in Canada are prohibited by law from selling insurance or paying for care already covered by the provincial plans. They can sell amenity services, such as private duty nursing, private room coverage, and other services not covered by the public plans. Of the 1,243 hospitals in Canada, all but 9 are not-for-profit institutions. Only in the field of nursing home services is there a sizable component of investor ownership. Canada, as described recently by the well-known Canadian economist Robert Evans, has a deep-rooted suspicion of class-based systems of any kind.[2] Private schools are a rarity in Canada, and private universities do not exist. Equality before the health care system is a political principle in Canada; in fact, in Canada the issues surrounding national health insurance have become apolitical because all political parties strongly favor the plans and support their expansion. In the field of health, at least, Canadians have become their brothers' and sisters' keepers.

The Bottom Line

The plans across the country are operated and financed primarily through the public purse. In the United States in 1990, 40 percent of national health expenditures will be publicly financed. In Canada, public funds will make up at least 75 percent of national health expenditures. At the federal level, the dollars come from the consolidated revenues of the country, primarily from the graduated income tax; at the provincial level, the money comes from the provincial income tax and sales taxes. Only two provinces still require premiums to be paid—Alberta and British Columbia. Most people appreciate the fact that still another public bureaucracy was avoided. The poor all over Canada fall into the mainstream of health care services because they are protected in the same fashion as all residents of Canada.

This year, 1990, it is estimated that Canada's national health expenditures will consume just under 9 percent of the gross national product, with everyone protected by a comprehensive system for paying hospital, medical, and certain other bills. In the United States this year, the best estimates are that just under 12 percent of the gross national product will be spent on health care, with at least 35 million persons totally uninsured and a further 20 million persons so scantily covered that they may be said to be severely underinsured in the face of serious illness.[3]

Trends in health care spending in the United States and Canada paralleled each other until the early 1960's when Canada's hospital plans were firmly in place. The gap has been widening ever since and currently stands at 3 percent of gross national product. For example, in Canada in 1985 just over 0.1 percent of the gross national product was spent on administrative costs of health insurance; in the United States in that same year, 0.655 percent of the gross national product was spent—a difference of 22 billion U.S. dollars for that item alone.[4]

The reasons for the difference in spending in both countries are worth elaborating on. In the Canadian system, insurance overhead is low because of the administrative simplicity of the provincial plans, and because all funding for covered services runs through the provincial plans, which are virtually the sole source for buying health care services. In the United States, in contrast, health insurance overhead is higher because of the hundreds of companies that sell coverage (the "Blues," the commercial insurers, the HMOs, the PPOs, etc., etc.), and health care dollars run through hundreds or thousands of pipes. The Canadian system has only a few pipes through which the money runs. Moreover, the Canadian system controls payments to physicians and hospitals through toughly and tightly negotiated fees and global budgeting.

An additional reason for the proportionately lower amount spent on health care in both countries may be its restraint on the distribution of some forms of technology. There is a noticeable separation in Canada between hospital operating expenses and capital spending. In addition to approving overall hospital budgets, the provinces must also approve the funding of new capital acquisitions. By controlling both capital and operating budgets, the provinces have effectively limited the growth of outlays for labor, supplies, and equipment. There have been sharp constraints on duplication of costly medical technologies. It is impossible in Canada to have a private magnetic resonance imaging (MRI) unit around the corner from an MRI unit based in a teaching hospital.

The Canadian argument is that costly new technologies should be regionally based and require doctors to judge carefully which patients can profit from their use; highly sophisticated tertiary technologies are exclusively diffused only in teaching hospitals. Such technologies as MRIs, lithotripsy, cardiac catheterization, and open-heart surgery are far more available on a per capita basis in the United States than in Canada. A recent study showed no evidence that substantial numbers of Canadians are seeking care at American medical centers; those that do travel to American medical centers—for example, from Windsor to Detroit—do so by agreement with the provincial health insurance plan.[5]

The original formula by which the provinces created their plans was based on federal-provincial cost-sharing arrangements on a 50-50 basis, with more dollars going to the poorer provinces—Newfoundland, Prince Edward Island, New Brunswick, and Nova Scotia. These formulas were built into the original hospital and medical care acts. Even though the poorer provinces receive far more than 50 percent, they do not have the fiscal resources to provide extra services beyond meeting the conditions for receiving federal dollars for the required coverages under the federal-provincial cost-sharing agreements. As a colleague and I wrote previously:

> Over the years, the Ottawa formulas to the provinces have not adequately compensated for lower provincial per capita incomes. For example, Alberta spends 3.9 percent of its gross domestic product for basic insured health services, Saskatchewan spends 5.1 percent, and Newfoundland and Prince Edward Island spend over 9 percent respectively. Poorer provinces have to spend a greater proportion of their domestic product to achieve a basic threshold of benefits under national health insurance. For example, as long ago as 1981, the federal per capita transfer to the provinces ranged from $541 for Alberta to $1,300 for Prince Edward Island; in turn, the federal transfers made up 12 percent of provincial revenues in Alberta and 56 percent of the provincial revenues in Prince Edward Island. Federal transfers have accounted for more than 50 percent of provincial revenues in all four maritime provinces. The poorer provinces have been less able to provide additional benefits, for example, pharmaceutical programs, dental programs, and alternatives to care in hospitals. These observations, of course, do not control for the philosophy and ideology of either provincial or federal governments in Canada.[6]

Thus, the poorer provinces spend far more of their gross domestic product on health care than do the wealthier provinces. There are wide disparities in per capita incomes in Canada, as there are all over the world.

As health care costs have escalated, Ottawa has stopped sharing equally with the provinces. Commencing with the 1977 Federal-Provincial Fiscal Arrangements and Established Programs Act, provincial programs and governments have been at greater risk of being hit with increases in the cost of medical care. The 1977 act linked the federal contribution to the provinces to the growth of gross national product, requiring the provinces to pick up more of the costs when their aggregate outlays for health care as a proportion of the provincial budgets were greater than that of their economies as a whole. Revisions of the act in 1987 and 1989 further restricted federal funding for health care to the provinces. In 1980, Ottawa provided 44.6 percent of provincial health care financing; the estimate for 1990 is 36.7 percent. By the year 2000, the federal contribution may be down to as low as 30 percent as a proportion of provincial health expenditures, leaving the provinces to make up the difference.[7]

During the same period in which health care costs were being shifted to the provinces, the Canada Health Act of 1984 was passed unanimously by the Canadian parliament to safeguard unlimited access to health care by patients. The provinces were forced to ban the practice of extra billing by doctors in excess of the amounts allowed by the provincial fee schedules as well as hospitals' insidious practice of charging for certain services to inpatients. Although there was a 25-day doctors' strike in Ontario, court challenges, and outcries from the Canadian Medical Association, every province has gone along with the ban on extra billing and user charges, because failure to do so means loss of federal dollars in proportion to the amounts of extra billing and user fees imposed on patients by both doctors and hospitals.

The Balance Sheet for NHI

We can draw several conclusions about the implementation of national health insurance in Canada. It has led to sharp narrowing of regional differences in distribution of hospitals, doctors, and other categories of health workers. Clear gains have been made in making primary care services uniformly available across the country. Accompanying this, infant mortality rates and longevity have leveled out regionally across the country. However, disparities have continued to exist in per capita spending on health. Poorer regions have poorer differential access, particularly to highly specialized tertiary care services.[8]

Most Canadians have made extensive use of hospital and medical care benefits under national health insurance, and access to services without opening your wallet has been a major step forward. But low-income groups have generated much less spending on health services than have higher-income groups, and long-established class disparities in the amount and types of health care received still characterize the use of health services. Lower-income families spend more of the total family income in out-of-pocket expenses for uninsured and other health services than do families with higher incomes. As before national health insurance, ill-health and disability remain more prevalent among the poor; those who are not poor also live longer, and that disparity is worsening.

The supply of Canadian doctors is ever increasing, and the number of Canadian graduates migrating to the United States is decreasing. For academic year 1988–89, there were four applications for every place in a medical school in Canada, compared to 1.6 for every place in a medical school in the United States. Fully 44.4 percent of Canadian medical students in that same year were women. In 1970 there was one practicing doctor to every 870 Canadians, compared to one to every 525 in 1988. These figures exclude residents in training programs. Although, as noted, Canada has an expanding supply of family practitioners, there are shortages in general surgery, in psychiatry, in oncology, and in the pediatric subspecialties. Medicine remains a highly attractive profession in Canada, and doctors are still highly regarded. They are by far the best-paid professionals in Canada. Doctors netted $84,700 in 1987, compared to $70,800 for dentists, $63,500 for lawyers, and $49,300 for accountants.[9] The net earnings of doctors in the early to the mid-1970s were at least four times the net earnings of other taxable Canadian workers.[10] I doubt if these figures have changed much in the intervening years.

While all in Canada have gained, pre-existing class-related disparities remain unaltered at the aggregate level. The Canadian experience tells us what we already know: that a single measure like national health insurance is insufficient to redistribute the inequitable allocation of services whose roots lie in the social and class structures of every country in the world.

Implications for the United States

To transpose the Canadian system to the United States, there has to be agreement on several key principles. First, everyone has to be covered. The United States has the technical ability to do this, but to date it lacks the political will. You have to agree once and for all that the right of access to needed health services applies to all residents of the country as a basic human right, like the right to public education or to police and fire department protection.

An analysis of the Canadian system in the 1970s by a group of experts from both the United States and Canada agreed that the application of the Canadian system in the United States would in most essential respects have the same effects.[11] However, the assumptions made by this group are not so easy to assume: that insurance payers and institutional and professional providers of services exercise more self-discipline, that government is willing to act in a manner consistent with protecting the public interest, not special interest groups. Legislators in the United States often appear to be partners with the insurance companies and the lobbyists for institutional and professional providers.

The second principle you have to agree on is to stop determining individuals' eligibility for benefits through means tests that create various bureaucracies of insensitive persons who try to block people from having access to sorely needed services. Third, you have to create a fund or funds to pay for services for everyone. The Canadian experience shows that public control of the payment process—and by that is meant not just regulatory control, but the actual responsibility for paying all the bills vested in a virtually sole-source funding mechanism—is sufficient to provide both universal and comprehensive coverage as well as control of costs. The 3 percent differential between proportions of gross national product devoted to health care in the two countries is testimony to that essential fact.

The only viable current proposal in the United States that takes at least some of these principles into account is the UNY*Care proposal of the New York State Department of Health, which is likely dead in the water anyway. All the other current proposals—with the exception of California Congressman Ronald Dellums' perennial proposal to enact a US national health service—will simply perpetuate the inadequacies and abuses associated with Medicare and Medicaid and with partly uninsured and inadequately insured populations. Any proposal that works properly has to remove the crushing tax burden from the backs of counties and cities with high levels of high-risk, poorly insured populations.

There are no ideal ways to pay doctors. The prevailing system in Canada, as in the United States, is payment by fee for service, which emphasizes procedures and downgrades counseling and talking, careful history taking, and thorough physical examinations. Fee-for-service leaves the problem of utilization-driven income untouched. The options are capitation payment (one-time flat fees, as in health maintenance organizations) and salaries for physicians, which also have their limitations. For example, in Saskatchewan, expenses for physician services increased by 153 percent between 1978 and 1986.[12] Close to 100 percent of this increase was due to increases in physicians' fees, and less than 1 percent was accounted for by increases in population growth.

Freezing or reducing payment levels to doctors is not an effective cost control, because doctors respond by increasing the quantity and complexity of their services. Fee controls that are not backed up by global caps on payments will not control costs. To maintain adequate cost controls, you have to address fee levels, rates and patterns of services provided per physician, and the number of physicians in the system.[13] In Canada today there is still professional control over the specifics of providing services, but public control over the total resources used, with, as I have pointed out, very little use of direct charges to patients and other market mechanisms. This has been satisfactory to date, but there have been escalating frictions, primarily due to the great expansion of the pool of doctors drawing money from the public purse, which leads to greater costs of the system or smaller incomes for doctors. In neither country have we faced up to the great expansion in the pool of doctors of the past two decades, and to the thousands each year that are still in the pipeline.

I am not optimistic that even such a minor social reform as universal financing for essential health services is imminent in the United States. The plans were enacted in Canada when there was a social democratic ferment across the country, and that moment has passed in Canada, at least at the present time; such a ferment does not exist in the United States.

But there are other indicators as well as causes for cautious optimism. First, the mass of uninsured and underinsured is not going to go away, and their numbers are increasing. Second, the middle class is being squeezed by health care, with increasing premiums, greater employee contributions, greater deductibles, and greater co-insurance. Third, in the face of the demographics of aging in the years ahead, the spectre of financing for long-term care is not going to disappear. Whether new coalitions can be mobilized to address these issues in a comprehensive rather than a piecemeal fashion remains to be seen.

NOTES

1. Wolfe, S., *National Health Insurance in Canada*, New York: Church and Society, 1977.

2. Evans, R. G., et al. "Controlling Health Expenditures—The Canadian Reality," *New England Journal of Medicine*, 1989:320, pp. 571–577.

3. "National Health Expenditures, 1986–2000," *HCFA Review*, 1987:8(4).

4. Evans, R. G., "Finding The Levers, Finding the Courage: Lessons from Cost Containment in North America," *Journal of Health Politics, Policy and Law*, 1986:11(4).

5. Iglehart, J. K., "Canada's Health Care System Faces Its Problems," *New England Journal of Medicine*, 1990:322, pp. 562–568.

6. Badgley, Robin F., and Samuel Wolfe, "Disparities on the Road to Equity in Health Services in Canada," paper presented at a meeting of the American Public Health Association, Montreal, Quebec, Canada, November 1982.

7. Iglehart, op. cit.

8. Badgley, Robin F., "Ethics and Equity in Canadian Health Care: The Data," paper presented at a meeting of the American Public Health Association, Chicago, October 1989; and Wolfe, Samuel, "Ethics and Equity in Canadian Health Care: Policy Implications of the Data," paper presented at a meeting of the American Public Health Association, Chicago, October 1989.

9. Iglehart, op. cit.

10. Wolfe, Samuel, and Robin F. Badgley, "How Much is Enough? The Payment of Doctors

—Implications for Health Policy in Canada," in Meilicke, C., and J. Starch, eds., *Perspectives on Canadian Health and Social Services Policy: History and Emerging Trends*, chapter 14, Ann Arbor, MI: Health Administration Press, 1980.

11. Andreopoulos, S., ed., *National Health Insurance: Can We Learn From Canada?* New York: Wiley, 1975.

12. Regina, N., "Study into the Growth of Use of Health Services," report of the Review Committee to the Minister of Health, January 1989.

13. Lomas, J., et al. "Paying Physicians in Canada," *Health Affairs*, 1989:8(1), pp. 80–102; and Barer, M. L., R. G. Evans, and R. Labelle, "Fee Controls as Cost Control: Evidence from the Frozen North," *Millbank Quarterly*, 1988:66(1).

CONTRIBUTORS

Kathryn Anastos, M.D., is Director of the AIDS Clinic at Bronx-Lebanon Hospital.

Ron J. Anderson, M.D., is President and CEO of Parkland Memorial Hospital in Dallas, Texas.

Byllye Y. Avery is founder of the National Black Women's Health Project.

Tony Bale is a sociologist at Bellevue Hospital in New York City and a member of the Health/PAC Board.

Ellen Baxter is Director of The Heights, five client-owned residences for homeless individuals in New York City.

Barbara Berney is a Pew Doctoral Fellow at Boston University.

Ellen Bilofsky is Editor of the *Health/PAC Bulletin*.

Thomas Bodenheimer, M.D., M.P.H., is a member of Physicians for a National Health Program Working Group.

Gwen Braxton is Director of the National Black Women's Health Project in Brooklyn, New York.

Durado D. Brooks, M.D., is Assistant Medical Director of Parkland Memorial Hospital's Community-oriented Primary Care Program in Dallas, Texas.

Rob Burlage, Ph.D., one of the founders of Health/PAC, is a member of the Health/PAC board and on the faculty of the Graduate Health Services program of the School of Urban Studies, New School for Social Research.

Michael Byrd, M.D., is a physician with the Department of Obstetrics and Gynecology and the Cancer Control Unit, Meharry Medical College, Nashville, Tennessee.

Christine Cassel, M.D., is a member of the Physicians for a National Health Program Working Group.

Barbara Caress is a health policy consultant in New York State and a former staff member of Health/PAC.

Frank Clancy, a writer in Venice, California, is working on a book on rural health care in Mississippi.

Linda Clayton, M.D., is a physician with the Department of Obstetrics and Gynecology and the Cancer Control Unit, Meharry Medical College, Nashville, Tennessee.

Geraldine Dallek is a health policy consultant in Los Angeles who writes widely on the problems of the poor and the elderly.

Karen Erdman is Project Director of the Survey of State Services, National Alliance for the Mentally Ill.

Carroll L. Estes, Ph.D., is a member of the Physicians for a National Health Program Working Group.

Marianne C. Fahs, Ph.D., M.P.H., is Director, Division of Health Economics and Associate Professor, Department of Community Medicine, Mt. Sinai School of Medicine.

Laurie M. Flynn has been the Executive Director of the National Alliance for the Mentally Ill since 1984.

Nick Freudenberg, Ph.D., is a Professor of Community Health Education and Executive Director of the Hunter College Center on AIDS, Drugs and Community Health of the City University of New York.

Emily Friedman, Ph.D., is a contributing editor for *Hospitals, Medical World News*, and the *Healthcare Forum Journal* and is a contributing writer for *Health Business, Health Progress*, and *JAMA*.

H. Jack Geiger, M.D., is Logan Professor of Community Health and Social Medicine at CUNY Medical School.

Bob Griss, Ph.D., is Director of Health Policy for the United Cerebral Palsy Associations of America.

Kevin Grumbach, M.D., is a member of Physicians for a National Health Program Working Group.

Sally Guttmacher, Ph.D., is an Associate Professor in the Department of Health Education at New York University and a member of the Health/PAC Board.

Martha Harnly, M.P.H., is a member of the Physicians for a National Health Program Working Group.

Charlene Harrington, R.N., Ph.D., is a member of the Physicians for a National Health Program Working Group.

David U. Himmelstein, M.D., is a member of the Physicians for a National Health Program Working Group.

Diana Holtzman wrote this as an editorial letter to the *New York Times*.

Eric Holtzman, Ph.D., is Chairman of the Department of Biological Sciences, Columbia University.

Gabrielle Immerman was an intern with the Women's Health Education Project and is now with the Center for Medical Consumers in New York City.

Bonnie J. Kay is a researcher specializing in women's reproductive health care.

Vicki Kemper is Associate Editor of *Common Cause Magazine*.

Louanne Kennedy, Ph.D., is Dean of Kean College in New Jersey and is a member of the Health/PAC Board.

David Kotelchuck, Ph.D., is Chairman of the Occupational Health and Safety Department at Hunter College and a member of the Health/PAC Board.

Ronda Kotelchuck, M.R.P., is Vice President for Strategic Planning, New York City's Health and Hospitals Corporation and a member of the Health/PAC Board.

Harry Krulewitch, M.D., a family physician, worked in participatory health centers from 1969 to 1982.

Bill Landis has written extensively about Times Square in New York City, the drug subculture, film and grey area lifestyles. His work appears in the *Village Voice, The Soho Weekly News, Sleazoid Express, Film Comment, Variety.*

Jeremy Leeds, Ph.D., is an Assistant Professor of Applied Psychology at New York University.

Arthur Levin, M.P.H., is Director of the Center for Medical Consumers and President of the Health/PAC Board.

Pam Lichty is the staff planner and legislative liaison for the Governor's Committee on AIDS in Honolulu, Hawaii, and wrote the initial draft of the needle exchange legislation for Hawaii.

Donald W. Light, Ph.D., is Professor of Sociology and Health Care Systems, University of Medicine and Dentistry of New Jersey, Graduate Faculty, Rutgers University, New Brunswick.

Stephan G. Lynn, M.D., is Director, Department of Emergency Medicine, St. Luke's-Roosevelt Hospital Center in New York City and Chair of the American College of Emergency Physicians Task Force on Hospital and Emergency Room Overcrowding.

Carola Marte, M.D., is Director of HIV Services, MMTP Program, Beth Israel Medical Center.

Dawn McGuire, M.D., is Director of the AIDS Neurology Clinics at San Francisco General Hospital and UCSF Medical Center.

Nancy F. McKenzie, Ph.D., is Executive Director of Health/PAC and the editor of *The Crisis in Health Care: Ethical Issues* and *The AIDS Reader: Social, Political and Ethical Issues.*

John B. McKinlay, Ph.D., is a Professor of Sociology and Research Professor of Medicine at Boston University.

Teresa McMillen, M.S.W., is a social worker at the Comprehensive Family Care Center at the Albert Einstein College of Medicine in the Bronx, New York.

Michele Melden is staff attorney at the National Health Law Program (NHELP) in Los Angeles, California.

Cheryl Merzel, Ph.D., is Assistant Research Specialist at the AIDS Research Group of the Institute for Health, Health Care Policy and Aging Research at Rutgers University and is a member of the Health/PAC Board.

Patricia Moccia, R.N., Ph.D., is Executive Vice President for Accreditation and Education of the National League for Nursing.

Regina Neal, M.U.P., is Senior Director, Office of Planning Services, New York City's Health and Hospitals Corporation and is a member of the Health/PAC Board.

Viveca Novak is senior staff writer at *Common Cause Magazine.*

Miriam Ostow, M.A., is a researcher in the Eisenhower Center for the Conservation of Human Resources at Columbia University.

Public Citizen is a non-profit citizen's research, lobbying, and litigation organization based in Washington, DC, founded by Ralph Nader in 1971.

Susan Reverby, Ph.D., is Professor of Women's Studies, Wellesley College.

Leonard Rodberg, Ph.D., is a Professor of Urban Studies at Queens College/CUNY.

Sumner M. Rosen, Ph.D., is Professor of Social Policy at Columbia University and Special Assistant to the Director, Center for Labor-Management Policy Studies, Graduate Center, City University of New York.

Cynthia Rudder, Ph.D., is Director of the Nursing Home Community Coalition of New York State.

J. Warren Salmon, Ph.D., is Professor and Head of the Department of Pharmacy Administration, College of Pharmacy, and Professor of Health Resources Management, School of Public Health, University of Illinois at Chicago.

Lisbeth Schorr, Ph.D., is a Lecturer in Social Medicine at Harvard University and lives in Washington, DC. This article is based on a presentation she made at a United Hospital Fund conference in Tuxedo, NY, September 1989.

Ruth Sidel, Ph.D., is Professor of Sociology at Hunter College.

Victor W. Sidel, M.D., is Distinguished University Professor of Social Medicine at Montefiore Medical Center and Albert Einstein College of Medicine.

David R. Smith, M.D., is formerly CEO and Medical Director of Parkland Memorial Hospital's Community-oriented Primary Care Program in Dallas, Texas, and is now Health Commissioner for the State of Texas.

Rod Sorge is the Director of the Needle Exchange Program of the Bronx AIDS Taskforce and former Assistant Editor of the *Health/PAC Bulletin*.

Jean Stewart is a disability activist and writer, author of *The Body's Memory*, St. Martin's Press. She lives in Kingston, New York.

John D. Stoeckle, M.D., is Professor of Medicine at Harvard Medical School and Chief of Medical Clinics at the Massachusetts General Hospital in Boston.

Hal Strelnick, M.D., is a family physician, Assistant Chairman of the Department of Family Medicine at the Montefiore Medical Center, and a Health/PAC Board member.

Milton Terris, M.D., M.P.H., is editor of the Journal of *Public Health Policy*.

E. Fuller Torrey, M.D., is a clinical and research psychiatrist in Washington DC who volunteers time and expertise to the Health Research Group. He is a long-time member of the National Alliance for the Mentally Ill.

Roderick Wallace, Ph.D., is a research scientist with the Epidemiology of Mental Disorders Research Department, New York State Psychiatric Institute, Columbia University.

Deborah Wallace, Ph.D., is President of the Public Interest Science Consulting Service of New York City.

David G. Whiteis, Ph.D., is Research Associate in the Center for Health Services Research in the School of Public Health, University of Illinois at Chicago.

Sam Wolfe, M.D., recently returned to Canada after being a physician and Professor of Public Health at the Columbia University School of Public Health for 20 years. From 1962 to 1966 he was a commissioner of health insurance in Saskatchewan, Canada.

Sidney Wolfe, M.D., is an internist who has been Director of the Public Citizen Health Research Group since 1971.

Steffie Woolhandler, M.D., M.P.H., is a member of the Physicians for a National Health Program Working Group.

Richard Younge, M.D., is Chair of Department of Family Health, State University of New York Health Science Center at Brooklyn (Downstate Medical Center), and a member of the Health/PAC Board.

ACKNOWLEDGMENTS

Section I. *Health Status in the United States: Communities at Risk*
Introduction by Sally Guttmacher and Dave Kotelchuck, Ph.D.

"The Uninsured: From Dilemma to Crisis," Emily Friedman, *Journal of the American Medical Association*, Vol. 265, No. 19, May 15, 1991, pp. 2491–2495, Copyright, 1991, American Medical Association. Reprinted by Permission of the Author and the American Medical Association.

(Charts) "Paying for Our Health System: $6,535 per family, 1991;" "Family Payments for Health Care, 1991, $4,296;" "Impact of Family Health Payments (1980–2000);" *Health Spending: The Growing Threat to the Family Budget*, Families USA Report, December 1991. Reprinted by Permission of The Families USA Foundation.

(Charts) "Number of People with Private Insurance, 1960–1990," "Number of People with Private Insurance and Total Insurance Premiums, 1960–1990," "Number of Uninsured Americans, 1976–1990," *The Vanishing Health Safety Net: New Data on Uninsured Americans*, David Himmelstein, et al. Reprinted by Permission of the Center for National Health Program Studies, Harvard Medical School/Cambridge Hospital.

(Chart) "Poverty," *Challenges in Health Care: A Chart Book*, Robert Wood Johnson Foundation, 1991. Reprinted by Permission of The Robert Wood Johnson Foundation.

"Women in Poverty," Ruth Sidel, "Democratic Socialists of America Newsletter," May/June 1992, pp. 4–6. Reprinted by Permission of The Institute for Democratic Socialism.

(Charts) "Homelessness;" "People with Chronic Mental Illness," *Challenges in Health Care: A Chart Book*, Robert Wood Johnson Foundation, 1991. Reprinted by Permission of The Robert Wood Johnson Foundation.

"Care of the Seriously Mentally Ill: Eight Current Crises," E. Fuller Torrey, Karen Erdman, Sidney M. Wolfe, Laurie M. Flynn, Public Citizen Research Group and the National Alliance for the Mentally Ill, 1990, pp. 1–17. Reprinted by Permission of The Public Citizen's Health Research Group and The National Alliance for the Mentally Ill.

"Healing the Delta," Frank Clancy, *America's Health*, November 1990, pp. 43–51. Reprinted by Permission of the Author.

"Burnout in L.A.," Frank Clancy, *America's Health*, November 1990, pp. 52–55. Reprinted by Permission of the Author.

"Lead, Race, and Public Health," Barbara Berney, Ph.D. *Health/PAC Bulletin*, Vol. 21, No. 1, 1991, pp. 30–31. Reprinted by Permission of the Author.

"Racial Comparison of Health Data" (chart), from "The Slave Health Deficit: Racism and Health Outcomes," Michael Byrd and Linda Clayton, *Health/PAC Bulletin*, Vol. 21, No. 2, Summer 1991, pp. 26–27.

(Chart) "Estimates of Types of Health Insurance Coverage by Race/Ethnicity," 1989; (excerpt) "Medicaid" pp. 17–20, GAO/PEMD 92–6.

"Women—The Missing Persons in the AIDS Epidemic," Kathryn Anatos and Carola Marte, *Health/PAC Bulletin*, Winter 1989, pp. 6–13.

"Abortion: Where We Came From, Where We're Going," Ellen Bilofsky, *Health/PAC Bulletin*, Summer 1991, pp. 37–38.

(Voice) "The Insurance Game," Diana Holtzman, *New York Times*, March 1, 1992.

(Voice) "Too Little, Too Late: A Child with AIDS," Teresa McMillen, *Health/PAC Bulletin*, Fall 1991, pp. 27–29.

Section II. *The Crisis in Provider Institutions: Issues and Areas for Reform*

Introduction by Nancy F. McKenzie

"Public Health in Crisis: The Economic Consequences of Inaction," Marianne C. Fahs, Prepared for Symposium: Imminent Peril: Public Health in a Declining Economy, Board of Health of New York City, August 1991. Reprinted by Permission of the Author.

"Worker Health and Safety in the 1990s," David Kotelchuck

"Shredding the Safety Net: The Dismantling of Public Programs," Nancy F. McKenzie and Ellen Bilofsky, *Health/PAC Bulletin*, Summer 1991, pp. 5–11.

"Frozen in Ice: Federal Health Policy During the Reagan Years," Geraldine Dallek, *Health/PAC Bulletin*, Vol. 18, No. 2, 1988, pp. 4–14.

"Contagious Urban Decay and the Collapse of Public Health," Rodrick Wallace and Deborah Wallace, *Health/PAC Bulletin*, Summer 1991, pp. 13–18.

(Chart) "NYC Homeless Families Count," *City Limits* 1991. New York Human Resources Administration.

"National Alert: Gridlock in the Emergency Department," Stephan G. Lynn, *Health/PAC Bulletin*, Spring 1991, pp. 5–8.

(Chart) "Percent of Aged Population Residing in Nursing and Related Care Homes;" "Percent Distribution of Nursing Homes . . . ;" "Percent Distribution of Expenditures for Nursing Home Care . . . ;" "National Expenditure for Home Care . . ." *Medical Care Chartbook*. Reprinted with Permission from *The Medical Care Chartbook*, 9th edition, edited by Leon Wyszewianski and Stephen S. Mick (Ann Arbor, MI: Health Administration Press, 1991).

"Testimony on Reforming Long-Term Care in New York State," Cynthia Rudder, Nursing Home Community Coalition of New York City, 1991, pp. 1–5.

"And What About the Patients?: Prospective Payment's Impact on Quality of Care," Ronda Kotelchuck, *Health/PAC Bulletin*, Vol. 17, No. 2, Jan/Feb 1987, pp. 13–18.

"Public Hospitals: Doing What Everyone Wants Done But Few Others Wish to Do," by Emily Friedman, *Journal of the American Medical Association*, March 20, 1987, Vol. 257, No. 11, 1437–1444. Copyright 1987, American Medical Association. Reprinted by Permission of the Author and the American Medical Association.

"Demise of Philadelphia General an Instructive Case; Other Cities Treat Public Hospital Ills Differently," Emily Friedman, *Journal of the American Medical Association*, March

27, 1987, Vol. 257, No. 12, 1571–1575. Copyright 1987, American Medical Association. Reprinted by Permission of the Author and the American Medical Association.

"Medicaid and Managed Care: Testimony Submitted to the House Subcommittee on Health and the Environment," Michele Melden. Reprinted by Permission of the Author.

"Medical Apartheid: An America Perspective," Durado D. Brooks, David R. Smith, Ron J. Anderson, *Journal of the American Medical Association*, Vol. 266, No. 19, November 20, 1991, pp. 2746–2749. Copyright, 1991, American Medical Association. Reprinted by Permission of the Authors and The American Medical Association.

(Insert) "Point of Return," by Bill Landis, *Village Voice*, 9/8/92. Reprinted by Permission of the Author and *The Village Voice*.

(Voice) "Medicine: A Bedside View," Dawn McGuire in *The Crisis in Health Care: Ethical Issues*, edited by Nancy F. McKenzie, Penguin Press, 1990, pp. 11–18. Reprinted by Permission of the Editor.

(Voice) "Washington Could Help Us Fight AIDS," Kathryn Anastos, *New York Times*, August 31, 1992. Editorial.

Section III. *The Changing Medical/Industrial Complex:*
The Bottom Line vs. The Public Agenda

Introduction by Hal Strelnick

(Chart) "Total US Gross Domestic Product and Percent of Expenditures for Health, Education and Defense . . ." *Challenges in Health Care: A Chart Book*, Robert Wood Johnson Foundation, 1991. Reprinted by the Permission of The Robert Wood Johnson Foundation.

(Chart) "Percent Distribution of Active Physicians . . . ;" "Average Net Income of Physicians . . ." *Medical Care Chartbook*. Reprinted with Permission from *The Medical Care Chartbook*, 9th edition, edited by Leon Wyszewianski and Stephen S. Mick (Ann Arbor, MI: Health Administration Press, 1991).

"The Proprietarization of Health Care and the Underdevelopment of the Public Sector," David G. Whiteis, and J. Warren Salmon, in *The Corporate Transformation of Medicine*, Baywood Publishers, 1990, pp. 117–131. Reprinted by Permission of the Authors.

"Corporatization and the Social Transformation of Doctoring," John B. McKinlay and John D. Stoeckle, *The Corporate Transformation of Health Care*, Baywood, 1990, pp. 133–149. Reprinted by Permission of Baywood Publishing Company.

"The Empires Strike Back," Regina Neal, *Health/PAC Bulletin*, Spring 1990, pp. 4–10.

"The Losses in Profits: How Proprietaries Affect Public and Voluntary Hospitals," Louanne Kennedy, *Health/PAC Bulletin*, Vol. 15, No. 6, 1984, pp. 5–13.

"Excluding More, Covering Less: The Health Insurance Industry in the United States," Donald W. Light, *Health/PAC Bulletin*, Vol. 22, No. 1, Spring 1992, pp. 7–13.

"The Threat and Promise of Medicaid Managed Care: A Mixed Review," Ronda Kotelchuck, *Health/PAC Bulletin*, Fall 1992.

"The Drug Manufacturing Industry: A Prescription for Profits," US Government Publications Office, September 1991, Serial No. 102F, pp. 7–31.

"The Commodification of Women's Health: The New Women's Health Centers," Bonnie J. Kay, *Health/PAC Bulletin*, Vol. 19, No. 4, Winter 1989, pp. 19–23.

(Chart) "Percent of Black and Hispanic Workers in Selected Health Care Occupations," *Medical Care Chartbook*. Reprinted with Permission from *Medical Care Chartbook*, 9th edition, editors, Leon Wyszewianski and Stephen S. Mick (Ann Arbor, MI: Health Administration Press, 1991).

"The Fall and Rise of the Hospital Workers Union," Sumner M. Rosen, *Health/PAC Bulletin*, Vol. 20, No. 3, Fall 1990, pp. 40–41.

(Chart) "Percent Distribution of Selected Health Care Practitioners by Gender," *Medical Care Chartbook*. Reprinted with Permission from *Medical Care Chartbook*, 9th Edition, editors Leon Wyszewianski and Stephen S. Mick (Ann Arbor, MI: Health Administration Press, 1991).

(Voice) "Ordered to Care: Demystifying Nursing" (review), Patricia Moccia, *Health/PAC Bulletin*, Vol. 18, No. 3, Fall 1988, pp. 15–18. "Nursing and Caring: Lessons From History" (interview), Susan Reverby, *Health/PAC Bulletin*, Fall 1988, pp. 20–23.

(Voice) "People Power vs. The Almighty Dollar," Harry Krulewitch, *Health/PAC Bulletin*, Vol. 18, No. 3, Fall 1988, pp. 24–27.

Section IV. *Community Response and Innovative Policy*
Introduction by Nancy F. McKenzie

"Activism in the New Urban Health Crisis" (editorial), Tony Bale, *Health/PAC Bulletin*, Vol. 21, No. 4, 1991, pp. 3–4.

"Rethinking Empowerment," Cheryl Merzel (convener) (panel presentations): "Empowerment," Sally Guttmacher and Jeremy Leeds; "Well-Being Is Our Birthright," Gwen Braxton; "Knowledge is Power," Gabrielle Immerman; and "Housing and Empowerment," Ellen Baxter, *Health/PAC Bulletin*, Vol. 21, No. 4, 1991, pp. 5–18.

(Chart) "Health Care Coverage for People Ages 16–64 by Disability Status . . . ;" "Days of Restricted Activity . . ." *Challenges in Health Care: A Chart Book*, 1991. Reprinted by Permission of The Robert Wood Johnson Foundation.

"The Role of the Disability Movement in Health Care Reform," Bob Griss, "Word From Washington," United Cerebral Palsy Associations, July/August/September 1991, pp. 16–18. Reprinted by Permission of the Author.

"The Fragile Rights of Sharon Kowalski," Ellen Bilofsky, *Health/PAC Bulletin*, Vol. 19, No. 1, Spring 1989, pp. 4–13; "Sharon Kowalski and the Rights of Nontraditional Families," Ellen Bilofsky, *Health/PAC Bulletin*, Vol. 20, No. 1, Spring 1990, pp. 29–31.

"Home is Where the Patients Are: New York's Home Care Workers' Contract Victory," Barbara Caress, *Health/PAC Bulletin*, Vol. 18, No. 3, Fall 1988, pp. 4–14.

"AIDS at the Beginning of the Second Decade," Nancy F. McKenzie, *Health/PAC Bulletin*, Fall 1990; "Teaching to Live: Learning from Ten Years of AIDS," Nick Freudenberg, *Health/PAC Bulletin*, Winter 1992, pp. 19–21; "Reassessing Communities," N. Freudenberg, *Health/PAC Bulletin*, Vol. 17, No. 5, November 1987, p. 30.

"Successful Strategies: Meeting the Health Needs of Children in Adversity," Lisbeth Schorr, *Health/PAC Bulletin*, Fall 1991, pp. 16–21.

"Media Scan: The View from Olympus," Hal Strelnick, *Health/PAC Bulletin*, Summer 1991, pp. 36–37.

"Harm Reduction: A New Approach to Drug Services," Rod Sorge, *Health/PAC Bulletin*, Vol. 21, No. 4, 1991.

(Voice) "Breathing Life Into Ourselves: The Evolution of the National Black Women's Health Project," Byllye Avery, in *Black Women's Health Book: Speaking for Ourselves*, edited by Evelyn White, The Seal Press, 1990, pp. 5–10. Reprinted by permission of the author.

(Voice) "The Troublesome Cripples of Orlando: Disability and Activism," Jean Stewart.

Section V. *Toward Adequate Policy in Health Care Delivery*
Introduction by Nancy F. McKenzie

(Sidebar) "Health Care: We Gotta Have it! Basic Principles," MADRE, Women's Campaign and Congress for Universal Health Care.

(Sidebar) "Principles for Health Care Reform from a Disability Perspective," Statement of the Consortium for Citizens with Disabilities Health Task Force, October 24, 1991, pp. 1–8.

"Civil Rights Issues Underlying Rejection of Oregon Medicaid Rationing Plan: Round One," Bob Griss, United Cerebral Palsy Associations, 1992. Reprinted by Permission of the Author.

"The Components of Care," Milton Terris, *Health/PAC Bulletin*, Vol. 17, No. 5, November 1987, pp. 12–17.

"A National Long-Term Care Program for the United States: A Caring Vision," Charlene Harrington, Christine Cassel, Carroll L. Estes, Steffie Woolhandler, David Himmelstein, Physicians for a National Health Program, 1991, pp. 3023–3029. Reprinted by permission of the author.

"In Search of a Solution: The Need for Community-Based Care," Barbara Caress, *Health/PAC Bulletin*, Summer 1989, pp. 17–24.

"Health Care for a Nation in Need," Victor Sidel, *Institute for Democratic Socialism*, January 1991. Reprinted by the Institute for Democratic Socialism.

"Another Kind of Bronx Cheer: Community Oriented Primary Care at the Montefiore Family Health Center," Hal Strelnick and Richard Younge, *Health/PAC Bulletin*, Winter 1992.

Section VI. *Proposals for a National Agenda*
Introduction by Arthur Levin

"What's Blocking Health Care Reform?" Vicki Kemper and Viveca Novak, *Common Cause Magazine*, January/February/March 1992, pp. 8–25. Reprinted by Permission of *Common Cause Magazine*.

"Taking Stock and Turning Corners," H. Jack Geiger, *Health/PAC Bulletin*, Vol. 17, no. 5, November 1987, pp. 7–12.

"Anatomy of a National Health Program: Reconsidering the Dellums Bill after 10 Years," Leonard S. Rodberg, *Health/PAC Bulletin*, Vol. 17, No. 6, December 1987, pp. 12–16.

"Managed Competition," Ronda Kotelchuck, *Health/PAC Bulletin*, Vol. 23, No. 1, Spring 1993.

"Achieving Effective Cost Control in Comprehensive Health Care Reform," Alain Enthoven, *Health-PAC Bulletin*, Vol. 23, No. 1, Spring 1993.

"California Health Care in the 21st Century," John Garamendi, *Health/PAC Bulletin*, Vol. 23, No. 1, Spring 1993.

"Managed Competition and Public Health," Nancy F. McKenzie, *Health/PAC Bulletin*, Vol. 23, No. 1, Spring 1993.

"Change the Health Care System?" Ken Frisof, *Health/PAC Bulletin*, Vol. 23, No. 1, Spring 1993.

"The American Health Security Act of 1993," *Health/PAC Bulletin*, Vol. 23, No. 1, Spring 1993.

"Organizations for Health Care Reform," *Health/PAC Bulletin*, Vol. 23, No. 1, Spring 1993.

"Universal Health Insurance: Who Should be the Single Payer?" Thomas Bodenheimer, *Health/PAC Bulletin*, Fall 1992.

"Liberal Benefits, Conservative Spending: The Physicians for a National Health Program Proposal," Kevin Grumbach, M.D., Thomas Bodenheimer, M.D., M.P.H., David Himmelstein, M.D., Steffie Woolhandler, M.D., M.P.H., et al, *Journal of the American Medical Association*, Vol. 265, No. 19, May 15, 1991, pp. 2549–2554. Copyright, 1991 American Medical Association. Reprinted by Permission of the Authors and the American Medical Association.

"Importing Health Care Reform: On Transposing Canada's Health Care System to the United States," Samuel Wolfe, *Health/PAC Bulletin*, Summer 1990, pp. 27–33.